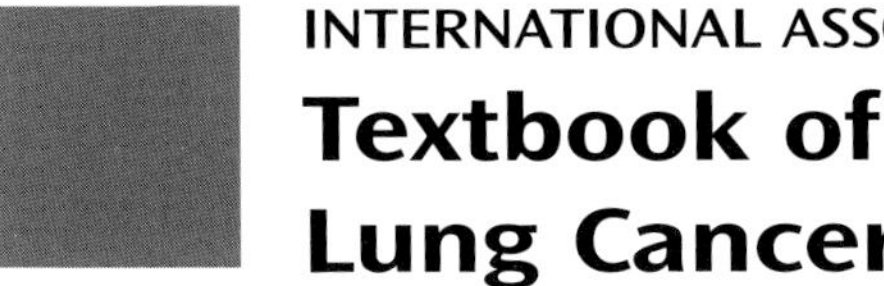

INTERNATIONAL ASSOCIATION FOR THE STUDY OF LUNG CANCER

Textbook of Lung Cancer

INTERNATIONAL ASSOCIATION FOR THE STUDY OF LUNG CANCER

Textbook of Lung Cancer

Edited by

Heine H Hansen, MD, FRCP

Professor of Medical Oncology
Executive Director, IASLC
The Finsen Center
National University Hospital
Copenhagen
Denmark

MARTIN DUNITZ

Although every effort has been made to ensure that drug doses and other information are presented accurately in this publication, the ultimate responsibility rests with the prescribing physician. Neither the publishers nor the authors can be held responsible for errors or for any consequences arising from the use of information contained herein.

First published in the United Kingdom in 2000 by
Martin Dunitz Ltd
The Livery House
7–9 Pratt Street
London NW1 0AE

A CIP catalogue record for this book is available from the British Library

ISBN 1-85317-708-3

Distributed in the United States by:
Blackwell Science Inc.
Commerce Place, 350 Main Street
Malden, MA 02148, USA
Tel: 1–800–215–1000

Distributed in Canada by:
Login Brothers Book Company
324 Salteaux Crescent
Winnipeg, Manitoba, R3J 3T2
Canada
Tel: 204–224–4068

Distributed in Brazil by:
Ernesto Reichmann Distribuidora de Livros, Ltda
Rue Coronel Marques 335, Tatuape 03440–000
São Paulo
Brazil

Composition by Scribe Design, Gillingham, Kent, UK
Printed and bound in Great Britain by Biddles Ltd,
Guildford and King's Lynn

Contents

Contributors

Hisao Asamura, MD
Attending Surgeon, Division of Thoracic Surgery
National Cancer Center Hospital
1-1, Tsukiji 5-Chome, Chuo-ku
Tokyo 104-0045
Japan

Jean-Marie Berthelot
Chief, Health Analysis, Social & Economic Studies Division
Statistics Canada, RH Coats Building 24R
Ottawa, Ontario K1A 0T6
Canada

Peter Boyle, PhD
Division of Epidemiology and Biostatistics
European Institute of Oncology
Via Ripamonti 435
20141 Milan
Italy

Paul A Bunn Jr, MD
University of Colorado Health Science Center
4200 East Ninth Avenue
Campus Box-B188
Denver, CO 80262
USA

Desmond N Carney, MD, PhD, FRCPI
Mater Misericordiae Hospital
Eccles Street
Dublin 7
Ireland

Daniel C Chan, PhD
University of Colorado Health Science Center
4200 East Ninth Avenue
Campus Box-B171
Denver, CO 80262
USA

Robert J Downey, MD
Assistant Professor of Surgery
Division of Thoracic Surgery
Department of Surgery
Memorial Sloan-Kettering Cancer Center
1275 York Avenue
New York, NY 10021
USA

William K Evans, MD, FRCPC
Chief Executive Officer
Ottawa Regional Cancer Center
501 Smyth Road
Ottawa, Ontario K1H 8L6
Canada

Sara Gandini, MSc
Division of Epidemiology and Biostatistics
European Institute of Oncology
Via Ripamonti 435
20141 Milan
Italy

Robert J Ginsberg, MD
Chief, Thoracic Service
Department of Surgery
Memorial Sloan-Kettering Cancer Center
1275 York Avenue
New York, NY 10021
USA

Peter Goldstraw, FRCS, FRCS Ed
Consultant Thoracic Surgeon, Director of Surgery
Head of Thoracic Surgery
Royal Brompton Hospital
Sydney Street
London SW3 6NP
UK

Nigel Gray, FRACP
Division of Epidemiology and Biostatistics
European Institute of Oncology
Via Ripamonti 435
20141 Milan
Italy

Anna Gregor, FRCR, FRCP Ed
Department of Clinical Oncology
Lothian University Hospitals NHS Trust
Crewe Road
Edinburgh EH4 2XU
UK

Heine H Hansen, MD, FRCP
Professor of Medical Oncology
Executive Director, IASLC
The Finsen Center
National University Hospital
Copenhagen
Denmark

Aage Haugen, PhD
Department of Toxicology
National Institute of Occupational Health
P0 Box 8149
N-0033 Oslo
Norway

Barbara Helfrich, MD
University of Colorado Health Science Center
4200 East Ninth Avenue
Campus Box-B171
Denver, CO 80262
USA

James R Jett, MD
Division of Pulmonary and Critical Care Medicine
Mayo Clinic and Mayo Foundation
200 First Street SW
Rochester, MN 55905
USA

Madeline A Kane, MD
University of Colorado Health Science Center
4200 East Ninth Avenue
Campus Box-B171
Denver, CO 80262
USA

Jean Klastersky, MD
Service de Médecine Interne &
Laboratoire d'Investigation Clinique et
d'Oncologie Expérimentale
Institut Jules Bordet
Rue Héger-Bordet 1
B-1000 Bruxelles
Belgium

Robert J Korst, MD
Clinical Assistant Surgeon
Thoracic Service, Department of Surgery
Memorial Sloan-Kettering Cancer Center
1275 York Avenue
New York, NY 10021
USA

Richard Lake, PhD
University Department of Medicine
Queen Elizabeth II Medical Centre
4th Floor, G Block
Nedlands
Perth, WA 6009
Australia

Isabelle Mancini, MD
Service de Médecine Interne &
Laboratoire d'Investigation Clinique et
d'Oncologie Expérimentale
Institut Jules Bordet
Rue Héger-Bordet 1
B-1000 Bruxelles
Belgium

Blair McLaren, MD
University Department of Medicine
Queen Elizabeth II Medical Centre
4th Floor, G Block
Nedlands
Perth, WA 6009
Australia

Vincenzo Minotti, MD
Medical Oncology Division
Policlinico, Monteluce
06122 Perugia
Italy

Sutapa Mukherjee, MD
University Department of Medicine
Queen Elizabeth II Medical Centre
4th Floor, G Block
Nedlands
Perth, WA 6009
Australia

James L Mulshine, MD
Department of Cell and Cancer Biology
Medicine Branch, Division of Clinical Sciences
National Cancer Institute
National Institutes of Health
Bethesda, MD 20892-1906
USA

Tsuguo Naruke, MD
Deputy Director
Chairman, Department of Surgery
Chief, Division of Thoracic Surgery
National Cancer Center Hospital
1-1, Tsukiji 5-Chome, Chuo-ku
Tokyo 104-0045
Japan

Eric J Olson, MD
Assistant Professor of Medicine
Division of Pulmonary and Critical Care Medicine
Mayo Clinic and Mayo Foundation
200 First Street SW
Rochester, MN 55905
USA

Marianne Paesmans, MSc
Service de Médecine Interne &
Laboratoire d'Investigation Clinique et
d'Oncologie Expérimentale
Institut Jules Bordet
Rue Héger-Bordet 1
B-1000 Bruxelles
Belgium

Ugo Pastorino, MD
Director
Division of Thoracic Surgery
European Institute of Oncology
Via Ripamonti 435
20141 Milan
Italy

Pieter E Postmus, MD
Department of Pulmonology
Free University Hospital
De Boelelaan 1117
1081 HV Amsterdam
The Netherlands

Bruce Robinson, MD
University Department of Medicine
Queen Elizabeth II Medical Centre
4th Floor, G Block
Nedlands
Perth, WA 6009
Australia

William T Sause, MD, FACR
Radiation Therapy Department
LDS Hospital
400 C Street
Salt Lake City, UT 84143
USA

Bernadette Scott, PhD
University Department of Medicine
Queen Elizabeth II Medical Centre
4th Floor, G Block
Nedlands
Perth, WA 6009
Australia

Jean-Paul Sculier, MD
Service de Médecine Interne &
Laboratoire d'Investigation Clinique et
d'Oncologie Expérimentale
Institut Jules Bordet
Rue Héger-Bordet 1
B-1000 Bruxelles
Belgium

Cristiana Sessa, MD
Oncology Institute of Southern Switzerland
Ospedale San Giovanni
6500 Bellinzona
Switzerland

Frances A Shepherd, MD, FRCP(C)
Princess Margaret Hospital
610 University Avenue, Suite 5-104
Toronto, Ontario MSG 2M9
Canada

Yukio Shimosato, MD
Visiting Professor
Department of Pathology
Keio University School of Medicine
35 Shinanomachi, Shinjukuku
Tokyo 160-0016
Japan

Ariel Soriano, MD
University of Colorado Health Science Center
4200 East Ninth Avenue
Campus Box-B171
Denver, CO 80262
USA

John D Stageberg, MD
Radiation Oncologist
LDS Hospital
400C Street
Salt Lake City, UT 84143
USA

Thomas G Sutedja, MD
Department of Pulmonology
Free University Hospital
De Boelelaan 1117
1081 HV Amsterdam
The Netherlands

Melvyn S Tockman, MD, PhD
Professor of Medicine
H.Lee Moffitt Cancer Center
University of South Florida
12902 Magnolia Drive
Tampa, FL 33612
USA

Maurizio Tonato, MD
Medical Oncology Division
Policlinico Monteluce
06122 Perugia
Italy

Philip Tønnesen, MD, Dr. Med. Sci
Chief, Department of Pulmonary Medicine
Gentofte University Hospital
Niels Andersenvej 65
DK-2900 Hellerup
Denmark

Ryosuke Tsuchiya, MD
Chief, Division of Thoracic Surgery
Department of Surgery
National Cancer Center Hospital
1-1, Tsukiji 5-Chome, Chuo-ku
Tokyo 104-0045
Japan

Anton JM van Boxem, MD
Department of Pulmonology
Free University Hospital
De Boelelaan 1117
1081 HV Amsterdam
The Netherlands

B Phyllis Will
Senior Research Analyst
Health Analysis, Social & Economic Studies Division
Statistics Canada, RH Coats Building 24R
Ottawa, Ontario K1A OT6
Canada

Introduction

The epidemiological features of smoking, and thus lung cancer, are rapidly changing. In some parts of the world, such as the USA, certain western European countries and Australia, the incidence of lung cancer among males is decreasing, while the disease continues to increase among females. In the USA, lung cancer now kills more women than breast cancer.

In southern and eastern parts of Europe, lung cancer is on a rapid rise, and unfortunately a similar pattern is being observed in highly populated countries like China, Indonesia and Japan. Other regions of the world, namely the Middle East, Africa and South America, also show the same dismal picture.

Worldwide, the annual number of new cases of lung cancer is estimated at one million and this is expected to increase to ten million in 2025. In spite of these figures, tobacco consumption continues to increase and the political endeavours to reduce the use of tobacco are lagging behind – even though efforts to inform the public are now proving fruitful in some countries.

In connection with these developments, the International Association for the Study of Lung Cancer (IASLC) is expanding its activities on a global basis. The organization has now existed for 25 years, and from a very small beginning, it is today a worldwide association with 1300 members in 60 countries. According to its Bylaws: "The purpose of the Association shall be to promote the study of the etiology, the epidemiology, the prevention, the diagnosis, the treatment, and all other aspects of lung cancer and to disseminate information about lung cancer to the members of the Association, to the medical community at large, and to the public."

The activities of the IASLC are centred around triannual world conferences on lung cancer (most recently in Dublin, Ireland), which attract 2500 participants. Other events include workshops, meetings on various aspects of lung cancer held around the world, and the monthly publication of the journal *Lung Cancer*, which has 1600 subscribers.

The most recent initiative from the IASLC consists of various educational symposia in some of the countries where lung cancer is emerging as a major health threat to the population. Up-to-date information is important in spreading knowledge about this man-made disease, and the IASLC has therefore decided to publish this comprehensive textbook, based on experience from worldwide meetings, for the use of the many physicians involved in this field.

Heine H Hansen
Executive Director, IASLC

Etiology of lung cancer

Aage Haugen

Contents Introduction • Carcinogens in tobacco smoke • Substances causatively associated with the use of tobacco products in the development of lung cancer • Environmental tobacco smoke • Genetic susceptibility in lung cancer etiology • Females and smoking

INTRODUCTION

Lung cancer, which was rare at the beginning of the 20th century, is now a global problem. It is the most frequent cancer in the world, and the epidemic of lung cancer is still continuing. The global incidence of lung cancer is increasing at 0.5% per year. A major contribution to this trend comes from the East European and developing countries. Consequently, lung cancer will remain a major cause of worldwide cancer death in the 21st century.

That lung cancer is caused by exposure to carcinogens in tobacco smoke is unquestionable. Other factors are of relatively minor importance. About 85–90% of lung cancer patients are smokers.[1] Inherited predisposition may, however, be an important component, since fewer than 20% of smokers will develop lung cancer in their lifetime.

CARCINOGENS IN TOBACCO SMOKE

Lung carcinogenesis is mediated through an interaction between several putative carcinogens. A smoker inhales gas-phase smoke (so-called 'mainstream smoke') as well as particulates (tar). Cigarette smoke is a complex mixture of compounds (almost 4000 compounds have been identified in tobacco mainstream smoke), and chemical analysis has identified a total of at least 50 known carcinogens in both the particulate and gas phases (Table 1.1).[2,3] Studies have led to the identification of carcinogenic polycyclic aromatic hydrocarbons (PAHs), nitrosamines, aromatic amines, aza-arenes, aldehydes, various organic compounds, inorganic compounds such as hydrazine and some metals, and free-radical species.[3] Cigarette smoke also contains certain chlorinated hydrocarbon pesticides. Table 1.2 lists likely causative agents for lung cancer.

Available evidence indicates that carcinogenic PAH compounds and nitrosamines are of major importance in lung cancer induction. Most studies on tobacco smoking genotoxicity in the lung have focused on these compounds. They are strong carcinogens, and tobacco contains relatively high amounts of PAHs and nitrosamines.

PAHs are formed by incomplete combustion of tobacco during smoking. PAHs, particularly benzo(*a*)pyrene (B(*a*)P), induce tumours of the lung in laboratory animals by various routes of administration.[4–6] Furthermore, studies have demonstrated that human lung tissue can metabolize PAHs to reactive metabolites that can interact with DNA, forming mutagenic DNA adducts.[7] Such DNA-adduct formation is thought to be the primary initiating event in carcinogenesis. Increased levels of PAH–DNA adducts in human

Table 1.1 Carcinogens in tobacco and cigarette smoke[a]

Compound[b]	IARC evaluation evidence of carcinogenicity[c] In laboratory animals	In humans
PAH		
Benz(*a*)anthracene	Sufficient	
Benzo(*b*)fluoranthene	Sufficient	
Benzo(*j*)fluoranthene	Sufficient	
Benzo(*k*)fluoranthene	Sufficient	
Benzo(*a*)pyrene	Sufficient	Probable
Dibenz(*a,h*)anthracene	Sufficient	
Dibenzo(*a,i*)pyrene	Sufficient	
Dibenzo(*a,l*)pyrene	Sufficient	
Indeno(1,2,3-*cd*)pyrene	Sufficient	
5-Methylchrysene	Sufficient	
Aza-arenes		
Quinoline		
Dibenz(*a,h*)acridine	Sufficient	
Dibenz(*a,j*)acridine	Sufficient	
7*H*-Dibenzo(*c,g*)carbazole	Sufficient	
N-Nitrosamines		
N-Nitrosodimethylamine	Sufficient	
N-Nitrosoethylmethylamine	Sufficient	
N-Nitrosodiethylamine	Sufficient	
N-Nitrosopyrrolidine	Sufficient	
N-Nitrosodiethanolamine	Sufficient	
N-Nitrososarcosine	Sufficient	
N-Nitrosonornicotine	Sufficient	
4-(Methylnitrosamino)-1-(3-pyridyl)-1-butanone		
N'-Nitrosoanabasine	Limited	
N-Nitrosomorpholine	Sufficient	
Aromatic amines		
2-Toluidine	Sufficient	Inadequate
2-Naphthylamine	Sufficient	Sufficient
4-Aminobiphenyl	Sufficient	Sufficient
N-Heterocyclic amines		
AaC	Sufficient	
MeAaC	Sufficient	
IQ	Sufficient	Probable

Table 1.1 Continued

Trp-P-1	Sufficient	
Trp-P-2	Sufficient	
Glu-P-1	Sufficient	
Glu-P-2	Sufficient	
PhIP	Sufficient	Possible
Aldehydes		
Formaldehyde	Sufficient	Limited
Acetaldehyde	Sufficient	Inadequate
Miscellaneous organic compounds		
1,3-Butadiene	Sufficient	Probable
Isoprene	Sufficient	Possible
Benzene	Sufficient	Sufficient
Styrene	Limited	Possible
Vinyl chloride	Sufficient	Sufficient
DDT[d]	Sufficient	
DDE[d]	Sufficient	
Acrylonitrile	Sufficient	Limited
Acrylamide	Sufficient	Probable
1,1-Dimethylhydrazine	Sufficient	
2-Nitropropane	Sufficient	
Ethyl carbamate	Sufficient	
Ethylene oxide	Sufficient	Limited
Di-(2-ethylhexyl)phthalate	Sufficient	
Furan	Sufficient	Inadequate
Benzo(*b*)furan	Sufficient	Inadequate
Inorganic componds		
Hydrazine	Sufficient	Inadequate
Arsenic	Inadequate	Sufficient
Nickel	Sufficient	Limited
Chromium	Sufficient	Sufficient
Cadmium	Sufficient	Limited
Lead	Sufficient	Inadequate
Polonium-210	Sufficient	Sufficient

[a]Modified from Hoffmann and Hoffmann.[3]

[b]PAH, polynuclear aromatic hydrocarbons; AaC, 2-amino-9*H*-pyrido[2,3-*b*]indole; MeAaC, 2-amino-3-methyl-9*H*-pyrido-[2,3-*b*]indole; IQ, 2-amino-3-methylimidazo[4,5-*b*]quinoline; Trp-P-1, 3-amino-1,4-dimethyl-5*H*-pyrido[4,3-*b*]indole; Trp-P-2, 3-amino-1-methyl-5*H*-pyrido[4,3-*b*]indole; Glu-P-1, 2-amino-6-methyl[1,2-*a*:3',2'-*d*]imidazole; Glu-P-2, 2-aminodipyrido-[1,2-*a*:3',2'-*d*]imidazole; PhIP, 2-amino-1-methyl-6-phenylimidazo[4,5-*b*]pyridine.

[c]No designation indicates that IARC has not evaluated the compound.

[d]During the last decade, DDT and DDE have been drastically reduced in US cigarette tobacco (<60 ng and <13 ng).

lung tissue of smokers and ex-smokers relative to nonsmokers have been reported in several studies.[8–10] The role of PAHs in lung cancer is consistent with recent data from mutational analysis of the *p53* gene, with the demonstration of a large number of G-to-T transversions in the gene.[11] Recent studies have shown a direct molecular link between B(*a*)P and the development of lung cancer. The reactive metabolites of this carcinogen were found to form adducts at mutational hotspots in the *p53*.[12]

The concentration of nitrosamines found in tobacco products is relatively high, and, except for some occupational exposure situations, heavy smokers have the highest levels of exposure to *N*-nitroso compounds. The so-called tobacco-specific *N*-nitrosamines (TSNA), principally 4-(methylnitrosamino)-1-(3-pyridyl)-1-butanone (NNK), are the strongest respiratory carcinogens identified in tobacco products.[13] NNK is derived from nicotine during tobacco processing. Adenocarcinoma of the lung is the main type of lung cancer induced by NNK. However, both benign and malignant tumours have been induced in rats, mice and hamsters.[14,15] Moreover, human lung tissue metabolically activates NNK, although less effectively than rodent lung tissue does. Metabolites of NNK have been reported in urine from smokers, and DNA adducts specific to NNK and *N′*-nitrosonornicotine (NNN) have been reported in smokers' lungs.[16,17] A high frequency of G-to-A transitions in the *p53* gene is consistent with the mutational spectrum expected from NNK.[11]

There are relatively high levels of metals in cigarette smoke. At least 30 metals have been identified.[2] Certain of these are also known respiratory carcinogens. Experimental evidence indicates that many metals are effective initiators of the carcinogenic process, but can also be potential promoters during carcinogenesis – especially in tobacco smoke, where exposure to multiple agents occurs. Chromium, cadmium and nickel are all present in tobacco smoke. It has been reported that chromates are carcinogenic in rats, inducing lung tumours after instillation;[18] cadmium chloride aerosols produce adenocarcinoma and squamous cell carcinoma in rats,[19] and nickel subsulfide yields lung cancer in rats upon inhalation.[20] Because of their relatively high levels in cigarette smoke, these metals may play some role in lung carcinogenesis. They are likely to contribute to lung cancer induction by multiple mechanisms and by causing a variety of DNA damage such as DNA strand breakage, crosslinking of DNA and proteins, and depurination. Many studies have demonstrated that reactive oxygen species are implicated in metal carcinogenesis.[21]

Table 1.2 lists some other (minor) constituents of tobacco smoke that could be involved in lung cancer induction. Less importance has been attributed to these compounds in comparison with PAH and NNK. Inhalation studies of formaldehyde and acetaldehyde have demonstrated that they are respiratory carcinogens in the rat.[22] These compounds are weak carcinogens, but their levels are relatively high in cigarette smoke.

Polonium-210 (^{210}Po) is a natural constituent of cigarette smoke, and will deposit in the lungs of smokers, emitting alpha particles. Radiation exposure may induce lung cancer both alone and in interactions with other carcinogens in tobacco. Animal studies have shown that ^{210}Po is a strong pulmonary carcinogen in rats and Syrian golden hamsters.[23]

DNA is an important target for reactive oxygen species (ROS). Cigarette smoke contains large amounts of free radicals and is known to induce oxidative damage. Both the gas and particulate phases are highly oxidized, and damage the lung. Alkenes (i.e. unsaturated aliphatic hydrocarbons), nitrosamines, aromatic and heterocyclic hydrocarbons, amines, and catechol and hydro-

Table 1.2 Causative agents in cigarette smoke

Carcinogens	Tumour promoters/ Co-carcinogens
Major risk factors	
PAHs	Catechol
Nitroso compounds	Phenol
	Aldehydes
	Oxidative radicals
Minor risk factors	
Polonium-210	
Aldehydes	
Butadiene	
Ni, Cd, Cr	
Oxidative radicals	

quinone are all well-known sources of reactive oxygen species such as hydroxyl radicals, superoxides and peroxides.[24] Damage can also result from the activation of phagocytic cells that generate ROS. Neutrophils play an important role in the defence of the lung through a variety of activities.[25] Myeloperoxidase, a lysosomal enzyme gene, is expressed at high levels in neutrophils. Neutrophils in the lung exposed to PAHs and aromatic amines generate oxidative radicals.[26] The oxidative capacity of neutrophils is therefore important as a potential cause of oxidative damage to the lung. In order for ROS to induce DNA damage, a sufficient concentration must be available to overwhelm the antioxidant capacity of the lung. Products that result from oxidative damage to both lipids and DNA have been detected in smokers, in whom their levels are higher than in non-smokers. Although the direct role of such products in carcinogenesis is unclear, 8-oxoguanine (8-oxo-G), a frequent product of oxidative damage, has miscoding properties associated with the cancer induction process.[27] Studies indicate that unrepaired 8-oxo-G gives rise to G-to-T transversions. Recent data indicate the existence of an 8-oxo-G DNA glycosylase gene (*hOGG1*) in human cells.[28] At least one allele of *hOGG1* (3p25/26) is commonly deleted in lung cancer, indicating that such cells may posses a reduced capacity to repair the mutagenic effect of ROS. The most abundant genetic change induced as a consequence of oxidative damage is a GC-to-AT transition. A recent study suggests a model for C-to-T oxidative mutagenesis in which initial cytosine oxidation is followed by deamination to a poorly repaired uracil derivative that is strongly miscoding during DNA replication.[29]

Nicotine is the agent in tobacco capable of producing addiction, or nicotine dependence. Direct involvement of nicotine in the development of lung cancer has not yet been shown, but nicotine does appear to play an important role and may have multiple sites of action. It is absorbed rapidly when smokers inhale. Specific high-affinity nicotine acetylcholine receptors are found on human lung cancer cells of all histological types, as well as in normal lung tissue.[30] Chronic exposure to nicotine can lead to the activation of growth-promoting pathways, and may also affect apoptosis.[31]

SUBSTANCES CAUSATIVELY ASSOCIATED WITH THE USE OF TOBACCO PRODUCTS IN THE DEVELOPMENT OF LUNG CANCER

The different incidence rates for lung cancer between different countries and among non-smokers suggest that environmental agents can modify the risk. Studies indicate that air pollution is a moderate risk factor for lung cancer. Numerous air pollutants may be important contributors to the incidence of lung cancer.

These pollutants include PAHs, benzene, ethylene oxide, petroleum vapours and metals. However, the etiological importance of air pollution as a contributory factor is still under debate. Association between lung cancer and air pollution has been reported in studies from cities with a high level of air pollution. Urban residents seem to have an increased incidence of lung cancer of 1.5–2.0 times that of rural residents. In a recent Danish study from Copenhagen, a city with relatively low air pollution, only a small effect on the incidence of lung cancer was demonstrated, indicating that the effect of air pollution on lung cancer is identifiable only above a certain threshold level.[32] However, analysis is complicated, because air pollution is a complex mixture with numerous components that also varies over time. Since the lung has a large respiratory volume (500–600 litres of air/h) with a large surface area (75–85 m^2) and a large blood perfusion, exposure to toxic compounds in the ambient air could lead to lung toxicity even at low levels.

Radon, a naturally radioactive but chemically inert gas, is found outdoors and in dwellings and sometimes reaching concentrations comparable to levels in uranium miners. Radon's carcinogenicity is attributable mainly to its short-lived alpha-emitting daughters, ^{214}Po and ^{218}Po.[33] Radon emanates from the soil and from building materials of terrestrial origin, such as stone, bricks and concrete. Studies have provided convincing evidence that radon causes lung cancer in miners.[34] Epidemiological evidence is also now beginning to emerge that exposure to lower levels found in homes and many workplaces may lead to lung cancer.[35] Available data suggest that the risks of lung cancer from exposure to radon and smoking are at least additive.

Workplace exposures play an important role in the causation of lung cancer. The evidence for lung cancer induction by occupational exposure to compounds of metals such as beryllium, chromium, nickel and arsenic is convincing and well documented.[36] High exposure to PAHs occurs in several occupations, such as aluminium production, coke production, coal gasification, iron and steel foundries, drivers (diesel engine exhaust), roofers and asphalt workers. The lung is the major target organ among PAH-exposed workers. There is a strong evidence regarding the synergistic relationship between smoking and asbestos exposure.[2]

ENVIRONMENTAL TOBACCO SMOKE

Recently, environmental tobacco smoke (ETS) has become a subject of concern. Cigarettes generate a great amount of ETS. Several studies have shown an increased risk of lung cancer among non-smokers living in the same household as smokers. A recent meta-analysis concluded that marriage to a smoker increased the risk of lung cancer by 26%.[37] ETS is a combination of sidestream smoke (smoke emitted between puffs of a burning cigarette) and smoke that is exhaled by the smoker. ETS contains essentially all the same carcinogenic agents (including benzene, aromatic amines, vinyl chloride, ethylene oxide, arsenic, chromium, nickel, cadmium, nitrosamines and PAHs) and toxic/irritating agents (including carbon monoxide, nicotine, hydrogen cyanide, ammonia and aldehydes) that have been identified in mainstream smoke inhaled by smokers. Sidestream smoke has higher concentrations of many of the possible carcinogenic compounds, such as benzene, formaldehyde, hydrazine, nitrosamines, 4-aminobiphenyl, benzo(*a*)pyrene, benzo(*a*)anthracene, and others.[38]

GENETIC SUSCEPTIBILITY IN LUNG CANCER ETIOLOGY

Do individuals have different capacities to respond to tobacco exposure? Some degree of

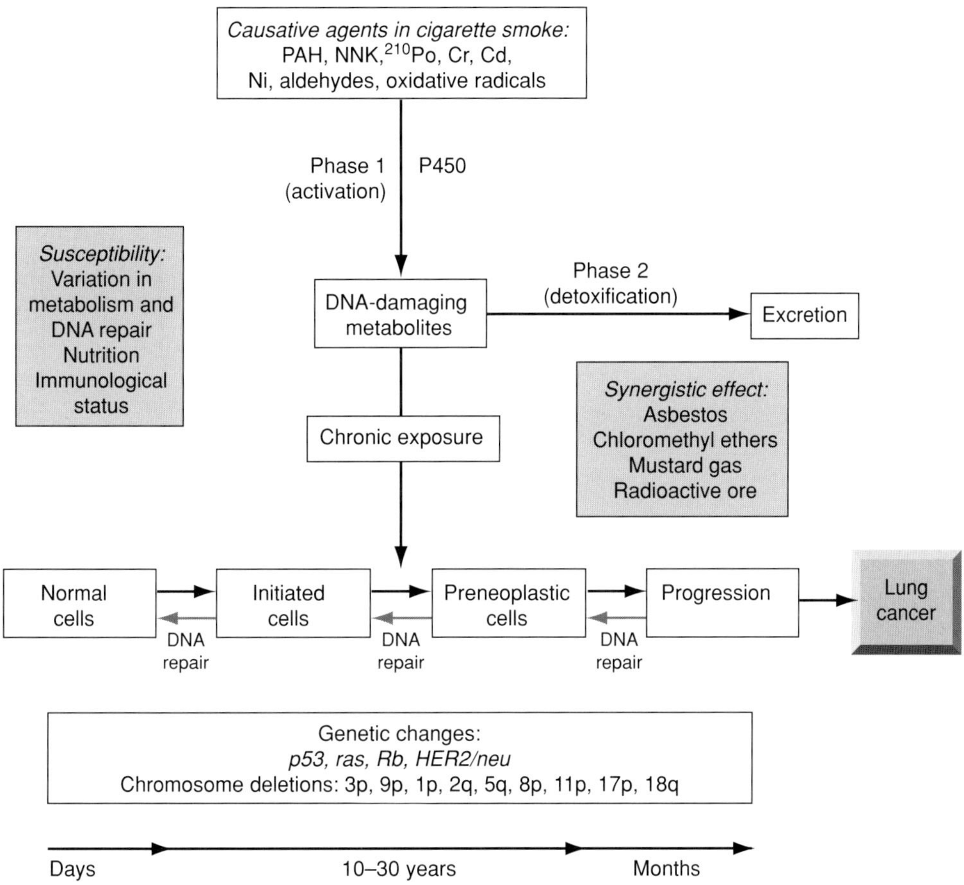

Figure 1.1
Lung carcinogenesis.

familial aggregation of lung cancer is evident in most family studies, so genetic factors are likely to be involved in susceptibility to lung cancer. This susceptibility may be modulated by host-specific factors, including differences in metabolism, DNA repair, and alterations in oncogenes and tumour suppressor genes. There is increasing knowledge of the allelic variants or genetic defects that give rise to the observed variation.

Most lung carcinogens require metabolic activation before binding to DNA (Figure 1.1). The role of metabolic genes in individual susceptibility to the carcinogenic effects of tobacco smoke has been studied. Procarcinogens in tobacco smoke are activated by several forms of cytochrome P450 (phase I) (Table 1.3) and detoxified by glutathione *S*-transferases (GST), NADPH:quinone oxidoreductase (NQO), *N*-acetyl-transferase (NAT), and others (phase II).[39] Generally, these enzymes play a central role in removing environmental toxins. Cytochrome P450 activity results in the insertion of an oxygen atom into the substrate, and the GST and NAT act on the products of the phase I enzymes by

Table 1.3 Tobacco-smoke carcinogens and P450 involvement

Compound	P450 family involved
PAH	CYP1A, CYP2C, CYP2E
NNK/nitrosamines	CYP2A, CYP2D, CYP2E
Acetaldehyde	CYP2E
Benzene	CYP2E
Nicotine	CYP2B
4-Aminobiphenyl	CYP1A

adding chemical groups to produce readily excretable compounds. PAHs in tobacco smoke are inert chemicals that are metabolized by various enzymes such as P450 and cyclooxygenases/peroxidases to carcinogenic metabolites. The CYP1 superfamily of cytochrome P450 isozymes are largely responsible for PAH activation. CYP1A1 activity is strongly induced by PAHs and by a variety of planar lipophilic xenobiotics.[40] Nitrosamines also require enzymatic activation, catalysed by members of the cytochrome P450 enzyme family (CYP2E1), to intermediates that bind to DNA to produce a variety of alkylated bases.[41] Molecular epidemiological studies indicate that smokers have a higher level of PAHs and alkylated DNA adducts in surgical lung non-neoplastic tissue than non-smokers, indicating that tobacco exposure is a source of B(*a*)P and nitrosamines.[8,10,42] However, large interindividual variation is found at the DNA-adduct level. The extent of DNA-adduct formation depends on the balance between the rate of oxidation and the rate of detoxification. Thus enhancement of monooxygenase enzymes or inhibition of conjugating enzymes enhances the covalent binding of B(*a*)P to DNA. On this basis, individuals with particular combinations of defects in the P450, GST and NAT enzyme systems may have a higher risk of contracting lung cancer. Certain of these enzymes have been shown to display genetic polymorphisms, and have been linked to altered susceptibility to lung cancer. In relation to lung cancer susceptibility, these supergene families have attracted recent interest. Many of these genes exhibit allelism, and there is accumulating evidence that some CYP, GST and NAT genotypes are associated with altered risks of various cancers, including lung. Investigations have focused on the CYP1A1 and GSTM1 enzymes. Japanese studies have shown that a high susceptibility to lung cancer is associated with *CYP1A1* gene polymorphisms (MspI and Ile–Val polymorphism).[43] This lung cancer susceptibility depends on cigarette dose, showing a high relative risk at a low level of cigarette smoking for individuals with susceptible genotypes. Furthermore, individuals with the susceptible genotype were shown to be at remarkably higher lung cancer risk, with an odds ratio of 16.0, when the genotype was combined with a deficient *GSTM1* genotype, *GSTM1*(–).[44] A deletion of both copies of the *GSTM1* gene is present in 40–60% of the general population, producing a complete lack of the GSTM1 enzyme. GSTM1 is particularly involved in detoxifying epoxides of PAH compounds. Previous studies have indicated that the homozygous null genotype is more common among patients with lung cancer than among healthy controls. A major GST protein in the human lung is GSTP1-1. This enzyme is also active against many epoxides of PAHs. A polymorphic site at codon 105 (Ile105Val substitution) in the *P1* gene is known that changes the kinetic properties of the enzyme. A recent study indicates that individuals with the low-activity alleles had a higher lung cancer risk and had a higher level of PAH–DNA adducts in the lung.[45]

These studies show that differences among individuals in enzymes that metabolize carcinogens may be important determinants of tobacco-induced cancer. Susceptibility to lung cancer may also be modulated by DNA repair. Recent findings suggest that individuals with reduced DNA repair capacity (DRC) are at an increased risk of lung cancer.[46]

Nicotine is metabolized to cotinine by CYP2A6. A recent study shows that individuals lacking fully functional CYP2A6, who therefore have impaired nicotine metabolism, are significantly protected against becoming tobacco-dependent smokers.[47] In addition, they smoke significantly fewer cigarettes than those with normal nicotine metabolism. Furthermore, nitrosamines in tobacco smoke can be activated by CYP2A6. So individuals carrying CYP2A6-null alleles may be less efficient in activating certain carcinogens. Recently, it was found that certain variant alleles of the D2 dopamine receptor gene appear to be related to differences in smoking behaviour and to play a role in determining nicotine addiction.[48] This gene affects the dopamine receptors in the brain, and certain versions of the gene have fewer receptors. Individuals with few receptors may experience a greater pleasure from smoking and therefore may be more vulnerable to tobacco use. However, other genes are certainly also involved in vulnerability to nicotine dependence.

FEMALES AND SMOKING

In several countries, lung cancer now kills more women each year than breast cancer, and for women in many countries (especially developing countries) the peak of the tobacco epidemic has yet to arrive. Furthermore, several recent epidemiological studies indicate that females may have a higher risk of lung cancer than males.[49,50] These studies are supported by experimental data on gender differences in metabolism and on the effect of hormones on tumour development.[51,52] A recent study of PAH–DNA adducts in the human lung found higher levels of adducts in females than in males, suggesting that susceptibility to DNA damage caused by PAH compounds may be higher among females.[53] Moreover, a higher frequency of G-to-T mutations in the *p53* gene in lung tumours of females than in males was observed.[54] More attention needs to be paid to the issue of smoking and women, since they are a main target for the tobacco industry.

In summary, lung carcinogenesis is mediated through an interaction between several putative carcinogens. Studies suggest that PAHs and nitrosamines are major risk factors. Genetic differences in carcinogen-metabolizing enzymes and DNA repair may be important determinants of lung cancer susceptibility.

REFERENCES

1. Mannino DM, Ford E, Giovono GA, Thun M, Lung cancer deaths in the United States from 1979 to 1992: an analysis using multiple-cause mortality data. *Int J Epidemiol* 1998; **27**: 159–66.
2. International Agency for Research on Cancer, Tobacco smoking. *IARC Monogr Eval Carcinogen Risk Chem Hum* 1986; **38**.
3. Hoffmann D, Hoffmann I, The changing cigarette, 1950–1995. *J Toxicol Environ Health* 1997; **50**: 307–64.
4. Wolterbeek APM, Schoevers EJ, Rutten AAJJL, Feron VJ, A critical appraisal of intratracheal instillation of benzo[a]pyrene to Syrian golden hamsters as a model in respiratory tract carcinogenesis. *Cancer Lett* 1995; **89**: 107–16.
5. Stanton MF, Miller E, Wrench C, Blackwell R, Experimental induction of epidermoid carcinoma in the lungs of rats by cigarette smoke condensate. *J Natl Cancer Inst* 1972; **49**: 867–77.

6. Thyssen J, Althoff J, Kimmerle G, Mohr U, Inhalation studies with benzo[*a*]pyrene in Syrian golden hamsters. *J Natl Cancer Inst* 1981; **66**: 575–7.
7. Harris CC, Frank A, van Haaften C et al, Binding of ^{3}H-benzo[*a*]pyrene to DNA in cultured human bronchus. *Cancer Res* 1976; **36**: 1011–18.
8. Phillips DH, Hewer A, Martin CM et al, Correlation of DNA adduct levels in human lung with cigarette smoking. *Nature* 1988; **336**: 790–2.
9. Perera F, Mayer J, Jaretzki A et al, Comparison of DNA adducts and sister chromatid exchange in lung cancer cases and controls. *Cancer Res* 1989; **49**: 4446–51.
10. Ryberg D, Hewer A, Phillips DH, Haugen A, Different susceptibility to smoking-induced DNA damage among male and female lung cancer patients. *Cancer Res* 1994; **54**: 5801–3.
11. Hainaut P, Hernandez T, Robinson A et al, IARC database of p53 gene mutations in human tumors and cell lines: updated compilation, revised formats and new visualisation tools. *Nucleic Acids Res* 1998; **26**: 205–13.
12. Denissenko MF, Pao A, Tang M, Pfeifer GP, Preferential formation of benzo[*a*]pyrene adducts at lung cancer mutational hotspots in *p53*. *Science* 1996; **274**: 430–2.
13. Hoffmann D, Rivenson A, Hecht SS, The biological significance of tobacco-specific *N*-nitrosamines: smoking and adenocarcinoma of the lung. *Crit Rev Toxicol* 1996; **26**: 199–211.
14. Rivenson A, Hecht SS, Hoffmann D, Carcinogenicity of tobacco-specific *N*-nitrosamines (TSNA): the role of the vascular network in the selection of target organs. *Crit Rev Toxicol* 1991; **21**: 255–64.
15. Hoffmann D, Brunnemann KD, Prokopczyk B, Djordjevic MV, Tobacco-specific *N*-nitrosamines: chemistry, biochemistry, carcinogenicity and relevance to humans. *J Toxicol Environ Health* 1994; **41**: 1–52.
16. Parsons WD, Carmella SG, Akerkal SA et al, A metabolite of the tobacco-specific lung carcinogen 4-(methylnitrosamino)-1-(3-pyridyl)-1-butanone in the urine of hospital workers exposed to environmental tobacco smoke. *Cancer Epidemiol Biomarkers Prev* 1998; **7**: 257–60.
17. Foiles PG, Akerkar SA, Carmella SG et al, Mass spectrometric analysis of tobacco-specific nitrosamine–DNA adducts in smokers and nonsmokers. *Chem Res Toxicol* 1991; **4**: 364–8.
18. Cohen MD, Kargacin B, Klein CB, Costa M, Mechanisms of chromium carcinogenicity and toxicity. *Crit Rev Toxicol* 1993; **23**: 255–81.
19. Waalkes MP, Oberdörster G, Cadmium carcinogenesis. In: *Biological Effects of Heavy Metals*, Vol 2 (Foulkes ED, ed). CRC Press: Boca Raton, FL, 1990: 129–58.
20. Oller AR, Costa M, Oberdörster G, Carcinogenicity assessment of selected nickel compounds. *Toxicol Appl Pharmacol* 1997; **143**: 152–66.
21. Klein CB, Frenkel K, Costa M, The role of oxidative process in metal carcinogenesis. *Chem Res Toxicol* 1991; **4**: 592–603.
22. International Agency for Research on Cancer, Formaldehyde. *IARC Monograph* 1982; **4**: 131–2.
23. Little JB, Kennedy AR, McCandy RB, Effect of dose rate on the induction of experimental lung cancer in hamsters by alpha radiation. *Radiat Res* 1985; **103**: 293–9.
24. Nakayama T, Kodama M, Generation of hydrogen peroxide and superoxide anion radicals from cigarette smoking. *Gann* 1984; **75**: 95–8.
25. Hunninghake GW, Crystal RG, Cigarette smoking and lung destruction: accumulation of neutrophils in the lungs of cigarette smokers. *Am Rev Respir Dis* 1990; **128**: 833–8.
26. London SJ, Lehman TA, Taylor JA, Myeloperoxidase genetic polymorphism and lung cancer risk. *Cancer Res* 1997; **57**: 5001–3.
27. Kasai H, Analysis of a form of oxidative DNA-damage, 8-hydroxy-2′-deoxyguanosine, as a marker of cellular oxidative stress during carcinogenesis. *Mut Res* 1997; **387**: 147–63.
28. Arai K, Morishita K, Shinmura K et al, Cloning of a human homolog of the yeast OGG1 gene that is involved in the repair of oxidative DNA damage. *Oncogene* 1997; **14**: 2857–61.

29. Kreutzer D, Essigmann JM, Oxidized, deaminated cytosines are a source of C → T transitions in vivo. *Proc Natl Acad Sci USA* 1998; **95**: 3578–82.
30. Maneckjee R, Minna JD. Opioid and nicotine receptors affect growth regulation of human lung cancer cell lines. *Proc Natl Acad Sci USA* 1990; **87**: 3294–8.
31. Heusch W, Maneckjee R, Signalling pathways involved in nicotine regulation of apoptosis of human lung cancer cells. *Carcinogenesis* 1998; **19**: 551–6.
32. Engholm G, Palmgren F, Lynge E, Lung cancer, smoking, and environment: a cohort study of the Danish population. *BMJ* 1996; **312**: 1259–63.
33. Phillips PS, Denman AR, Radon: a human carcinogen. *Sci Prog* 1997; **80**: 317–36.
34. Hornung RW, Deddens JA, Roscoe RJ, Modifiers of lung cancer risk in uranium miners from the Colorado Plateau. *Health Phys* 1998; **74**: 12–21.
35. Cohen BL, Lung cancer risk from residential radon: meta-analysis of eight epidemiologic studies. *J Natl Cancer Inst* 1997; **89**: 664.
36. Searle CE, Teale OJ, Occupational carcinogens. In: *Chemical Carcinogenesis and Mutagenesis I*. Vol 94/I (Cooper CS, Grover PL, eds). Springer-Verlag: Berlin, 1990: 103–51.
37. Hackshaw AK, Law M, Wald NJ, The accumulated evidence on lung cancer and environmental tobacco smoke. *BMJ* 1997; **315**: 980–8.
38. Dockery DW, Trichopoulos D, Risk of lung cancer from environmental exposures to tobacco smoke. *Cancer Causes Control* 1997; **8**: 333–45.
39. Spivack SD, Fasco M, Walker VE, Kaminsky LS, The molecular epidemiology of lung cancer. *Crit Rev Toxicol* 1997; **27**: 319–65.
40. Swanson HI, Bradfield CA, The Ah receptor, genetics, structure and function. *Pharmacogenetics* 1993; **3**: 213.
41. Hecht SS, Approaches to cancer prevention based on an understanding of *N*-nitrosamine carcinogenesis. *Proc Soc Exp Biol Med* 1997; **216**: 181–91.
42. Hecht SS, Carmella SG, Foiles PG, Murphy SE, Biomarkers for human uptake and metabolic activation to tobacco-specific nitrosamines. *Cancer Res* 1994; **54**: 1912.
43. Hayashi S, Watanabe J, Nakachi K, Kawajiri K, Genetic linkage of lung cancer-associated *Msp*I polymorphisms with amino acid replacement in the human cytochrome P450IA1 gene. *J Biochem* 1991; **110**: 407.
44. Hayashi S, Watanabe J, Kawajiri K, High susceptibility to lung cancer analyzed in terms of combined genotypes of P4501A1 and mu-class glutathione S-transferase genes. *Jpn J Cancer Res* 1992; **83**: 866.
45. Ryberg D, Skaug V, Hewer A et al, Genotypes of glutathione transferase M1 and P1 and their significance for lung DNA adduct levels and cancer risk. *Carcinogenesis* 1997; **18**: 1427–31.
46. Wei Q, Cheng L, Hong WK, Spitz MR, Reduced DNA repair capacity in lung cancer patients. *Cancer Res* 1996; **56**: 4103–7.
47. Panezza ML, Sellers EM, Tyndale RF, Nicotine metabolism defect reduces smoking. *Nature* 1998; **393**: 750.
48. Spitz MR, Shi H, Yang F et al, Case-control study of the D2 dopamine receptor gene and smoking status in lung cancer patients. *J Natl Cancer Inst* 1998; **90**: 358–63.
49. Engeland A, Haldorsen T, Andersen A, Tretli S. The impact of smoking habits on lung-cancer risk; twenty-eight years' observation of 26 000 Norwegian men and women. *Cancer Causes Control* 1996; **7**: 366–76.
50. Brownson RC, Chang JC, Davis JR, Gender and histologic type variations in smoking-related risk of lung cancer. *Epidemiology* 1992; **3**: 61–4.
51. Singhal SS, Saxena M, Ahmad H, Awasthi YC, Glutathione S-transferase of mouse-liver: sex-related differences in the expression of various isozymes. *Biochim Biophys Acta* 1992; **1116**: 137–46.
52. Singhal SS, Saxena M, Awasthi S et al, Gender related differences in the expression and characteristics of glutathione *S*-transferases of human colon. *Biochim Biophys Acta* 1992; **1171**: 19–26.
53. Ryberg D, Hewer A, Phillips DH, Haugen A, Different susceptibility to smoking-induced

DNA damage among male and female lung-cancer patients. *Cancer Res* 1994; **54**: 5801–3.

54. Kure EH, Ryberg D, Hewer A et al, *p53* mutations in lung tumours: relationship to gender and lung DNA adduct levels. *Carcinogenesis* 1996; **17**: 2201–5.

Epidemiology of lung cancer: A century of great success and ignominious failure

Peter Boyle, Sara Gandini, Nigel Gray

Contents

INTRODUCTION

The present century has witnessed a remarkable epidemic of lung cancer. The words of Adler,[1] published in 1912, today make salutary reading:

> Is it worthwhile to write a monograph on the subject of primary malignant tumours of the lung? In the course of the last two centuries an ever-increasing literature has accumulated around this subject. But this literature is without correlation, much of it buried in dissertations and other out-of-the-way places, and, with but a few notable exceptions, no attempt has been made to study the subject as a whole, either the pathological or the clinical aspect having been emphasised at the expense of the other, according to the special predilection of the author. On one point, however, there is nearly complete consensus of opinion, and that is that primary malignant neoplasms of the lungs are among the rarest forms of the disease. This latter opinion of the extreme rarity of primary tumours has persisted for centuries.

Lung cancer is currently the most common form of cancer worldwide. It is the most common cause of cancer death in men in North America and in virtually all European countries, west and east, and it is increasingly common as a cause of death in developing populations in Asia, Latin American and Africa, although comparable high-quality data are not available from many of these populations. From being virtually an unknown and rare disease at the beginning of this century, public health has documented the development of a true epidemic of lung cancer this century, and has failed to alleviate the situation by positive actions. Knowing the cause, which has been the case for lung cancer for at least the second half of this century, has been of little value in public health terms, since there has been no real action taken to reduce the impact of this serious disease.

In viewing the century of lung cancer epidemiology, there are a number of distinct phases that can be identified. Initially (phase I), there was the great success of epidemiology, the basic science of public health, in establishing the causal link between cigarette smoking and lung cancer risk. Following this period, from the mid-1950s onwards, there was a period (phase II) where there was an increasing understanding of the etiology of lung cancer, and simultaneously public health began losing ground as smoking rates led to great increases in the incidence and mortality of the disease, particularly among men in developed countries. The association between tobacco smoking and lung cancer became widely known, and many groups actively took up the movement towards tobacco control. During this period (phase III), the situation stabilized while activists and scientists united to try to bring the adverse effects of tobacco smoking to general attention and thereby to take actions designed to reduce smoking and its harmful side-effects. It quickly became clear that a great deal of ground had been lost, and during phase IV large increases in lung cancer among women became apparent, indicating the great failure of public health to curb the development of the habit among women.

PHASE I: PUBLIC HEALTH SUCCESS, 1930s ONWARDS

The association between tobacco smoking and the development of lung cancer appears to have been suggested in the UK in 1927.[2] The first interview study on tobacco smoking and lung cancer seems to have been reported from Vienna,[3] where lung cancer rates had risen dramatically. Fleckseder[3] found 51 smokers among 54 patients with lung cancer. Thirty-seven of these smoked between 20 and 90 cigarettes daily, while excessive smoking of pipes, cigars or both was rarer.

The same association was alluded to in a report from the USA[4] on a study primarily of a series of 79 patients treated by total pneumonectomy. A report from Cologne followed one year later,[5] based on the postmortem records of 96 patients. The patients (or more usually the relatives of fatal cases) were interviewed as to patient's occupation, tobacco consumption and exposure to specific 'inhalants'.

Reanalysis of Muller's[5] data shows a relative risk of 3.1 among moderate smokers, 2.7 among heavy smokers, 16.8 among very heavy smokers and 29.16 among excessive smokers. Within the limitations of the study (e.g. small numbers, especially among non-smoking cases, and possible inaccuracies in elucidation of precise smoking histories), these results were noticeably similar to results obtained from later case–control studies in the USA and, apart from a lack of increase among heavy smokers, there is the possible appearance of a dose–response relationship.

A study of smoking habits and occupation based on 195 postmortem records of lung cancer cases from the Pathology Institute at Jena for the years 1930–1941 was reported: usable replies were obtained from relatives of 93 men and 16 women. Of the women, 13 were non-smokers.[6] The authors attempted to collect control information by interviewing 700 men in Jena between the ages of 53 and 54, the average age of the lung cancer patients at death (53.9 years). This was a study performed in Germany towards the end of the Second World War, and only 270 men from Jena responded to the questionnaire. The authors showed great insight in concluding that wartime conditions (particularly the rationing system) may have favoured results from non-smokers.

They reported a statistically significant difference between non-smokers and heavy smokers among lung cancer patients on the one hand and normal patients on the other. Realizing the possible errors on their material, they concluded that there was a considerable probability that lung cancer was far more frequent among non-smokers than expected. Their data are such that an approximate relative risk can be calculated: the risk relative to non-smokers was 1.90 among light smokers, 9.05 among moderate smokers and 11.34 among heavy/excessive smokers. Again there appears to be a moderate dose–response relationship.

The rapid escalation in lung cancer during the 1940s reached a level that permitted more and larger studies to be conducted and, in 1950, five major contributions were made to the literature.[7–11]

The data presented by Wynder and Graham[10] are capable of transformation to calculate the relative risks (the concept of which was unknown for a few more years). Setting the risk among non-smokers at 1.0, there is to some extent or other a dose–response relationship with increasing levels of smoking in all age groups. Together with the study of Wynder and Graham,[10] the fifth paper published on this subject during the year represented a significant contribution not only to knowledge about smoking and cancer but also to the methodology of retrospective epidemiological studies.[11]

This well-planned, controlled and well-conducted study was initially reported,[11] and completed and published more extensively two years later. It is this latter report[12] that we shall discuss here. Doll and Hill[12] did not discuss cigar smoking, but calculated that use of one ounce of pipe tobacco was the equivalent of 26.5 cigarettes, and one ounce per week was equivalent to smoking four cigarettes per day. Non-smokers were defined as people who had never consistently smoked as much as one cigarette per day for as long as one year.[11]

The strongest difference between cases and controls (for both males and females) was found to be the average amount smoked daily over the 10 years preceding the patient's illness. Qualitatively similar results were also obtained using the amount smoked immediately before the patient's illness, the maximum amount ever smoked regularly, the total smoked since smoking began, and the average amount smoked daily over the 10 years preceding the patient's illness, over the penultimate 10 years and over the whole of the patient's life since the age of 15 (even after allowance had been made for recorded changes in smoking habit).

Patients who recognized that they inhaled were found no more frequently in the lung cancer group than in the control group, although those cases with growths of central origin inhaled less frequently than normal. It also appeared that lung cancer patients more frequently had a history of preceding pneumonia or chronic bronchitis, while other respiratory illnesses were referred to with approximately equal frequency by the two groups.

Doll and Hill's reports[11,12] contained a remarkable amount of information, but the fundamental finding in men was a highly significant difference between the proportions of non-smokers and of smokers in the disease group and in the control group. A less marked series of differences was reported for women. Highly significant differences were also shown between the proportions of both groups smoking different average amounts, i.e. between heavy and light smokers, and this result held for males and females. It is apparent from the raw data that there is a dose–response relationship present.

Less marked but nevertheless distinct differences were found when the duration of smoking was considered rather than the amount smoked. Lung cancer cases, as a group, began to smoke earlier; they continued to smoke longer and gave up less often and, when they did, did so for shorter periods. In males, all these differences were statistically significant, but, although the differences were in the same direction in women, they did not reach the commonly accepted (5%) level of statistical significance.

These five studies,[7–11] but mainly the impact of two,[10,11] alerted the medical and scientific community to the serious health hazards associated with cigarette smoking. Once alerted, the public response to these studies was a significant, but brief, drop in the per capita consumption of cigarettes in both the USA and the UK.

PHASE II: UNDERSTANDING ETIOLOGY, LOSING GROUND IN INCIDENCE AND MORTALITY

Throughout the 1950s, a mass of information was published demonstrating the association between lung cancer and cigarette smoking, using data derived from retrospective studies. Many concentrated on inhalation and, while some studies demonstrated a higher occurrence of inhalation among lung cancer patients than among controls, others failed to detect this association.

The US Surgeon General was moved by the weight of evidence associating smoking with cancer of the lung, as well as of other sites, to produce an official statement on 'Smoking and Health' on behalf of the US Government.[13] This created a worldwide reaction, since it implicated a frightening link between cigarette smoking and a variety of fatal diseases in a document of impeccable scientific authority.

This report weighed the available evidence, and considered that it had been established that cigarette smoking was causally related to lung cancer in men, and judged cigarette smoking in the USA a sufficiently important health hazard to warrant remedial action.

In the 15 years that passed from that initial report, the body of evidence increased, and extended to include women,[14] in whom lung cancer had increased fivefold in two decades in the USA. The Secretary for Health of the time (Mr Joseph Califano) concluded 'that smoking is the largest preventable cause of death in America'.

An important factor in the causal relationship between smoking and lung cancer is the demonstrated dose–response relationship. In epidemiological studies, the dose has been measured by:

- the number of cigarettes smoked per day at interview;
- the maximum number of cigarettes smoked per day;
- the age when smoking commenced;
- the degree of inhalation of tobacco smoke;
- the total number of years smoked;
- the total lifetime number of cigarettes smoked;
- the tar and nicotine levels of the brand of cigarettes used;
- the number of puffs per cigarette;
- the length of the unburned portion of cigarette.

A variety of combinations of these variables can be converted into dosage scores.

Lung cancer mortality ratios exhibit an inverse relationship with the age of initiation of the smoking habit. Those who develop the habit at school have a much higher risk of lung cancer than those who begin smoking at age 25+, in whom the risk is only four to five times that of non-smokers.

Available data show a strong dose–response relationship between self-reported inhalation of cigarette smoke and lung cancer mortality. Those who inhale deeply have risks double those of smokers who do not. The American Cancer Society 25 State Study[15] reported a mortality ratio among non-smokers of 1.0, a mortality ratio of 8.0 among smokers who stated that they did not inhale, and elevations in this risk among those who inhaled slightly (8.9), moderately (13.1) and deeply (17.0). Similar results were reported from a Swedish study:[16] although the mortality ratios among non-smokers (1.0), non-inhalers (3.7), light inhalers (7.8) and deep inhalers (9.2) were smaller in magnitude, the same steady pattern was found.

Although it has been suggested for some time that the risk of developing lung cancer increases with the tar and nicotine content of cigarettes, there has not been any substantial evidence to suggest that individuals who switch to lower-tar and lower-nicotine cigarettes experience less lung cancer mortality.[17] It has been proposed that, if the tar and nicotine contents of tobacco were reduced, smokers might increase the number of cigarettes smoked per day and effectively vitiate any benefit. On the other hand, those who switch to low-tar and low-nicotine brands might inhale smoke more deeply than smokers of high-tar and high-nicotine cigarettes, and thus exposure to tar and nicotine might be reduced.

The relationship of tar and nicotine was carefully examined with respect to lung cancer in a major study,[18] in which 897 825 men and women were classified by levels of tar and nicotine smoked. Brands were considered to be high in nicotine if they contained between 2.0 and 2.7 mg of nicotine and high in tar if they contained between 25.8 and 35.7 mg of tar. The medium levels of tar and nicotine were set at 17.6 and 25.7 mg and at 1.2 and 1.9 mg respectively. Low tar and nicotine levels were all those below these limits.

The risk in the high-tar and high-nicotine group of makes was set at 1.0, and the relative risks in the medium group (risk ratio, RR = 0.95) and low group (RR=0.81) were appreciably lower. Similar results were found for females: high (RR = 1.0), medium (RR=0.79) and low (RR=0.60). These results take into account the daily cigarette consumption.

In other words, for men smoking the same number of cigarettes per day, there appears to be an almost 20% reduction in the risk of developing lung cancer with the use of cigarettes low in tar and nicotine. In females, keeping the number of cigarettes smoked per day constant, there appears to be a 40% reduction in risk. The amount of tar and nicotine taken into the body per day obviously depends on the number of cigarettes smoked as well as on the tar and nicotine content of individual cigarettes. Hammond therefore performed a second analysis comparing subjects who smoked 1–19 high-tar and -nicotine cigarettes per day with those who smoked 20–39 low-tar and -nicotine cigarettes per day. Setting the risk to be 1.0 among the high categories of both males and females, Hammond found risks of 1.6 (males) and 2.1 (females) among the groups who smoked 20–39 low-tar and -nicotine cigarettes. He concluded that the number of cigarettes smoked per day was relatively more important than the tar and nicotine content.[15,18]

All these early observations were regarding forms of cancer and forms of tobacco smoking that were the most common at the period. Cigarette smoking increased heavily in Europe during the last years of Napoleon,[19] and the habit spread during the Crimean War, accelerated around 1900 and reached many men, and increasingly women, during the First World War (1914–1918). In many countries, such as the USA and the UK, women began to reach the same smoking levels as men during the Second World War (1939–1945).

Subsequent to this period, cancer was becoming more frequent, and was developing into an international disease that was to become, by the latter part of the 20th century, a significant global public health problem. An increasing number of forms of cancer became linked with cigarette smoking: initially oral cancers, then lung cancer, bladder cancer, laryngeal cancer, oesophageal cancer, pancreatic cancer, acute myeloid leukaemia, cervical cancer, kidney cancer and gastric cancer. Several of these are of unusually high frequency in international populations.[20]

PHASE III: DESCRIPTIVE EPIDEMIOLOGY OF LUNG CANCER

The main tobacco-related site is the lung. Lung cancer rates in self-reported non-smokers from various studies are of the order of only 10–15 per 100 000. The IARC monograph *Tobacco Smoking*[21] gave estimates of the proportions of lung cancer deaths attributable to tobacco smoking in five developed countries (Canada, England and Wales, Japan, Sweden and the USA): these ranged between 83% and 92% for males, and between 57% and 80% for females.

The most recent, international, cancer incidence data are available for the period around 1990. The highest incidence rate in men is recorded among the Afro-American population of New Orleans in the USA, where the average, annual, age-standardized rate per 100 000 person-years is 110.8 (Table 2.1). Other Afro-American populations in the USA also have remarkably high lung cancer rates in men. Rates are also high among the Maori population of New Zealand, where the incidence rate is 99.7 per 100 000 (Table 2.1). The incidence rate is high in Lower Silesia (Poland) and in the west of Scotland (Table 2.1). There are virtually no regions of the world where the annual incidence rates are *low*: the lowest incidence rates are reported from a variety of population groups from the developing world (Table 2.2).

Among women, the highest rates are found in the Maori population group of New Zealand (72.9 per 100 000) (Table 2.3). High rates are also found among a variety of populations of North America – both Afro-American and Caucasian. Notably high rates are reported from the west of Scotland, where incidence rates are high in men as well as in women (Table 2.3). The finding of the incidence rate among women in Tianjin, China, among the 15 highest incidence

Table 2.1 Highest incidence rates of cancer of the trachea, bronchus and lung in men circa 1990

Registry	Cases	ASR[a]
USA, New Orleans: Black (1988–1992)	842	110.81
USA, Central Louisiana: Black (1988–1992)	172	105.62
USA, Detroit: Black (1988–1992)	2263	103.23
USA, San Francisco: Black (1988–1992)	1003	101.49
New Zealand: Maori (1988–1992)	387	99.73
USA, SEER:[b] Black (1988–1992)	4964	99.11
USA, Atlanta: Black (1988–1992)	892	97.26
Poland, Lower Silesia (1988–1992)	7213	95.52
Canada, Northwest Territories (1983–1992)	126	90.26
UK, Scotland, west (1988–1992)	8877	88.90
USA, Los Angeles: Black (1988–1992)	1925	88.74
USA, Connecticut: Black (1988–1992)	422	86.15
Italy, Ferrara (1991–1992)	597	85.73
USA, New Orleans: White (1988–1992)	1707	84.01
Italy, Trieste (1989–1992)	897	82.73

[a]Average, annual, age-standardized rate per 100 000 person-years.
[b]Surveillance Epidermiology and End Results Program (National Cancer Institute).

Table 2.2 Lowest incidence rates of cancer of the trachea, bronchus and lung in men circa 1990

Registry	Cases	ASR[a]
India, Karunagappally (1991–1992)	58	17.04
Thailand, Kohn Kaen (1990–1993)	355	17.02
Peru, Lima (1990–1991)	635	15.89
Costa Rica (1988–1992)	686	15.63
India, Bombay (1988–1992)	1867	14.48
Singapore: Indian (1988–1992)	83	14.33
India, Madras (1988–1992)	789	12.64
Peru, Trujillo (1988–1990)	47	11.93
India, Trivandrum (1991–1992)	69	10.63
USA, New Mexico: American Indian (1988–1992)	24	10.32
Ecuador, Quito (1988–1992)	172	10.13
India, Bangalore (1988–1992)	495	8.06
Mali, Bamako (1988–1992)	38	5.28
Uganda, Kyadondo (1991–1993)	20	4.24
India, Barshi, Paranda and Bhum (1988–1992)	11	1.26

[a]Average, annual, age-standardized rate per 100 000 person-years.

Table 2.3 Highest incidence rates of cancer of the trachea, bronchus and lung in women circa 1990

Registry	Cases	ASR[a]
New Zealand: Maori (1988–1992)	326	72.93
Canada, Northwest Territories (1983–1992)	80	65.56
Canada, Yukon (1983–1992)	39	47.62
USA, San Francisco: Black (1988–1992)	562	44.33
USA, Detroit: Black (1988–1992)	1213	42.02
USA, New Orleans: White (1988–1992)	1115	41.19
USA, San Franciso: non-Hispanic White (1988–1992)	3906	40.42
USA, Detroit: White (1988–1992)	4772	40.17
USA, Central California: non-Hispanic White (1988–1992)	2267	39.48
USA, Los Angeles: non-Hispanic White (1988–1992)	6674	38.58
UK, Scotland, west (1988–1992)	5086	38.47
USA, SEER:[b] Black (1988–1992)	2558	38.46
USA, Hawaii: White (1988–1992)	340	37.94
USA, Seattle (1988–1992)	4413	37.62
China, Tianjin (1988–1992)	3870	37.00

[a]Average, annual, age-standardized rate per 100 000 person-years.
[b]Surveillance Epidermiology and End Results Program (National Cancer Institute).

Table 2.4 Lowest incidence rates of cancer of the trachea, bronchus and lung in women circa 1990

Registry	Cases	ASR[a]
Malta (1992–1993)	18	3.35
France, La Réunion (1988–1992)	46	3.34
France, Tarn (1988–1992)	60	3.19
Spain, Albacete (1991–1992)	19	3.14
Spain, Tarragona (1988–1992)	72	3.09
Algeria, Setif (1990–1993)	33	2.88
Spain, Granada (1988–1992)	92	2.71
Spain, Zaragoza (1986–1990)	116	2.66
India, Karunagappally (1991–1992)	10	2.59
India, Madras (1988–1992)	142	2.37
India, Trivandrum (1991–1992)	14	1.89
India, Bangalore (1988–1992)	103	1.67
Mali, Bamako (1988–1992)	13	1.53
Uganda, Kyadondo (1991–1993)	4	0.41
India, Barshi, Paranda and Bhum (1988–1992)	3	0.33

[a]Average, annual, age-standardized rate per 100 000 person-years.

rates recorded, is the first clear indication of the rising epidemic of lung cancer, and other cancers, resulting from the increasing prevalence of cigarette smoking during recent decades (Table 2.3). There are some regions of the world where the incidence rate among women is still truly low (Table 2.4).

In men in all European countries, except Portugal, lung cancer is now the leading cause of cancer death. In the USA (and in all European countries except a few Scandinavian countries), it is also the commonest tumour in terms of incidence (although the recent inflation of prostate cancer incidence figures with very early detection of cases is taking prostate cancer above lung cancer in terms of the incidence of the disease). The range of geographical variation in lung cancer mortality in Europe is threefold in both sexes – the highest rates being observed in the UK, Belgium, the Netherlands and the former Czechoslovakia, and the lowest rates being reported in southern Europe and in Norway and Sweden.[22] This overall pattern of age-standardized lung cancer mortality rates does not reveal the important and diverging cohort effects occurring in various countries: for instance, some of the countries in which there are now low rates, such as those in southern Europe and parts of eastern Europe, experienced a later uptake and spread of tobacco use, and now appear among the most elevated rates in the younger age groups. This suggests that these same countries, including Italy, Greece, France, Spain and several countries in eastern Europe, will have the highest lung cancer rates in men at the beginning of the next century, in the absence of rapid intervention.

The importance of adequate intervention is shown by the low lung cancer rates in Scandinavian countries, which have adopted, since the early 1970s, integrated central and local policies and programmes against smoking.[23,24] These policies may have been enabled by the limited influence of the tobacco lobby in these countries. The experience in Finland provides convincing evidence of the favourable impact, after a relatively short delay, of well-targeted large-scale interventions on the most common cause of cancer death and of premature mortality in general.

With specific reference to women, current rates in most European countries (except the UK and Ireland) are still substantially lower than in the USA, where lung cancer is now the leading cause of cancer death in females. In several countries, including France, Switzerland, Gernnany and Italy, where smoking is now becoming commoner in young and middle-aged women, overall national mortality rates are still relatively low, although appreciable upward trends have been registered over the last two decades. This is particularly worrisome in perspective, since smoking prevalence has continued to increase in subsequent generations of young women in these countries. Thus the observation that lung cancer is still relatively rare in women, with smoking at present accounting for only approximately 40–60% of all lung cancer deaths, cannot constitute a reason for delaying efficacious interventions against smoking by women. The currently more favourable situation in Europe compared with the USA, together with the observation that smoking cessation reduces lung cancer risk after a delay of several years, should, in the presence of adequate intervention, enable a major lung cancer epidemic in European women to be avoided.

A proportion of lung cancers, varying in various countries and geographical areas, may be due to exposures at work, and a small proportion to atmospheric pollution.[25] The effect of atmospheric pollution in increasing lung cancer risk appears to be chiefly confined to smokers. Lung cancer risk is elevated in atomic bomb survivors,[26] in patients treated for ankylosing spondylitis,[27] and in underground miners whose bronchial mucosa was exposed to radon gas and its decay products: this last exposure was reviewed and it was concluded that there was 'sufficient evidence' that this occupational exposure caused lung cancer.[28] A greater risk of lung cancer is generally seen for individuals who are exposed at an older age. Investigation of the interaction with cigarette smoking among atomic bomb survivors suggests that it is additive,[29] but the data from underground miners in Colorado are consistent with a multiplicative effect.[30]

In conclusion, the overwhelming role of tobacco smoking in the causation of lung cancer has been repeatedly demonstrated over the past 50 years. Current lung cancer rates reflect cigarette smoking habits of men and women over past decades,[31–33] but not necessarily current smoking patterns, since there is an interval of several decades between the change in smoking habits in a population and its consequences on lung cancer rates. Over 90% of lung cancer may be avoidable simply through avoidance of cigarette smoking. Rates of lung cancer in central and eastern Europe at present are higher than those ever before recorded elsewhere; lung cancer has increased tenfold in men and eightfold in women in Japan since 1950; there is a worldwide epidemic of smoking among young women,[34] which will be translated into increasing rates of tobacco-related disease, including cancer, in the coming decades; there is another epidemic of lung cancer and tobacco-related deaths building up in China as the cohorts of men in whom tobacco smoking became popular reach ages at which cancer is an important hazard.[35] Many solutions have been attempted to reduce cigarette smoking, and increasingly many countries are enacting legislation to curb this habit.[36]

PHASE IV: PUBLIC HEALTH FAILURE, 1960s ONWARDS

Thus it has been clear for the entire second half of the 20th century that cigarette smoking causes lung cancer. Current low levels of smoking among physicians and research scientists in many countries have led many of them unconsciously to overlook tobacco smoking as an important cause of cancer.[37] There is, however, a very substantial body of evidence from many sources that indicates the carcinogenicity of tobacco smoking. Not only does cigarette smoking greatly increase the risk of lung cancer in smokers, but the risk of oral cavity cancer, laryngeal cancer, oesophageal cancer, bladder cancer, pancreatic cancer and kidney cancer is also increased. The risk of cancer of the cervix and stomach may also be increased, although the evidence for this is much less consistent.[38] These forms of cancer can be expected to rise in women as a result of their increased levels of cigarette smoking.

There is at present a worldwide epidemic of tobacco-related disease: not only does smoking cause increased levels of many different common forms of cancer, it also increases the risk of cardiovascular disease. As mentioned in the previous section, deaths from lung cancer, the tumour most strongly linked to cigarette smoking, have increased in Japan by a factor of 10 in men and 8 in women since 1950. In central and eastern Europe, more than 400 000 premature deaths are currently caused each year by tobacco smoking. In young men in all countries of central and eastern Europe, there are current levels of lung cancer that are greater than anything seen before in the Western countries, and these rates are still rising. In Poland – a country severely hit by the tobacco epidemic – the life-expectancy of a 45-year-old man has been falling for over a decade now owing to the increasing premature death rates from tobacco-related cancers and cardiovascular disease.[39] Tragically, cigarette smoking is still increasing in central and eastern Europe and also in China, where an epidemic of tobacco-related deaths is building up quickly. Tobacco smoking is also the most easily avoided risk factor for cancer.

The most important determinant of risk of lung cancer is the duration of smoking: long-term cigarette smokers have a 100-fold increased risk compared with never-smokers. The content of cigarettes (*low tar*) produces only a threefold variation in risks between the extremes. ('Low tar' is frequently taken to include a number of features, including filter-tips as well as the active tar yield.) Lung cancer is the major tobacco-related tumour and the leading cause of cancer death in men in almost every developed country. Incidence rates are around 10–15 per 100 000 in non-smokers and between 80 and 100 per 100 000 in the highest-incidence population groups such as Afro-Americans, and rates exceeding 200 per 100 000 have been reported in cities of central and eastern Europe. Since lung cancer is frequently fatal, mortality rates are high, and consequently so are the social costs.

Women around the world have taken up the cigarette smoking habit with gusto. For many years, it appeared that their lung cancer rates were low and that tobacco was not having the same effect as on men. This complacency, which crept in during the two decades from the mid-1960s especially, is now exposed as false: nor is there evidence that the effect of cigarette smoking on lung cancer risk is greater in women than in men. The dominance of the effect of duration of smoking means that a long period of time will pass between the exposure (large numbers of women smoking) and the effect (high levels of lung cancer). Lung cancer now exceeds breast cancer as the leading cancer cause of death in women in the USA, Canada, Scotland and several other countries. In Canada, breast cancer mortality has remained at least constant for nearly four decades, while lung cancer death rates have increased between three- and fourfold during the same period. While the higher case-fatality of lung cancer may be one factor in the mortality rates overtaking breast cancer, there is, increasingly, evidence that there are regions of the world where the gap in the incidence rate is now closing. For example, in Glasgow, an area where lung cancer has been historically high, by 1990 the incidence rate for lung cancer (115 per 100 000) exceeded that for breast cancer (105 per 100 000) in 1990.[40] Among international cancer registries, there are some where the incidence of lung cancer now exceeds the incidence of breast cancer, and others where there is still a gap. In the SEER (Surveillance Epidemiology and End Results) Program of the US National Cancer Institute, the incidence of lung cancer in both Black and White women increased by over 90% between 1973–1977 and 1988–1992: the increase in the incidence of breast cancer was around 25% in both racial groups (comparison made between incidence rates age-adjusted using the 1970 US population). It is a great worry that there does not appear to be any end in sight to this increase in lung cancer risk internationally: it is programmed to continue for several decades to come.

Part of the complacency over the effect on women was also due to the strong tendency for women to smoke brands of cigarettes that were lower in tar and nicotine content than those smoked by men: it was assumed that these would have less of a risk for lung cancer than the higher-tar cigarettes that men generally smoked. Marked changes in the rates of the major histological cell types of lung cancer can now be seen, with particular increases in the risk of adenocarcinoma.[41,42] The changes seen are compatible with increased risk adenocarcinoma due to increasing levels of smoking of 'light' cigarettes (low-tar, low-nicotine). It appears that abandoning high-tar cigarettes (15–45 mg tar) may have some impact on reducing squamous-cell carcinoma risk, but this is now being balanced by 'light' cigarettes increasing the risk of adenocarcinoma.

Cigarette smoking kills half of all those who adopt the habit, with 50% of these deaths occurring in middle age and each losing an average of 20 years of non-smoker's life expectancy.[43] It kills in over 24 different ways, with the lung being the commonest cancer site.[43] Lung cancer rates have been declining in men and increasing in women: cigarette smoking in men has been declining while it has been increasing in women. These two trends are closely related. The move to 'light' cigarettes, which is increasingly common, now appears to be linked to increases in adenocarcinoma of the lung, and shows no sign of being linked to a reduced risk overall. There is no such thing as a 'safe cigarette'. Smokers should be urged and helped to stop smoking; children and young adults should be convinced not to smoke. Tobacco can become an addictive drug: it should be left alone.[20]

ACKNOWLEDGEMENTS

It is a pleasure to acknowledge that this work was conducted within the framework of support from the Associazione Intaliana per la Ricerca sul Cancro (Italian Association for Research on Cancer).

REFERENCES

1. Adler I, *Primary Malignant Growths of the Lungs and Bronchi: A Pathological and Clinical Study*. Longmans, Green and Co: London, 1912.
2. Tylecote FE, Cancer of the lung. *Lancet* 1927; **ii**: 256–7.

3. Fleckseder R, Ueber den Bronchialkrebs und einge seiner Entstehungsbedingungen. *Munch Med Wochenschr Nr* 1936; **36**: 1585–93.
4. Ochsner A, Debakey M, Primary pulmonary malignancy. Treatment by total pneumonectomy. Analysis of 79 collected cases and presentation of 7 personal cases. *Surg Gynecol Obstet* 1939; **68**: 435–51.
5. Muller FH, Tabaksmisbrauch und Lungenkarzinom. *Z Krebsforsch* 1940; **49**: 57–85.
6. Schairer E, Schöniger E, Lungenkrebs und Tabaksverbrauch. *Z Krebsforsch* 1943; **54**: 261–9.
7. Schrek R, Baker LA, Ballard GP, Dolgoff S, Tobacco smoking as an etiologic factor in disease. *Cancer Res* 1950; **10**: 49–58.
8. Levin ML, Goldstein H, Gerhardt PR, Cancer and tobacco smoking. *JAMA* 1950; **143**: 336–8.
9. Mills CA, Porter MM, Tobacco smoking habits and cancer of the mouth and respiratory system. *Cancer Res* 1950; **10**: 539–42.
10. Wynder EL, Graham EA, Tobacco smoking as a possible etiologic factor in bronchiogenic carcinoma. *JAMA* 1950; **143**: 329–36.
11. Doll R, Hill AB, Smoking and carcinoma of the lung. *BMJ* 1950; **ii**: 739–48.
12. Doll R, Hill AB, A study of the aetiology of carcinoma of the lung. *BMJ* 1952; **ii**: 1271–86.
13. US Public Health Services, *Smoking and Health. Report of the Advisory Committee to the Surgeon General of the Public Health Service*. US Department of Health, Education and Welfare, Public Health Service, Center for Disease Control, DHEW Publication 1103: Washington, DC, 1964.
14. United States Surgeon General, *Smoking and Health. A Report of the Surgeon General*. US Department of Health, Education and Welfare, Public Health Service, DHEW Publication (PHS) 79-50066: Washington, DC, 1979.
15. Hammond EC, Smoking in relation to death rates of one million men and women. *Natl Cancer Inst Monogr* 1966; **19**: 127–204.
16. Cederlof R, Friberg L, Hrubec Z, Lorich U, *The Relationship of Smoking and Some Social Covariates to Mortality and Cancer Morbidity. A Ten Year Follow-up in a Probability Sample of 55,000 Swedish Subjects Age 18–69*, Parts 1 and 2. Karolinska Institute: Stockholm, 1975.
17. Bross IDJ, Gibson R, Risks of lung cancer in smokers who switch to filter cigarettes. *Am J Publ Health* 1968; **58**: 1396–403.
18. Hammond EC, Garfinkel L, Seidman H, Lew EA, Some recent findings concerning cigarette smoking. In: *Origins of Human Cancer*. Book A: *Incidence of Cancer in Humans* (Hiatt HH, Watson JD, Winsten JA, eds). Cold Spring Harbor Laboratory: New York, 1977: 101–12.
19. Bouisson J, Du cancer buccal chez les fumeurs. *Montpellier Med* 1859; **2**: 539–99.
20. Boyle P, Veronesi U, Tubiana M et al, School of Oncology Advisory Report to the European Commission for the 'Europe Against Cancer Programme' European Code Against Cancer. *Eur J Cancer* 1995; **9**: 1395–405.
21. IARC (International Agency for Research on Cancer), *Monographs on the Evaluation of Carcinogenic Risk to Humans*. Vol 38. *Tobacco Smoking*. IARC: Lyon, 1986.
22. Levi F, Maisonneuve P, Filiberti R et al, Cancer incidence and mortality in Europe. *Sozial-Präventivmedizin* 1989; **34**(Suppl 2): 1–84.
23. Bjartveit K, Legislation and political activity. In: *Tobacco: A Major International Health Hazard* (Zaridze DG, Peto R, eds). IARC: Lyon, 1986: 285–98.
24. Della-Vorgia P, Sasco AJ, Skalkidis Y et al, An evaluation of the effectiveness of tobacco-control legislative policies in European Community countries. *Scand J Soc Med* 1990; **18**: 81–9.
25. Tomatis L, *Air Pollution and Human Cancer*. European School of Oncology Monograph. Springer-Verlag: Berlin, 1990.
26. Shimizu Y, Kato H, Schull WJ et al, *Life Span Study Report 11*, Part 1: *Comparison of Risk Coefficients for Site Specific Cancer Mortality Based on the DS86 and T65DR Shielded Kerma and Organ Doses*. Radiation Effects Research Foundation Technical Report 12-87. Radiation Effects Research Foundation: Hiroshima, 1987.
27. Smith PG, Doll R, Mortality among patients with

ankylosing spondylitis after a single treatment course with X-rays. *BMJ* 1982; **284**: 449–54.

28. IARC (International Agency for Research on Cancer), *Monographs on the Evaluation of Carcinogenic Risk to Humans*. Vol 44. *Alcohol Drinking*. IARC: Lyon, 1988.
29. Kopecky KJ, Yamamoto T, Fujikura T et al, *Lung Cancer, Radiation Exposure and Smoking Among A-Bomb Survivors, Hiroshima and Nagasaki, 1950–1980*. Radiation Effects Research Foundation Technical Report 13-86. Radiation Effects Research Foundation: Hiroshima, 1987.
30. Whittemore AS, McMillan A, Lung cancer mortality among US uranium miners: a reappraisal. *J Natl Cancer Inst* 1983; **71**: 489–99.
31. Boyle P, Robertson C, Statistical modelling of lung cancer and laryngeal cancer incidence data in Scotland, 1960–1979. *Am J Epidemiol* 1987; **125**: 731–44.
32. Le Vecchia C, Franceschi S, Italian lung cancer death rates in young males. *Lancet* 1984; **ii**: 406.
33. La Vecchia C, Levi F, Decarli A et al, Trends in smoking and lung cancer mortality in Switzerland. *Prev Med* 1988; **17**: 712–24.
34. Chollat-Traquet C, *Women and Tobacco*. World Health Organization: Geneva, 1992.
35. Boyle P, The hazards of passive and active smoking. *N Engl J Med* 1993; **328**: 1708–9.
36. Roemer R, *Legislative Action to Combat the World Tobacco Epidemic*. World Health Organization: Geneva, 1993.
37. Boyle P, The hazards of passive and active smoking. *N Engl J Med* 1993; **329**: 1581.
38. Boyle P, Cancer, cigarette smoking and premature death in Europe. A review including the recommendations of European Cancer Experts Consensus Meeting. Helsinki, October 1996. *Lung Cancer* 1997; **17**: 1–60.
39. Zatonski WA, Boyle P, Health transformations in Poland after 1988. *J Epidemiol Biol* 1996; **1**: 183–97.
40. Gillis CR, Hole DJ, Lamont DW et al, The incidences of lung cancer and breast cancer in women in Glasgow. *BMJ* 1994; **305**: 1331.
41. Zheng T, Holford T, Boyle P et al, Time trend and age–period–cohort effect on the incidence of histologic types of lung cancer in Connecticut, 1960–1989. *Cancer* 1994; **74**: 1556.
42. Levi F, Franceschi S, La Vecchia C et al, Lung carcinoma trends by histologic type in Vaud and Neuchatel, Switzerland, 1974–1994. *Cancer* 1997; **79**: 906–14.
43. Doll R, Peto R, Wheatley K et al, Mortality in relation to smoking: 40 years' observations on make British doctors. *BMJ* 1994; **309**: 901–11.

3 Biology of lung cancer

Daniel C Chan, Ariel Soriano, Madeleine A Kane, Barbara Helfrich, Paul A Bunn, Jr

Contents Introduction • Growth factors in lung cancer • Invasion and metastasis • Cell surface molecules in lung cancer • Genetic abonormalities in lung cancer

INTRODUCTION

Knowledge of the molecular and biologic underpinning of lung cancer and its preneoplastic lesions has expanded exponentially over the last decade. This chaper will focus on growth factors, invasion and metastases, cell surface antigens and molecular changes. We shall attempt to illustrate how understanding the biologic and molecular changes will lead to new detection, prevention and treatment strategies for the future.

Lung cancers are heterogeneous. Pathologists divide lung cancers into four histologic types. Our understanding of the biology may lead to other groupings in the future. For example, Table 3.1 illustrates the major growth factors of lung cancer. They can be divided into two groups: those predominantly stimulated by receptor tyrosine kinases and those predominantly stimulated by peptide growth factors. Among the non-small cell lung cancers, some overexpress ErbB-2 (HER2/Neu) and some have *ras* mutations. We may have different therapies for these specific subgroups.

GROWTH FACTORS IN LUNG CANCER

Peptide growth factor signaling in small cell lung cancer and some non-small cell lung cancers

Neuropeptide production by small cell lung cancer (SCLC) has been recognized for many years. All SCLC cells produce one or more of the

Table 3.1 Growth factors in lung cancer

Small cell lung cancer	Non-small cell lung cancer
1. Neuropeptides	1A. Epidermal growth factor (EGF)
2. Insulin-like growth factor I (IGF-I)	1B. Transforming growth factor α (TGF-α)
3. Transferrin	2. Neuropeptides
4. Hematopoietic growth factors	3. IGF-I
	4. Nerve growth factor (NGF)
	5. Hepatocyte growth factor (HGF)

Table 3.2 Neuropeptide growth factors

Gastrin-releasing peptide (GRP)	Neurotensin
Bradykinin (BK)	Motilin
Arginine vasopressin (AVP)	Neurophysin
Cholecytokinin	Litorin
Gastrin	Somatostatin
Galanin	Adrenomedullin
Opioids	Atrial natriuretic peptide

neuropeptides listed in Table 3.2 and generally produce multiple peptides, although there is remarkable heterogeneity of peptide production by different SCLC cell lines and tumors.[1–7] Non-small cell lung cancer (NSCLC) cell lines and tumors may also produce peptides.[3,5] This is more common in adenocarcinomas and in large cell carcinomas than in squamous carcinomas.

SCLC cell lines and tumors also express neuropeptide receptors.[1,2,8–10] All SCLC cell lines/tumors express one or more of these receptors, and there is also great heterogeneity of receptor expression. Essentially all neuropeptide receptors have a similar structure: seven-membrane spanning portions coupled at the intracellular carboxyl terminus to G protein.[2] Most peptide receptors exist in more than one form. For example, there are at least three forms of receptors for gastrin-releasing peptide,[8] two forms of the bradykinin receptor[11] and two forms of the cholecystokinin receptor.[9] SCLC cells may express only one form of multiple forms of a receptor.[8–11]

The signal transduction pathway excited by peptide–receptor binding is essentially identical for each peptide, and is summarized in Figure 3.1.[2,4] The peptide receptors are coupled to heterotrimeric G proteins of both the $G_{q,11}$ and $G_{12,13}$ classes. Activation of G protein occurs when ligand–receptor binding produces guanosine diphosphate (GDP) dissociation from the G-protein α subunit, allowing guanosine triphosphate (GTP) to bind. The α–GTP complex dissociates from the G-protein βγ subunits, and is then capable of activating downstream effectors.

As shown in Figure 3.1, G_q activation leads to stimulation of phospholipase Cβ (PLCβ). Activated PLCβ hydrolyzes phosphatidylinositol 4,5-bisphosphate (PIP_2) to generate diacylglycerol (DAG) and inositol trisphosphate (IP_3), which lead to activation of protein kinase C (PKC) and release of intracellular calcium respectively. These in turn lead to activation of downstream effectors, including calmodulin kinase II (CaMKII). Activation of the βγ subunits of both G_q and $G_{12,13}$ proteins leads to activation of the Ras p42/p44 MAPK sequential protein kinase pathway. The βγ subunits also activate the specific phosphatidylinositol 3-kinase (PI3-K) γ isoform. Ligand–receptor binding also activates the α subunit of $G_{12,13}$, which in turn activates the Rac, MEKK pathway as shown in Figure 3.1.

Epidermal growth factor receptor signaling in NSCLC

Epidermal growth factor (EGF) and transforming growth factor α (TGF-α) bind to and activate the EGF receptor (EGFR).[3,4,12–15] EGFR is expressed or overexpressed in nearly all squamous carcinomas and some adeno/large cell carcinomas, but

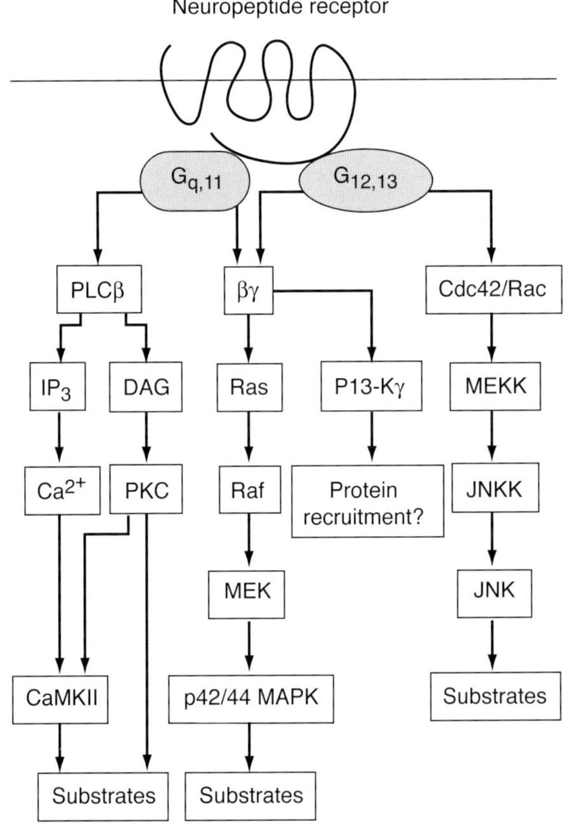

Figure 3.1
Neuropeptide receptor coupling to $G_{q,11}$ and $G_{12,13}$ heterotrimeric G proteins and recruitment of signal transduction proteins. CaMKII, calmodulin kinase II; DAG, diacylglycerol; IP_3, inositol trisphosphate; JNK, Jun N-terminal kinase; JNKK, JNK kinase; MAPK, mitogen-activated protein kinase; MEK, MAPK/Erk kinase; MEKK, MEK kinase; PI3-Kγ, phosphatidylinositol 3-kinase γ isoform; PKC, protein kinase C; PLCβ, phospholipase Cβ. (Reproduced with permission of Marcel Dekker, Inc from Biology of Lung Cancer. Lung Biology in Health and Disease, Vol 122 (Kane MA, Bunn PA Jr, eds). 1998: 378.)

is rarely expressed in small cell carcinomas.[12–15] Ligand (EGF or TGF-α) binding leads to dimerization of EGFR, autophosphorylation of EFGR, and subsequent tyrosine phosphorylation of specific proteins, as illustrated in Figure 3.2.[3,4] Some of the tyrosine autophosphorylation sites on EGFR function as high-affinity binding sites for the Src homology 2 (SH2) domain sequences. Examples of proteins with SH2 domains that bind to the EGFR include PLCγ, PI3-K, Grb2, GTPase-activating protein (GAP), P91 and protein tyrosine phosphatase 1b (PTP1b, Syp), as illustrated. Grb2 is an adapter protein that binds Sos, which is an exchange catalyst that stimulates GDP dissociation from Ras, allowing GTP to bind and activate Ras.

EGFR (ErbB-1) is a member of the ErbB family of receptors, which also includes ErbB-2 (also known as HER2/Neu), ErbB-3 (HER3) and ErbB-4 (HER4). ErbB-2 is overexpressed in many NSCLCs, especially in adenocarcinomas, and may impart a poor prognosis.[3,4] Herceptin, a monoclonal antibody that binds ErbB-2, has been shown to increase response rate and survival when given in conjunction with certain chemotherapeutic agents (paclitaxel and doxorubicin) in breast cancer patients.[16] Clinical trials of Herceptin in lung cancer are currently in progress.

Another ligand of the EGF family, amphiregulin (AR), was expressed in 92% of lung adenocarcinomas.[4] There are few, if any, data regarding expression of ErbB-3 and ErbB-4 in lung cancer.[3,4] NSCLCs frequently overexpress EGFR and/or have activating Ras mutations.[4] Autocrine stimulation of EGFR and constitutively activated Ras both result in persistent activation of the p42/p44 MAPK pathway. This pathway provides important targets for lung cancer prevention and treatment strategies, as discussed below.

Growth factors in the development of lung cancer

Tobacco smoke and other carcinogens initiate the process of malignant transformation, beginning with inflammation and proliferation. The growth

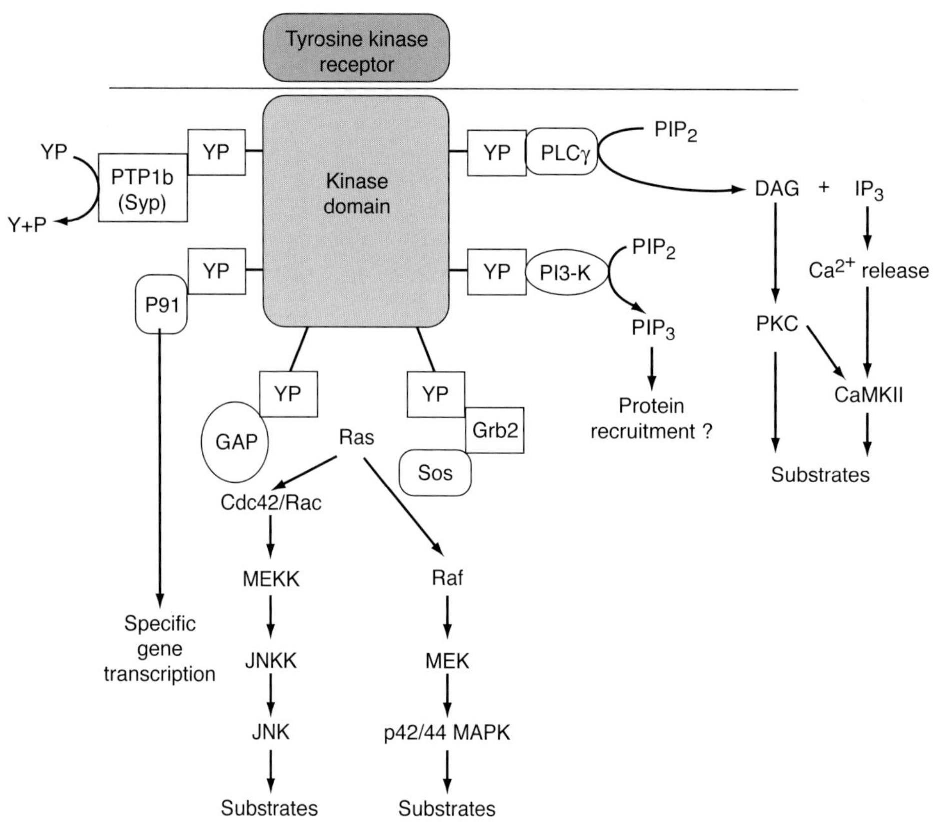

Figure 3.2
Recruitment of signal transduction proteins to the EGFR in response to tyrosine kinase activation and autophosphorylation. Abbreviations as in Figure 3.1, plus: GAP, GTPase-activating protein; P, phosphate group; PIP_2, phosphatidylinositol 4,5-bisphosphate; PIP_3 phosphatidylinositol 3,4,5-trisphosphate; PLCγ, phospholipase Cγ; PTP1b, protein tyrosine phosphatase 1b; Y, tyrosine; YP, phosphorylated tyrosine. (Reproduced with permission of Marcel Dekker, Inc from Biology of Lung Cancer. Lung Biology in Health and Disease, Vol 122 (Kane MA, Bunn PA Jr, eds). 1998: 376.)

factors described above are involved with the pathogenesis of lung cancer as well as its progression. Overexpression of EGFR is found in metaplasia and dysplasia, which are precursors of lung cancer.[14] EGFR also appears to play a role in the autocrine growth of many transformed bronchial epithelial cells.[17] The role of the neuropeptides in the pathogenesis of SCLC is less clear – largely because the identification of the premalignant cell is not possible at present. Hyperplasia of pulmonary neuroendocrine cells may lead to interstitial lung disease,[18] but such a role has not been proven in the pathogenesis of SCLC. However, the gastrin-releasing peptide receptor confers a growth response in immortalized human bronchial epithelial cells.[19]

Other growth factors

Insulin-like growth factor I (IGF-I)

This is a 70-amino-acid growth factor that stimulates the growth of both SCLC and NSCLC cell lines. IGF-I has been shown to be produced by SCLC cells, and its receptor has been shown to be expressed by the same cell lines.[20,21] An IGF-I receptor monoclonal antibody inhibited the growth of several SCLC cell lines.[26]

Transferrin

This is an 80 kDa cell surface protein that transports iron from the plasma to the cytoplasm. SCLC cells proliferate in response to exogenous transferrin, and express large amounts of transferrin receptors.[22–24] Growth of SCLC cell lines has been inhibited by an anti-transferrin receptor monoclonal antibody.[2]

Hepatocyte growth factor (HGF)

HGF (also known as c-Met) is widely overexpressed in human NSCLC cell lines, tumors and cultures of normal bronchial epithelium.[3,25,26] These cells also display a proliferative response to HGF. HGF appears to be produced more by lung fibroblasts than by tumor cells, so it may act more in a paracrine than in an autocrine manner.[3]

Hematopoietic growth factors

SCLC cells may express receptors for granulocyte (G-CSF) or granulocyte–macrophage (GM-CSF) colony-stimulating factors and for interleukin-3 (IL-3). c-Kit is the receptor for the hematopoietic growth factor, stem cell factor (SCF).[3] Expression of both SCF and c-Kit has been reported for SCLC cells.[26–29] These growth factors have been reported to stimulate the growth of a few SCLC cell lines. This raises the concern that their use to reduce chemotherapy-induced neutropenia could stimulate tumor growth. The clinical studies reported to date have shown no evidence of lower response rates or tumor stimulation with the use of these growth factors. These clinical results are consistent with the lack of in vitro effects of most growth factors on proliferation of SCLC cell lines.[30]

Anti-growth-factor strategies for prevention and treatment

There are many potential targets for growth-inhibitory or apoptosis-stimulating agents based on the signal pathways of the growth factors described above. Examples of these strategies will be discussed below.

Anti-ligand antibodies

Effective removal of the growth factor by a monoclonal antibody would be predicted to inhibit tumor growth, and there are examples of where this is the case. Gastrin-releasing peptide (GRP), the human analog of amphibian bombesin, was one of the first peptide growth factors described for SCLC.[31] Monoclonal antibodies that bind GRP and bombesin produced growth-inhibitory effects in vitro and in some instances in athymic nude mice bearing human SCLC xenografts.[31] In human clinical trials, a complete response was observed in 1 of 12 treated patients.[32] These studies established the proof of the principle that tumor responses could be observed, but the failure to produce responses in the majority of instances is probably due to the heterogeneity of peptide production and receptor expression.

Peptidases that inactivate growth factors

Several studies have demonstrated that lung cancers have low expression of neutral endopeptidase (NEP, EC24.11, CD10, CALLA).[33,34] NEP degrades all peptides reported to be growth factors for SCLC. Shipp et al[34] reported that exogenous porcine NEP inhibited the growth of NCI-H345 SCLC cells, which lack cell surface

NEP and which are sensitive to multiple peptides. We have studied the effects of recombinant human NEP (rNEP) on a series of lung cancer cell lines both in vitro and in vivo in athymic nude mice.[35] We have shown that rNEP inhibited the growth of most lung cancer cell lines in vitro – but only at high concentrations and with continued exposure to rNEP.[35] Growth inhibition is more problematic in vivo. There was no growth inhibition with treatment of large established tumors. Some growth inhibition/growth delay was observed when the rNEP was given three times daily at the highest concentrations, starting before tumors became well established. Huge amounts of rNEP would be required in humans to sustain the concentrations required for such growth inhibition.

Anti-receptor monoclonal antibodies

The largest amount of data has accumulated on antibodies directed against EGFR.[36–40] Such antibodies have been shown to inhibit the growth of cell lines expressing EGFR in vitro and in nude mouse models. The presumed mechanism is blockade of EGFR function, rather than by an immunological effect.[36] These preclinical studies have led to human trials with unlabeled antibody alone,[37] radiolabeled antibodies,[38] and antibody plus cisplatin.[39] Problems identified in these studies are high uptake in liver and other sites, low antibody concentrations in tumor, and the development of immune reactions to the antibody. Studies are in progress to overcome these problems.

Specific growth factor antagonists

Several modifications in the amino acid sequences of specific peptides convert agonist activity to antagonist activity. Specific antagonists have been developed for many peptide growth factors, including GRP, cholecystokinin, gastrin, arginine vasopressin, bradykinin and others.[11,40–42] These specific receptor antagonists have very poor growth-inhibitory effects against lung cancer cell lines, even when modified to increase potency and serum stability. The heterogeneity of peptide production and receptor expression is the likely reason for the failure of these agents in most instances.

Broad-spectrum antagonists/biased agonists

Several substance P derivatives (SPDs) were shown to block the activity of multiple peptides, and were thought to act as broad-spectrum antagonists.[42–45] More recent studies have shown that these agents and some bradykinin antagonist dimers interact with receptor G proteins to produce 'biased agonist' effects, including apoptosis and growth inhibition.[42–45] These agents are discussed in detail below.

Toxin-conjugated growth factors

Both the *GRP* and the *EGF* genes have been fused to the catalytic domain of the diphtheria toxin gene to produce toxic fusion proteins termed DAB_{389}GRP and DAB_{389}EGF.[46,47] These fusion proteins inhibit the growth of squamous and SCLC cell lines expressing EGFR and GRPR respectively.[47] Phase I clinical trials of DAB_{389}EGF are in progress. An advisory committee of the US Federal Drug Administration (FDA) recently recommended a similar fusion protein, DAB_{389}IL2, for approval for cutaneous T-cell lymphomas. Hypoalbuminemia, capillary leak and constitutional symptoms were the most frequent toxicities, as they are with most toxin products.

Agonist or receptor ribozymes or antisense constructs

Several groups have made ribozymes that block production of EGFR[48] or antisense constructs that block production of IGF-I.[49] These constructs have been shown to inhibit the growth of tumor cell lines in vitro. However, in vivo delivery of these constructs remains a significant problem to overcome before there is widespread clinical testing.

Specific tyrosine kinase inhibitors

Several small molecules that inhibit EGFR activation have been developed.[50] These compounds inhibit the in vitro growth of human tumor cells in a receptor-number-dependent manner. Clinical trials of such compounds are planned.

Tyrphostin AG825, a selective tyrosine kinase inhibitor, enhanced the chemosensitivities to doxorubicin, etoposide and cisplatin in NSCLC cell lines that overexpress ErbB-2 (HER2/Neu).[51] Emodin, another tyrosine kinase inhibitor, has been shown to synergistically inhibit the proliferation of ErbB-2-overexpressing NSCLC cells when combined with paclitaxel, cisplatin, doxorubicin or etoposide.[52]

Mechanism of biased agonists to peptide growth factor-coupled G proteins

Substance P derivatives (SPDs) have been shown to block the intracellular response to several exogenous peptides and to inhibit the growth of SCLC cell lines.[42–45] These SPDs blocked binding of these peptides to their receptors, leading to the initial conclusion that competitive antagonism of ligand is the principal mechanism of action. Subsequent studies have shown the mechanism of growth inhibition to be more complex. As expected, SPDs inhibited activation of $G_{\alpha q}$ subunit and downstream effectors (see Figure 3.1) and inhibited proliferation. Surprisingly, Johnson and co-workers[44,45] showed that SPDs stimulate, rather than inhibit, the $G_{\alpha 12,13}$ subunit. This activation leads to activation of downstream effectors such as the Jun kinase cascade, and this stimulates apoptosis. Thus the SPDs have a split action, inhibiting $G_{\alpha q}$ and downstream effectors, and stimulating $G_{\alpha 12,13}$ downstream effectors. We have coined the term 'biased agonist' to describe these discordant effects. The SPDs inhibit both the in vitro and the in vivo growth of human SCLCs. However, high concentrations are required for optimal inhibition in both settings.

Recently, we have described more potent biased agonists, the bradykinin antagonist dimers.[11] Bradykinin (BK) is a nonapeptide that stimulates the highest percentage of lung cancer cell lines. Potent BK antagonists that are stable and long-acting have been developed and shown to inhibit the intracellular signal pathway stimulated by BK. These compounds failed to inhibit cell growth, presumably owing to heterogeneity of receptor production and the ability of other peptides to stimulate growth. When homodimers of two peptide chains are created with crosslinkers of the appropriate length, the resultant BK antagonist dimers act as biased agonists. These compounds are potent inhibitors of lung cancer cell growth in vitro and in vivo. Clinical trials of such agents are being planned.

Inhibitors of activated Ras

Both EGF and activating Ras mutations activate the p42/p44 MAPK pathway as summarized in Figure 3.2. It might be predicted that disruption of the function of activated Ras could prevent transformed cell growth. Transformation by activated Ras requires carboxyl-terminal farnesylation or geranylation of the cysteine within the CAAX sequence. The farnesyltransferases (FT) and geranyltranferases that modify the Ras proteins are thus novel targets for new therapeutic agents. Potent inhibitors of farnesylation have been developed and shown to inhibit the growth of lung cancer cell lines in vitro and in vivo.[53] Several of these FT inhibitors have recently entered clinical trial.

INVASION AND METASTASIS

Introduction: the spread of cancers

Metastases are the major cause of morbidity and death in cancer patients.[54] Cancer cells invade parenchymal tissue, and spread through the vascular and lymphatic channels to different organs and to different regions of the same organ, making curative treatment by local measures such as surgery or radiation impossible.[54] Metastases are especially common in lung cancer, where two-thirds of SCLC cases and one-third of NSCLC cases have metastases to distant organs at diagnosis.[1,54] The cure rate for all lung cancer patients is only 14%, largely because of early spread.[55] The lung is a common ground of metastasis because of:[56–60]

- the physiology and anatomy of the bronchial and pulmonary circulation system (first-pass organ);
- the adhesive characteristic of lung endothelial cells;
- preferential interactions between adhesion molecules of metastatic cells with lung endothelium and subendothelial matrix;
- the growth-permissive environment of lung tissue.

Since lymphatic vessels and blood vessels are widely interconnected, the actual routes of metastatic spread should not be separated into independent vascular and lymphatic systems. The most common distant sites of metastases from primary lung cancers are lung, brain, liver, adrenal and bone (marrow).[1,56] For lung cancer patients without distant metastatic disease at diagnosis, lymph node involvement is the greatest predictor of subsequent failure.

Molecular mechanisms of invasion and metastasis

Metastasis is an inefficient process.[61] It is a non-random phenomenon, and may depend to some extent on multiple survival factors associated with traversing the various stages of the metastatic processes.[56,61] These stages are each rate-limiting and interdependent, and a failure to complete any of the steps prevents tumor cells from metastasis. The major steps involved in the process of invasion and metastasis in all tumors are:[54,56]

(1) detachment from the primary tumor;
(2) invasion and migration through the basement membrane and extracellular matrix underlying the tumor;
(3) penetration of the vascular or lymphatic channels;
(4) survival within the circulating blood or lymph;
(5) exit from the circulation and arrest in a new tissue site;
(6) finally, the ability to initiate neovascularization (angiogenesis) and grow as a metastasis at a new site.

Figure 3.3 is a schema of invasion and metastasis.[62]

Understanding both the steps involved in the invasion process and the molecular mechanism of metastasis is crucial for the development of novel therapeutic agents and strategies to prevent and treat metastatic disease. Here, we shall first examine the current understanding of the crucial steps involved in the metastatic cascades, such as:

(a) proteolysis of the extracellular matrix in the invasion process;
(b) cell–cell adhesion in the tumor-specific organ homing step;
(c) angiogenesis and neovascularization of metastases at distant sites.

Next, we shall review the current development of novel agents for the treatment of human cancers through:

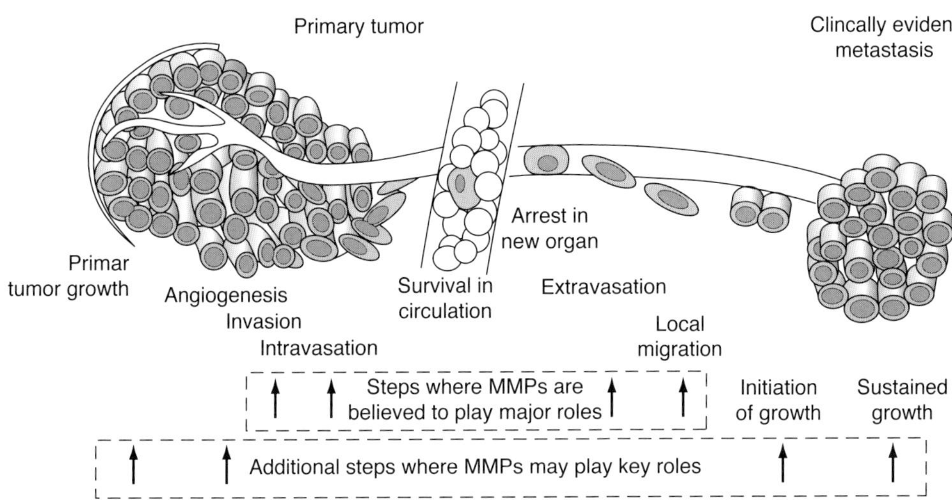

Figure 3.3
Tumor invasion and metastasis. It is believed that, in a sequential manner, tumor cells detach from the primary tumor, invade and migrate through the basement membrane and extracellular matrix, enter and survive in the circulation, arrest in a new organ, and initiate growth as a clinically detectable metastasis. The arrows indicate the roles of matrix metalloproteinases (MMPs) that involve matrix degradation, including invasion, intravasation, extravasation and local migration. MMPs may also play key roles in a number of other steps, as indicated. (Reproduced with permission of Oxford University Press from Chambers AF, Matrisian LM, Changing views of the role of matrix metalloproteinases in metastasis. J Natl Cancer Inst 1997; **89**: 1260–70.)

(a) inhibition of extracellular matrix degradation;
(b) inhibition of cell–cell adhesion;
(c) inhibition of angiogenesis or neovascularization.

Degradation of the extracellular matrix in the invasion process

Malignant carcinomas arise from the epithelium, which is supported by the basement membranes (BM) and the extracellular matrix (EM). The BM and EM separate normal or malignant epithelial cells from the surrounding connective tissues, muscles, blood capillaries and lymphatic vessels. Invasion of normal tissue surrounding the primary tumor, and passage through the BM and EM represent the first crucial steps of the metastatic cascade. The thin-walled blood vessels (venules), capillaries and lymphatic vessels show little resistance to penetration by cancer cells, and provide the most common routes for such cells to enter the circulatory system. The major components of BM and EM are type IV collagen, laminin, fibronectin, vitronectin and heparan sulfate proteoglycan, as well as thrombospondin, entactin, elastin, hyaluronan and von Willebrand's factor.[54,56] Tumor cells produce a number of proteolytic enzymes that degrade the BM and EM, including matrix metalloproteinases (MMPs), collagenases, urokinase plasminogen activator (uPA), plasmin, cathepsin B, tumor-associated trypsinogen 2 (TAT2), heparanases and invadolysin.[62–64]

Table 3.3 Matrix metalloproteinase (MMP) family proteins

MMP	Substrates
Interstitial collagenase (MMP-1)	Types I, II and III fibrillar collagens
Collagenase-III (MMP-13)	Types I, II and III fibrillar collagens
Stromelysin-1 (MMP-3)	Fibronectin, laminin, proteoglycans, types IV, V, VII and IX collagens
Stromelysin-2 (MMP-10)	Fibronectin, laminin, proteoglycans, types IV, V, VII and IX collagens
Stromelysin-3 (MMP-11)	Serpin, laminin, fibronectin
Metrilysin (MMP-7)	Fibronectin, laminin, elastin, types IV, V, VII and X collagens
Gelatinase A (MMP-2)	Types IV and V collagens, gelatin
Gelatinase B (MMP-9)	Types IV and V collagens, gelatin
PMN collagenase (MMP-8)	Types I, II and III collagens
Metalloelastase (MMP-12)	Elastin
MT1-MMP (MMP-14)	Progelatinase A, type IV collagen, proteoglycan
MT2-MMP (MMP-15)	Not defined
MT3-MMP (MMP-16)	Progelatinase A
MT4-MMP (MMP-17)	Not defined

Among these proteinases, MMPs play a major functional role in the metastatic spread of lung cancers,[65] and a wide range of other cancers, including breast,[66] skin,[67] ovarian,[68] colon[69] and bladder cancer.[70] MMPs are a family of structurally related zinc-dependent endopeptidases, either secreted or membrane-bound, which are capable of digesting the broad class of BM and EM proteins that constitute connective tissue around the tumor beds.[62,64] Some MMPs and their substrates are listed in Table 3.3. MMPs are involved in both local invasion and distant metastasis, and they tend to increase in the later stages of tumor progression. Chambers' group demonstrated that, besides facilitating the breakdown of BM and EM, MMPs also play a role as important regulators in creating and maintaining an environment that supports the initiation and maintenance of growth of both primary and metastatic tumors.[56] A better understanding of the involvement of these MMPs in the invasion and regulation of growth of both primary and metastatic tumors may provide insight into the development of MMP inhibitors as therapeutic agents to fight metastases. Because of the importance of MMPs in lung cancer progression, several MMP inhibitors are now in clinical trial for both SCLC and NSCLC.

Adhesion molecules and tumor cell interaction with endothelium and subendothelial matrix in the tumor homing process

After penetration into the circulation, the vast majority of the cancers cells are rapidly eliminated.[61,71,72] Factors that influence the survival of tumor emboli in the circulation can be attributed to cell surface adhesion molecules,[73] macrophages,[74] platelets,[73] natural killer (NK) cells,[75] blood turbulence[72] and nitric oxide (NO) produced by cytokine-activated endothelial cells.[76] The surviving cancer cells or emboli arrest in the capillary beds of the first-pass organ or of distant organs through the interaction of specific cell surface adhesion molecules with the endothelium and the exposed subendothelial basement membrane or extracellular matrix. This constitutes the most crucial factor in determining the organ preference of metastastic cells.[54] A lung-specific endothelial cell adhesion molecule (Lu-ECAM-1) localized on endothelia of distant branches of lung blood vessels has been implicated in the arrest of blood-borne cancer cells in selective, secondary metastases.[77] Cell surface adhesion molecules, present on both cancer cells and host cells, in particular the target-organ microvascular endothelial cells, represent a group of cell surface structures encompassing four major superfamilies. The families of cell surface adhesion molecules are the integrins, cadherins, immunoglobulins, CD44, and many other unclassified molecules that are involved in cell–cell and cell–matrix interactions.[54,59]

Integrins

Integrins are heterodimers, comprising non-covalently associated α and β subunits, each of which spans the plasma membrane and possesses a short cytoplasmic domain.[78] The cytoplasmic domain of the integrin β subunit is thought to interact directly with proteins of the actin cytoskeleton, such as actin and talin. The extracellular domains form widely expressed transmembrane receptors that interact and bind to the tripeptide sequence Arg-Gly-Asp (RGD), which is commonly detected on extracellular matrix proteins such as fibronectin, laminin, vitronectin and collagens.[78] There are 16 α and 9 β subunits, forming at least 24 functioning heterodimeric integrins.[78] During the progression of tumor cells from a low to a high metastatic phenotype, the expression of integrin receptors changes markedly. Expression of integrin $\alpha_v\beta_3$ or $\alpha_4\beta_1$ generally leads to a more metastatic phenotype, especially in the case of $\alpha_v\beta_3$, which has been identified as a marker of angiogenic vascular tissue.[54,79] Expression of integrin subunits that bind to collagen and laminin (α_2, α_3, $\alpha_6\beta_4$) and subunits that bind to fibronectin and fibrinogen (α_5, α_v, β_3, β_6) has been reported in NSCLC.[80] Changes in $\alpha_2\beta_1$, $\alpha_5\beta_1$ and β_2 have been found in human lung cancer cells.[81,82] An increase in integrin α_v and decreases in α_2 and α_3 subunits has been detected in nodal metastases of lung adenocarcinomas.[84] Furthermore, reduced expression of the integrin α_3 subunit has been found to be a poor-prognosis factor for patients with adenocarcinomas.[84] In general, aggressive lung cancer cells adhere strongly to the EM and to endothelial cells through integrins, especially the β_1 subfamily, which constitutes a crucial factor in metastasis.[85]

Cadherins

Cadherins are calcium-dependent transmembrane glycoproteins that bind to one another by homophilic cell–cell adhesion.[54,59] There are approximately 20 cadherins and protocadherins, which can be divided into three major subclasses: epithelial cadherin (E-cadherin, LCAM), neutral cadherin (N-cadherin, ACAM) and placental cadherin (P-cadherin). Cadherins have five extracellular domains, a transmembrane domain and a cytoplasmic domain that interacts with microfilaments via catenins, or with intermediate filaments through desmoplakins and plakoglobin.[59] Cadherins utilize a tripeptide His-Ala-Val (HAV), located in the first extracellular domain closest to the amino terminus, as the cell adhesion recognition (CAR) sequence.[54,59,86] There is evidence that E-cadherins are involved in the suppression of tumor invasion and metastasis. Downregulated E-cadherin expression correlates with loss of cell–cell contact,[87] and is associated with increased lymph node metastasis and unfavorable prognosis in NSCLC.[88]

Adhesion molecules of the immunoglobulin superfamily

Members of the immunoglobulin superfamily (IgSF) are involved in both homophilic and heterophilic cell–cell adhesion interactions.[54,59,86] These interactions are *independent* of divalent cations such as calcium. Adhesion molecules of the IgSF are divided into several subgroups: neural (NCAM, NgCAM, NrCAM), vascular (VCAM-1), intercellular (ICAM-1, ICAM-2, ICAM-3), tumor antigen immunoglobulins (carcinoembryonic antigen (CEA), deleted in colon carcinoma (DCC)), and platelet endothelial (PECAM-1).[54,59,86] IgG adhesion molecules, such as NCAM, may promote tumor cell dissociation, invasion and cancer metastasis through overexpression, dysfunction or loss.[89] The presence of NCAM is indicative for poor prognosis for patients with SCLC.[90,91] The tumor antigen CEA is overexpressed in many lung cancers, colon and breast carcinomas, and correlates with poor prognosis in these patients.[92]

CD44 hyaluronate-binding proteins

CD44 is a ubiquitous multistructural and multifunctional cell surface glycoprotein involved in cell–cell and cell–matrix interactions, cell traffic, lymph node homing, presentation of chemokines and growth factors to traveling cells, and transmission of growth signals.[93] It is a single-chain molecule composed of a distal extracellular domain (containing the ligand-binding sites), a membrane-proximal region, a transmembrane-spanning domain and a cytoplasmic tail. The amino-terminal extracellular region binds to hyaluronate of the extracellular matrix through a disulfide bond-stabilized loop structure, while the cytoplasmic domain interacts with action filaments through ankyrin, ezrin, radexin and moesin.[93] CD44 also interacts with other extracellular matrix compounds, including collagen, fibronectin, laminin and chondroitin sulfate. Many lung cancers and others, including breast, bladder and gastrointestinal cancers, gliomas and non-Hodgkin's lymphomas, as well as their metastases, express high levels of CD44 or CD44 variants.[93] CD44 undergoes complex changes in tumor cells, characterized by alternative splicing, increased expression and cellular redistribution.[94] CD44 isoforms, especially CD44v8–10 in NSCLC, are involved in tumor invasion and metastasis.[95] Furthermore, CD44 and its isoforms promote micrometastasis of murine fibrosarcoma cells to the lungs and facilitate their retention in the lung vasculature during the very early stage of invasion.[96]

Tumor angiogenesis

Angiogenesis and tumor-associated neovascularization play a central role tumor growth, invasion and metastasis.[97] The exact mechanism by which tumors switch to the angiogenic phenotype is unknown, but is dependent on the local balance between positive and negative regulatory factors.[97] In the absence of the acquired angiogenic phenotype, a tumor remains in a dormant state and is unable to grow in size beyond a few millimeters, since the rate of cellular proliferation is balanced by apoptosis.[98] The process of angiogenesis is very complex, and is similar to many of the steps of tumor cell invasion. Angiogenesis involves interactions among the tumor cells, activation of the endothelial cells of a mature vessel, degradation of the surrounding basement membrane, and invasion and migration of endothelial cells through such a breach into the surrounding connective tissue stroma. Here, the endothelial cells proliferate and eventually form capillary tubular structures, which join to form a network of new blood vessels.[97] Thus tumor-associated neovascularization, by establishing continuity with the systemic circulation, allows the tumor cells to receive the necessary nutrients and oxygen to survive and grow, and facilitates further metastatic spreading.

A large number of molecules that initiate angiogenesis have been identified. These include heparin-binding proteins such as basic and acidic fibroblast growth factors (bFGF and aFGF), and vascular endothelial cell growth factor/vascular permeability factor (VEGF/VPF). Non-heparin-binding angiogenic proteins include transforming growth factors α and β (TGF-α and -β), platelet-derived endothelial cell growth factor (PD-ECGF), platelet-derived growth factor (PDGF), placental growth factor, insulin-like growth factor (IGF), epidermal growth factor (EGF), substance P, proliferin and polyamines. Mitogenic factors that initiate angiogenesis are hepatocyte growth factor (HGF), scatter factor, interleukin-8 (IL-8), granulocyte–macrophage colony-stimulating factor (GM-CSF), angiogenin, angiotensin II, ceruloplasmin, platelet-activating factor (PAF) and prostaglandins E_1 and E_2.[54,59,97] A non-mitogenic factor involved in angiogenesis is tumor necrosis factor α (TNF-α). Of these molecules, many act as paracrine or autocrine growth factors, and mediate signals through receptor tyrosine kinases. With the exception of VEGF, most of these molecules have a broad spectrum of target cells, and therefore are not specific to vascular endothelial cells.

VEGF is a homodimeric heparin-binding glycoprotein that exists in at least four variants of 121, 165, 189 and 206 amino acid residues because of alternative mRNA splicing.[99] $VEGF_{121}$ and $VEGF_{165}$ are secreted and soluble factors, where $VEGF_{189}$ and $VEGF_{206}$ are secreted but bound to the extracellular matrix.[99] VEGF activates only endothelial cells, through selective binding to two high-affinity cell surface receptors: Flt-1 (Fms-like tyrosine kinase), also called VEGFR1, on 'activated' endothelial cells; and Flk-1 (fetal liver kinase 1), also called VEGFR2 (in mice) or KDR (kinase domain region) (in humans).[99] The receptors are tyrosine kinases, having seven extracellular immunoglobulin-like globular domains and an intracellular kinase domain.[99] These receptors are not detectable in resting endothelial cells of mature blood vessels or in most other cell types in the body, but are found in blood vessels within or near tumors.[99]

VEGF and its specific receptor systems (Flt-1 and Flk-1/KDR) are clearly involved in tumor angiogenesis in vivo.[99] VEGF increases vascular permeability – a crucial step in tumor angiogenesis. VEGF is one of the most important prognostic factors in NSCLC, especially in adenocarcinoma and squamous cell carcinoma.[100,101] Co-expression of VEGF and its receptor Flt-1 promotes angiogenesis and metastasis in pulmonary adenocarcinoma. Because VEGF and its receptors play such an important role in tumor angiogenesis, they serve as an obvious target for the development of anti-angiogenic agents. Approximately 100 tumor cells may be supported by the length of a capillary blood vessel occupied by one endothelial cell; thus suppression of the growth of one endothelial cell could inhibit the growth of approximately 100 tumor cells. Several endogenous inhibitors of angiogenesis have been identified, many of which are proteolytically cleaved fragments of various proteins, including plasminogen, fibronectin, platelet factor 4 (PF-4), prolactin, EGF, thrombospondin (TSP) and collagen-XVIII.[97] The use of these endogenous protein fragments as well as many other exogenous inhibitors for anti-angiogenic therapy will be discussed in the following section.

Strategies for anti-metastatic and anti-angiogenic therapy

The process of tumor invasion and metastasis relies heavily on:

(a) extracellular matrix degradation;
(b) cell–cell adhesion;
(c) angiogenesis and tumor-associated neovascularization.

These three steps offer potential targets for the development of strategies for anti-metastatic and anti-angiogenic therapy. Since metastasis is angiogenic-dependent, and the processes of tumor invasion and angiogenesis are very much alike in several steps, many agents that inhibit extracellular matrix degradation or cell–cell adhesion are known to be anti-metastatic and anti-angiogenic as well, and vice versa.

Inhibition of extracellular matrix/basement membrane degradation

Matrix metalloproteinase inhibitors (MMPIs) block the activity of many MMPs used by cancer cells to break down the remodelled tissue matrices during the process of metastatic spread and angiogenesis. Many agents that inhibit extracellular matrix degradation have been identified, including broad-spectrum MMPIs (batimastat, marimastat, AG3340), tissue inhibitors of MMP (TIMP-1, TIMP-2, TIMP-3), urokinase (uPA) inhibitors (4-substituted benzo(*b*)thiophene-2-carboxamidines, which are synthetic uPA antagonists), a collagenase IV inhibitior (Ubenimex), a stromelysin inhibitor (dimethyl sulfoxide), a proteinase inhibitor (leupeptin), tissue plasminogen activators (PAI-1, PAI-2, PAI-3), a chelator (Razoxane), a semisynthetic tetracycline (minocycline), a fumagillin analog (FR111142), a sulfated polysaccharide (SCM-chitin III) and retinoic acid.[68,69,103]

The MMPIs such as batimastat and marimastat are by far the most advanced MMPI compounds in terms of preclinical and clinical development.[103,104] These compounds are collagen peptide-based hydroxamic acids, and specifically mimic the substrate of the MMPs (such as collagenase EC3.4.24.7). The drugs work by competitive, potent but reversible inhibition.[105] They are broad-spectrum MMPIs with potent activities against several major MMPs, including MMP-1, MMP-2, MMP-3, MMP-7 and MMP-9.[105] Batimastat is very insoluble and has very poor bioavailability orally, while marimastat is orally active and has a favorable pharmacokinetic profile in humans. In vivo efficacy of these two compounds has been demonstrated in small animals, and both are currently in clinical phase I, II and III trials.[103,104] AG3340 is another novel MMPI, which selectively inhibits MMP-2, MMP-3 and MMP-13. It is also in preclinical and clinical trials. It is envisioned that these broad-spectrum MMPIs will have low toxicity, with the potential to halt tumor progression while complementing current chemotherapeutic regimens.

Anti-adhesion therapies

Once the tumor cells enter the circulation, interference of tumor cell interactions with endothelium, platelets and subendothelial matrix represent a logical and potentially effective way to block the tumor-homing step ('docking' to organ-specific vascular endothelium) in the process of metastasis. Blocking endothelial adhesion molecules, such as Lu-ECAM-1, integrin $\alpha_v\beta_3$, $\alpha_{II}b_{\beta 3}$, $\alpha_5\beta_1$, α_6 or β_1 subunits, and CD44 with specific antibodies has been found to significantly reduce tumor metastasis.[59,73,79–81] Alternatively, the tripeptide Arg-Gly-Asp (RGD) sequence, which is present in most extracellular matrix proteins such as fibronectin, laminin, vitronectin and collagens, serves as a potential target for interference with cell–cell adhesion interactions in the tumor vasculature. Many polymeric or cyclic peptides containing the RGD sequence, with or without polyethylene glycol conjugation, strongly inhibit tumor cell adhesion and tumor progression in experimental animals.[106,107] When coupled to the anticancer drug doxorubicin, a peptide containing the RGD or Asn-Gly-Arg (NGR) motif enhanced the efficacy of doxorubicin against human breast cancer xenografts in nude mice.[108] Several RGD mimetics with structures containing guanidinium and carboxylic acid groups separated by an 11-carbon atom backbone have been found to inhibit cell adhesion and reduce metastasis.[109] Apart from RGD-containing peptides, multimeric forms of the Tyr-Ile-Gly-Ser-Arg (YIGSR) sequence, which is derived from the laminin B1 chain, have been shown to decrease tumor growth and metastasis.[110]

Anti-angiogenesis

Many new *exogenous* inhibitors of angiogenesis have been discovered or developed. These include fungus-derived angiogenesis inhibitors such as TNP-470 (AGM1470, a fumagillin analog) and bacteria-derived angiogenesis inhibitors such as CM101 (a streptococcal polysaccharide) and tecogalan (a bacterial sulfated polysaccharide peptidoglycan complex). Polysulfate inhibitors of angiogenesis include DS4152 (a sulfated polysaccharide peptidoglycan complex), SCM-chitin III (a sulfated polysaccharide), suramin and pentosan polysulfate. Antibiotics and therapeutic angiogenesis inhibitors include thalidomide, methotrexate, trimetrexate, herbimycin, erbstatin, staurosporine, paclitaxel, minocycline, D-penicillamine, gold thiomalate, batimastat, marimastat, heparin adipic hydrazide, guaiaconic acid and derivatives, quinoline-3-carboxamide linomide, vitamin D_3 analogues, and cortisone acetate. Anti-angiogenic antibodies and conjugates include VEGF (A4.6.1, MV833), VEGF receptors, bFGF, Vitaxin (a humanized anti-integrin $\alpha_v\beta_3$ antibody), VEGF– toxin conjugates and many other polymeric and cyclic peptides containing the RGD or YIGSR sequences.[54,56,97,99,106,107] Many of these compounds have been shown to inhibit angiogenesis by inhibiting endothelial cell proliferation and migration, blocking cell–cell adhesion, or inhibiting MMP proteolysis. Among these compounds, anti-VEGF neutralizing antibodies have been found to completely inhibit angiogenesis and growth of tumors without affecting the normal vessels in animals.[111] Many of these exogenous anti-angiogenic agents are currently in clinical trials.

Endogenous angiogenesis inhibitors have also been identified. Many of these are proteolytically cleaved fragments of larger proteins, such as angiostatin (a plasminogen fragment generated by elastase) and endostatin (a proteolytic fragment of collagen XVIII). Other endogenous inhibitors of angiogenesis include TIMP-1, -2 and -3, TSP-1, PF-4, EGF fragments, IL-12 and interferon (IFN)-β and -γ.[97] Among this group, angiostatin and endostatin have recently received much attention. Both compounds effectively inhibit endothelial cell proliferation and angiogenesis by an unknown mechanism. One possible explanation is that the fragments may act as 'dominant-negative' proteins that disrupt contact with 'weakened' basement membranes and interfere with the already sparse association between endothelial and periendothelial support cells. The interaction between the endothelium and periendothelium is critical for vascular stability.[114] Repeated cycles of therapy with endostatin in tumor-bearing mice did not lead to acquired resistance, whereas repeated cycles of conventional chemotherapeutic agents rapidly cause multidrug resistance.[113] More interestingly, after two to six cycles of endostatin therapy (the exact number being characteristic of the tumor cell type), the tumors shrank and did not recur upon cessation of therapy.[113] These studies represent a landmark achievement in anti-angiogenic therapy of human cancers, and set the course for the development of more novel and potent anti-angiogenic agents.

CELL SURFACE MOLECULES IN LUNG CANCER

The cell surface is a complex network of protein, carbohydrate and lipid molecules that defines the boundary of the intact cell, and also provides the means by which the cell communicates with its external environment. Dysregulated cellular communication with the external environment as well as aberrant intracellular signal transduction result from alterations in the surface features of cancer cells, as well as other internal changes. The malignant properties of lung cancer cells that result in part from changes in the phenotype of the cell surface include unregulated growth, failure of contact inhibition, invasion into normal tissues, metastasis and paraneoplastic syndromes. Alterations in growth factor receptors, as well as surface adhesion molecules, may affect growth properties. Adhesion molecules and surface glycolipids may impact upon density-dependent inhibition of growth ('contact inhibition'), as well as metastatic properties. Invasion and metastasis are promoted by alterations in adhesion molecules as well as proteolytic and glycolytic enzymes. Expression of tumor-specific cell surface antigens (neoantigens, oncofetal antigens) may result in degenerative neuronal paraneoplastic syndromes as a result of production of cross-reacting antibodies. Decreased expression of MHC antigens may contribute to lung cancer cell evasion of normal immune surveillance. Table 3.4 summarizes some of the cell surface alterations observed in lung cancer.

Receptors

Cell surface receptors are integral membrane proteins that exhibit specific, saturable, high-affinity binding to smaller molecules called ligands. Ligands may themselves be proteins, peptides or a variety of hormones. Cell surface receptors fall into two broad groups, depending upon the major way in which they initiate signal transduction as a result of ligand binding. Receptor tyrosine kinases begin signal transduction by dimerization and autophosphorylation, initiating a cascade of sequential binding of adaptor molecules and activation of subsequent protein kinases. These receptors consist of one or more subunits, each of which usually has a single transmembrane domain, as well as one extracellular and one cytosolic domain, as discussed above for the EGFR. G-protein-coupled receptors initiate signal transduction by activation of heterotrimeric G proteins, which consist of α and $\beta\gamma$ subunits that associate with the cytosolic surface of the cell membrane. Activated G proteins activate either adenylate cyclase or phospholipid hydrolysis, which leads to intracellular Ca^{2+} release and activation of protein kinase C isoenzymes. Receptors of this type usually consist of a single polypeptide chain with multiple extracellular, transmembrane (usually seven) and cytosolic domains; these receptors have been discussed above.

Table 3.4 Cell surface changes in NSCLC and SCLC

Cell surface molecules	Lung cancer subtype	
	NSCLC	SCLC
Receptors	EGFR (+, a) HGFR (+) VIPR (+, a) Fas (–)	BLP receptors (+, a) IGF-IR (+, a) Transferrin receptor (+, a) Opioid receptor (+) Acetylcholine receptor (+) Vasopressin receptor (+) Bradykinin receptor (+) Serotonin receptor (+, a)
Adhesion molecules	E-cadherin (–) Connexin-43 (–) ICAM-1 (–) Integrin α_3 (–) Integrin β_6 (+)	NCAM (+)
Enzymes	MT1-MMP (+) Stromelysin-3 (+) Gelatinase B (+) Collagenase-I (+) TIMP (–/+) NEP (–)	NEP (–)
Glycoproteins	A (better prognosis) α(1,3)-Fuc-T (+) Sialyl Le^x (+)	
Glycolipids	G_{D3} (–)	9-*O*-AcG_{D3} (+)
Autoantibodies		Anti-Hu Anti-Ca channel
MHC antigens	Class I and II (– with metastases)	Class I (–)

Abbreviations: R, receptor; EGF, epidermal growth factor; HGF, hepatocyte growth factor; VIP, vasoactive intestinal peptide; BLP, bombesin-like peptide; IGF-I, insulin-like growth factor I; ICAM-1, intercellular adhesion molecule 1; NCAM, neural cell adhesion molecule; MMP, metalloproteinase; TIMP, tissue inhibitor of MMP; NEP, neutral endopeptidase; α(1,3)-Fuc-T, α(1,3)-fucosyltransferase; Sialyl Le^x, sialylated Lewis x antigen; + , increased expression; – , decreased expression; a, autocrine system.

In contrast to receptors associated with enhanced proliferation, Fas (also known as CD95 and APO-1) is a transmembrane receptor that plays a key role in initiation of an apoptotic pathway together with Fas ligand. Fas is frequently expressed in normal cells, but may be lost in malignant cells, theoretically contributing to their unregulated growth by the loss of one mechanism of apoptosis. In normal lung, cell surface Fas protein is normally expressed on ciliated cells and goblet cells of the trachea and on alveolar cells. Soluble forms of Fas lacking the transmembrane domain have also been identified in some cancer cells and in patient serum. In a recent study of resected pulmonary adenocarcinomas, Fas protein was detected in approximately half of the tumors.[115] In all cases, however, Fas was found in a soluble form in the cytoplasm, and not on the cell surface. Findings were similar in human pulmonary adenocarcinoma A549 cells, which did not undergo apoptosis after treatment with anti-Fas antibody.

Cell adhesion molecules

The following cell adhesion molecules (CAMs) have been discussed above: cadherins, neural cell adhesion molecule (NCAM), intracellular adhesion molecule 1 (ICAM-1) and integrins.

Enzymes

The cell surface degradative enzymes of the matrix metalloproteinase (MMP) family and the cell-surface-associated peptidase neutral endopeptidase (NEP), which degrades all the known SCLC neuropeptide growth factors, have been discussed above.

Glycoproteins

ABH blood group antigen expression may be altered in NSCLC, and these alterations may affect prognosis.[116] Patients with tumors expressing blood group antigen A had a better prognosis than those whose tumors did not express the A antigen. Expression of B or O blood group antigens did not correlate with prognosis. NSCLC cells with a greater degree of invasiveness could be predicted by expression of the carbohydrate structure Fucα1→2Galβ1-R, an epitope shared among blood group antigen H, Lewis-Y and Lewis-H antigens. Lewis-Y antigen is expressed during normal embryonal lung development, and its expression in lung cancer suggests a loss of dedifferentiation. In a recent study comparing various forms of Lewis antigens (Le^x, sialyl Le^x, sialyl Le^x dimeric, Le^a, sialyl Le^a) and levels of the five α(1,3)-fucosyltransferases (α(1,3)-Fuc-T), which control the synthesis of these molecules, in metastatic and nonmetastatic sublines of a human pulmonary adenocarcinoma, the metastatic subline expressed all five Lewis antigens and higher levels of all five α(1,3)-Fuc-T genes than the nonmetastatic subline.[117] In addition, only the metastatic cell line bound to E-selectin on human endothelial cells, and binding was inhibited by antibodies to E-selectin and to sialyl Le^x.

Glycolipids

Gangliosides are complex glycolipids that are located in the outer leaflet of the plasma membrane and participate in cell–cell recognition, cell matrix attachment, cell growth regulation and differentiation. Limited studies of the ganglioside components of the cell surface have been performed in lung cancer.[118] Cell surface G_{D3} expression was observed in SCLC but not in NSCLC cell lines. G_{D1a}, G_{D2}, G_{M1}, G_{M2} and G_{M3} were expressed, and G_{D1b} was not expressed, in both SCLC and NSCLC. This study also found high levels of 9-*O*-AcG_{D3} expression in classic SCLC cell lines, but in only one of four NSCLC (a squamous cell carcinoma) cell lines. Gangliosides (e.g. G_{D2}/G_{D3}) help mediate integrin binding to its ligands such as vitronectin – so altered expression could predispose to invasion and metastasis. Enhanced ganglioside expression could provide a target for specific therapy with antiganglioside toxin-conjugated monoclonal antibodies, which are currently being studied in melanoma. An anti-idiotypic vaccine to G_{D2} is being tested in SCLC patients.

Paraneoplastic syndromes

Two well-described neurological paraneoplastic syndromes in patients with SCLC result from the production of antibodies that bind to neuronal tissues. Eaton–Lambert syndrome, which mimics myasthenia gravis, but spares bulbar or extraocular muscles, results from antibodies directed against presynaptic neuronal calcium channels, impairing stimulus-induced acetylcholine release.[119] Antibodies can be detected in the serum of 75% of lung cancer patients with this clinical syndrome, and 10% of lung cancer patients without it. Regression of the neurologic symptoms has been reported to accompany tumor reduction, but this is not usually the case. Other treatments, such as plasmapheresis, immunosuppression and acetylcholinesterase inhibitors, may provide benefit.

Peripheral neuropathy characterized by progressive impairment of all sensory modalities with areflexia and marked sensory ataxia may also result from autoantibodies. Subacute, sensory neuropathy, the most common subtype, result from type 1 antineuronal nuclear antibodies (ANNA-1), which are distinguished from lupus antinuclear antibodies by their selective binding to neuronal tissues.[120] Other rarer and more severe degenerative neurologic syndromes have been associated with specific antibodies directed against specific nervous system antigens. Progressive blindness has been associated with antibodies cross-reacting with retinal antigens.

Major histocompatibility complex

HLA class I antigens of the major histocompability complex (MHC) are essential for antigenic presentation to cytotoxic T lymphocytes, and are expressed on most cells. SCLC cell lines have low or absent class I MHC antigens, and the majority of SCLC tumors ($n = 32$) lacked β_2-microglobulin expression, although most NSCLCs ($n = 79$) expressed it.[121] However, both MHC class I and II antigen expression was significantly reduced in tumors from NSCLC patients with modal micrometastases.[122] Thus loss or reduction of MHC antigens may result in escape from immune surveillance, with greater metastatic tendency resulting. Interferon-γ (IFN-γ) exposure upregulates MHC expression in some NSCLC tumor cells.[123] IFN-γ and transfection with the MHC-encoded *TAP1* gene increased class I antigen expression in SCLC cell lines as well.[124]

GENETIC ABNORMALITIES IN LUNG CANCER

Remarkable advances in understanding lung cancer molecular genetics have occurred over the past decade. Lung cancer arises after a series of morphological changes, progressing from normal epithelium to hyperplasia, metaplasia, dysplasia, carcinoma in situ, invasive cancer, and finally to metastatic cancer.[125,126] In this multistage process of tumorigenesis, multple genetic lesions must accumulate to produce the final malignant phenotype. Genetic abnormalities in cancer cells affect genes classified into two broad categories: proto-oncogenes (dominant) and tumor suppressor genes (recessive). Table 3.5 lists reported abnormalities and their frequencies in the various histologic types of lung cancer. Proto-oncogenes are genes that when activated via genetic changes lead to the production of dysregulated or abnormal protein products that

Table 3.5 Molecular and genetic abnormalities in lung cancer

Genes	Chromosome location	Abnormal mutation or expression (frequency, %)		References
		NSCLC	SCLC	
Oncogenes				
K-ras	6p–q13	26	0	128, 130, 131, 134, 136, 137
c-*myc*	8q24	8	25	154–158
c-*erb*B-1 (*EGFR*)	7p13	63	0	177, 181
c-*erb*B-2 (*HER2/neu*)	17q21	31	0	131, 180, 184, 185, 187
bcl-2	18q21	38	55	131, 170, 171, 173
Tumor suppressor genes				
Rb	13q14	22	88	131, 193–197, 202
p53	17p13	48	80	131, 173, 196, 214, 218, 219
CDKN2A (p16INK4A)	9p21	31[a]	100[a]	198, 199, 201–203
3p LOH	3p	46	90	246, 251

[a]p16 expression increased in SCLC samples compared with NSCLC, where it is decreased.

act in a dominant fashion. Typically, the product increases a particular metabolic or transcriptional process in the cell. Activation can occur by several mechanisms: point mutations, gene amplification or overexpression, chromosomal translocations, and chromosomal inversions. Tumor suppressor genes are genes in which a genetic change leads to decreased activity of a protein product that ordinarily plays a role in restraining cellular growth. Unlike oncogenes, where an abnormality in one of the two alleles is sufficient to lead to an abnormal function, both tumor suppressor alleles must be abnormal – both deleted, both mutated or one of each. Common types of oncogenes and suppressor genes involved in lung cancer will be discussed. Genetic alterations occur before a histologic diagnosis of lung cancer can be established. Table 3.6 shows the frequencies of various genetic abnormalities in preneoplasia, and Table 3.7 indicates the proposed timing by which changes occur in the development of cancer.

Table 3.6 Molecular and genetic abnormalities in premalignant lesions (percentages in parentheses)

Refs	Marker	Normal mucosa	Metaplasia/ atypia	Mild dysplasia	Moderate dysplasia	Severe dysplasia	Carcinoma in situ	Microinvasive cancer	Invasive cancer[a]
181	EGFR	—	12/33 (36)	←	10/17 (59%)	→	8/12 (67)	—	18/34 (53)
180	EGFR	5/13 (38)	—		—		—	—	9/16 (56)
180	c-ErbB-2	3/13 (23)	—		—		—	—	6/16 (38)
142	K-*ras*	0/4 (0)	0/2 (0)	←	1/12 (8)	→	4/5 (80)	—	21/21 (100)[b]
174	Bcl-2 protein	0/42 (0)		←	56/56 (100)	→	—	—	18/29 (62)
204	*Rb*	2/10 (20)	—	←	12/19 (63)	→	0/4	—	9/33 (27)
233	p53 protein	0/22 (0)	1/15 (6.7)	3.25/11 (29.5)	4.6/17 (27)	11/18 (60)	15/25 (58)	6.8/10 (68)	8.75/11 (80)
232, 234, 235, 238	p53 protein	0/1 (0)	—	1/5 (20)	1/2 (50)	15/19 (79)	1/3 (33)	1/1 (100)	20/27 (74)
181	p53 protein	—	0/32 (0)	←	2/17 (12)	→	8/12 (67)	—	19/34 (56)
239	p53 protein	—	1/1 (100)	←	3/8 (38)	→	—	—	7/9 (78)
238	3p LOH[c]	—		←	3/3 (100)	→	—	—	6/6 (100)
239	3p LOH	—	1/1 (100)	←	6/8 (75)	→	—	—	7/9 (78)
256	3p LOH	—	13/17 (76)	←	6/7 (86)	→	4/4 (100)	—	6/6 (100)
207	3p21 LOH	—	0/9 (0)	3/9 (33)	7/18 (39)	—	6/6 (100)	4/4 (100)	7/7 (100)
207	9p21 LOH	—	0/7 (0)	1/2 (50)	4/14	—	5/6 (83)	4/4 (100)	5/5 (100)
207	5q21 LOH	—	1/9 (16)	1/7 (14)	8/20 (40)	—	2/5 (40)	3/4 (75)	4/6 (67)
NCI and literature data combined	p53 protein	0/23 (0)	1/15 (6.7)	4.25/16 (26.5) (20–29.5)	5.6/19 (29.5) (27–50)	26/37 (70) (60–79)	16/28 (57) (33–58)	7.8/11 (71) (68–100)	28.75/38 (75.6) (74–80)

[a]Study involved both NSCLC and SCLC samples.
[b]All samples taken from six cancer cases containing the *ras* mutation.
[c]LOH, loss of heterozygosity.

Table 3.7 Development of lung carcinogenesis

	Normal	Mild dysplasia	Moderate dysplasia	Severe dysplasia	Carcinoma in situ	Invasive cancer
EGFR	+	+	++	++	+++	++++
c-erbB-2	+	+	++	++	+++	++++
3p		+	++	+++	++++	++++
9p			+	++	+++	++++
p53				+	+++	++++
ras				+	+++	++++
bcl-2				++	+++	++++

Oncogenes

ras

The *ras* dominant oncogenes play an important role in signal transduction and cellular proliferation. The *ras* gene family includes K-*ras* (homologous to the Kirsten murine sarcoma virus oncogene), H-*ras* (homologous to the Harvey murine sarcoma virus oncogene), and N-*ras* (initially isolated from a neuroblastoma cell line). The *ras* genes code for 21 kDa proteins that are anchored to the inner leaflet of the cytoplasmic membrane via farnesylation. Ras proteins are homologous to G proteins, and play a key role in signal transduction by linking tyrosine kinases to downstream serine/threonine kinases such as Raf and mitogen-activated protein kinase (MAPK).[127] Ras and G proteins can be viewed as molecular switches. When bound to guanosine triphosphate (GTP), they are in their active configuration, allowing the transduction of a growth signal to the cell nucleus. The Ras proteins are inactivated by GTPase-activating protein (GAP), which hydrolyzes GTP to guanosine diphosphate (GDP). Activation can occur by point mutations at codons 12, 13 or 61. As a result of these mutations, Ras proteins can no longer be inactivated by GAP, resulting in a constitutive growth signal being sent to the cell nucleus.

The *ras* genes are mutated in approximately 30% of all NSCLCs, but rarely in SCLC. In a series of 61 NSCLC and 42 SCLC cell lines, Mitsudomi et al[128] found *ras* mutations in 36% of NSCLC cell lines, but none in the SCLC cell lines. K-*ras* mutations were the most frequent (20/22, 91%), especially at codon 12 (13/22, 59%). Of the K-*ras* mutations, 76% were G-to-T transversions, involving the substitution of the normal glycine with either cysteine or valine. G-to-T transversions are characteristic of lung cancers, in contrast to the frequent G-to-A transitions present in colorectal carcinomas.[129] Similar G-to-T transversions also affect the *p53* gene in lung cancer, and represent the type of DNA damage expected from bulky DNA adducts caused by the polycyclic hydrocarbons and nitrosamines in tobacco smoke. In a study of 80 resected lung cancer specimens, *ras* mutations were found exclusively in adenocarcinoma (15/80, 19%), with 90% of these mutations occurring in the K-*ras* gene.[130] In a large study involving 244 stage I NSCLC patients, K-*ras* mutations were detected in 48 of 140 (34%) adenocarcinomas and in 11 of 40 (27%) large cell or mixed histology cancers, but in only three of 62 (5%) squamous cell carcinomas.[131]

The significance of *ras* mutations for prognosis remains controversial. Several studies showed that *ras* mutations and increased Ras expression correlated with decreased survival, especially in resectable cases.[132–135] Slebos et al[132] demonstrated that activation of the K-*ras* oncogene correlated with a poorer survival prognosis in resected adenocarcinoma of the lung. With a median follow-up of 36 months, 12 of the 19 patients (63%) with a K-*ras* point mutation died, compared with only 16 of 50 patients (32%) without a point mutation. The associations between K-*ras* mutations and tumor size, stage, nodal status or tumor differentiation were not significant. Mitsudomi et al[133] demonstrated that patients from whom *ras* mutation-positive cell lines had been established had significantly shorter survival durations than those from whom *ras* mutation-negative cell lines were obtained (one-year survival rate of 12% versus 25%). K-*ras* mutations were noted in 24% (16/66) of NSCLC cell lines. *ras* mutations were shown to adversely affect patient survival, irrespective of disease extent. Sugio et al[134] evaluated 115 patients with surgically resected NSCLC specimens, without lymph node metastases, and showed a worse prognosis for the patients with *ras* mutations (five-year survival rate of 53.3% versus 83.6%). Cho et al[135] also showed that the presence of K-*ras* mutations in tissue from patients who received treatment for curative intent was associated with a shorter survival (9 months versus 30 months). A significant association between K-*ras* mutations and tumor stage (i.e. the higher the stage, the higher the mutation rate) was noted in this study. Two larger studies, however, showed no correlation between the presence of K-*ras* mutations and survival.[131,136] Keohavong et al[136] showed no difference in overall survival for adenocarcinomas with K-*ras* mutations (43/173) compared with K-*ras*-negative adenocarcinomas, with a two-year survival rate of about 60%. A trend, however, was noted for shorter survival times for stage I patents with K-*ras* mutations (two-year survival rate of 68% versus 78%), but was not statistically significant. Kwiatkowski et al[131] showed that the presence or absence of *ras* mutations alone did not correlate with surival. K-*ras* codon 12 mutations were an independent prognostic factor in this population, conferring a higher risk of recurrence.

Other studies showed that overexpression of the Ras protein, p21, correlated with an unfavorable prognosis. Harada et al[137] analyzed 116 surgically treated patients with NSCLC for immunohistochemical staining using an anti-Ras p21 monoclonal antibody. Survival among patients with p21$^-$ tumors (64% five-year survival rate) was superior to those with p21$^+$ tumors (38% survival rate) and those with p21^{++} tumors (11% survival rate).[137] When the analysis was restricted to stage I and II tumors, patients with p21$^-$ tumors survived significantly longer than those with p21$^+$ tumors. Cox multivariate analysis showed that enhanced Ras p21 expression was a major determinant of survival and was independent of stage, histology and nodal status.

ras mutations may affect chemotherapy response, as noted from in vitro studies showing decreased sensitivity to radiation and cisplatin in the mouse fibroblast cell line NIH-3T3 transfected with mutated *ras* genes.[138,139] Rodenhuis et al[140] showed that the presence of a *ras* mutation does not confer a worse prognosis for patients with advanced disease (inoperable stage III or stage IV) treated with chemotherapy. The presence or absence of an activated *ras* gene appeared to have little, if any, clinical significance in advanced adenocarcinoma of the lung.

Fukuyama et al,[141] looking at K-*ras* and *p53* mutations in NSCLC, showed a worse prognosis in the *ras*$^+$ group compared with the *ras*$^-$ group in all cases, including early stage cases (stage I and II); *p53*$^{+}$ had a worse prognosis in the early stage patients, but no statistically significant difference in advanced disease. Of note, *p53* and *ras* mutations were unfavorable prognostic factors for patients with adenocarcinoma, but were of no statistical significance in cases involving squamous cell carcinoma. Combined immunohistochemical analysis of p53 and Ras p21 expression demonstrated that patients without *p53* or *ras* mutations (*p53*$^{-}$/*ras*$^{-}$) tumors survived the longest among patients with different p53 and Ras p21 features. There was a five-year survival rate of 87% in patients with *p53*$^{-}$/*ras*$^{-}$, compared with 43%, 26 % and 23% for *p53*$^{+}$/*ras*$^{-}$, *p53*$^{-}$/*ras*$^{+}$ and *p53*$^{+}$/*ras*$^{+}$, respectively. In *p53*$^{+}$ patients, a higher survival rate was noted in the *ras*$^{-}$ group, but was not statistically significant. More studies need to be done before a definite conclusion can be made.

Sugio et al[142] investigated preneoplastic lesions associated with lung cancer to determine at what stage in lung carcinogenesis K-*ras* mutations appear. Six cases positive for *ras* mutations and having extensive areas of preneoplastic changes were analyzed. They noted that K-*ras* mutations were evident in a later event in lung tumorigenesis, occurring in the carcinoma in situ stage. All samples of invasive and metastatic cancers had K-*ras* mutations, as did four of five lesions of non-invasive cancer. Mutations were detected in only one of twelve dysplastic lesions, and were absent from hyperplastic and normal-appearing cells.

Strategies involving gene therapy, using antisense oligonucleotides (ASOs) and ribozymes have been attempted. ASOs have been used to downregulate mRNA expression by annealing to a specific region of an mRNA, thus inhibiting its translation.[143] In a lung cancer cell line with a K-*ras* mutation, transfection of an antisense construct resulted in inhibition of K-*ras* mRNA expression and p21 protein.[144] This translated into a threefold suppression of cancer growth. The mutated K-Ras p21 protein synthesis was also downregulated by 95% after antisense therapy. The growth of H460 tumors in nu/nu mice was also substantially reduced by K-*ras* antisense RNA expression. Furthermore, intratracheal instillation of a retroviral antisense K-*ras* construct into irradiated nude mice inoculated intratracheally with carcinoma cells resulted in 87% of the ASO-treated mice remaining tumor-free, compared with 10% of the control mice treated with K-*ras* sense, DNA vector or medium alone.[145]

Another well-characterized means of interfering with the translation of mRNA is the use of ribozymes. These are small catalytic RNAs that possess both site specificity and cleavage capability for an mRNA substrate.[146] Anti-*ras* ribozymes have been tested in several settings. An anti-*ras* ribozyme, transfected into EJ bladder carcinoma cells, resulted in decreased H-*ras* gene expression and inhibition of cell growth. In athymic nude mice, the EJ ribozyme transfectants exhibited reduced tumorigenicity, which resulted in non-invasive, non-metastatic tumors.[147,148] Another study in bladder cancer demonstrated blunting of the invasive phenotype of a human bladder cancer cell line with the anti-*ras* ribozyme, delaying but not abolishing the metastatic phenotype.[149]

Another strategy to inhibit cancer growth involves the use of farnesylation inhibitors. Localization of the Ras oncoprotein to the cytoplasmic face of the plasma membrane via farnesylation is essential for efficient cell-transforming ability. Thus inhibition of the Ras farnesylation reaction can inhibit cancer growth. Strategies to inhibit Ras farnesylation include inhibition of isoprenoid biosynthesis and inhibition of farnesyl-protein transferase (FPTase), the enzyme that catalyzes the farnesylation reaction. Inhibitors of 3-hydroxy-3-methylglutaryl coenzyme. A reductase, the rate-limiting enzyme in isoprenoid biosynthesis, such as lovastatin, block the post-translational modification of Ras and other farnesylation proteins by blocking the synthesis of farnesyl diphosphate (FPP).[150] However, it is unlikely that the anti-proliferative effect of lovastatin is due to inhibition of Ras farnesylation, since cells transformed by viral Raf, an oncoprotein whose function is not dependent on farnesylation, are similarly growth-inhibited.[151] Compounds that inhibit FPTase were found to block the farnesylation of Ras proteins in cell culture and to block then anchorage-independent growth of Ras-transformed cells and human tumor cell lines. These compounds also suppressed the growth of tumors arising from Ras-transformed cells in nude mice.[152,153]

myc

The *myc* dominant oncogenes include c-*myc* (cellular), N-*myc* (originally isolated from neuroblastoma cells) and L-*myc* (originally isolated from SCLC cells). They encode for nuclear DNA-binding proteins, which are involved in transcriptional regulation. Myc may heterodimerize with proteins such as Max, Mad and Mx11. The formation of heterodimers with Max results in the transcriptional activation of the *myc* gene, whereas Mad and Mx11 bound to Max compete with the Myc/Max heterodimer for binding to the target site, resulting in transcriptional repression.[154] Max thus appears to be the control player in this scheme, where, depending on whether it binds to Myc or to Mad/Mx11, it can cause activation or repression respectively.

In contrast to *ras* genes, which are activated by point mutations, activation of *myc* genes occurs via gene amplification and transcriptional dysregulation, with resultant protein overexpression. In SCLC, the *myc* gene is amplified in about 30–50% of cell lines and 11–24% of tumors, and is overexpressed in 89% of cell lines and 83% of tumors, compared with NSCLC, where the *myc* gene is amplified in 8% of tumors.[155] Of the well-characterized *myc* genes, c-*myc* is the most frequently activated in SCLC and NSCLC, whereas abnormalities of N-*myc* and L-*myc* usually only occur in SCLC. In a study of 291 specimens (183 tumors and 108 tumor cell lines) from patients with SCLC from 15 different studies, 35 of 108 (32%) cell lines and 37 of 183 (20%) tumors had *myc* family DNA amplification.[156] When evaluating these cell lines and tumors in relation to chemotherapy, *myc* family DNA amplification occurred more commonly in specimens from treated than in those from untreated patients. DNA amplifications were seen in 16 of 44 (36%) treated specimens, compared with 7 of 52 (11%) untreated.[157] This study confirmed a prior study that showed DNA amplification in 19 of 67 (28%) treated specimens compared with 3 of 40 (8%) untreated.[158] c-*myc* amplification is associated with the variant form of SCLC that is characterized by altered morphology, rapid in vitro growth, radioresistance and shortened survival. NSCLC infrequently showed amplification of c-*myc* (2/47), and these two cases were adenocarcinomas with normal *ras* genes.[159] Thus c-*myc* amplification is associated not only with a particular class of lung tumor (SCLC) but also with exposure to chemotherapy and a particular subtype of SCLC (variant) and poor survival. In premalignant lesions, abnormal expression of c-*myc* is rare.

Modulation of gene expression using oligonucleotides has been targeted at different levels of the cellular machinery. Triplex-forming oligonucleotides, as well as peptide nucleic acids, have been used to limit gene expression at the level of transcription by binding to DNA, resulting in a conformational change in the DNA's helical structure and preventing any further DNA–protein interaction necessary for transcription. One target for triplex DNA is the c-*myc* gene. Studies have shown that exposure to the triplex

DNA led to reduced transcriptional levels of c-*myc* and to growth suppression of ovarian and cervical carcinomas.[160,161] The use of antisense oligonucleotides against c-*myc* transcription has also been shown to inhibit the proliferation of Burkitt's lymphoma cell lines without any adverse effects on normal cells.[162] In NSCLC cell lines, Robinson et al[163] demonstrated inhibition of proliferation of all cell lines as well as reduction of c-*myc* protein expression with antisense c-*myc*.[162] In mice bearing human melanoma xenografts, the combination of c-*myc* antisense oligodeoxynucleotides with cisplatin therapy resulted in a higher inhibition of tumor growth, a reduction in the number of lung metastases and an increase in lifespan compared with those treated with either agent alone.[164]

bcl-2

Bcl-2 expression has also been found to be abnormal in lung cancer. The *bcl*-2 gene was first identified in follicular lymphomas with a t(14;18) translocation. Bcl-2 is a negative regulator of cell death, prolonging the survival of non-cycling cells and inhibiting apoptosis of cycling cells. There are a number of proteins identified that regulate apoptosis and belong to the *bcl*-2 family.[165] Some are negative regulators of apoptosis, such as Bcl-2, and some are enhancers of apoptosis, such as Bax. Members of the Bcl-2 family are capable of forming homodimers, heterodimers or both, and these complexes are tightly controlled. Under normal conditions, many of the Bcl-2 family members bind to Bax as heterodimers, since homodimers of Bax induce apoptosis. Bcl-2 expression is negatively regulated by p53.[166] Upon radiation injury, p53 protein induces more expression of Bax in the cell and drives the equilibrium of interaction toward Bax homodimers, thereby inducing apoptosis. It has been suggested that Bcl-2 expression is directly involved in the emergence of drug resistance by disrupting or delaying the apoptotic program and promoting tumor survival. Expression of Bcl-2 prevents apoptosis from a wide variety of cell stresses and cytotoxic chemicals, including heat shock, ionizing radiation and a range of chemotherapeutic agents.[167] In acute myeloid leukemia, patients with high expression of *bcl*-2 mRNA achieved lower complete response rates and shorter survival than those with no or low expression.[168] In ovarian cancer, cisplatin-resistant ovarian cell lines overexpressed Bcl-2, resulting in protection from drug-induced apoptosis and a delay in drug-mediated S-phase arrest.[169]

Fifty-five per cent of SCLC cell lines express relatively high levels of Bcl-2, compared with only 25% in NSCLC.[170,171] As with other malignant states, high levels of Bcl-2 expression in SCLC cells may be associated with resistance to chemotherapy and radiotherapy, resulting in poor survival. Takayama et al[170] investigated the correlation between Bcl-2 expression and prognosis, including response to chemotherapy in SCLC patients. Of 38 patients, 21 (55%) were found to have abnormal Bcl-2 expression. Response rates were similar for positive Bcl-2 expression and for negative Bcl-2 expression (62% versus 76%). Survival time was, however, shorter for patients with Bcl-2$^+$ tumors (median survial of 7 months versus 12 months). In NSCLC, abnormal Bcl-2 expression was associated with a longer survival in four studies.[131,171–173] Pezzella et al[171] showed that patients with Bcl-2$^+$ tumors (20/80 squamous and 5/42 adenocarcinoma) have a better survival rate at five years, reaching statistical significance only for patients with squamous cell carcinoma (five-year survival rate of 78% versus 48%). The suggested reason was less aggressive growth of tumors with Bcl-2 expression. Studies by Fontanini et al[172] and Kwiatowski et al[131] confirmed significantly better prognosis for patients with Bcl-2 expression. There is a possibility that increased Bcl-2 involved in the pathogenesis of some cases of lung cancer confers a survival advantage through its anti-apoptotic effects. This may occur by inhibiting the selection of further genetic mutants. Further studies are needed to prove this hypothesis. Ohsaki et al[173] analyzed Bcl-2 and p53 expression in NSCLC in correlation with survival time. The Bcl-2 protein was expressed in 19.2% of NSCLCs (19/99 cases), 30.4% of stage I and II carcinomas and in 36.8% of squamous cell carcinomas. Bcl-2 expression correlated with prolonged survival, with a 65.6% five-year survival rate and a median survival of 50 months compared with a 33% five-year survival rate and 23-month median survival in Bcl-2$^-$ patients. When only stage I and II patients were considered, the five-year survival rate of 80.8% and median survival of 62 months in Bcl-2$^+$ patients were significantly superior to the 49.5% five-year survival rate and 49-month median survival in the Bcl-2$^-$ group. p53 protein was found in 44.4% (44/99 cases), and did not correlate with survival time. However, patients who were both Bcl-2$^+$ and p53$^-$ survived significantly longer than those who were Bcl-2$^-$ or p53$^+$. Thus the role of Bcl-2 expression in SCLC and NSCLC remains unclear in relation to survival and response to chemotherapy.

Although expression of the Bcl-2 protein has been investigated in a number of non-hematologic malignancies, little is known of its distribution in premalignant lesions. Walker et al[174] investigated the expression of Bcl-2 in biopsies of normal and dysplastic bronchial epithelium, as well as in 31 bronchial resection margins and their corresponding carcinomas. Strong expression was observed in over 90% of the epithelial cells in 11 cases, all of which were severe dysaplasias. An increasingly aberrant pattern of Bcl-2 expression correlated with an increasing grade of dysplasia. Sixty-five percent of the carcinomas contained Bcl-2$^+$ cells.

Antisense oligonucleotides to *bcl-2* have also been shown to inhibit cancer growth.[163] In lymphoma and lymphocytic leukemia cell lines, Reed et al[175] demonstrated reduction in Bcl-2 protein levels with *bcl-2* antisense oligodeoxynucleotides, and subsequent enhanced sensitivity to anticancer drugs. Ziegler et al[176] demonstrated decreased cell viability of several SCLC cell lines with antisense oligodeoxynucleotides. Viability was reduced through apoptosis, corresponding to a reduction in Bcl-2 levels.

c-erbB-1

Proto-oncogenes that encode components of cell signaling pathways can become abnormally activated in lung cancer. The *c-erbB-1* proto-oncogene encodes the EGFR with tyrosine kinase activity, which has been discussed above.

In a summary of studies evaluating EFGR expression in lung cancers, 86% (100/116) of squamous carcinomas, 50% (97/193) of adenocarcinomas, 55% (17/31) of large cell carcinomas and 0% (0/37) of small cell carcinomas expressed EGFR.[177] Data involving increased expression of *c-erbB-1* and survival are conflicting. Volm et al[178] investigated the correlation of the expression of the proto-oncogene-encoded proteins c-ErbB-1, c-ErbB-2, c-Myc and c-Fos and the suppressor gene product p53 in 81 human squamous cell carcinomas of the lung with clinical parameters of the patient (survival, presence of metastases and tumor stage). By immunohistochemistry, expression of c-ErbB-1 oncoprotein was detected in 79% of the tumors, c-ErbB-2 proteins in 35% and c-Myc proteins in 48%. Patients with c-ErbB-1$^+$ tumors had a poor prognosis when compared with patients with c-ErbB-1$^-$ tumors (three-year survival rate of 31% versus 61%). Expression of c-ErbB-1 also conferred resistance. No significant relationship was found with the other oncoproteins and survival. However, Scagliotti et al[179] noted no relationship between EGFR expression and age, sex, disease extent, squamous versus non-squamous histology or survival in 163 NSCLC samples obtained at the time of radical surgery for operable disease.

Overexpression of EGFR has also been found in premalignant bronchial epithelium. In a study evaluating aberrant expression of p53 and EGFR in NSCLC and associated bronchial lesions, 18 (53%) of the invasive carcinomas and 30 (48%) of the bronchial lesions showed positive staining for EGFR.[180] Aberrant EGFR expression occurred as frequently in metaplasia and atypia as it did in dysplasia and carcinoma. However, the staining was more intense and involved more of the superficial layers of the epithelium in areas of dysplasia and carcinoma in situ than in metaplasia and atypia, suggesting the presence of more receptors as lesions progress from metaplasia to dysplasia to carcinoma in situ to invasive tumors.

c-erbB-2 (HER2/neu)

A related proto-oncogene, *c-erbB-2*, encodes another growth factor receptor, a 185 kDa protein that appears to be homologous to the EGFR. (*c-erbB-2* is also known as *HER2*, and is the human homolog of the *neu* oncogene, originally identified in rat neuroblastomas.) Like the EGFR, the c-ErbB-2 (HER2/Neu, or p185neu) protein was found to regulate cell adhesion and the invasive growth of cancer through its association with the cadherin–catenin complex.[182] c-ErbB-2 has also been shown to contribute to tumor angiogenesis by upregulating VEGF/VPF.[183] Treatment of c-ErbB-2$^+$ SKBR-3 human breast cancer cells in vitro with an anti-c-ErbB-2 monoclonal antibody (4D5) resulted in a dose-dependent reduction of VEGF/VPF protein expression. Abnormal expression of c-ErbB-2 is present in about 25% of NSCLCs but has not been reported in SCLC. Expression of c-ErbB-2 is abundant in some tumors and tumor cell lines from patients with NSCLC, particularly adenocarcinomas: in the study by Hern et al,[184] involving 55 NSCLC tumors, 5/16 (36%) squamous and 10/29 (38%) adenocarcinomas overexpressed c-ErbB-2, compared with none in the large cell tumors. Overexpression of c-ErbB-2 in patients with adenocarcinoma resulted in a shorter survival duration (83.7 weeks versus 188.5 weeks), in contrast to patients with squamous cell carcinoma, where c-ErbB-2 overexpression did not correlate with prognosis. In a study by Tateishi et al,[185] involving 119 patients with adenocarcinoma and 84 patients with squamous cell carcinoma of the lung, 28% of adenocarcinomas stained positive for c-ErbB-2, compared with only 2% of squamous carcinomas. c-ErbB-2 expression was correlated with more advanced disease and poorer survival for the group with adenocarcinoma (five-year survival rate 30% versus 52%).[185] Its expression also correlated with resistance to chemotherapy.[186]

Kern et al[187] reported that c-ErbB-2 was expressed in 15 of 44 adenocarcinomas (34%), and also found K-*ras* mutations in 16 of 44 (36%). Univariate analysis identified c-ErbB-2 expression as a negative prognostic factor, with a 2.4-fold increase in the patient's relative risk of dying. The presence of a K-*ras* mutation was not found to be statistically associated with survival. c-ErbB-2 was identified as an independent negative prognostic factor, while a K-*ras* mutation approached significance in multivariate analysis. K-*ras* mutations and c-ErbB-2 expression were additive in their effect on survival, with a hazard ratio of 4.4. In a study of 271 stage I patients, c-ErbB-2 expression had a significant impact on survival, and the group that expressed both p53 and c-ErbB-2 had a very poor survival.[188] Two studies, however, did not show a correlation between c-ErbB-2 expression and survival.[131,179] More studies are needed before c-ErbB-2 expression can be used as a prognostic factor.

Like EGFR, c-ErbB-2 overexpression has been found in both normal bronchial epithelium and in epithelium tumors.[180] Overexpression of c-ErbB-2 was observed in 3 of 13 normal epithelium and 6 of 16 lung tumors. Thus chronic damage of the bronchial epithelial cells can result from either a cytogenetic instability or a misregulation of the normal growth factor. Progression toward full tumorigenicity can then be accomplished by further genomic changes that occur during the multistep pathogenesis of lung cancer.

Tumor suppressor genes

Tumor suppressor genes cause dysregulated growth primarily through loss of function (classically by allele loss of one and point mutation of the other allele), which contributes to malignant transformation.

The retinoblastoma gene (Rb)

Altered expression of the retinoblastoma gene *Rb* has been identified in SCLC and NSCLC. *Rb*, located at chromosomal region 13q14, encodes a nuclear phosphoprotein that regulates the G_1/S boundary, a checkpoint in cell cycle regulation as summarized in Figure 3.4. Phosphorylation of the Rb protein is one of the most critical determinants of progression through the various phases. Rb is dephosphorylated at the end of mitosis and during most of G_0/G_1. Hypophosphorylated Rb is complexed to the transcription factor E2F. In this state, Rb actively suppresses the transition from G_1 phase to S phase by binding to E2F. When phosphorylated by cyclin-dependent kinases (CDKs), Rb dissociates from E2F, which then binds to E2F sites in cell cycle-regulating genes and induces the expression of genes encoding for proteins such as dihydrofolate reductase, thymidine kinase, thymidylate synthase and DNA polymerase, which are needed for S phase. This process therefore drives the cell into completing the cell cycle. The activity of

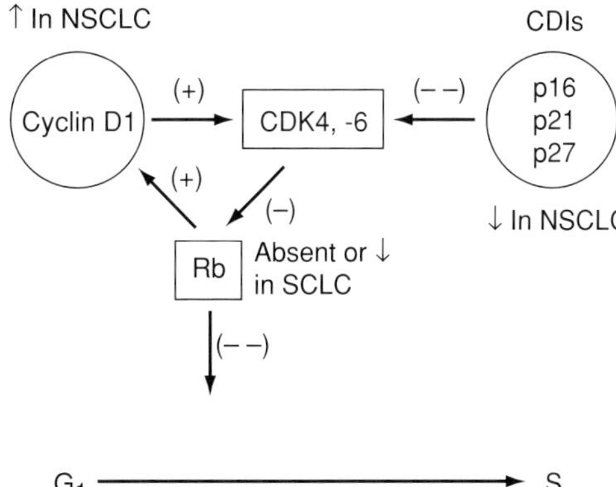

Figure 3.4
Cell cycle regulation of Rb by cyclin-dependent kinase (CDK)–cyclin D1 and CDK inhibitors (CDIs). During the cell cycle, CDKs are activated by the binding of cyclins and inhibited by the binding of CDIs. Rb is an inhibitor of the G_1-to-S transition of the cell cycle. +, activation; – and – –, inhibition. Changes in lung cancer: ↑, increased; ↓, decreased.

CDKs requires cyclin binding. Several inhibitors, such as p16INK4A, p15INK4B and p21,[189] suppress the activity of CDKs.

In SCLC cell lines, there is rearrangement of chromosome 13, directly affecting the 13q14 locus where *Rb* is located (see Figure 3.4). Up to 70% of SCLC cell lines have a structural alteration in the *Rb* gene or abnormal mRNA expression, thereby leading to absent expression of the protein. In more than 90% of SCLC tumors, the Rb protein is either absent or is aberrantly expressed, through hypophosphorylation, thus losing its ability to bind viral oncoproteins or cellular proteins, or through deletion or mutation of the pocket domain.[190–192] Shimizu et al[193] detected absent or aberrant Rb protein expression in 66/75 (88%) SCLC. Unlike SCLC, altered or absent Rb transcript was detected in only 10% (22/219) of NSCLC cases.[194] Absent or aberrant

Rb protein expression was detected in about 15–32% of NSCLC.[193–195] In NSCLC, the Rb-mediated growth control pathway is inactivated through alternate mechanisms instead of alteration in the *Rb* gene (see Figure 3.4). Cyclin D1, which regulates the activity of Rb by stimulating its phosphorylation by CDK4, can be overexpressed and cause disruption of this pathway. Another mechanism for inactivating the Rb-mediated pathway is through the mutational inactivation of the CDK inhibitor p16INK4A.

Xu et al,[196] in a study of 119 patients with stage I and II NSCLC, demonstrated that Rb and p53 were synergistic prognostic factors. Absent Rb nuclear staining indicating loss of Rb function occurred in 19 (16%) of the cases studied, whereas expression of a putative mutant p53 nuclear protein ($p53^+$) was found in 54 (45%) of the tumors. Median survival was longer for patients with Rb^+ tumors (39 months versus 12 months) and no expression of mutant p53 (41 months versus 24 months). Individuals with $Rb^-/p53^+$ tumors had a significantly shorter median survival compared with those with $Rb^+/p53^-$ tumors (12 months versus 41 months). Dosaka-Akita et al[197] evaluated the prognostic significance of the loss of Rb protein expression alone and in combination with Ras p21 status and p53 protein status. Ninety-one patients with NSCLC underwent potentially curative resection, with 65 also receiving postoperative chemotherapy. Nineteen (21%) showed negative Rb protein expression. The five-year survival for patients who had absence of protein expression was lower than for patients with Rb^+ tumors. This comparison did not reach statistical significance. In patients with adenocarcinomas, when combined with either Ras p21 status or p53 status, absence of Rb expression combined with either mutated Ras or p53 correlated with a poor survival (13% five-year survival rate versus 82% in Rb^+/Ras^- tumors and 20% five-year survival rate versus 73% in $Rb^+/p53^-$ tumors). No significant correlation was found in patients with squamous cell carcinoma. However, a third study involving 244 patients did not confirm the negative prognostic factor of abnormal Rb expression.[131] Abnormal Rb expression, which is evident in 79 of 242 patients (33%), did not show a statistically significant survival difference (five-year cancer-free survival rate of 73% versus 65%).

Chromosome 9p and CDKN2A (p16INK4A)

p16 regulates the activity of Rb by inhibiting CDK4:cyclin D1 kinase activity, and therefore the absence of p16 allows uncontrolled CDK4 phosphorylation of Rb and transcription factor activation (see Figure 3.4). Alteration in p16 expression can thus affect regulation of the cell cycle at the G_1 checkpoint. Its gene, *CDKN2A* (also known as *MTS1*), which is situated on chromosome 9p21, is frequently mutated in lung and other cancers.[198] De Vos et al[198] noted a higher frequency of either deletions or mutations in the *CDKN2A* gene in NSCLC cell lines (6/9, 67%) compared with primary tumor samples (7/34, 21%). *CDKN2A* is inactivated by deletions (commonly), point mutations (less commonly) or hypermethylation (occasionally), which downregulates its expression in more than 40% of NSCLC, but is only infrequently mutated in SCLC. It appears that *CDKN2A* inactivation is the most common mechanism inactivating the *Rb/CDKN2A*/cyclin D1 growth control pathway in NSCLC, whereas *Rb* mutation is the most frequent in SCLC. Shapiro et al[199] examined cyclin D1 and p16 expression in NSCLC (predominantly Rb^+) and SCLC (Rb^-), and demonstrated reciprocal *Rb* inactivation and p16 expression in both primary lung cancers and cell lines. In NSCLC samples, cyclin D1 protein was overexpressed in 15 of 27 (56%) samples and in 6 of 9 (67%) NSCLC cell lines compared with controls. In SCLC samples, cyclin D1 was overexpressed in 4 of 5 (80%) SCLC resection samples and in 2 of 5 (40%) SCLC cell lines compared with matched controls. This suggests that cyclin D1 overexpression and Rb loss may both be involved in SCLC. In contrast to cyclin D1 expression, p16 expression was not detected in 18 of 27 (67%) NSCLC samples and in 6 of 9 (67%) Rb^+ NSCLC cell lines, compared with 1 of 5 (20%) SCLC tumors and 0 of 5 (0%) SCLC cell lines. In contrast to Rb^+ cell lines, Rb^- cell lines showed abundant levels of p16 (5 of 5 SCLC and one Rb^- NSCLC cell line). Thus this confirms the proposed theory of Serrano et al[200] that physiological inactivation of Rb during G_1 leads to increased p16 expression in order to limit CDK4 activity. Rb^- tumors, as predicted, would have high levels of p16, while Rb^+ tumors might require decreased amounts of functional p16 in order to achieve levels of CDK4 activity sufficient for Rb inactivation.

Taga et al[201] evaluated the prognostic significance of p16 alteration. In 115 NSCLC specimens, 31 (27%) showed negative p126 staining, with a higher frequency noted in squamous cell carcinoma (39.5%) compared with adenocarcinoma (20.3%). Negative p16 expression was a significant prognostic factor, with patients surviving for a shorter period of time compared with those with positive p16 expression. This difference was more evident for patients with early-stage disease. In a study involving 125 NSCLC samples (71 cell lines and 56 tumors), Nakagawa et al[202] examined the relationship of *CDKN2A* gene alterations and those of the related gene *MTS2* (*CDKN2B*/p15INK4B) with patient stage and site of cancer. Mutations were observed more frequently in tumors or cell lines from patients with stage III or IV disease. *CDKN2A* alterations were noted in 37% (26/71) of the NSCLC cell lines and 39% (22/56) of the tumors, with all the alterations occurring in stage III and IV disease.

Kinoshita et al[203] examined fresh frozen specimens of 114 resected NSCLCs for loss of p16 and Rb expression together with aberrant accumulation of p53 protein and the proliferative activity measured by Ki-67 antibody. Of 111 tumors, 30 (27%) lacked p16 expression and 10 (9%) lost Rb expression. No tumor showed coincident loss of both proteins, supporting the hypothesis that they function in a single pathway. Loss of p16 expression did not correlate with any clinical factors, whereas loss of Rb expression correlated with heavy smoking (pack years $\geq$ 20). Aberrant accumulation of p53 protein was observed in 41% of tumors, and did not correlate with the loss of p16 or Rb. Proliferative activity was higher in $p53^+$ tumors than in $p53^-$ tumors. Loss of p16 or Rb expression was associated with a further increase in proliferative activity in the $p53^+$ tumors, but no significant change in the $p53^-$ tumors, suggesting that derangement of the p16/Rb pathway might synergistically increase cell proliferation with altered p53 protein. Alteration of both p16/Rb and p53 pathways may be linked to poor prognosis because of its association with an extremely high proliferative activity.

Positive Rb staining is normally found within bronchial epithelia in patients without lung tumors and who had never smoked, as opposed to NSCLC patients, where abnormal expression of cyclin D1 (*CCND1*) and *Rb* gene expression was detected in the resection margins.[204] Examination of the resection margins revealed four carcinomas in situ, 19 hyperplasias and 10 sections showing apparently normal bronchial epithelium. Increased cyclin D1 and diminished Rb expression were found in 76% and 27% of the resection margins respectively, and both cyclin D1 and Rb expression were altered in 12%. Abnormal expression of Rb was noted in 63% (12/19) of the samples showing hyperplasia/dysplasia. In the corresponding tumors, 48%

were normal, while altered expression was found for cyclin D1 in 33%, Rb in 27% and both in 9% of cases. In another study, Ferron et al[205] noted the frequency of p53$^+$ and Rb$^-$ microscopic fields to be directly related to the morphological grading of lesions.

The *CDKN2A* tumor suppressor gene is located on 9p along with another CDK inhibitor p15 (*CDKN2B/MTS2*/p15INK4B). Loss of genetic material at a certain chromosomal locus resulting in loss of heterozygosity (LOH) is frequently seen in various types of human malignancies, and is considered a hallmark of a tumor suppressor gene. Merlo et al[206] were able to detect LOH at loci on 9p in 67% of NSCLC and 52% of SCLC tumors. LOH at 9p has been evident in premalignant epithelial lesions. Thiberville et al[207] showed evidence of cumulative gene losses with progression from premalignant epithelial lesions to carcinoma. They showed an increase in prevalence of 9p deletions, from no deletions in the hyperplasia/metaplasia samples to 31% in the dysplasia samples, 83% for the carcinoma in situ and 100% in the invasive cancers. Kishimoto et al[208] noted that LOH at 9p loci occurred at the earliest stage of hyperplasia, when comparing sequential appearance of 3p LOH, 9p LOH and *ras* gene mutations in the pathogenesis of NSCLC. In hyperplastic lesions, LOH at 9p occurred in 38% of the cases. In a prospective study in current and former smokers, LOH at 9p21 occurred in 57% of the tissue samples tested in healthy chronic smokers compared with none in the lifetime non-smokers.[209] Ookawa et al[210] reported that reconstitution of *Rb* inhibited the growth of SCLC, and Jiu et al[211] showed that direct injection of *CDKN2A* gene vectors into NSCLC cells in athymic nude mice inhibited their growth.

p53

The *p53* gene, which has been studied extensively in SCLC, is mutated in all types of lung cancer. *p53*, located at chromosome 17p13.1, encodes a 53 kDa nuclear protein that acts as a transcription factor, blocks the progression of cells through the cell cycle late in the G_1 phase and can trigger apoptosis. Normally, p53 (wild type) is a tumor suppressor protein, binding to the promoter region of the *WAF1* gene encoding the CDK inhibitor p21WAF1, and incuding p21WAF1 expression. Once the cyclin/CDK complex has been inhibited by p21WAF1, Rb cannot be phosphorylated. Hypophosphorylated Rb binds E2F, preventing DNA synthesis, and the cell cycle is blocked before S phase.[212] In lung cancer, however, p21WAF1 is usually expressed at higher than normal levels, independent of the status of p53, suggesting a p53-independent pathway for its induction.[213] p53 can also induce apoptosis in response to DNA damage. p53 levels, upon response to DNA damage such as that from radiation, rise, and the p53 protein binds to the *bax* promoter, increases *bax* transcription and drives the cell toward apoptosis.[165]

Abnormalities of *p53* in NSCLC have been studied both by analysis of protein expression (immunostaining) and by analysis of gene mutations (single-strand conformation polymorphism (SSCP) gel analysis and DNA sequencing). *p53* mutations in lung cancer occur throughout the gene, and include deletions, point mutations and overexpression. The most common *p53* mutations in lung cancer are the G–T transversions related to adducts of benzo(*a*)pyrene from cigarette smoking.[214] The frequency of mutations may be up to 50% in NSCLC and 80% in SCLC.[215]

The presence of *p53* mutations has an uncertain relationship with clinical outcome. Two studies showed no significant correlation between *p53* mutations and overall survival.[216,217] Carbone and co-workers evaluated the correlation of *p53* abnormalities and survival in 85 resected NSCLC patients. p53 overexpression was present in 55%

and mutant sequences in 54%. There was no correlation between the presence of gene mutations and survival.[214] A significant decrease in survival resulted with p53 overexpression but not with *p53* mutations. Chiba et al[217] noted no significant correlation between the presence of *p53* mutations and survival. However, two studies noted a shorter survival for patients having these mutations.[218,219] Mitsudomi et al[218] reported that mutations of *p53* (43%) in 120 resected patients with NSCLC resulted in a shorter survival rate (28% in three years, compared with 51%). Horio et al[219] demonstrated mutations in *p53* in 49% of 71 cases of NSCLC in stage I to IIIA. The presence of *p53* mutations correlated with a shorter survival time in all patient groups.[218]

Studies have used expression of p53 detected with immunostaining as a marker for mutation, since normal cellular levels are far too low to be detected. Increased expression has been noted in 38–68% of NSCLC tumors.[52,215,220–225] As with *p53* mutations, data correlating survival with p53 expression are conflicting. Several studies showed expression to be associated with a shortened survival.[52,220–224] Nuclear p53 overexpression was shown to be an independent prognostic parameter in node-negative NSCLC.[223] Survival analysis showed no difference in clinical outcome between $p53^+$ and $p53^-$ tumors in node-positive tumors, in contrast to node-negative tumors, where patients with $p53^-$ tumors had a significantly better survival time. Another study showed that patients with altered p53 expression had a shorter survival after surgery compared with those without p53 expression (five-year survival rate of 24% versus 50%).[224] For those who underwent potential curative surgery, $p53^+$ patients had a shorter survival than $p53^-$ patients, with five-year survival rates of 36% and 63% respectively. In the study by Kwiatkowski et al,[131] abnormal p53 expression was evident in 108 of 242 samples (44%), and was associated with decreased cancer-free survival in a univariate analysis. An improved survival with p53 overexpression was noted in three studies,[215,225,226] and no effect on survival in two studies.[227,228] The reasons for the conflicting results are unclear, and may be due to small numbers of samples, heterogeneous groups of patients studied or different monoclonal antibodies used to detect mutated p53 protein.

In a small study involving 18 patients with NSCLC, Kawasaki et al[229] demonstrated that the immunohistochemical expression of p53 correlated with unresponsiveness to chemotherapy. This process may be due to the stimulatory effect of mutant p53 on the *MDR1* promoter, resulting in expression of the human *MDR1* multidrug-resistance gene, which encodes an energy-dependent efflux pump, responsible for drug resistance.[230] In stage III patients treated with radiotherapy, the response to radiotherapy was slightly better in the $p53^-$ cases (65% versus 42%).[231] Overall survival between $p53^-$ and $p53^+$ cases did not differ; however, the disease-specific survival was found to be worse in the $p53^+$ cases than in the $p53^-$ cases (median survival 8.4 months versus 14.4 months).

p53 protein overexpression and *p53* gene mutations have also been reported in bronchial dysplasia and carcinoma in situ.[232–235] Bennett et al[233] noted abnormal p53 accumulation in 71% (24/34) of cases of early bronchial neoplasia. They noted an increasing frequency of p53 accumulation from normal mucosa to invasive tumors: 0% in normal mucosa, 6.7% in squamous metaplasia, 29.5% in mild dysplasia, 26.9% in moderate dysplasia, 59.7% in severe dysplasia, 58.5% in carcinoma in situ, 67.5% in microinvasive carcinomas and 79.5% in invasive tumors. *p53* mutations and p53 overexpression have also been seen in premalignant lesions associated with other tobacco-related tumors, including head and neck and esophageal squamous cell carcinomas.[236,237] One study found aberrant expression of p53 in preneoplastic bronchial lesions but not in reactive or metaplastic epithelium associated with squamous cell carcinoma.[181] Sundaresan et al[238] demonstrated mutation and allele loss in *p53* in severe bronchial dysplasia adjacent to invasive tumors. Chung et al[239] demonstrated that damage to *p53* occurred after allele loss on chromosome 3p, with damage to chromosome 3p being sequential and progressive, as discussed below. In the study by Mao et al,[209] LOH at 17p13 was only observed in 18% in tissues from chronic smokers, compared with none in non-smokers.

Therapeutic strategies involving *p53* have been initiated using gene therapy. Cai et al[240] showed that expression of wild-type *p53* in tumors lacking *p53* or having mutant *p53* suppresses proliferation. Restoration of wild-type *p53* function is also associated with enhanced radiosensitivity and chemosensitivity.[241] In a clinical study, Roth et al[242] locally injected retrovirus-containing wild-type *p53* into patients with relapsed NSCLC with *p53* mutations. They demonstrated that gene expression was achieved and that the treatment was capable of inducing an objective response. Regression of the treated lesion was seen in three patients, and tumor growth was stabilized in a further three cases. A recent phase I trial of adenoviral *p53* gene replacement in 21 patients with advanced NSCLC produced little toxicity.[243] Expression of the *p53* transgene was evident along with clinical reponses. Disease stabilization lasting up to six months and greater than 50% tumor regression were seen for patients receiving adenoviral *p53* alone or with cisplatin.

MDM2

MDM2 is an oncoprotein that inhibits the p53 tumor suppressor protein. Amplification of the *MDM2* gene and overexpression of its protein have been observed in some human malignancies, and these abnormalities have a role in tumorigenesis through inactivation of p53 function. Higashiyama et al[244] analyzed *MDM2* gene amplification and protein expression as well as *p53* mutations in 201 surgically resected NSCLC patients. Of the 30 patients tested, only 2 (7%) showed amplification, while MDM2 protein was found immunohistochemically in a total of 48 (24%) of 201 samples. MDM2 protein expression was found more frequently in patients with adenocarcinoma. There was no association with clinical stage or tumor differentiation. p53 protein accumulation was seen in a total of 91 patients (45%), but there was no correlation between MDM2 protein expression and p53 protein accumulation. In relation to survival, patients with MDM2 protein expression showed a marginally better prognosis than patients without it. When survival was analyzed in relation to p53 status, MDMS$^+$ patients showed a significantly more favourable prognosis than MDM2$^-$ patients in the p53$^-$ group. This was also evident when stage I patients were evaluated separately. However, among the p53$^+$ group, there was no difference in the postoperative survival curve associated with the MDM2 protein status. Thus it can be speculated that *MDM2* abnormalities may have little or no effect on the p53-mediated pathway if *p53* itself is mutated.

3p

The first non-random chromosomal abnormality identified in human lung cancer was 3p deletion.[245] This deletion has been shown to be the most frequent alteration in lung cancers, occurring even in mild dysplasia, an early precursor lesion. Loss of alleles at 3p is observed in more than 90% of SCLC tumors and approximately 50% of NSCLC tumors.[246] Three distinct chromosomal regions, 3p25, 3p21.3 and 3p12–p14, are suspected locations for tumor suppressor genes.[247] The *VHL* (von Hippel–Lindau disease) gene at 3p25 was found to play a role in the tumorigenesis of renal cancer and hemangioblastoma.[248] Recently, the *FHIT* (fragile histidine triad) gene has been localized to 3p14.2, and in one study approximately 80% of SCLC tumors showed this genetic abnormality.[249] Loss of the *FHIT* gene results in the accumulation of diadenosine tetraphosphate, which could lead to the stimulation of DNA synthesis and proliferation.

The relationship of 3p LOH to prognosis in NSCLC is unclear. Two studies suggested that 3p LOH was associated with less differentiated histology or with the advanced stage in adenocarcinoma of the lung and with a trend toward a poor prognosis.[219,250] One study showed 3p LOH to be more prevalent in squamous cell carcinoma (24/35, 69%) than in adenocarcinoma (18/52, 35%).[251] There was no significant association with sex, tumor stage or grade of differentiation. However, 3p LOH was associated with a significantly poor survival for patients with adenocarcinoma, but not for patients with squamous cell carcinoma. Another study showed the presence of abnormalities in transcripts of the *FHIT* gene in at least 80% of SCLCs and 40% of NSCLCs, with 76% of the informative cases also exhibiting loss of one *FHIT* allele.[249] A recent study evaluated the biologic activity of the *FHIT* gene product as a potential tumor suppressor.[252] Overexpression of the protein product, pFHIT, had no effect on cell morphology, cellular proliferation or colony formation of several tumor cell lines not expressing this protein. The investigators concluded that the effect of *FHIT* loss or inactivation during tumorigenesis is distinct from that of the 'classic' suppressor genes such as in the p16/Rb or p53 pathways.

Studies involving normal bronchial epithelium exposed to carcinogens have noted genetic abnormalities on chromosome 3 in histologically normal bronchial epithelium.[253–255] Frequent LOH at 3p14 has been observed in oral premalignant lesions and in normal-appearing bronchial epithelia of smokers, supporting the notion that loss of the 3p14 region occurs early and frequently in tissue exposed to carcinogens.[209,254] LOH affecting at least one locus of the *FHIT* gene was observed in 41 of 51 (80%) tumors in the smokers group, compared with only 9 of 40 (22%) tumors in non-smokers.[255] In a study involving current and former smokers, 75% (27/36) of assessable patients showed LOH at 3p14.[209] Thiberville et al[207] showed an increase in prevalence of 3p deletions, from no deletions in the hyperplasia/metaplasia samples to 37% of the informative cases in the dysplasia samples, to 100% for carcinoma in situ and the invasive cancers. Kishimoto et al[208] noted extensive deletions of the short arm of chromosome 3 in the early stages at the stage of hyperplasia when comparing sequential appearance of 3p LOH, 9p LOH and *ras* gene mutations in the pathogenesis of NSCLC. In hyperplastic lesions, LOH occurred at a higher frequency at 3p (76%) than at 9p (38%), suggesting that the presence of LOH at 3p may be an earlier event. Chung et al[239] demonstrated that allele loss on chromosome 3p precedes damage to the *p53* gene, with damage to chromosome 3p being sequential and progressive. Damage to 3p may be progressive, as indicated by the incomplete loss of allele in dysplastic cells compared with the loss in tumor cells. In a comparison of adenocarcinoma of the lung and associated preinvasive lesions, Hung et al[256] also noted sequential loss of 3p markers. This suggests that a number of distinct regions (and therefore presumably genes) are involved in establishing the fully malignant phenotype, and that as tumor development progresses through the premalignant states, the genes located on 3p are inactivated in a sequential manner. The incidence of the deletion increases as the lesions advance from hyperplasia to dysplasia to carcinoma in situ to invasive cancer. This sequential process is discussed in a review of the above studies.[257]

Genetic changes in the pathogenesis of lung cancer

In the multistage process of lung cancer tumorigenesis, genetic lesions accumulate to produce the final malignant phenotype (see Tables 3.6 and 3.7). These abnormalities appear to occur in a sequential manner. Abnormalities involving growth factor receptors are detected in the earliest stages, setting the scene for further changes. Deletions in chromosome 3p and 9p subsequently occur, with allele loss at 3p preceding loss at 9p. As the grade of dysplasia increases, sequential losses in both chromosomes 3p and 9p are noted, along with the detection of abnormalities involving *ras*, *p53* and *bcl-2*, which are evident in the severe dysplasia/carcinoma in situ stage. These genetic abnormalities become cumulative, driving the cell to become malignant, and immune to the effects of local control. New strategies involving gene therapy and monoclonal antibodies to EGFR and c-ErbB-2 are continuing to be developed, and will be an important factor in the fight against cancer.

REFERENCES

1. Cook RM, Miller YE, Bunn PA Jr, Small cell lung cancer: etiology, biology, clinical features, staging and treatment. *Curr Prob Cancer* 1993; **17**: 69–141.
2. Moody TW, Growth factors and growth factor receptors in small cell lung cancer. In: *Biology of Lung Cancer. Lung Biology in Health and Disease*, Vol 122 (Kane MA, Bunn PA Jr, eds). Marcel Dekker: New York, 1998: 337–70.
3. Siegfried JM, Davis AJ, Gubish CT et al, Growth factors and receptors in non-small cell lung cancer. In: *Biology of Lung Cancer. Lung Biology in Health and Disease*, Vol 122 (Kane MA, Bunn PA Jr, eds). Marcel Dekker: New York, 1998: 317–36.
4. Heasley LE, Johnson GL, Signal transduction abnormalities in lung cancer. In: *Biology of Lung Cancer. Lung Biology in Health and Disease*, Vol 122 (Kane MA, Bunn PA Jr, eds). Marcel Dekker: New York, 1998: 371–90.
5. Bunn PA Jr, Chan D, Dienhart DG, Neuropeptide signal transduction in lung cancer: clinical implications of bradykinin sensitivity and overall heterogeneity. *Cancer Res* 1992; **52**: 24–31.
6. Bunn PA Jr, Dienhart DG, Chan D et al, Neuropeptide stimulation of calcium flux in human lung cancer cells: delineation of alternative pathways. *Proc Natl Acad Sci USA* 1990; **87**: 2162–6.
7. Sethi T, Rozengurt E, Multiple neuropeptides stimulate clonal growth of small cell lung cancer. *Cancer Res* 1993; **51**: 3621–3.
8. Corjay MJ, Dobrzanski DJ, Way JM, Two distinct bombesin receptor subtypes are expressed and functional in human lung carcinoma cells. *J Biol Chem* 1991; **226**: 18771–9.
9. Sethi T, Herget T, Wu SV et al, CCKA and CCKB receptors are expressed in small cell lung cancer cell lines and mediate Ca^{2+} mobilization and clonal growth. *Cancer Res* 1993; **53**: 5208–13.
10. Moody TW, Staley J, Zia F et al, Neuromedin B receptors are present on small cell lung cancer cells. *J Pharmacol Exp Ther* 1992; **262**: 311–17.
11. Chan D, Gera L, Bunn PA Jr et al, Novel bradykinin antagonist dimers for the treatment of human lung cancers. *Immunopharmacology* 1996; **33**: 201–4.
12. Hader M, Rotsch M, Bepler G et al, Epidermal growth factor receptor expression in human lung cancer cell lines. *Cancer Res* 1998; **48**: 1132–6.
13. Dazzi H, Haselton PS, Thatcher N et al, Expression of epidermal growth factor receptor (EGF-R) in non-small cell lung cancer. *Br J Cancer* 1989; **59**: 746–9.
14. Rusch V, Baselga J, Cordon-Cardo C et al, Differential expression of the epidermal growth factor receptor and its ligands in primary non-small cell lung cancers and adjacent benign lung. *Cancer Res* 1993; **53**: 2379–85.

15. Rachival WJ, Expression and activation of erb B-2 and epidermal growth factor receptor in lung adenocarcinomas. *Br J Cancer* 1995; **72**: 56–64.
16. Slamon D, Leyland-Jones B, Shak S et al, Addition of Herceptin™ (humanized anti-Her2 antibody) to first line chemotherapy for Her2 overexpressing metastic breast cancer markedly increases anticancer activity: a randomized multinational controlled phase III trials. *Proc Am Soc Clin Oncol* 1998; **17**: 98a.
17. Tsao MS, Zhu H, Viallet J, Autocrine growth loop of the epidermal growth factor receptor in normal and immortalized human bronchial epithelial cells. *Exp Cell Res* 1996; **223**: 268–73.
18. Aguayo SM, Miller YE, Waldron JR et al, Idiopathic diffuse hyperplasia of pulmonary neuroendocrine cells and airways disease. *N Engl J Med* 1992; **327**: 1285–8.
19. Minuto F, Del MP, Barreca A et al, Expression of the gastrin releasing peptide receptor confers a growth response to bombesin in immortalized human bronchial epithelial cells. *Cancer Res* 1995; **45**: 1853–5.
20. Jacques G, Rotsch M, Wegmann C et al, Production of insulin-like binding proteins by small cell lung cancer cell lines. *Exp Cell Res* 1989; **184**: 396–406.
21. Nakanishi Y, Cuttitta F, Kasprzyk PG, Evidence for autocrine mitogenic stimulation by somatomedin/insulin like growth factor I in established human lung cancer cell lines. *Cancer Res* 1988; **48**: 3716–19.
22. Nakanishi Y, Cuttitta F, Kasprzyk PG et al, Growth factor effects on small cell lung cancer cells using a colorimetric essay: Can a transferrin-like factor mediate autocrine growth? *Exp Cell Res* 1988; **56**: 74–85.
23. Vostrejs M, Moran PL, Seligman PA, Transferrin synthesis by small cell lung cancer cells acts as an autocrine regulator of cellular proliferation. *J Clin Invest* 1988; **82**: 331–9.
24. Cavanaugh PG, Nicholson GL, Lung-derived growth factor that stimulates the growth of lung-metastasizing tumor cell identification as transferrin. *J Cell Biochem* 1991; **47**: 261–71.
25. Tsao MS, Zhu H, Giaid A et al, Hepatocyte growth factor/scatter factor is an autocrine factor for human normal bronchial epithelial and lung carcinoma cells. *Cell Growth Differ* 1993; **4**: 571–9.
26. Rygaard K, Nakamura T, Spang-Thomsen M, Expression of the proto-oncogene c-met and c-kit and their ligands, hepatocyte growth factor/scatter factor and the stem cell factor in SCLC cell lines and xenografts. *Br J Cancer* 1993; **67**: 37–46.
27. Hibi K, Takahashi T, Selodo Y et al, Coexpression of the stem cell factor and the c-kit genes in small cell lung cancer. *Oncogene* 1991; **6**: 2291–6.
28. Sekido Y, Takashi T, Ueda R et al, Recombinant human stem cell factor mediates chemotaxis of small cell lung cancer cell lines aberrantly expressing the c-kit proto oncogene. *Cancer Res* 1993; **53**: 1709–14.
29. Pedrazzoli P, Bacciocchi G, Bergamasdi B, Effects of granulocyte–macrophage colon stimulating factor and interleukin-3 on small cell lung cancer cells. *Cancer Invest* 1994; **12**: 283–8.
30. Twentyman PR, Wright KA, Failure of GM-CSF to influence the growth of small cell and non-small cell lung cancer cell lines in vitro. *Eur J Cancer* 1991; **27**: 6–8.
31. Cuttitta F, Carney DN, Mulshine J et al, Bombesin-like peptides can function as autocrine growth factors in human small-cell lung cancer. *Nature* 1985; **316**: 823–6.
32. Kelley MJ, Linnoila RI, Avis IL et al, Antitumor activity of a monoclonal antibody directed against gastrin-releasing peptide in patients with small cell lung cancer. *Chest* 1997; **112**: 256–61.
33. Cohen AJ, Bunn PA Jr, Franklin W et al, Variable expression in human lung inactivation in lung cancer, and modulation of peptide-induced calcium flux. *Cancer Res* 1996; **56**: 831–9.
34. Shipp MA, Tarr GE, Chen CY et al, CD10/neutral endopeptidase 24.11 hydrolyzes bombesin-like peptides and regulates the growth of small cell carcinomas of the lung. *Proc Natl Acad Sci USA* 1991; **88**: 10662–6.
35. Bunn PA, Chan D, Helfrich B et al, Recombinant

neutral endopeptidase inhibits the in vitro and in vivo growth of human lung cancers with neuroendocrine features. *Lung Cancer* 1997; **18**: 147–9.

36. Fan Z, Masui H, Atlas F et al, Blockade of epidermal growth factor receptor function by bivalent and monovalent fragments of 225 anti-epidermal growth factor receptor monoclonal antibodies. *Cancer Res* 1993; **53**: 4322–8.
37. Bos M, Mendelsohn J, Bowden D et al, Phase I studies of anti-epidermal growth factor receptor (EGFR) chimeric monoclonal antibody C225 in patients with EGFR overexpressing tumors. *Proc Am Soc Clin Oncol* 1996; **15**: 443.
38. Divigi CR, Welt S, Dris M et al, Phase I and imaging trial of indium 111-labeled anti-epidermal growth factor receptor monoclonal antibody 225 in patients with squamous cell lung carcinoma. *J Natl Cancer Inst* 1991; **83**: 97–104.
39. Falcey J, Pfister D, Cohen R et al, A study of anti-epidermal growth factor receptor (EGFr) monoclonal antibody C225 and cisplatin in patients with head and neck or lung carcinomas. *Proc Am Soc Clin Oncol* 1997; **16**: 383a.
40. Layton JE, Scanlon DB, Soveny C et al, Effects of bombesin antagonists on the growth of small cell lung cancer cells in vitro. *Cancer Res* 1988; **48**: 4783–9.
41. Trepel JB, Moyer JD, Cuttitta F et al, A novel bombesin receptor antagonist inhibits autocrine signals in a small-cell lung carcinoma cell line. *Biochem Biophys Res Commun* 1988; **156**: 1383–9.
42. Woll PJ, Rozengurt EA, (D-Argl, D-Phe5, D-Trp7, 9, Leu 11) substance P, a potent bombesin antagonist in murine Swiss 3T3 cells, inhibits the growth of human small cell lung cancer in vitro. *Proc Natl Acad Sci USA* 1988; **85**: 1859–63.
43. Langdon SP, Sethi T, Ritchie A et al, Broad spectrum neuropeptide antagonist inhibit growth of small cell lung cancer in vitro. *Cancer Res* 1992; **52**: 4554–7.
44. Mitchell FM, Heasley LE, Qian NX et al, Differential modulation of bombesin-stimulated phospholipase C and mitogen-activated protein kinase activity by (D-Argl, D-Phe5, D-Trp7, 9, Leu 11) substance P. *J Biol Chem* 1995; **270**: 8623–8.
45. Jarpe MB, Knall C, Micthell FM et al, (D-Argl, D-Phe5, D-Trp 7, 9, Leu 11) substance P acts as a biased agonist toward neuropeptide and chemokine receptors. *J Biol Chem* 1998; **273**: 3097–104.
46. VanderSpek JC, Sutherland JA, Zeng H et al, Inhibition of protein synthesis in small cell lung cancer induced by the diphtheria toxin-related fusion protein DAB389 GRP. *Cancer Res* 1997; **57**: 290–4.
47. Shaw JP, Akiyoshi DE, Arrigo D et al, Cytotoxic properties of DAB_{486}EGF and DAB_{389}EGF, epidermal growth factor (EGF) receptor-targeted fusion toxins. *J Biol Chem* 1991; **51**: 21118–24.
48. Yamazaki H, Kijima H, Ohnishi Y et al, Inhibition of tumor growth by ribozyme-mediated suppression of aberrant epidermal growth factor receptor gene expression. *J Natl Cancer Inst* 1998; **90**: 581–7.
49. Lee CT, Wu S, Gabrilovich D et al, Antitumor effects of an adenovirus expressing antisense insulin-like growth factor I receptor on human lung cancer cell lines. *Cancer Res* 1996; **56**: 3038–41.
50. Bos M, Mendelsohn J, Kim Y et al, PD 153035, a tyrosine kinase inhibitor, prevents epidermal growth factor activation and inhibits growth of cancer cells in a receptor number-dependent manner. *Clin Cancer Res* 1997; **3**: 2099–106.
51. Tsai CM, Levitzki A, Wu LH et al, Enhancement of chemosensitivity by tyrphostin AG825 in high-p185neu expressing non-small cell lung cancer (NSCLC). *Proc Ann Meet Am Assoc Cancer Res* 1996; **37**: A2882.
52. Zhang L, Hung MC, Sensitization for Her-2/neu-overexpressing cancer cells to chemotherapeutic drugs by tyrosine kinase inhibitor emodin. *Proc Ann Meet Am Assoc Cancer Res* 1996; **37**: A2854.
53. Sun J, Qian Y, Hamilton AD et al, Ras CAAX peptidomimetic FTI 276 selectively blocks tumor growth in nude mice of a human lung carcinoma with K-ras mutation and p53 deletion. *Cancer Res* 1995; **55**: 4243–7.

54. Fidler IJ, Molecular biology of cancer: invasion and metastasis. In: *Cancer: Principles and Practice of Oncology*, 5th edn (De Vita, VT, Hellman S, Rosenberg SA, eds). Lippincott-Raven: Philadelphia, 1997: 135–52.
55. Landis SH, Murray T, Bolden S, Wingo PA, Cancer statistics 1998. *CA Cancer J Clin* 1998; **48**: 6–29.
56. Chambers AF, Hill RP, Tumor progression and metastasis. In: *The Basic Science of Oncology*, 3rd edn (Tannock IF, Hill RP, eds). McGraw-Hill: New York, 1998: 219–39.
57. Johnson RC, Zhu D, Augustin-Voss HG, Pauli BU, Lung endothelial dipeptidyl peptidase IV is an adhesion molecule for lung-metastatic rat breast and prostate carcinoma cells. *J Cell Biol* 1993; **121**: 1423–32.
58. El-Sabban ME, Pauli BU, Adhesion-mediated gap junctional communication between lung-metastatic cancer cells and endothelium. *Invasion Metastasis* 1994; **14**: 164–76.
59. Honn KV, Tang DG, Adhesion molecules and tumor cell interaction with endothelium and subendothelial matrix. *Cancer Metastasis Rev* 1992; **11**: 353–75.
60. Nicolson GL, Paracrine and autocrine growth mechanisms in tumor metastasis to specific sites with particular emphasis on brain and lung. *Cancer Metastasis Rev* 1993; **12**: 325–43.
61. Weiss L, Metastatic inefficiency. *Adv Cancer Res* 1990; **54**: 159–211.
62. Chambers AF, Matrisian LM, Changing views of the role of matrix metalloproteinases in metastasis. *J Natl Cancer Inst* 1997; **89**: 1260–70.
63. Nakajima M, Chop AM, Tumor invasion and extracellular matrix degradative enzymes: regulation of activity by organ factors. *Semin Cancer Biol* 1991; **2**: 115–17.
64. Mignatti P, Rifkin DB, Biology and biochemistry of proteinases in tumor invasion. *Physiol Rev* 1993; **73**: 161–95.
65. Brown PD, Bloxodge RE, Sturart NSA et al, Association between expression of activated 72-kilodalton gelatinase and tumor spread in non-small cell lung carcinoma. *J Natl Cancer Inst* 1993; **85**: 574–8.
66. Davies B, Miles DW, Happerfield LC et al, Activity to type IV collagenases in benign and malignant breast disease. *Br J Cancer* 1993; **67**: 1126–31.
67. Hamdy FC, Fadlon D, Cottam D et al, Localization of messenger RNA for MW 72,000 and 92,000 type IV collagenases in human skin cancers by in situ hybridization. *Cancer Res* 1994; **52**: 1336–41.
68. Poole C, Adams M, Barley V et al, A dose-finding study of marimastat, an oral matrix metalloproteinase inhibitor, in patients with advanced ovarian cancer. *Ann Oncol* 1996; **7**(Suppl 5): 68.
69. Wang X, Fu X, Brown PD et al, Matrix metalloproteinase inhibitor BB-94 (batimastat) inhibits human colon tumor growth and spread in a patient-like orthotopic model in nude mice. *Cancer Res* 1994; **54**: 4726–8.
70. Davies B, Waxman J, Wasan H et al, Levels of matrix metalloproteinases in bladder cancer correlate with tumor grade and invasion. *Cancer Res* 1993; **53**: 5365–9.
71. Glaves D, Correlation between circulating cancer cells and incidence of metastases. *Br J Cancer* 1983; **48**: 665–73.
72. Weiss L, Biomechanical interactions of cancer cells with the microvasculature during hematogenous metastasis. *Cancer Metastasis Rev* 1992; **11**: 227–35.
73. Karpatkin S, Pearlstein E, Ambrogio C, Coller BS, Role of adhesive proteins in platelet tumor interaction in vitro and metastasis formation in vivo. *J Clin Invest* 1988; **81**: 1012–19.
74. Fidler IJ, Macrophages and metastasis: a biological approach to cancer therapy: presidential address. *Cancer Res* 1985; **45**: 4714–26.
75. Hanna N, Fidler IJ, The role of natural killer cells in the destruction of circulating tumor emboli. *J Natl Cancer Inst* 1980; **65**: 801–9.
76. Li L, Kilbourn RG, Adams J, Fidler IJ, Role of nitric oxide in lysis of tumor cells by cyto-activated endothelial cells. *Cancer Res* 1991; **51**: 2531–5.
77. Zhu DZ, Cheng CF, Pauli BU, Mediation of lung metastasis of murine melanomas by a lung-

specific endothelial cell adhesion molecule. *Proc Natl Acad Sci USA* 1991; **88**: 9568–72.

78. Hynes RO, Integrins: versatility, modulation, and signaling in cell adhesion. *Cell* 1992; **69**: 11–25.
79. Brooks PC, Clark RAF, Cheresh DA, Requirement of vascular integrin avb3 for angiogenesis. *Science* 1994; **264**: 569–71.
80. Smythe WR, LeBel E, Bavaria JE et al, Integrin expression non-small cell carcinoma of the lung. *Cancer Metastasis Rev* 1995; **14**: 229–39.
81. Feldman LE, Shin KC, Natale RB, Todd RF et al, b1 integrin expression on human small cell lung cancers. *Cancer Res* 1991; **51**: 1065–70.
82. Chen FA, Repasky EA, Bankert RB, Human lung tumor associated antigen identified as an extracellular matrix adhesion molecule. *J Exp Med* 1991; **173**: 1111–19.
83. Clarke MR, Landreneau RJ, Finkelstein SD et al, Extracellaular matrix expression in metastasizing and nonmetastasizing adenocarcinomas of the lung. *Hum Pathol* 1997; **28**: 54–9.
84. Adachi M, Taki T, HUang C et al, Reduced integrin alpha 3 expression as a factor of poor prognosis of patients with adenocarcinoma of the lung. *J Clin Oncol* 1998; **16**: 1060–7.
85. Hirasawa M, Shijubo N, Uede T, Abe S, Integrin expression and ability to adhere to extracellular matrix proteins and endothelial cells in human cancer cell lines. *Br J Cancer* 1994; **70**: 466–73.
86. Blaschuk OW, Sullivan R, David S, Pouliot T, Identification of a cadherin cell adhesion recognition sequence. *Dev Biol* 1990; **139**: 227–9.
87. Schipper JH, Frixen UH, Behrens J et al, E-cadherin expression in squamous cell carcinoma of head and neck: inverse correlation with tumor dedifferentiation and lymph node metastasis. *Cancer Res* 1991; **51**: 6328–37.
88. Sulzer MA, Leers MP, van Noord JA et al, Reduced E-cadherin expression is associated with increased lymph node metastasis and unfavorable prognosis in non-small cell lung cancer. *Am J Respir Crit Care Med* 1998; **157**: 1319–23.
89. Johnson JP, Cell adhesion molecules of the immunoglobulin supergene family and their role in malignant transformation and progression to metastatic disease. *Cancer Metastasis Rev* 1991; **10**: 11–22.
90. Vangsted A, Drivsholm L, Andersen E, Bock E, New serum markers for small cell lung cancer. The neural cell adhesion molecule, NCAM. *Cancer Detect Prev* 1994; **18**: 291–8.
91. Michalides R, Kwa B, Springall D et al, NCAM and lung cancer. *Int J Cancer Suppl* 1994; **8**: 34–7.
92. Benchimol S, Juks A, Jothy S et al, Carcinoembryonic antigen, a human tumor marker, functions as an intercellular adhesion molecule. *Cell* 1989; **57**: 327–34.
93. Naor D, Sionov RV, Ish-Shalom D, CD44: structure, function and association with the malignant process. *Adv Cancer Res* 1997; **71**: 241–319.
94. Screaton GR, Bell MV, Jackson DG et al, Genomic structure of DNA encoding the lymphocyte homing receptor CD44 reveals at least 12 alternatively spliced exons. *Proc Natl Acad Sci USA* 1992; **89**: 12160–4.
95. Sasaki JI, Tanabe KK, Takahashi K et al, Expression of CD44 splicing isoforms in lung cancers: dominant expression of CD44v8–10 in non-small cell lung carcinomas. *Int J Oncol* 1998; **12**: 525–33.
96. Kogerman P, Sy MS, Culp LA, Overexpressed human CD44s promotes lung colonization during micrometastasis of murine fibrosarcoma cells: facilitated retention in the lung vasculature. *Proc Natl Acad Sci USA* 1997; **94**: 13233–8.
97. Folkman J, Tumor angiogenesis: a possible control point in tumor growth. *Ann Intern Med* 1995; **82**: 96–100.
98. Holmgren L, O'Reilly MS, Folkman J, Dormancy of micrometastasis: balanced proliferation and apoptosis in the presence of angiogenesis suppression. *Nature Med* 1995; **1**: 149–53.
99. Ferrara N, Davis-Smyth T, The biology of vascular endothelial growth factor. *Endocrine Rev* 1997; **18**: 4–25.
100. Imoto H, Osaki T, Taga S et al, Vascular endothelial growth factor expression in non-small cell lung cancer: prognostic significance in squamous cell carcinoma. *J Thorac Cardiovasc Surg* 1998; **115**: 1007–14.

101. Takahama M, Tsutsumi M, Tsujiuchi T et al, Frequent expression of the vascular endothelial growth factor in human non-small cell lung cancers. *Jpn J Clin Oncol* 1998; **28**: 176–81.
102. Takanami I, Tanaka F, Hashizume T, Kodaira S, Vascular endothelial growth factor and its receptor correlate with angiogenesis and survival in pulmonary adenocarcinoma. *Anticancer Res* 1997; **17**: 2811–14.
103. Talbot DC, Brown PD, Experimental and clinical studies on the use of matrix metalloproteinase inhibitors for the treatment of cancer. *Eur J Cancer* 1996; **32A**: 2528–33.
104. Sledge GW, Qulali M, Goulet R et al, Effect of matrix metalloproteinase inhibitor batimastat on breast cancer growth and metastasis in athymic mice. *J Natl Cancer Int* 1995; **87**: 1546–50.
105. Rasmussen H, McCann P, Matrix metalloproteinase inhibition as a novel anticancer strategy: a review with special focus on batimastat and marimastat. *Pharmacol Ther* 1997; **75**: 69–75.
106. Gehlsen KR, Argaves WS, Pierschbaccher MD, Rouslahti E, Inhibition of in vitro tumor cell invasion by Arg-Gly-Asp-containing synthetic peptides. *J Cell Biol* 1988; **106**: 925–30.
107. Saiki I, Yoneda J, Igarashi Y et al, Antimetastatic activity of polymeric RGDT peptides conjugated with poly(ethylene glycol). *Jpn J Cancer Res* 1993; **84**: 558–65.
108. Arap W, Pasqualini R, Rouslahti E, Cancer treatment by targeted drug delivery to tumor vasculature in a mouse model. *Science* 1998; **279**: 377–80.
109. Greenspoon N, Hershkoviz R, Alon R et al, Structural analysis of integrin recognition and the inhibition of integrin-mediated cell functions by novel nonpeptidic surrogates of the Arg-Gly-Asp sequence. *Biochemistry* 1993; **32**: 1001–8.
110. Sakamoto N, Iwahana M, Tanaka N, Osada Y, Inhibition of angiogenesis and tumor growth by a synthetic laminin peptide, CDPGYIGSR-NH_2. *Cancer Res* 1991; **51**: 903–6.
111. Kim KJ, Li B, Winer J et al, Inhibition of vascular endothelial growth factor-induced angiogenesis suppresses tumor growth in vivo. *Nature* 1993; **362**: 841–4.
112. O'Reilly MS, Holmgren L, Chen C, Folkman J, Angiostatin induces and sustains tumor dormancy of human primary tumors in mice. *Nature Med* 1996; **2**: 689–92.
113. Boehm T, Folkman J, Browder T, O'Reilly MS, Antiangiogenic therapy of experimental cancer does not induce acquired drug resistance. *Nature* 1997; **390**: 404–7.
114. Hanahan D, A flanking attack on cancer. *Nature Med* 1998; **4**: 13–14.
115. Nambu Y, Hughes SJ, Rehemtulla A et al, Lack of cell surface Fas/APO-1 expression in pulmonary adenocarcinomas. *J Clin Invest* 1998; **101**: 1102–10.
116. Stahel RA, Antigens, receptors and dominant oncogenes and the prognosis of non-small cell lung cancer. *Lung Cancer* 1994; **11**(Suppl 3): S31–8.
117. Martin-Satue M, Marrugat R, Cancelas JA, Blanco J, Enhanced expression of $\alpha(1,3)$-fucosyltransferase genes correlates with E-selectin-mediated adhesion and metastatic potential of human lung adenocarcinoma. *Cancer Res* 1998; **58**: 1544–50.
118. Fuentes R, Allman R, Mason MD, Ganglioside expression in lung cancer cell lines. *Lung Cancer* 1997; **18**: 21–33.
119. Leys K, Lang B, Johnston I et al, Calcium channel autoantibodies in the Eaton–Lambert myasthenic syndrome: a review of 50 cases. *Ann Neurol* 1991; **29**: 307–12.
120. Dalmau J, Graus F, Rosenblum MK, Posner JB, Anti-Hu associated encephalomyelitis/sensory neuronopathy. A clinical study of 71 patients. *Medicine* 1992; **71**: 59–72.
121. Funa K, Gazdar AF, Minna JD, Linnoila RI, Paucity of beta 2 microglobulin expression on small cell lung cancer, bronchial carcinoids and certain other NE tumors. *Lab Invest* 1986; **55**: 186–93.
122. Passlick B, Pantel K, Kubuschok B et al, Expression of MHC molecules and ICAM-1 on non-small cell lung carcinomas: association with early lymphatic spread of tumour cells. *Eur J Cancer* 1996; **32A**: 141–5.
123. Yamo T, Fukuyam Y, Yokoyama H et al, HLA class I and class II expression of pulmonary

adenocarcinoma cells and the influence of interferon gamma. *Lung Cancer* 1998; **20**: 185–90.

124. Singal DP, Ye M, Bienzle D, Transfection of TAP 1 gene restores HLA class I expression in human small-cell lung carcinoma. *Int J Cancer* 1998; **75**: 112–16.

125. Shimosato Y, Sobin LH, Spencer H et al, The World Health Organization histological typing of lung tumors, second edition. *Am J Clin Pathol* 1982; **77**: 1123–36.

126. Saccomanno G, Archer VE, Auerbach O et al, Development of carcinoma of the lung as reflected in exfoliative cells. *Cancer* 1974; **33**: 256–70.

127. De Vries J, ten Kate J, Bosman F, p21ras in carcinogenesis. *Pathol Res Pract* 1996; **192**: 658–68.

128. Mitsudomi T, Viallet J, Mulshine JL et al, Mutations of ras gene distinguished a subset of non-small cell lung cancer cell lines from small cell lung cancer cell lines. *Oncogene* 1991; **6**: 1353–62.

129. Bos J, Ras oncogene in human cancer: a review. *Cancer Res* 1989; **49**: 4682–9.

130. Rodenhuis S, Slebos RJC, Boot AJM et al, Incidence and possible significance of K-ras oncogene activation in adenocarcinoma of the human lung. *Cancer Res* 1988; **48**: 5738–41.

131. Kwiatkowski DJ, Harpole DH, Godleski J et al, Molecular pathologic substaging in 244 stage I non-small cell lung cancer patients: clinical implications. *J Clin Oncol* 1998; **16**: 2468–77.

132. Slebos RJ, Kibbelaar RE, Dalesio O et al, K-ras oncogene activation as a prognostic marker in adenocarcinoma of the lung. *N Engl J Med* 1990; **323**: 561–5.

133. Mitsudomi T, Steinberg SM, Oie HK et al, Ras gene mutations in non-small cell lung cancers associated with shortened survival irrespective of treatment intent. *Cancer Res* 1991; **51**: 4999–5002.

134. Sugio K, Ishida T, Yokoyama T et al, Ras gene mutations as a prognostic marker in adenocarcinoma of the human lung without lymph node metastasis. *Cancer Res* 1992; **52**: 2903–6.

135. Cho JY, Kim JH, Lee YH et al, Correlation between K-ras gene mutation and prognosis of patients with non-small cell lung cancer. *Cancer* 1997; **79**: 462–7.

136. Keohavong P, DeMichele MA, Melacrinos AC et al, Detection of K-ras mutations in lung carcinomas: relationship to prognosis. *Clin Cancer Res* 1996; **2**: 411–18.

137. Harada M, Dosaka-Akita H, Miyamoto H et al, Prognostic significance of the expression of ras oncogene product in non-small cell lung cancer. *Cancer* 1992; **69**: 72–7.

138. Sklar MD, The ras oncogenes increase the intrinsic resistance of NIH 3T3 cells to ionizing radiation. *Science* 1988; **239**: 645–7.

139. Sklar MD, Increased resistance to *cis*-diamminedichloroplatinum(II) in NIH 3T3 cells transformed by ras oncogenes. *Cancer Res* 1988; **48**: 793–7.

140. Rodenhuis S, Boerrigter L, Top B et al, Mutational activation of the K-ras oncogene and the effect of chemotherapy in advanced adenocarcinoma of the lung: a prospective study. *J Clin Oncol* 1997; **15**: 285–91.

141. Fukuyama Y, Mitsudomi T, Sugio K et al, K-ras and p53 mutations are an independent unfavorable prognostic indicator in patients with non-small cell lung cancer. *Br J Cancer* 1997; **75**: 1125–30.

142. Sugio K, Kishimoto Y, Virmani AK et al, K-ras mutations are a relatively late event in the pathogenesis of lung carcinomas. *Cancer Res* 1994; **54**: 5811–15.

143. Neckers L, Whitesell L, Rosolen A et al, Antisense inhibition of oncogene expression. *Crit Rev Oncol* 1992; **3**: 175–231.

144. Mukhopadhyay T, Tansky M, Cavender A et al, Specific inhibition of K-ras expression and tumorigenicity of lung cancer cells by antisense RNA. *Cancer Res* 1991; **51**: 1744–8.

145. Georges RN, Mukhopadhyay T, Zhang Y et al, Prevention of orthotopic human lung cancer growth by intratracheal instillation of a retrovirus antisense K-ras construct. *Cancer Res* 1993; **53**: 1743–6.

146. Symons RH, Ribozymes. *Curr Opin Struct Biol* 1994; **4**: 322–30.
147. Tone T, Kashani-Sabet M, Funato T et al, Suppression of EJ cells tumorigenicity. *In Vivo* 1993; **7**: 471–6.
148. Feng M, Cabrera G, Deshane J et al, Neoplastic reversion accomplished by high efficiency adenoviral mediated delivery of anti-ras ribozymes. *Cancer Res* 1995; **55**: 2024–8.
149. Eastham JA, Ahlering TE, Use of an anti-ras ribozyme to alter the malignant phenotype of a human bladder cancer cell line. *J Urol* 1996; **156**: 1186–8.
150. Alberts AW, Discovery, biochemistry and biology of lovastatin. *Am J Cardiol* 1988; **62**: 10J–15J.
151. DeClue JE, Vass WC, Papageorge AG et al, Inhibition of cell growth by lovastatin is independent of Ras function. *Cancer Res* 1991; **51**: 712–17.
152. Gibbs JB, Kohl NE, Koblan KS et al, Farnesyltransferase inhibitors and anti-Ras therapy. *Breast Cancer Res Treat* 1996; **38**: 75–83.
153. Gibbs JB, Oliff A, Kohl NE, Farnesylation inhibitors: ras research yields a potential cancer therapeutic. *Cell* 1994; **77**: 175–8.
154. Eisenman RN, Myc, Max and Mad: a regulatory network. *Adv Oncol* 1994; **10**: 3–6.
155. Giaccone G, Oncogenes and antioncogenes in lung tumorigenesis. *Chest* 1996; **109**: 130S–4S.
156. Johnson BE, Brennan JF, Ihde DC et al, Myc family DNA amplification in tumors and tumor cell lines from patients with small cell lung cancer. *J Natl Cancer Inst Monogr* 1992; **13**: 39–43.
157. Johnson B, Ihde D, Makuch R et al, Myc family oncogene amplification in tumor cell lines established from small cell lung cancer patients and its relationship to clinical status and course. *J Clin Invest* 1987; **79**: 1629–34.
158. Brennan J, O'Connor T, Makuch KW et al, Myc family DNA amplification of 107 tumors and tumor cell lines from patients with small cell lung cancer treated with different combination chemotherapy regimens. *Cancer Res* 1991; **51**: 1708–12.
159. Slebos R, Evers S, Wagenaar S et al, Cellular protooncogenes are infrequently amplified in untreated non-small cell lung cancer. *Br J Cancer* 1989; **59**: 76–80.
160. Cooney M, Czernuszewicz G, Postel EH et al, Site-specific oligonucleotides binding represses transcription of the human c-myc gene in vitro. *Science* 1988; **241**: 456–9.
161. Helm CW, Shrestha K, Thomas S et al, A unique c-myc targeted triplex-forming oligonucleotide inhibits the growth of ovarian and cervical carcinomas in vitro. *Gynecol Oncol* 1993; **49**: 339–43.
162. McManaway ME, Neckers LM, Loke SL et al, Tumor-specific inhibition of lymphoma growth by an anti-sense oligonucleotide. *Lancet* 1990; **335**: 808–11.
163. Robinson LA, Smith LJ, Fontaine MP et al, c-myc antisense oligonucleotides inhibit proliferation of non-small cell lung cancer. *Ann Thorac Surg* 1995; **60**: 1583–91.
164. Citro G, D'Agnano I, Leonetti C et al, c-myc antisense oligodeoxynucleotides enhance the efficacy of cisplatin in melanoma chemotherapy in vitro and in nude mice. *Cancer Res* 1998; **58**: 283–9.
165. Farrow S, Brown R, New members of the bcl-2 family and their protein partners. *Curr Opin Genet Dev* 1996; **6**: 45–9.
166. Miyashita T, Reed J, Tumor suppressor p53 is a direct transcriptional activator of the human bax gene. *Cell* 1995; **80**: 293–9.
167. Lotem J, Sachs L, Regulation by bcl-2, c-myc, and p53 susceptibility to induction of apoptosis by heat shock and cancer chemotherapy compounds in differentiation-competent and defective myeloid leukemia cells. *Cell Growth Diff* 1993; **4**: 41–7.
168. Karakas T, Maurer U, Weidmann E et al, High expression of bcl-2 mRNA as a determinant of poor prognosis in acute myeloid leukemia. *Ann Oncol* 1998; **9**: 159–65.
169. Eliopoulos AG, Kerr DJ, Herod J et al, The control of apoptosis and drug resistance in ovarian cancer: influence of p53 and Bcl-2. *Oncogene* 1995; **11**: 1217–28.
170. Takayama K, Ogata K, Nakanishi Y et al, Bcl-2 expression as a predictor of chemosensivities and

survival in small cell lung cancer. *Cancer J Sci Am* 1996; **2**: 213–16.

171. Pezzella F, Turley H, Kuzu I et al, Bcl-2 protein in non-small cell lung carcinoma. *N Engl J Med* 1993; **329**: 690–4.

172. Fontanini G, Vignati S, Bigini D et al, Bcl-2 protein: a prognostic factor inversely correlated to p53. *Br J Cancer* 1995; **71**: 1003–7.

173. Ohsaki Y, Toyoshima E, Fujiuchi S et al, bcl-2 and p53 protein expression in non-small cell lung cancers: correlation with survival time. *Clin Cancer Res* 1996; **2**: 915–20.

174. Walker C, Robertson L, Myskow M et al, Expression of the Bcl-2 protein in normal and dysplastic bronchial epithelium and in lung carcinomas. *Br J Cancer* 1995; **72**: 164–9.

175. Reed J, Kitada S, Takayama S et al, Regulation of chemoresistance by the bcl-2 oncoprotein in non-Hodgkin's lymphoma and lymphocytic leukemia cell lines. *Ann Oncol* 1994; **5**(Suppl 1): 61–5.

176. Ziegler A, Luedke GH, Fabbro D et al, Induction of apoptosis in small-cell lung cancer cells by an antisense oligodeoxynucleotide targeting the Bcl-2 coding sequence. *J Natl Cancer Inst* 1997; **89**: 1027–36.

177. Bunn PA Jr, The biology of lung cancer. In: *Lung Cancer: Frontiers in Science and Treatment* (Motta G, ed). Grafica LP: Italy, 1994: 49–56.

178. Volm M, Efferth T, Mattern J, Oncoprotein (c-myc, c-erbB1, c-erbB2, c-fos) and suppressor gene products (p53) expression in squamous cell carcinomas of the lung. Clinical and biological correlations. *Anticancer Res* 1992; **12**: 11–20.

179. Scagliotti GV, Leonardo E, Cappia S et al, Epidermal growth factor receptor and neu oncogene expression in lung cancer. *Proc Am Soc Clin Oncol* 1993; **12**: 328.

180. Sozzi G, Miozzo M, Tagliabue E et al, Cytogenic abnormalities and overexpression of receptors for growth factors in normal bronchial epithelium and tumor samples of lung cancer patients. *Cancer Res* 1991; **51**: 5811–15.

181. Rusch V, Klimstra D, Linkov I et al, Aberrant expression of p53 or the epidermal growth factor receptor is frequent in early bronchial neoplasia, and coexpression precedes squamous cell carcinoma development. *Cancer Res* 1995; **55**: 1365–72.

182. Ochiai A, Akimoto S, Kanai Y et al, c-erbB-2 gene product associates with catenins in human cancer cells. *Biochem Biophys Res Commun* 1994; **205**: 73–8.

183. Petit AM, Rak J, Hung MC et al, Neutralizing antibodies against epidermal growth factor and ErbB-2/neu receptor tyrosine kinases down-regulate vascular endothelial growth factor production by tumor cells in vitro and in vivo: angiogenic implications for signal transduction therapy of solid tumors. *Am J Pathol* 1997; **151**: 1523–30.

184. Kern JA, Schwartz DA, Nordberg JE et al, p185neu expression in human lung adenocarcinomas predicts shortened survival. *Cancer Res* 1990; **50**: 5184–7.

185. Tateishi M, Ishida T, Mitsudomi T et al, Prognostic value of c-erbB2 protein expression in human lung adenocarcinoma and squamous cell carcinoma. *Eur J Cancer* 1991; **27**: 1372–5.

186. Tsai CM, Chang KT, Wu LH et al, Correlations between intrinsic chemoresistance and HER-2/neu gene expression, p53 gene mutations, and cell proliferation characteristics in non-small cell lung cancer cell lines. *Cancer Res* 1996; **56**: 206–9.

187. Kern J, Slebos R, Toop B et al, c-erbB-2 expression and codon 12 K-ras mutations both predict shortened survival for patients with pulmonary adenocarcinomas. *J Clin Invest* 1994; **93**: 516–20.

188. Harpole DH, Herndon JE, Wolfe WG et al, A prognostic model of recurrence and death in stage I non-small cell lung cancer utilizing presentation, histopathology and oncoprotein expression. *Cancer Res* 1995; **55**: 51–6.

189. Sellers WR, Kaelin WG, Role of the retinoblastoma protein in the pathogenesis of human cancer. *J Clin Oncol* 1997; **15**: 3301–12.

190. Kaelin W, Ewen M, Livingstone D, Definition of the minimal simian virus 40 large t antigen- and adenovirus E1A-binding domain in the

retinoblastoma gene product. *Mol Cell Biol* 1990; **10**: 3761–9.

191. HU Q, Dyson N, Harlow E, The regions of the retinoblastoma protein needed for binding to adenovirus or SV40 large T antigen are common sites for mutations. *EMBO J* 1990; **9**: 1147–55.
192. Huang S, Wang N, Tseng B et al, Two distinct and frequently mutated regions of retinoblastoma protein are required for binding to SV40 T antigen. *EMBO J* 1990; **9**: 1815–22.
193. Shimizu E, Coxon A, Otterson G et al, RB protein status and clinical correlation from 171 cell lines representing lung cancer, extrapulmonary small cell carcinoma and mesothelioma. *Oncogene* 1994; **9**: 2441–8.
194. Reissmann PT, Koga H, Takahashi R et al, Inactivation of the retinoblastoma susceptibility gene in non-small cell lung cancer. The Lung Cancer Study Group. *Oncogene* 1993; **8**: 1913–19.
195. Higashiyama M, Doi O, Kodama K et al, Retinoblastoma protein expression in lung cancer: an immunohistochemical analysis. *Oncology* 1994; **51**: 544–51.
196. Xu H, Cagle P, Hu S et al, Altered retinoblastoma (RB) and p53 protein status as a synergistic prognostic factor in non-small cell lung carcinoma. *Proc Am Assoc Cancer Res* 1995; **36**: 246.
197. Dosaka-Akita H, Hu SX, Fujino M et al, Altered retinoblastoma protein expression in non small cell lung cancer. *Cancer* 1997; **79**: 1329–37.
198. deVos S, Miller CW, Takeuchi S et al, Alterations of CDKN2 (p16) in non-small cell lung cancer. *Genes Chromosome Cancer* 1995; **14**: 164–70.
199. Shapiro GI, Edwards CD, Kobzik L et al, Reciprocal Rb inactivation and p16INK4 expression in primary lung cancers and cell lines. *Cancer Res* 1995; **55**: 505–9.
200. Serrano M, Hannon GJ, Beach D, A new regulatory motif in cell-cycle control causing specific inhibition of cyclin D/CDK4. *Nature* 1993; **166**: 704–7.
201. Taga S, Osaki T, Ohgami A et al, Prognostic value of the immunohistochemical detection of p16INK4 expression in non small cell lung carcinoma. *Cancer* 1997; **80**: 389–95.
202. Nakagawa K, Conrad NK, Williams JP et al, Mechanism of inactivation of CDKN2 and MTS2 in non-small cell lung cancer and association with advanced stage. *Oncogene* 1995; **11**: 1843–51.
203. Kinoshita I, Dosaka-Akita H, Mishina T et al, Altered p16INK4 and retinoblastoma protein status in non-small cell lung cancer: potential synergistic effect with altered p53 protein on proliferative activity. *Cancer Res* 1996; **56**: 5557–62.
204. Betticher DC, Heighway J, Thatcher N et al, Abnormal expression of CCND1 and Rb1 in resection margin epithelia of lung cancer patients. *Br J Cancer* 1997; **75**: 1761–8.
205. Ferron PE, Bagni I, Guidoboni M et al, Combined and sequential expression of p53, Rb, Ras and Bcl-2 in bronchial preneoplastic lesions. *Tumori* 1997; **83**: 587–93.
206. Merlo A, Gabrielson E, Askin F et al, Frequent loss of chromosome 9 in human primary non-small cell lung cancer. *Cancer Res* 1994; **54**: 640–2.
207. Thiberville L, Payne P, Vielkinds J et al, Evidence of cumulative gene losses with progression of premalignant epithelial lesions to carcinoma of the bronchus. *Cancer Res* 1995; **55**: 5133–9.
208. Kishimoto Y, Sugio K, Hung J et al, Allele-specific loss in chromosome 9p loci in preneoplastic lesions accompanying non small cell lung cancers. *J Natl Cancer Inst* 1995; **87**: 1224–9.
209. Mao L, Lee JS, Kurie JM et al, Clonal genetic alterations in the lungs of current and former smokers. *J Natl Cancer Inst* 1997; **89**: 857–62.
210. Ookawa K, Shiseki M, Takahashi R et al, Reconstitution of the Rb gene suppresses the growth of small cell lung carcinoma cells carrying multiple genetic alterations. *Oncogene* 1993; **8**: 2175–82.
211. Jiu X, Nguyen D, Zhang WW et al, Cell cycle arrest and inhibition of tumor cell proliferation

by the p16INK4 gene mediated by an adenovirus vector. *Cancer Res* 1995; **55**: 3250–3.

212. el-Deiry W, Tokino T, Velculescu V et al, WAF1, a potential mediator of p53 tumor suppression. *Cell* 1993; **75**: 817–25.
213. Marchette A, Doglioni C, Barbareschi M et al, p21 RNA and protein expression in non-small cell lung carcinomas: evidence of p53 independent expression and association with tumoral differentiation. *Oncogene* 1996; **12**: 1319–24.
214. Carbone D, The biology of the lung cancer. *Semin Oncol* 1997; **24**: 388–401.
215. Volm M, Mattern J, Immunohistochemical detection of p53 in non-small cell lung cancer. *J Natl Cancer Inst* 1994; **86**: 1249.
216. Sidransky D, Hollstein M, Clinical implications of the p53 gene. *Annu Rev Med* 1996; **47**: 285–301.
217. Chiba I, Takahashi T, Nau MM et al, Mutations in the p53 gene are frequent in primary, resected non-small cell lung cancer. *Oncogene* 1990; **5**: 1603–10.
218. Mitsudomi T, Oyama T, Kusano T et al, Mutation of the p53 gene as a predictor of poor prognosis in patients with non-small cell lung cancer. *J Natl Cancer Inst* 1993; **85**: 2018–23.
219. Horio Y, Takahashi T, Kurosishi T et al, Prognostic significance of p53 mutations and 3p deletions in primary resected non-small cell lung cancer. *Cancer Res* 1993; **53**: 1–4.
220. Carbone DP, Mitsudomi T, Chiba I et al, p53 immunostaining positivity is associated with reduced survival and is imperfectly correlated with gene mutations in resected non-small cell lung cancer. *Chest* 1994; **106**: 377S 81S.
221. Quinlan DC, Davidson AG, Summers CK et al, Accumulation of p53 correlates with a poor prognosis in human lung cancer. *Cancer Res* 1992; **52**: 4828–31.
222. Ebina M, Steinberg SM, Mulshine JL et al, Relationship of p53 expression and upregulation of proliferating cell nuclear antigen with the clinical course of non-small cell lung cancer. *Cancer Res* 1994; **54**: 2496–503.
223. Dalquen P, Sauter G, Tohorst J et al, Nuclear p53 overexpression is an independent prognostic parameter in node-negative non-small cell lung carcinoma. *J Pathol* 1996; **178**: 53–8.
224. Fujino M, Dosaka-Akita H, Harada M et al, Prognostic significance of p53 and ras p21 expression in non-small cell lung cancer. *Cancer* 1995; **76**: 2457–63.
225. Passlick B, Izbicki JR, Haussinger K et al, Immunohistochemical detection of p53 protein is not associated with a poor prognosis in non-small cell lung cancer. *J Thorac Cardiovasc Surg* 1995; **109**: 1205–11.
226. Lee JS, Yoon A, Kalapurakal SK et al, Expression of p53 oncoprotein in non-small cell lung cancer: a favorable prognostic factor. *J Clin Oncol* 1995; **13**: 1893–903.
227. McLaren R, Kuzu I, Dunnill M et al, The relationship of p53 immunistaining to survival in carcinoma of the lung. *Br J Cancer* 1992; **66**: 735–8.
228. Top B, Mooi WJ, Klaver SG et al, Comparative analysis of p53 gene mutations and protein accumulation in human non-small cell lung cancer. *Int J Cancer* 1995; **64**: 83–91.
229. Kawasaki M, Nakanishi Y, Yatsunami J et al, p53 immunostaining predicts chemosensitivity in non-small cell lung cancer: a preliminary report. *Cancer J Sci Am* 1996; **2**: 217–20.
230. Chin KV, Ueda K, Pastan I et al, Modulation of activity of the promoter of the human MDR1 gene by Ras and p53. *Science* 1992; **2**: 459–62.
231. Langendijk JA, Thunnissen FB, Lamers RJ et al, The prognostic significance of accumulation of p53 protein in stage III non-small cell lung cancer treated by radiotherapy. *Radiother Oncol* 1995; **36**: 218–24.
232. Nuorva K, Soini Y, Kamel D et al, Concurrent p53 expression in bronchial dysplasias and squamous cell lung carcinoma. *Am J Pathol* 1993; **142**: 725–32.
233. Bennett WP, Colby TV, Travis WD et al, p53 protein accumulates frequently in early bronchial neoplasia. *Cancer Res* 1993; **53**: 4817–22.
234. Vahakangas KH, Samet JM, Metcalf RA et al,

Mutations of p53 and ras gene in radon-associated lung cancer from uranium miners. *Lancet* 1992; **339**: 576–80.

235. Sozzi G, Miozzo M, Donghi R et al, Deletions of 17p and p53 mutations in preneoplastic lesions of the lung. *Cancer Res* 1992; **52**: 6079–82.
236. Dolcetti R, Doglioni C, Maestro R et al, p53 overexpression is an early event in the development of human squamous cell carcinoma of the larynx: genetic and prognostic implications. *Int J Cancer* 1992; **52**: 178–82.
237. Bennett WP, Hollstein MC, Metcalf RA et al, p53 mutation and protein accumulation during multistage human esophageal carcinogenesis. *Cancer Res* 1992; **52**: 6092–7.
238. Sundaresan V, Ganly P, Hasleton P et al, p53 and chromosome 3 abnormalities, characteristic of malignant lung tumors, are detectable in preinvasive lesions of the bronchis. *Oncogene* 1992; **7**: 1989–97.
239. Chung G, Sundaresan V, Hasleton P et al, Sequential molecular genetic changes in lung cancer development. *Oncogene* 1995; **11**: 2591–8.
240. Cai D, Mukhopadhyay T, Liu Y et al, Stable expression of the wild-type p53 gene in human lung cancer cells after retrovirus-mediated gene transfer. *Hum Gene Ther* 1993; **4**: 617–24.
241. Lowe S, Bodis S, McClatchey A et al, p53 status and the efficacy of cancer therapy in vivo. *Science* 1994; **266**: 807–10.
242. Roth JA, Nguyen D, Lawrence DD et al, Retrovirus-mediated wild-type p53 gene transfer to tumors of patients with lung cancer. *Nature Med* 1996; **2**: 985–91.
243. Roth JA, Swisher SG, Merritt JA et al, Gene therapy for non-small cell lung cancer: a preliminary report of a phase I trials of adenoviral p53 gene replacement. *Semin Oncol* 1998; **25**(Suppl 8): 33–7.
244. Higashiyama M, Doi O, Kodama K et al, MDM2 gene amplification and expression in non-small cell lung cancer: immunohistochemical expression of its protein is a favourable prognostic marker in patients without p53 protein accumulation. *Br J Cancer* 1997; **75**: 1302–8.
245. Whang-Peng J, Kao SC, Lee EC et al, A specific chromosome defect associated with human small cell lung cancer. *Science* 1982; **215**: 181–5.
246. Otterson G, Lin A, Kaye F, Genetic etiology of lung cancer. *Oncology* 1992; **6**: 97–112.
247. Hibi K, Takahashi T, Yamakawa K et al, Three distinct regions involved in 3p deletion in human lung cancer. *Oncogene* 1992; **7**: 445–9.
248. Linehan WM, Lerman MI, Zbar B, Identification of the von Hippel–Landau (VHL) gene. Its role in renal cancer. *JAMA* 1995; **273**: 564–70.
249. Sozzi G, Veronese M, Negrini M et al, The FHIT gene at 3p14.2 is abnormal in lung cancer. *Cell* 1996; **85**: 17–26.
250. Yokoyama S, Yamakawa K, Tsuchiya E et al, Deletion mapping on the short arm of chromosome 3 in squamous cell carcinoma and adenocarcinoma of the lung. *Cancer Res* 1992; **52**: 873–7.
251. Mitsudomi T, Oyama T, Nishida K et al, Loss of heterozygosity at 3p in non-small cell lung cancer and its prognostic implication. *Clin Cancer Res* 1996; **2**: 1185–9.
252. Otterson GA, Xiao GH, Geradts J et al, Protein expression and functional analysis of the FHIT gene in human tumor cells. *J Natl Cancer Inst* 1998; **90**: 426–32.
253. Sundaresan V, Heppell-Patron A, Coleman N et al, Somatic genetic changes in lung cancer and precancerous lesions. *Ann Oncol* 1995; **6**(Suppl 1): 27–31.
254. Mao L, Lee JS, Fan YH et al, Frequent microsatellite alterations at chromosomes 9p21 and 3p14 in oral premalignant lesions and their value in cancer risk assessment. *Nature Med* 1996; **2**: 682–5.
255. Sozzi G, Sard L, De Gregorio L et al, Association between cigarette smoking and FHIT gene alterations in lung cancer. *Cancer Res* 1997; **57**: 2121–3.
256. Hung J, Kishimoto Y, Sugio K et al, Allele specific chromosome 3p deletions occur at an early stage in the pathogenesis of lung carcinomas. *JAMA* 1995; **273**: 558–63.
257. Wiest J, Franklin W, Otstot J et al, Identification of a novel region of homozygous deletion on chromosome 9p in squamous carcinoma of the lung: the location of a putative tumor suppressor gene. *Cancer Res* 1997; **57**: 1–6.

Prevention of lung cancer

Ugo Pastorino

Contents Introduction • Primary prevention • Pharmacological prevention • Randomized chemoprevention trials • Conclusions

INTRODUCTION

Lung cancer survival in the general population, calculated on all incident cases, ranges between 10% and 15%, with values as low as 6% in some European countries such as the United Kingdom. Despite optimal use of therapeutic resources, the overall improvement in survival during the last decade has been modest, and major reductions of mortality for this disease can only come from prevention, early detection and truly innovative treatments.

Lung cancer prevention covers different areas of experimental and clinical research:

- primary prevention, aimed at eliminating or reducing the environmental exposure to known carcinogens;
- early diagnosis and treatment of preneoplastic or preinvasive lesions;
- chemoprevention, aimed at inhibiting the process of carcinogenesis by the administration of drugs or other natural substances.

While there is no doubt that widespread control of tobacco consumption represents the most effective way of preventing lung cancer, selective pharmacological intervention could offer a useful support to primary prevention. In fact, with the success of tobacco-control policies, an expanding cohort of ex-smokers will remain at high risk of lung cancer for 15–20 years.[1] Therefore strategies aimed at reducing cancer mortality in individuals who have stopped smoking represent an undisputable priority. Experimental data have proved that chemoprevention of upper aerodigestive tract cancer is feasible in the laboratory,[2] but the evidence of a beneficial effect in humans is still limited and controversial, and the first generation of randomized trials ended up with no proof of efficacy – if not detrimental results. Better selection of high-risk individuals and identification of more effective preventive agents remain the most critical aspects of chemoprevention.

PRIMARY PREVENTION

Tobacco and lung cancer

The worldwide consequences of present tobacco smoking trends on mortality over the next two to three decades are alarming.[3,4] Overall mortality attributable to tobacco has already reached two million per year in developed countries and one million in developing countries, but worldwide figures are expected to double in the next 30 years, with a sevenfold increase in the developing countries (Figure 4.1).

Smokers have a much higher risk of developing various cancers[5] and chronic cardiovascular or pulmonary diseases (Table 4.1). One in two heavy smokers dies prematurely because of his

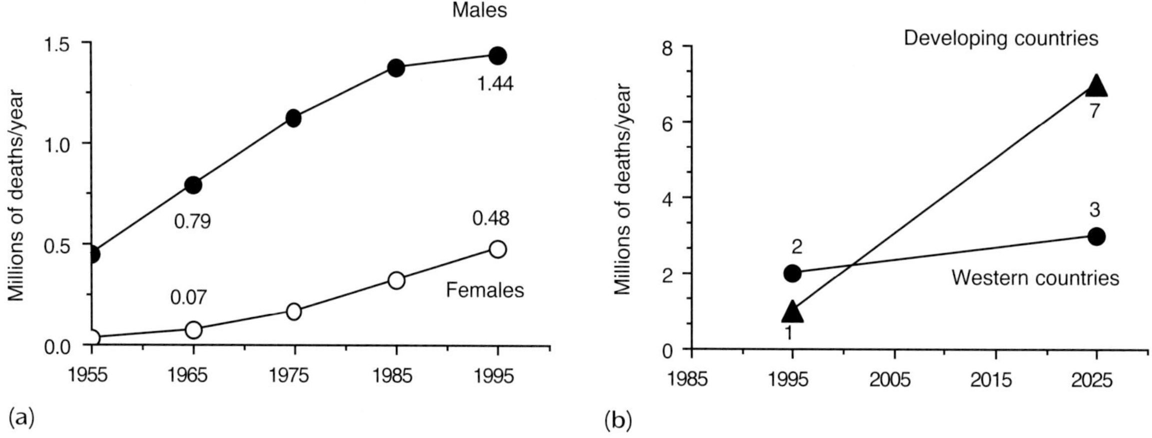

Figure 4.1
(a) Evolution of mortality for diseases attributable to tobacco smoking in developed countries by sex, and (b) comparison with expected mortality in developing countries over the next 30 years (estimates expressed in millions of deaths per year). (Modified with permission from Peto R, Smoking and death: the past 40 years and the next 40. BMJ 1994; **309**: 937–9.)

Table 4.1 Smoking and risk of death for common diseases: average annual mortality rate per 100 000 males between 35 and 69 years of age in the USA. Prospective study of the American Cancer Society, 1984–88[a]

Disease	Never-smokers	Chronic smokers	Relative risk of smokers
Neoplastic	122	412	× 3.4
Lung	8	196	× 24.5
Oral cavity, larynx, oesophagus	5	28	× 5.6
Other sites	109	188	× 1.7
Respiratory	9	62	× 6.9
Cardiovascular	176	446	× 2.5
Other	39	81	× 2.1
Total	382	1083	× 2.8

[a]Modified from US Department of Health and Human Services.[5]

habit, and the average shortening of life is 20–25 years. Approximately 90% of lung cancers and other malignancies arising in the upper aero-digestive tract are due to tobacco smoking (Table 4.2).[6] The relative risk of lung cancer in smokers of 20 or more cigarettes a day is 20–30 times

Table 4.2 Annual incidence and mortality for tumours related to tobacco smoking and percentage of cases attributable to smoking among the male population of the European Community (1978–82)[a]

	Incidence (cases/year)	Mortality (cases/year)	Percentage attributable to smoking
Lung	135 200	117 100	80–90
Larynx	24 600	11 000	80–90
Oral cavity	27 300	14 800	80–90
Oesophagus	11 900	13 500	80–90
Bladder	41 600	18 000	30–40
Kidney	16 300	8 400	30–40
Pancreas	16 100	15 800	20
Stomach	55 100	40 000	20
Leukaemia	16 600	12 600	20
Total	344 700	251 200	

[a] Modified from Jensen et al.[6]

higher, but declines constantly in those who quit, to reach the risk of never-smokers after 20–25 years from cessation.

In the USA and northern Europe, where the magnitude of the tobacco epidemic was first recognized and large-scale prevention programmes were adopted from the early 1970s, a significant reduction in tobacco consumption has already been achieved, with a concurrent decline in lung cancer mortality in males. The US National Cancer Institute estimated that approximately 800 000 tobacco-related deaths were either posponed or prevented by primary prevention measures, between 1964 and 1985.[7] In Scotland, mortality started to decline in males 20 years ago, although in females it is still on the rise; in southern European countries such as Italy, mortality rates are similar to those observed in England 30 years ago (Table 4.3).[8]

Recent studies have elucidated better the complex pharmacological interactions among the various components of tobacco, in particular between nicotine and carcinogens or promoters (Table 4.4). In addition to polycyclic aromatic hydrocarbons (PAHs) generated by combustion, substances such as nitrosamines have shown their carcinogenic effect in other forms of tobacco consumption (e.g. snuff) that are becoming more popular in the USA (over 10 million addicts). Knowledge of the essential role of nicotine in maintaining the smoking habit offers new tools for primary prevention. It has been demonstrated that the average smoker can absorb 1–3 mg of nicotine out of the 6–11 mg contained in one cigarette, but the level of 1 mg is crucial to maintain the addiction.[9] This evidence explains why tobacco companies have categorically refused to set nicotine levels below the threshold of 1 mg,

Table 4.3 Mortality trends for lung cancer in Scotland and Italy from 1955 to 1989 (standardized annual rates per 100 000)

		1955–59	1965–69	1975–79	1985–89
Scotland	Males	59.3	79.9	84.2	75.8
	Females	8.2	12.3	19.8	27.2
Italy	Males	17.5	33.3	48.0	58.7
	Females	3.4	4.6	5.6	7.1

Modified from La Vecchia et al.[8]

Table 4.4 Carcinogenic substances in tobacco smoke

Carcinogenic agents	Risk modifiers
Nitrosamines: 4-methylnitrosamino-1-(3-pyridyl)-1-butanone (NNK), methylnitros-aminobutanone	Promoters (e.g. phenols)
	Toxic aldehydes (e.g. acrolein)
Polycyclic aromatic hydrocarbons (PAHs): benzopyrene, benzo-fluoranthene, methyl-chrysene, dibenz-anthracene	Diet
Oxidative stress and free radicals	
Metals: chromium, cadmium, nickel	
Aldehydes	

which would significantly reduce the risk of cardiovascular disease.

A best-selling myth of the last 20 years is that there is a much-reduced risk from low-tar or ultralight cigarettes, whose share in the market has jumped from 20% to 60%. Epidemiological studies have demonstrated, however, that smokers shifting to light cigarettes adopt compensatory mechanisms (deeper and more frequent inhalation) in order to achieve sufficient blood levels of nicotine.[96] Therefore the ultimate risk reduction is by no means proportional to the decrease in tar concentration.

Environmental tobacco smoking (ETS) or passive smoking has been a source of increasing concern in developed countries, with positive effects on tobacco control policies. Even though the relative risk of lung cancer is low (about 1.5 with respect to non-exposed subjects), the enormous number of individuals involved may result in a significant social impact. It has been estimated that in the USA approximately 50 000 deaths per year are attributable to involuntary smoking. Moreover, about 200 000 cases of acute bronchitis or pneumonia occurring in children below 18 months of age may be due to ETS.

Doctors and health workers have a fundamental role in the social perception of damage related to smoking, but other professionals (mass media, public officers, teachers) may influence the market development to a greater extent by promoting specific behavioural models that are perceived as successful or desirable. A specific field of cultural intervention involves teenagers, particularly young females, who represent today the target of a most aggressive advertising campaign. This campaign has been very successful, in that many women still consider tobacco smoking a valid alternative to rational diet and physical exercise to keep slim and active, and ignore the dangerous effects of smoking during pregnancy and the early life of the child. A measure of this cultural gap (at least in Europe) is the higher number of nurses who still smoke at the workplace, in comparison with other health professionals. Preventing the onset of addiction among children and adolescents is the key point of every programme, taking into account that the vast majority of chronic smokers start before the age of 16. Smoking prevention should start at primary school with systematic programmes of continuous education.

Medical intervention aimed at current adult smokers, with therapeutic support of different intensity, has in the past achieved limited but still appreciable results. It has been estimated that approximately 2.5% of the total number of smokers quit every year, and the individual decision is strongly influenced by the clear and unequivocal advice of the family doctor.

In fact, with the optimal use of all available resources, it is now possible to improve significantly the success of individual cessation programmes.[10] For instance, randomized prospective trials have demonstrated that nicotine patches can double the proportion of subjects still refraining from smoking at 6 and 12 months compared with placebo – a much better result than that obtained with oral tabs. The success rate at 6 months is about 25–30% for an integrated treatment combining nicotine patches and psychological support.[9] In order to improve long-term results it is essential to give the chronic smoker a realistic perception of the benefit associated with stopping, which is inversely related to age and duration of habit but is substantial in every condition. While the risk of myocardial infarction and stroke drops within a few months, the risk of cancer declines very slowly over the years. It is crucial, however, to inform younger adults that stopping smoking before the age of 40 prevents chronic damage almost completely, and keeps the mortality curve within the expected range for lifelong non-smokers. Legislative measures aimed at restriction of smoking in public have proven to be a very effective way to control the production, distribution and consumption of tobacco. If applied systematically worldwide, they could extend to the majority of developing countries the benefits already achieved in the USA and northern Europe, and reduce the extent of the tobacco epidemic.

Increasing taxation is the other form of economic leverage that can reduce consumption with marginal effect on government income. Such a measure is particularly effective among those social groups that are less sensitive to educational programmes (teenagers, the poorly educated and ethnic minorities). In southern European countries (France, Italy, Greece, Spain and Portugal), the average cost per pack of cigarettes is still too low to represent a real deterrent, and should be increased substantially.

Professional exposure

Workplaces in particular conditions represent a strong source of exposure to chemical and physical carcinogenic agents (Table 4.5), which may drastically increase the risk of cancer at specific target sites. Progressive clearance from the working environment of those substances that represent a proven danger, protection of potentially exposed individuals, and prevention of dispersion in the atmosphere, water or soil are goals within the reach of modern technology, and should be pursued as a first priority.

Table 4.5 Carcinogenic agents associated with professional exposure

Tumour	Carcinogen
Lung	Asbestos Arsenic compounds Chromium Nickel Bis(chloromethyl) ether Tar, mineral oils Mustard gas Ionizing radiation
Bladder	Aromatic amines Tar, mineral oils Rubber manufacture
Paranasal sinuses	Isopropyl alcohol
Liver	Vinyl chloride
Leukaemia	Benzene Rubber manufacture

Often, professional exposure interacts synergistically with tobacco smoking, and concurrent exposure to these two factors causes a multiplicative increase in the risk of cancer. For example, the risk of lung cancer among non-smokers exposed to asbestos is five times higher than that of non-exposed individuals, while the risk of lung cancer among smokers exposed to asbestos is 50 times higher. People exposed to significant amounts of known carcinogens should be properly informed of the multiplicative effect of simultaneous use of tobacco on their risk of cancer.

Diet and lung cancer

On the basis of evidence of geographical and historical trends in cancer incidence, human epidemiological studies have correlated the risk of lung cancer with environmental factors other than tobacco consumption. Among these, dietary deficiencies in vitamins, micronutrients or specific foods have emerged as potential modifiers of lung cancer risk. A relative protection against lung cancer has been hypothesized for β-carotene and other substances belonging to the group of antioxidants, such as selenium and vitamin E (α-tocopherol), in terms of both dietary consumption and serum levels.

A major limitation in defining individual habits is represented by the low accuracy of dietary questionnaires, and the poor specificity of epidemiological instruments with respect to the individual substances with biological anticancer activity.

Overall, the epidemiological data support the hypothesis that a different intake of common dietary components could modulate the risk of lung cancer, but unequivocal confirmation can only be provided by prospective trials testing the effects of specific dietary measures.[11]

PHARMACOLOGICAL PREVENTION

Latency and intervention

Human epidemiology and experimental carcinogenesis indicate that the development of invasive lung cancer requires a complex sequence of critical events. Most epidemiological studies on time trends and human cohorts, as well as analytical case–control studies, have demonstrated that the interval between the beginning of the exposure to known carcinogens and the occurrence of lung cancer ranges from 20 to 30 years. Such a long phase of latency suggests a large potential space for intervention. From the theoretical point of view, it would be possible to combine various chemopreventive agents to antagonize early carcinogenesis (metabolic activation, formation of DNA adducts, DNA repair) as well as tumour promotion and progression to invasive cancer. The damage induced by inhaled carcinogens affects the respiratory and upper digestive epithelium diffusely, thereby inducing multiple areas of premalignant changes and in some individuals the occurrence of multiple primary cancers. Biological and clinical research related to chemoprevention is now trying to identify the preclinical steps of lung carcinogenesis and the genetic basis of individual susceptibility to tobacco exposure.

Experimental evidence

Lung cancer can be pharmacologically prevented in vitro and in vivo. Substances with potential chemopreventive properties, such as retinoids and antioxidants, have been investigated using nearly all the available systems for testing anticarcinogenic activity.[12] Retinoids exert a strong regulatory effect upon the physiological mechanisms of cell proliferation and differentiation, being able to inhibit malignant transformation and suppress tumour promotion, particularly in the presence of indirect carcinogens such as benzopyrene or methylcholanthrene.[2]

The discovery of specific nuclear retinoid receptors has improved our knowledge on the mechanisms of action of retinoids.[13,14] These receptors belong to the superfamily of ligand-activated nuclear receptors for steroid and thyroid hormones. They are DNA-binding, transcription-modulating proteins, whose expression may be induced by retinoic acid administration.[15,16] Unlike other members of this family, there are two classes of retinoid receptors namely RARs and RXRs, each having α, β and γ subtypes. Upregulation or downregulation of RARs and RXRs may explain how retinoids can interfere with epithelial cell growth, differentiation and apoptosis, or inhibit progression of premalignant cells to cancer, and offers a rational basis for the selection of receptor-specific retinoids in chemoprevention.[17] Different retinoids bind to the different receptor classes and subclasses with different affinities. Retinoid receptors are active only as dimers, in the forms of RAR/RXR heterodimers or RXR/RXR homodimers, which bind to specific DNA sequences, causing induction or suppression of gene transcription.[15] Nuclear receptor subclasses are not evenly distributed in the various tissues: while RARγ is mainly expressed in the skin, RARβ expression is of key relevance for the respiratory and upper digestive epithelia. Their concentration in target tissues also varies in pathological conditions, thus making them a suitable marker of carcinogenic damage.

Antioxidants, including selenium, β-carotene, α-tocopherol (vitamin E) and *N*-acetylcysteine, may inhibit the process of carcinogenesis at various steps: from metabolic inactivation or detoxification of chemical carcinogens to prevention of DNA damage by free radical scavenging. Interest has arisen in particular in *N*-acetylcysteine (NAC), an aminothiol and synthetic precursor of intracellular cysteine and glutathione (GSH), which has been widely used in the past as a mucolytic drug and antidote against paracetamol (acetaminophen)-induced hepatotoxicity. NAC has proven effective in decreasing the direct mutagenicity of several chemical compounds, inhibiting the in vivo formation of carcinogen–DNA adducts and DNA damage, as well as urethane-induced lung tumours in mice.[18] Further promising agents with preclinical and early clinical data include folate, vitamin B_{12}, tea polyphenols, selenium and non-steroidal anti-inflammatory drugs (NSAIDs).

Development of preventive agents

Among the various substances with potential preventive activity (Table 4.6), retinoids have been the most extensively investigated, especially

Table 4.6 Potentially active chemopreventive agents

Natural vitamin A	Retinol Retinyl palmitate
Synthetic retinoids	All-*trans*-retinoic acid (ATRA) 13-*cis*-Retinoic acid (isotretinoin) Etretinate Fenretinide (4-HPR) 9-*cis*-Retinoic acid
Antioxidants	β-Carotene Vitamin C (ascorbic acid) Vitamin E (α-tocopherol) N-Acetylcysteine (NAC)
Micronutrients	Calcium Selenium Zinc
Antiinflammatory (NSAIDs)	Aspirin Piroxicam Sulindac Ibuprofen
Ornithine decarboxylase (ODC) inhibitors	Difluoromethylornithine (DFMO)
Dithiolthiones	Oltipraz
Isothiocyanates	Phenethyl isothiocyanate (PEITC)
Polyphenols	Ellagic acid (EA)

in view of their proven clinical efficacy against skin cancer.[19] Of the hundreds of synthetic retinoids tested in the laboratory, only a few have ultimately entered thorough clinical investigation: retinyl esters (palmitate, acetate), all-*trans*-retinoic acid (ATRA), 13-*cis*-retinoic acid (isotretinoin), etretinate and 4-HPR (fenretinide). This is a heterogeneous group of substances, with specific individual properties in terms of resorption, metabolism, pharmacokinetics, bioavailability and toxicity. Significant interest and expectations were generated by the studies in oral leukoplakia where 13-*cis*-retinoic acid achieved clinical and pathological regression of premalignancy in a high proportion of patients. Unfortunately, most patients would not tolerate the treatment for more than six months, and relapse occurred in most cases after the interruption of treatment. Clinical side-effects such as dry skin, itching, flaking, xerostomia and cheilitis, observed in patients receiving 13-*cis*-retinoic acid at full dosage, were a limiting factor for chemoprevention studies. In the group of antioxidants, β-carotene, α-tocopherol and *N*-acetylcysteine showed excellent long-term tolerability.

In the USA, the National Cancer Institute has invested considerable resources in identifying and testing specific dietary components and drugs for chemoprevention purposes, through a comprehensive programme covering preclinical screening of new agents, assessment of efficacy and safety, and conduct of clinical trials in humans.[20] The results of such a large effort may not be fully established before the next decade.

Design of clinical studies

Primary chemoprevention trials have been designed for individuals at high risk of developing lung cancer because of previous heavy exposure to tobacco smoke, asbestos or other carcinogens, or for volunteers with a high level of cultural motivation, such as physicians or nurses. These studies have tried to counteract a hypothetical deficiency of putative protective agents, such as β-carotene, retinol (vitamin A) or α-tocopherol (vitamin E). Many thousands of people have had to be recruited, with a long period of observation (5–10 years), to reach an adequate number of events. The doses selected for preventive agents have been relatively low, in order to avoid any side-effects and to obtain high recruitment and compliance rates. A second level of intervention involved subjects affected by precancerous or preinvasive lesions such as oral leukoplakia, bronchial metaplasia or dysplasia. The aim of the intervention was to induce regression of preneoplastic disease and thereby prevent progression to invasive cancer. The third level of intervention was focused on the prevention of new primary tumours in patients cured for a prior cancer.

Clinical aspects of field cancerization

Multiple primary tumours may arise in the lung, as well as in the upper aerodigestive tract, as a result of generalized exposure of this epithelium to the multiplicity of carcinogens contained in tobacco smoke – sometimes in association with other environmental risk factors. The theory of 'field cancerization' is that repeated exposure of the entire epithelial surface to carcinogenic insults may result in the occurrence of multiple, independent, premalignant or malignant foci.[21] In support of this concept is the demonstration that significant genetic changes may be detectable, with various degrees of severity, in bronchial dysplasia as well as in pathologically normal mucosa of patients with lung cancer.[22,23] In a prospective series of 163 cases of resected non-small cell lung cancer, we have shown that multiple genetic abnormalities can be detected in the normal bronchial epithelium at distant sites from the primary tumour in 55% of cases (Figure 4.2),

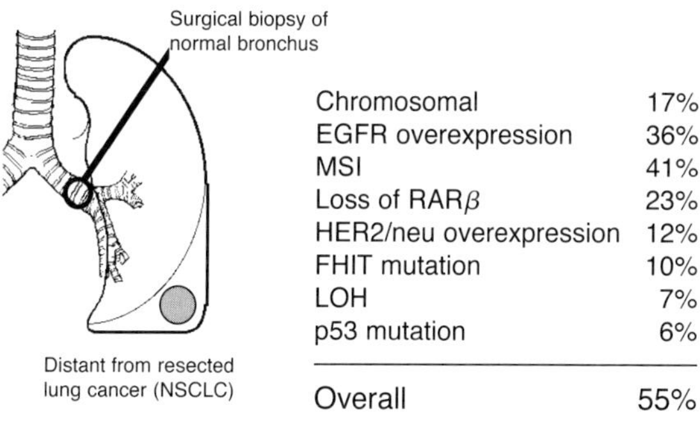

Figure 4.2
Frequency of genetic abnormalities observed in the normal bronchial mucosa of patients resected for early stage non-small cell lung cancer (NSCLC). EGFR, epidermal growth factor receptor gene; MSI, microsatellite instability; RARβ, retinoic acid receptor β gene; FHIT, fragile histidine triad gene; LOH, loss of heterozygosity.

including a rearranged karyotype (mainly 3p, 7p, 17), microsatellite instability, overexpression of specific oncogenes (*EGFR*, *HER2/neu*) or loss of *RARβ*.[24–26]. The frequency of genetic changes in the normal mucosa was higher in patients with multiple tumours of the upper aerodigestive tract, as compared with those with single tumours (69% versus 48%; $p=0.019$). Whether these or other abnormalities, detected in the distant bronchi of tumour-bearing patients, are just an indicator of accumulated damage, or whether they may represent a specific marker of individual genetic predisposition to lung cancer, remains to be clarified. In this respect, the interaction between exogenous carcinogens contained in tobacco smoke and individual tumour susceptibility is a crucial field of research.

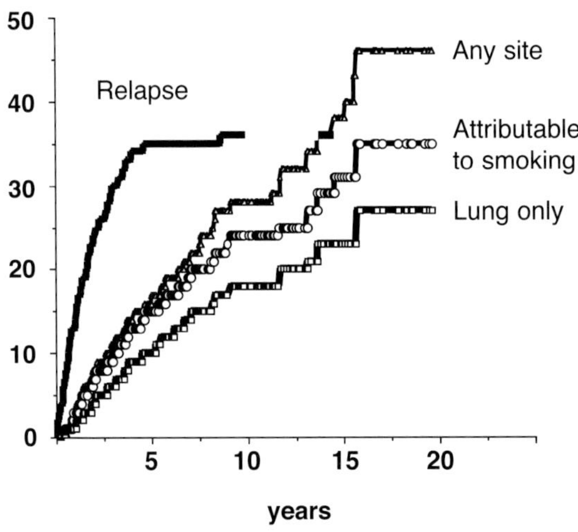

Figure 4.3
Long-term incidence of relapse and second primary tumours in a cohort of 659 patients resected for stage I NSCLC who underwent intense follow-up with four-monthly chest X-rays and sputum cytology.

Frequency and curability of second primaries in the field

In lung cancer patients, the problem of second primary tumours has often been underestimated because of inaccurate follow-up and misclassification of solitary relapses in the lungs. None the less, a few prospective studies on screening and/or patterns of failure after surgery[27–29] have shown a frequency of second primary tumours (all sites) of 10–25%, or 2–3% per year.[27–29] The majority of second primary tumours occurred in the lung (8–20% overall).

In a cohort of 659 patients resected for stage I non-small cell lung cancer (NSCLC) who underwent intense follow-up with four-monthly chest X-rays and sputum cytology, after a median observation time of 64 months a total of 213 (32%) independent primary cancers were detected in 170 (26%) patients, either prior to (59), synchronous with (23) or after (131) resection of the index tumour.[30] The gross frequency of second primary tumours was 20% (131/659), and 82% of second primaries occurred in the tobacco-related field (77 lung, 11 bladder, 10 larynx, 5 oesophagus and 4 oral cavity). These figures are remarkably similar to those reported recently by Martini et al,[31] based on 598 patients treated at Memorial Hospital. Figure 4.3 illustrates the long-term incidence of relapse and second primary tumours in the cohort of 659 patients: while the vast majority of relapses occurred within three years of surgery, the incidence of second primaries was constant up to 20 years. Differential diagnosis between locoregional recurrence and second primary cancer may be difficult in the presence of solitary lesions. Traditional criteria based on the anatomical site (distance from prior cancer), histological type (same versus different) and temporal sequence (time elapsed from prior cancer) have proven inadequate, and in our experience 60% of new primaries showed the same histological type as the previous lung cancer.

Recent studies suggest that biological markers such as *p53* mutations may improve the differential diagnosis of multiple primary tumours occurring in the same area.[32] Even in multiple synchronous lung cancers, a different pattern of genetic abnormalities was found in the various neoplastic foci, providing genetic evidence for an independent origin of these preneoplastic and neoplastic lung lesions.[33] The observed discordance involved at least one of the following markers: 3p deletion, loss of heterozygosity (LOH 3p), *p53* mutation, and K-*RAS* mutation. Interestingly, these data were obtained from tumours with identical histological type and/or occurring in the same pulmonary lobe.

If intense clinical follow-up is adopted after the first lung resection, nearly half of metachronous lung cancers are amenable to complete resection. In our experience, the overall five-year survival from the time of diagnosis of metachronous tumour was 27%; it was 45% after complete resection versus 16% after radiotherapy ($p<0.01$). None of the 22 patients receiving palliative treatment survived more than three years. Both resectability and survival rates were very similar to those reported by other recent series.[31,34]

RANDOMIZED CHEMOPREVENTION TRIALS

High-risk individuals

Within the comprehensive chemoprevention programme funded by the US National Cancer Institute (Table 4.7), three large prospective trials designed to prevent lung cancer with β-carotene supplementation have recently been completed and their results published.[35–37] The first study was conducted in cooperation with the National Public Health Institute of Finland, to test the effects of dietary supplementation of β-carotene (20 mg/day) and α-tocopherol (vitamin E, 50 mg/day) in a population of heavy smokers with low expected intake of crucial micronutrients.[35] The study accrued 29 133 men, aged 50–69, randomized with a two-by-two factorial design into four separate treatment groups, to receive β-carotene, α-tocopherol, both substances or none. The factorial design was selected to evaluate the effect of the two intervention plans in a single large trial. Unfortunately, this trial did not show any protective effect of either α-tocopherol or β-carotene. α-Tocopherol supplementation failed to reduce the incidence and mortality for lung cancer or for the other sites combined. There was indeed a reduction (99% versus 151% = –34%) of prostate cancer, whose significance, however, is unclear. In contrast, β-carotene supplementation was associated with a statistically significant *increase* in lung cancer incidence (56.3% versus 47.5% = +18%) and mortality rate (35.6% versus 30.8%). Mortality rate from ischaemic heart disease was also higher in the group receiving β-carotene (77.1% versus 68.9%), thus contributing to the overall excess in mortality rate of 8%. The trial also showed that dietary supplementation of low doses of the two agents caused significant increases in the serum levels of both, thus ruling out a potential defect of compliance. A critical aspect, however, is the fact that the trial enrolled only active smokers, the vast majority of whom (79%) continued to smoke throughout the intervention.

The detrimental effect of β-carotene was confirmed by the other large trial (CARET) conducted on 13 629 heavy smokers and 4277 asbestos-exposed individuals, showing a 28% increase in lung cancer incidence in the treated group compared with the placebo group.[36] Even in this trial, the initial proportion of current smokers was very high (60%), and as many as 48% of the total were still active smokers at the end of the intervention.

Table 4.7 Randomized trials on primary lung cancer chemoprevention

Investigator	Population	Agent	Dose	Number of subjects	Endpoint
Hennekens (Harvard)	Male physicians aged 40–84 years	β-Carotene	50 mg/ alternate days	22 071	Epithelial cancer, mortality
Buring (Harvard)	Female nurses aged ≥ 45 years	β-Carotene Aspirin α-Tocopherol	50 mg/day 100 mg/day 600 IU/day	40 000	Epithelial cancer, cardiovascular mortality
Albanes (Finland)	Smokers aged 50–69 years	β-Carotene α-Tocopherol	20 mg/day 50 mg/day	29 133	Lung cancer, mortality
Goodman (Seattle)	Smokers aged 50–69 years	β-Carotene Retinol	30 mg/day 25 000 IU/day	13 629	Lung cancer
Omenn (Seattle)	Asbestos workers, smokers, aged 45–69 years	β-Carotene Retinol	30 mg/day 25 000 IU/day	4 277	Lung cancer
McLarty (Tyler)	Asbestos workers	β-Carotene Retinol	50 mg/day 25 000 IU/day	755	Lung cancer
Xuan (Cina)	Tin miners	Retinol β-Carotene α-Tocopherol Selenium	25 000 IU/day 50 mg/day 800 IU/day 400 μg/day	7 000	Lung cancer

On the other hand, the third trial (PHS), conducted in the USA on 22 000 male physicians aged 40–84 (taking 50 mg β-carotene every other day for many years), could not demonstrate any effect of β-carotene administration.[37] The main difference is likely to be due to the different smoking habits of that population: in fact, 61% of the participants were lifelong non-smokers, and only a small minority (11%) were current smokers. These data suggest a unfavourable interaction between current smoking and β-carotene treatment; however, a residual confounding effect of

Table 4.8 Lung cancer incidence and overall mortality (10 000 person-years) and proportion of smokers at entry

	β-Carotene[a]	Control	Smokers at entry (%)	
			Current	Former
ATBC trial[35]				
Lung cancer incidence	56	47	100	0
Total mortality	218	201		
CARET trial[36]				
Lung cancer incidence	59	46	60	39
Total mortality	144	119		
PHS trial[37]				
Lung cancer incidence	6	6	11	39
Total mortality	74	73		

[a]Combined with retinol in the CARET trial.

the quantity and duration of smoking during the trial cannot be completely ruled out, since the difference in lung cancer incidence (6 versus 47) and overall mortality (73 versus 201) among the control arms of the three studies is much larger than that observed between cases and controls of each trial (Table 4.8).[38]

While a definitive judgement on the carcinogenic effect of β-carotene will require further investigations, it is clear that vitamin supplementation cannot replace primary prevention, and it is reasonable to exclude current smokers from chemoprevention studies.

Patients with prior cancer

The potential benefit of retinoids as adjuvant treatment, to reduce the occurrence of second primary tumours, was indicated by two independent randomized trials. The first study was conducted on 103 patients with previously treated head and neck cancer, randomized to receive either 13-*cis*-retinoic acid (isotretinoin) or placebo for 12 months.[39] The incidence of second primary tumours was significantly lower in the treatment arm after a median follow-up of 32 months (4% versus 24%), and persisted at a later analysis with 54 months of median follow-up (14% versus 31%).

The second trial was conducted on 307 patients with early stage lung cancer, randomized after complete surgical resection to receive high-dose retinyl palmitate (300 000 IU/day) for 12–24 months or no further treatment.[40] After a median follow-up of 46 months, we observed a significant difference in the frequency of second primaries (12% versus 21%) and total cancer failures (37% versus 48%) in favour of the treatment arm. Despite our initial concerns and a very intense monitoring of side-effects in the pilot phase of the study, the toxicity and tolerabilty profile of high-dose retinyl palmitate were excellent. A high proportion of patients presented typical side-effects such as skin desquamation or dryness of mucosae, but only in a very few patients did the treatment have to be discontinued because of toxicity.[41]

Based on this favourable pilot experience, a series of trials has been designed with the purpose of preventing new primary malignancies after curative resection. The EUROSCAN cooperative study was set up in 1988 as a joint venture of the European Organization for Research and Treatment of Cancer (EORTC) Lung Cancer and Head and Neck Cancer Cooperative Groups,[42] to test the efficacy of retinyl palmitate and NAC, given for two years with a two-by-two factorial design to patients with previous cancer of the larynx, oral cavity and lung (NSCLC). The accrual was closed in 1994, with 2595 patients entered; the analysis is ongoing and results will be published in 1999. A reassuring aspect of the EUROSCAN trial is the fact that only a minority (11%) of randomized patients with prior lung cancer continued or resumed smoking throughout the intervention period. The early analysis of smoking habits provided evidence that, regardless of the intervention programme, smoking after treatment of the initial cancer was associated with a significant worsening of long-term survival. Another chemoprevention trial on resected stage I NSCLC was launched by the US Intergroup in 1992.[43] This study has randomized over 600 patients per arm, to receive low-dose oral 13-*cis*-retinoic acid (30 mg/day) or placebo in a double-blind scheme.

Future prospects of intervention

After 15 years of clinical investigation, the evidence of a beneficial effect of pharmacological prevention of human lung cancer is still scarce.

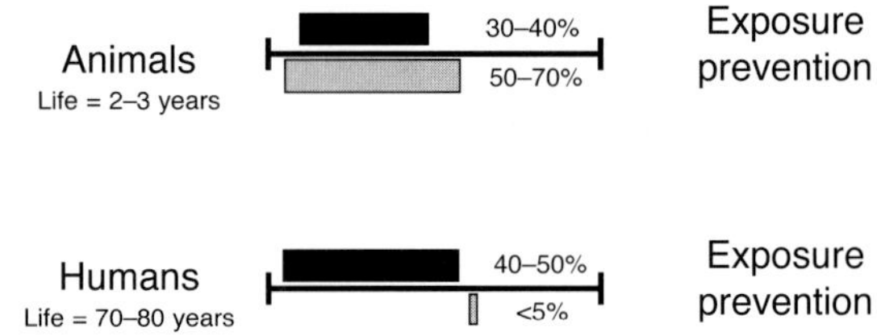

Figure 4.4
Schematic representation of the discrepancy between experimental chemoprevention in animals and human trials: duration of exposure to carcinogenic agents and preventive treatment in relation to the average life.

The first generation of clinical trials has served as a test of whether various experimental and epidemiological hypotheses are realistic, but the failure of most randomized studies emphasizes the limits of initial experience in humans and represents a great challenge for future research and developments.

Many problems remain open: simplistic interpretation of epidemiological data on diet and cancer, low predictivity of animal models (Figure 4.4), unfavourable efficacy/toxicity profile of retinoids, reversibility of biological effects, lack of intermediate biological endpoints, difficulty in designing proper phase II trials, low risk of cancer requiring prolonged intervention and a huge number of subjects, and persisting exposure to known carcinogens such as tobacco smoking.

Ideally, a new generation of clinical trials should be based on innovative preclinical studies providing fresh data on the efficacy of new substances, alone and in combination with older agents, against bronchial premalignancy defined by new biomarkers. Unfortunately, more human-orientated experimental models are still beyond our reach, and the difficulty of inducing lung carcinomas in animals by tobacco smoking appears an insurmountable paradox.

Several new agents are in the pipeline, and a few of them have gone through clinical toxicological investigation. Natural dietary components such as genistein or curcumin appear to be very attractive on safety grounds, but new retinoids such as 4-HPR and 9-*cis*-retinoic acid are also promising.

Topical application of retinoids is a logical way to circumvent systemic toxicity and increase pharmacological levels in target tissues. This is particularly sound for substances like retinol and other retinoids with a view to their well-established capacity to induce complete regression of skin cancer (and other dermatological diseases) by topical application. Pilot studies on inhalation of aerosolized retinoids are ongoing in the USA and Europe using all-*trans*- and 13-*cis*-retinoic acids via aerosol.[44]

After the experience of the ATBC and CARET trials, overwelming scientific and ethical problems have led to the strong recommendation that chemoprevention programmes should focus on former smokers or other individuals who are at high risk because of previous cancer or genetic susceptibility.

Biological markers and intermediate endpoints

To increase the cost/benefit ratio of intervention plans, specific subpopulations of very high-risk individuals must be identified on the basis of constitutive or acquired abnormalities detectable in the target tissues. Intermediate biomarkers are the hypothetical instrument to select high-risk populations on the basis of tissue-specific genetic damage rather than non-specific carcinogenic exposure.[43] In addition, biological intermediate endpoints could satisfy the crucial need to monitor the efficacy of preventive strategies on premalignant lesions, well before the actual occurrence of invasive cancer.[22,23,45]

A number of genetic abnormalities have been consistently observed in lung cancer, premalignant lesions and normal bronchial mucosa, and represent potential biomarkers for chemoprevention. Some of the new biomarkers, such as RARβ and the *FHIT* gene, display some very promising features: a high specificity for lung cancer, early occurrence in bronchial metaplasia and even microscopically normal mucosa, and detectability through routine sputum samples.[45–47] In practical terms, it is now conceivable to use a panel of specific markers (3p deletion, *p53*, *EGFR*, K-*RAS*, microsatellite instability, *FHIT*) to select candidates for chemoprevention. In fact, with the present developments in research technology, such as immunocytochemistry, fluorescence in situ hybridization (FISH) and polymerase chain reaction (PCR), even small samples collected through bronchoscopic biopsies, brushing or sputum cytology will become suitable for systematic screening of high-risk individuals.[45]

More recent data on the expression of the FHIT protein by immunohistochemistry on a series of 474 pathological stage I NSCLC patients indicate that loss of FHIT protein is the most frequent alteration in NSCLC (73%) and precancerous lesions (93%), is significantly higher in tumours of smokers (76%) versus non-smokers (46%), and is an independent and more frequent event than *p53* overexpression in tumours (73% versus 46%) and precancerous lesions (93% versus 55%). This represents a useful diagnostic tool for the early detection of lung cancer.[48]

A considerable amount of effort will be required in the coming years to test and validate such a large group of biomarkers through purpose-designed, small-scale, controlled studies. In order to justify their systematic use, intermediate endpoints will have to prove specific for the process of lung carcinogenesis, correlate quantitatively or qualitatively with the stage of progression towards invasive tumour, show a low rate of spontaneous regression, and be modulated by the selected preventive agent. Such biomarkers should also be easily measurable on small specimens, and the process of sampling tolerable at repeated intervals with minimal side-effects.

CONCLUSIONS

Notwithstanding all the problems encountered so far, research on cancer chemoprevention has provided a new insight and better comprehension of the mechanisms of human carcinogenesis, and represents a indisputable priority, particularly in those diseases such as lung cancer that are common and poorly curable. Second primary lung cancers are a suitable endpoint to test the efficacy of preventive agents, but differential diagnosis is critical. Retinoids, β-carotene and other vitamins or antioxidants, widely tested in randomized clinical trials, have failed to demonstrate a significant effect against lung cancer. The use of these substances for cancer chemoprevention has still to be considered experimental, and they should be administered with this purpose only in the framework of controlled studies. There is an urgent need for greater investments in cancer chemoprevention programmes exploiting the new resources provided by recent molecular biological findings.

REFERENCES

1. Greenwald P, Stern HR, Role of biology and prevention in aerodigestive tract cancers. *J Natl Cancer Inst Monogr* 1992; **13**: 3–14.
2. Lotan R, Effects of vitamin A and its analogs (retinoids) on normal and neoplastic cells. *Biochim Biophys Acta* 1980; **605**: 33–91.
3. Peto R, Smoking and death: the past 40 years and the next 40. *BMJ* 1994; **309**: 937–9.
4. Peto R, Lopez AD, Boreham J et al, Mortality from smoking worldwide. *Br Med Bull* 1996; **52**: 12–21.
5. US Department of Health and Human Services, *Reducing the Health Consequences of Smoking: 25 Years of Progress. A Report of the Surgeon General 1989*. US DHHS Office of Smoking and Health: Washington, DC, 1989.
6. Jensen OM, Esteve J, Moller H, Renard H, Cancer in the European Community and its member states. *Eur J Cancer* 1990; **26**: 1167–256.
7. National Cancer Institute, *Smoking, Tobacco, and Cancer Program 1985–89 Status Report*. US DHHS, PHS NIH Publication 90-3107.
8. La Vecchia C, Lucchini F, Negri E et al, Trends of cancer mortality in Europe, 1955–1989: I, Digestive sites. *Eur J Cancer* 1992; **28**: 132–235.
9. Cinciripini PM, Hecht SS, Henningfield JE et al, Tobacco addiction: implications for treatment and cancer prevention. *J Natl Cancer Inst* 1997; **89**: 1852–67.
10. Henningfield JE, Nicotine medications for smoking cessation. *N Engl J Med* 1995; **333**: 1196–203.
11. Greenwald P, Sondik E, Lynch BS, Diet and chemoprevention in NCI's research strategy to achieve national cancer control objectives. *Annu Rev Public Health* 1986; **7**: 267–91.
12. Sporn MB, Newton DL, Chemoprevention of cancer with retinoids. *Fed Proc* 1979; **38**: 2528–34.
13. Lotan R, Clifford JL, Nuclear receptors for retinoids: mediators of retinoid effects on normal and malignant cells. *Biomed Pharmacother* 1990; **45**: 145–56.
14. Chambon P, The retinoid signalling pathway: molecular and genetic analyses. *Semin Cell Biol* 1994; **5**: 115–25.
15. de Thé H, Marchio A, Tiollais P, Dejean A, Differential expression and ligand regulation of the retinoic acid receptor α and β genes. *EMBO J* 1989; **8**: 429–33.
16. Clifford J, Petkovich M, Chambon P, Lotan R, Modulation by retinoids of mRNA levels for nuclear retinoic acid receptors in murine melanoma cells. *Mol Endocrinol* 1990; **4**: 1546–55.
17. Lehman JM, Dawson MI, Hobbs PD et al, Iden-

tification of retinoids with nuclear receptor-subtype-selective activities. *Cancer Res* 1991; **51**: 4804–9.

18. De Flora S, Izzotti A, D'Agostini F et al, Chemopreventive properties of *N*-acetylcysteine and other thiols. In: *Cancer Chemoprevention* (Wattenberg L, Lipkin M, Boone CW, Kelloff GJ, eds). CRC Press: Boca Raton, FL, 1992: 183–94.
19. Lippman SM, Kessler JF, Meyskens FL, Retinoids as preventive and therapeutic anticancer agents (part II). *Cancer Treat Rep* 1987; **71**: 493–515.
20. Kelloff GJ, Boone CW, Crowell JA et al, Chemopreventive drug development: perspectives and progress. *Cancer Epidemiol Biomarkers Prev* 1994; **3**: 85–98.
21. Slaughter DP, Southwick HW, Smejkal W, 'Field cancerization' in oral stratified squamous epithelium: clinical implications of multicentric origin. *Cancer* 1953; **6**: 963–8.
22. Sozzi G, Miozzo M, Tagliabue E et al, Cytogenetic abnormalities and overexpression of receptors for growth factors in normal bronchial epithelium and tumour samples of lung cancer patients. *Cancer Res* 1991; **51**: 400–4.
23. Sundaresan V, Ganly P, Hasleton P et al, p53 and chromosome 3 abnormalities, characteristic of malignant lung tumours, are detectable in preinvasive lesions of the bronchus. *Oncogene* 1992; **7**: 1989–97.
24. Sozzi G, Miozzo M, Donghi R et al, Deletions of 17p and p53 mutations in preneoplastic lesions of the lung. *Cancer Res* 1992; **52**: 6079–82.
25. Pastorino U, Sozzi G, Miozzo M et al, Genetic changes in lung cancer. *J Cell Biochem* 1993; **17F**: 237–48.
26. Xu XC, Sozzi G, Lee JS et al, Suppression of retinoic acid receptor beta in non small cell lung cancer in vivo: implications for lung cancer development. *J Natl Cancer Inst* 1997; **89**: 624–9.
27. Fontana RS, Early diagnosis of lung cancer. *Am Rev Respir Dis* 1977; **116**: 399–2.
28. Pairolero P, Williams DE, Bergstrahl EJ et al, Postsurgical stage I bronchogenic carcinoma: morbid implications of recurrent disease. *Ann Thorac Surg* 1984; **38**: 331–8.
29. Shields TW, Robinette CD, Long-term survivors after resection of bronchial carcinoma. *Surg Gynecol Obstet* 1973; **136**: 759–68.
30. Andreani S, Pastorino U, Ante M et al, Second primary tumours in resected stage I lung cancer. *Lung Cancer* 1994; **11**: 167 (Abst 644).
31. Martini N, Bains MS, Burt ME et al, Incidence of local recurrence and second primary tumours in resected stage I lung cancer. *J Thorac Cardiovasc Surg* 1995; **109**: 120–9.
32. Chung KY, Mukhopadhyay T, Kim J et al, Discordant p53 gene mutations in primary head and neck cancers and corresponding second primary cancers of the upper aerodigestive tract. *Cancer Res* 1993; **53**: 1676–83.
33. Sozzi G, Miozzo M, Pastorino U et al, Genetic evidence for an independent origin of multiple preneoplastic and neoplastic lung lesions. *Cancer Res* 1995; **55**: 135–40.
34. Rosengart TK, Martini N, Ghosn P, Burt M, Multiple primary lung carcinomas: prognosis and treatment. *Ann Thorac Surg* 1991; **52**: 773–8.
35. The Alpha-Tocopherol, Beta-Carotene Cancer Prevention Study Group, The effect of vitamin E and beta-carotene on the incidence of lung cancer and other cancers in male smokers. *N Engl J Med* 1994; **330**: 1029–35.
36. Omenn GS, Goodman GE, Thornquist MD et al, Effects of a combination of beta-carotene and vitamin A on lung cancer and cardiovascular disease. *N Engl J Med* 1996; **334**: 1150–5.
37. Hennekens CH, Buring JE, Manson JE et al, Lack of effect of long-term supplementation with beta-carotene on the incidence of malignant neoplasms and cardiovascular disease. *N Engl J Med* 1996; **334**: 1145–9.
38. Pastorino U, Re: B-carotene and the risk of lung cancer [letter]. *J Natl Cancer Inst* 1997; **89**: 456–7.
39. Hong WK, Lippman JM, Itri L et al, Prevention of second primary tumours with isotretinoin in squamous cell carcinoma of the head and neck. *N Engl J Med* 1990; **323**: 795–801.
40. Pastorino U, Infante I, Maioli M et al, Adjuvant treatment of stage I lung cancer with high dose vitamin A. *J Clin Oncol* 1993; **11**: 1216–22.

41. Pastorino U, Chiesa G, Infante M et al, Safety of high-dose vitamin A. Randomized trial on lung cancer chemoprevention. *Oncology* 1991; **48**: 131–7.
42. De Vries N, Van Zandwijk N, Pastorino U, The EUROSCAN Study. *Br J Cancer* 1991; **64**: 985–9.
43. Lee JS, Lippman SM, Hong WK et al, Determination of biomarkers for intermediate end points in chemoprevention trials. *Cancer Res* 1992; **52**(9 Suppl): 2707–10s.
44. Brooks AD, Benedetti F, Tong WP et al, Chemoprevention of respiratory tract cancers. *Proc Am Assoc Cancer Res* 1997; **38**: 86 (Abst 574).
45. Miozzo M, Sozzi G, Musso K et al, Microsatellite alterations in bronchial and sputum specimens of lung cancer patients. *Cancer Res* 1996; **56**: 2285–8.
46. Sozzi G, Veronese ML, Negrini M et al, The FHIT gene at 3p14.2 is abnormal in lung cancer. *Cell* 1996; **85**: 117–26.
47. Sozzi G, Tornielli S, Tagliabue E et al, Absence of FHIT protein in primary lung tumours and cell lines with FHIT gene abnormalities. *Cancer Res* 1997; **57**: 5207–12.
48. Sozzi G, Pastorino U, Moiraghi L et al, Loss of FHIT function in lung cancer and preinvasive bronchial lesions. *Cancer Res* 1998; **58**: 5032–7.

5 Tobacco policy

Nigel Gray

Contents Introduction • Basic policy • Developing countries • The future

INTRODUCTION

The single global public health objective in this field is to reduce consumption of tobacco by all possible means as quickly as possible. Major successes such as the decline in British consumption and mortality are currently matched by the steep ascent of these two indices in developing countries, particularly China,[1] which illustrates the urgency of policy action.

It is reasonable to assert that the implementation of policy lags – sometimes decades – behind policy development, which lags similarly behind the development of knowledge. In a number of sophisticated countries, among which are the UK, Norway, Sweden, Australia, Canada and the USA, the proportion of the population that continues to smoke has fallen from over a half to about a quarter. Mortality declines have usually followed, but at very different rates. So it is wrong to be pessimistic – but important to be impatient. Pressing for activist policies, on the grounds that outcomes take a long time, seems to be an integral part of the duty of the health professions.

Comprehensive tobacco policy has been well established and understood since the mid-1970s.[2] The recommendations in this chapter are informed by long experience of successful and unsuccessful policies in many diverse countries. Many of the important policy issues and outcomes have never been the subject of refereed articles in the technical press, so the reader must be satisfied with basic references and must be willing to search newspaper archives for historical detail.

Tobacco use has been, and is, perhaps the most difficult issue faced by public health workers in the 20th century. Historic diseases, such as smallpox, polio, measles, diphtheria, tetanus, whooping cough, rubella and scarlet fever, were conquered in developed countries within a decade or so of the arrival of effective control systems. When vaccines and antibiotics worked, they were used. Failures in developing countries relate to the failure of national and international social organization and rarely to organized opposition. The reappearance of malaria and tuberculosis, depressing though it is, is due partly to these factors and partly to the lack of really effective means of control.

The singular feature of the tobacco problem is that someone is selling it. No one is selling tuberculosis. To this can be attributed the fact that, five decades after discovering its carcinogenicity, tobacco consumption worldwide is rising. Comparisons with the other industries selling toxic products are unsatisfactory. There is no pretence that asbestos does not cause asbestosis, nor that drunken driving is merely a pleasurable habit. The international tobacco industry is unique in its stubborn refusal to concede the side-effects of its product, despite recent revelations[3] that make it clear that the industry knew of the carcinogenic and addictive properties of tobacco some decades ago. Once having retreated into its legal bunker, it is now in the difficult position of facing enormous legal and financial consequences if it makes concessions or tells the truth. Thus the forces of public health and the global tobacco industry are locked in continuous warfare, and prospects for peace are slight.

While no form of tobacco use has been discovered to be safe, the cigarette is the most ubiquitous, widely used and best-studied product. The myriad forms of tobacco use seen in India and other parts of Asia are carcinogenic in many different ways, and, with the tobacco being personally grown or based on cottage industry production, each poses specific individual problems. Certainly it is easier to develop policies to control cigarette smoking than tobacco/betel chewing, since the product is factory-made, taxed, exported and imported, and often the subject of retail licensing.

The unrepentant nature of the global tobacco industry, which is controlled by relatively few major manufacturers, is reflected in the sales statistics. Sales are in decline in the most developed countries, and the expected indices follow. Lung cancer in males, especially younger ones, is declining, as is heart disease.[1] By contrast, tobacco exports from the USA are climbing, and the antique tobacco monopolies of the previously communist world are being replaced by modern mass production systems owned by the same people. Marketing measures forbidden in the USA, the UK and Europe are rampant in many developing countries.

Consideration of tobacco policy may conveniently focus first on the cigarette. Such consideration should take note that smoking is a *learned habit*, which is *initiated* by social forces but *sustained* by the development of *addiction* in persistent users

BASIC POLICY

This is theoretically simple:

- change the cultural background;
- change the smoker;
- change the cigarette;
- protect the children.

Changing the cultural background

The cultural background against which tobacco smoking must be considered is a mixture of community law and community norms. Laws usually arise as a result of public opinion at a point in time and are an important reflection of community norms, although they do not always mirror public opinion in those countries where the tobacco industry is strongest. The failed battle to introduce strong tobacco legislation in the USA in 1998 shows the difficulties in the path of lawmakers that are posed by the organized and well-funded opposition of tobacco manufacturers. This situation, while obvious in the USA, arises in most countries when tobacco policy requires lawmaking, although the opposition may be less obvious and behind the scenes.

An important element in the interaction between government, parliaments and popular opinion may be non-government organizations. Policy frequently arises in the non-government sector, as may the drive for legislation. Thus the interactive process of introducing legislation may be an important part of providing a driving force for implementation. Popular laws are more likely to be implemented. Opposition to standard comprehensive laws is to be expected, and is routinely led by those with vested interests, supported by the industry, using arguments now outdated and often ugly when exposed to public gaze.

Model legislation

- *Health warnings* These should state government policy and the facts. Rotating, explanatory warnings are the first step. Warnings researched for understandability and offering a telephone number to an information service are better.

- *Packet labelling* There is a powerful case for generic packaging as a way of interfering with global brand advertising. Packaging should declare yields of known major carcinogens and other substances, which may be specified as knowledge develops. Packet inserts are a way of providing the sort of comprehensive information that is given with such substances as aspirin. Tobacco industry claims for the right to compete for adult markets are specious, as adults and children coexist in society and measures to protect or attract children often impinge on adults and vice versa.
- *Abolition of promotion – in every form* Tobacco brand names need to be forbidden in advertisements for any other product. Direct and indirect advertising needs to be specifically addressed. This issue remains difficult because of the cross-border abilities of satellite media. It should be understood that there is no case that can be made in favour of tobacco promotion, since the product is seriously and chronically toxic when used as the manufacturers intend. Evasion of promotional restrictions is the profession of a large number of people, all of whose arguments should be ignored. Even at the point of sale, advertisement should be forbidden.
- *Availability* Sales to children, defined as age 16–18 in most countries, need to be prohibited and the prohibition policed. Such legislation is widespread – but policing is not. Vending machine sales need to be supervised in places inaccessible to children, or forbidden. This policy measure is widely adopted, but almost nowhere has policing been tried. Until that experiment is done and shown to fail, this issue remains high on the agenda for developing countries.
- *Smoke-free environments* These need encouragement for exemplary as well as risk-avoidance reasons. As a minimum, schools, hospitals, workplaces and public transport should be smoke-free. Smokers in many countries have been remarkably accepting of this policy. It is an important downward pressure on smoking rates in all age groups, and probably reduces daily dose as well as encouraging quitting.
- *Tax* This should be high in the context of individual income and should be regularly increased; a set proportion should be allocated to health purposes, including tobacco education.[4] Tobacco tax is among the only taxes demonstrated to be popular. There is good reason why the price of a packet of cigarettes should be several times that of a hamburger
- *Regulation of the product* It is unacceptable that a product as dangerous as tobacco should be unregulated. Additives need to demonstrated to be non-toxic in both burnt and unburnt form; and upper limits should be set, and continuously reviewed, for major carcinogens and toxins. Public health advisors and departments have been slow to act in this field, possibly because of perceived complexities. However, the establishment of upper limits for cigarette emissions is relatively straightforward, and is in need of urgent implementation.

The importance of legislation is underlined by the experience of Norway, the pioneer, in 1975, of comprehensive tobacco legislation. Tobacco consumption peaked in the mid-1970s, having by that time risen by about 25% since the mid-1950s. Since then it has declined by approximately the same amount. The original legislation in Norway was from a unanimous parliament, but was surrounded by much discussion and public interaction. This early legislation did not include severe workplace and public place restrictions, and Norwegian prices have risen only slightly, in real terms, since the 1980s.[5] While it is possible to argue over the potential benefits of more aggressive pricing, public education and smoking opportunity restrictions, the Norwegian experience is a testimony to the efficacy of good legislation as the basis for a comprehensive anti-tobacco programme.

Community norms are usually well reflected in public opinion. A comprehensive tobacco policy would include regular surveys of tobacco consumption, public opinion, relevant attitudes among smokers and non-smokers, and evaluation of education programmes. Opinion may move slowly, but it does move with time and in the presence of well-directed education programmes. It is both logical and true that parental attitudes and example flow through to youth behaviour, and so changing the cultural background implies measuring beliefs and recruiting all the potential role models of society as well as removing the tobacco industry's ability to promote its product. It is also logical to believe that education programmes work better without opposition, further underlining the importance of complete eradication of promotion.

In summary, changing the cultural background requires an activist and persistent approach to legislation and community involvement. This means that a well-organized and coordinated antismoking movement is a necessary basis. Such movements are not always large; efficiency and coordination are the keys.

Changing the smoker

Changing the smoker to become a non-smoker is a complex multifaceted process requiring analysis of individual society's smoking patterns. It is accepted that addiction to tobacco is the major force in maintaining smoking status. Progress towards becoming a non-smoker may be generally and simply summarized:

Rational information → dissonance → attempts to quit → success → maintenance

Dissonance may be defined as dissatisfaction with one's own smoking behaviour, and affects a majority of smokers in the USA, for example, but probably a minority in less well-informed societies. Clearly dissonance is more likely to occur if the victim/person is well informed, so the place of varied education programmes, targeted to the subgroups as well as the totality of smokers, cannot be doubted, but is country-specific, at least to a degree. Other factors can be expected to stimulate dissonance: the smoke-free workplace and public places; peer group and family pressure; negative peer group experiences such as deaths or disease; societal attitudes and levels of information. Such factors reflect the cultural background, and vary from country to country.

Attempts to quit occur frequently in sophisticated countries and policy should encourage and provide support for smokers who make them.

The role of nicotine replacement therapy (NRT) is crucial, and is in need of considerable development. Its value is well established, although results are generally disappointing by comparison with expectations. Better products are needed, as are greater availability and more support services. It is bizarre that cigarette content is virtually unregulated, while bureaucratic restrictions on alternative sources of clean nicotine are widespread. The general global failure of health professionals, especially physicians, in support of patients and provision of therapy is a disturbing reflection of health priorities, which at least means there is hope for potential improvement.

The debate over nicotine addiction[6] per se ought not to hold back the development of better products and services. Tobacco is a uniquely toxic way of delivering the desired dose of nicotine, while NRT appears to be safe or relatively so. Up to the present time, there is no evidence of mass addiction to nicotine chewing gum, although the lack of competitive products that will deliver the quick, efficient 'fix' of the cigarette might well explain this. Nevertheless, policy should be aimed at providing support, NRT and whatever other pharmaceutical aids may be developed, because the status quo is an ongoing disaster that justifies greater effort than it receives. Continuing use of NRT in smokers who cut down but do not abstain is a sensible form of harm reduction, although the obvious goal is abstinence.

Policy makers should note that the costs of helping smokers are infinitely less than those of treating them and that, while the most immediate mortality, morbidity and cost benefits are achieved by attention to long-duration heavy smokers, every smoker is at risk sooner or later, and early intervention is always best.

Changing the cigarette

The cigarette is a uniquely efficient nicotine delivery device, which has so far escaped significant production controls worldwide. This is in contrast to motor vehicles, pharmaceuticals, food, houses and even sewage systems. While the reasons for this disparity are interesting, since they include corruption on a global scale, there can be no excuse for continuing to allow the tobacco industry alone to decide what will go into the product, and therefore what is present in mainstream smoke.

First it is necessary to state that the policy of the 1960s, which favoured reduction of tar and nicotine levels over time, has not produced the benefits anticipated. Changes in cigarette design[7] have brought about reductions in some carcinogens and increases in others. Mortality benefit, if present, is small, and adenocarcinoma has increased in the USA and elsewhere. Since tar measurement takes no account of the qualitative changes that have occurred in smoke, it is misleading. Over the same time, bioavailability of nicotine has been increased, and, together with compensatory smoking, this means that machine-measured levels of nicotine are also misleading.

It can therefore be unequivocally stated that tar and nicotine measures as currently used should be abolished – the policy question is what they should be replaced with.

It must be recognized that cigarette design is best understood by the tobacco industry and is clouded by commercial secrecy, and that no governments have applied the necessary research resources to know enough to tell manufacturers how to make their product. However, it is certainly possible to apply the principles learned in reducing vehicle emissions to the cigarette, and to base regulations upon it.

It is known[8,9] that there is great diversity in the levels of major carcinogens in mainstream smoke yields on the world market, so the evidence that cigarettes with lower carcinogen levels can be made and sold is indisputable – cigarettes low in nitrates and nitrosamines are made and sold.

The policy issues then become the following:

- Governments must claim power to regulate the content of cigarette smoke – this power already exists in some countries.
- Health authorities require suitable advisory systems involving independent scientists and with mandatory access to industry information.
- Initially, major carcinogens such as benzo(*a*)pyrene, 4-(methylnitrosamino)-1-(3-pyridyl)-1-butanone (NNK) and *N*-nitrosonornicotine (NNN) should be

targeted. Market analysis would show the range of yields. Those cigarettes yielding above the median should be removed from the market, or modified, within a standard period such as 12 months.

- Over time, this process would allow progressive reduction in carcinogens and other toxins, since the starting point is a level found to exist on the market and already achieved by at least some manufacturers.
- Nicotine needs special treatment. The first essential is a new measurement system. However, a measure of smoke content will not accurately reflect what gets into the smoker's bloodstream, since it cannot control for compensatory smoking practices. Therefore, while control of smoke yield can be exerted by a measure such as nicotine content per litre of smoke, the decision-making process that sets the yield levels needs to be informed by behavioural experiment and analysis.

The ultimate policy decision – whether mass weaning of nicotine-dependent populations should be attempted by regulatory reduction of dose per cigarette – cannot be made in the light of knowledge in 1999. However, the goal of reduction in the addictiveness of the cigarette is a proper one, and should be pursued as a matter of policy.

In facing the decision to control nicotine yields, policy makers must understand that the rise of cigarette smoking was a vast unplanned experiment performed by the tobacco industry, initially ignorant of its product's toxicity. Long-term decisions on nicotine policy will require similarly large experiments based on sensibly considered probabilities. The decision to reduce tar and nicotine was sensible when conceived, but was subverted by industry manipulation. This mistake should not be made again, but should not prevent innovative regulatory policies.

- New products containing tobacco ought also to be regulated and only tested in situations similar to those that are used for the testing of new pharmaceuticals. So far the tobacco industry has not produced a successful alternative to the standard cigarette. They should not be discouraged from doing so, but should not receive marketing advantages over NRT and other nicotine alternatives.

Protecting the children

As social norms and fashions have changed over time, so have the specific stimuli that trigger or contribute to initiation of the smoking habit. Age of onset of initiation varies around the world, beginning earlier in developed countries. Cultural differences play an important role, as exemplified by the great diversity in smoking rates between men and women in countries such as China. Whereas the factors contributing to initiation in particular societies differ, the policy question concerns what can be done to interfere with the pressures towards initiation – or, in simple terms, what can be done to protect the children.

The first policy approach is to remove or reduce all the pro-smoking pressures that can be controlled. Formal and informal promotion of tobacco has been dealt with above. Nevertheless, it must be re-emphasized that children are extremely sensitive to promotional pressures and that any presentation of a tobacco brand name needs to disappear from the social environment. This has been substantially achieved in a number of countries, but has been subverted to a variable degree by cross-border advertising of events such as motor races and cricket matches sponsored by tobacco interests. Global control of this phenomenon will not be achieved easily, but the battle, slowly being won in developed countries, needs to be fought in developing countries as the industry seeks to source such events from them.

Local social pressures need policy attention. The role of parents, siblings, peer groups, and local and international role models should be the subject of education programmes and local campaigns with the specific objective of reducing initiating pressures wherever they exist. What happens in schools, homes, workplaces and public places needs detailed consideration. The rights of ongoing smokers need to be related to those of children to a smoke-free and promotion-free environment.

Policy is not only about prohibitions and restraints. There is a clear need for experimentally based, expensive, education programmes aimed at children. The fact that few of these have been developed outside a few richer countries, and even fewer adequately funded, is not an excuse for failure to change. Every society that spends money on treating sick smokers would be well advised to spend funds of the sort spent on promotion of cola drinks on campaigns aimed at discouraging smoking.

DEVELOPING COUNTRIES

Tobacco use is already built in to many developing countries, and takes many forms. No form of tobacco use has been shown to be free of risk, and the fact that snuff use in Sweden is less hazardous than tobacco/betel chewing in India is not sufficient to allow fantasies of safe tobacco products to intrude on public policy.

The principles set out above are applicable to some degree with most forms of tobacco use. However, local cultures in which the many and strange variants of tobacco smoking and chewing persist need to be considered individually. The broad-brush weapons of education, warning labels, taxation and restriction where relevant can be considered by policy makers, and locally suitable policies can be developed and tried. The after-effects of tobacco use as known are such that no variant of use can be neglected.

The reappearance of the cigar as a social status symbol in the USA should warn against complacency.

THE FUTURE

The basic principles of tobacco policy discussed here have been tested and appraised in real societies, and have been shown to work to a greater or lesser degree. The degree usually depends on the enthusiasm with which policies are implemented. The force of the vested interests of the tobacco industry has been able to slow policy implementation, but the fact remains that tobacco use in developed countries had declined substantially – and the tobacco industry is now seeking to replace its lost, dying and dead smokers in developed countries with new users in the poor and developing world.

The political battle over the proposed tobacco settlement in the USA in 1998, although seemingly lost at that time, is a serious and important indication of the degree to which the international tobacco industry has declined in power and influence. It is to be expected that the public health principles espoused here will be applied progressively and more rapidly over the next decade. The result can only minimize the tobacco mortality epidemic already set in train by past events, but while tobacco remains one of the largest causes of avoidable death and disease, it remains one of the major global public health targets for all countries.

REFERENCES

1. Peto R, Lopez AD, Boreham J, Mortality from smoking world wide. *Br Med Bull* 1996; **52**: 12–21.
2. Gray N (ed), *Lung Cancer Prevention; Guidelines for Smoking Control*. Union Internationale Contre le Cancer: Geneva, 1977.
3. Glantz SA, Slade J, Bero LA et al, *The Cigarette Papers*. University of California Press: Berkeley, 1996.
4. Manley M, Glynn TJ, Shopland D, *The Impact of Cigarette Excise Taxes on Smoking Among Children and Adults: Summary Report of a National Cancer Institute Expert Panel*. National Cancer Institute: Bethesda, MD, 1993.
5. Bjartveit K, Lund KE, *The Norwegian Ban on Advertising of Tobacco Products. Has it Worked?* Norwegian Cancer Society: Oslo, 1996.
6. Benowitz NL, Henningfield JE, Establishing a nicotine threshold for addiction. *N Eng J Med* 1994; **331**: 123–4.
7. Hoffmann D, Hoffmann I, The changing cigarette, 1950–1995. *J Toxicol Environ Health* 1997; **50**: 307–64.
8. Fischer S, Speigelhalder B, Preussmann R, Tobacco specific nitrosamines in commercial cigarettes; possibilities for reducing exposure. In: *Relevance to Human Cancer of* N-*Nitroso Compounds, Tobacco Smoke and Mycotoxins*. International Agency for Research on Cancer Monograph 105: Lyon, 1991: 489–93.
9. Gray N, Boyle P, Zatonzki W, Tar concentrations in cigarettes and carcinogen content. *Lancet* 1998; **352**: 787–8.

6 Smoking cessation programmes

Philip Tønnesen

Contents

INTRODUCTION

This chapter focuses on the proper use of nicotine replacement therapy (NRT), golden rules in smoking cessation, predictors of success and the new concept of harm reduction. It should be remembered that cigarette smoking is an addiction, and for that reason smoking cessation cannot be compared with treatment of other medical conditions. NRT will produce low success rates when used without adjunctive behavioural support; however, since most smokers quit on their own and using over-the-counter (OTC) NRT, even these low success rates will have an important influence on public health. The degree of supportive adjunctive behavioural therapy parallels the actual success rate, while the relative success rate (i.e. the odds ratio between NRT and placebo) remains more or less unchanged at around a factor of two.[1]

As a preventive tool, smoking cessation is very cost-effective. Smoking cessation with NRT is approximately eight times more cost-effective per saved year compared with 300 medical treatments.[2] Also, smoking is the most important etiological factor in the development of lung cancer, accounting for almost 85% of all lung cancer cases, and has been strongly correlated with other cancers, including oral, laryngeal and bladder cancer. Around one-third of all cancer deaths are attributed to tobacco.[3] Also, tobacco use is a major contributor to chronic obstructive pulmonary disease (COPD) and coronary arteriosclerosis – diseases that often prevent lung cancer patients from undergoing curative surgery.

CLINICAL APPROACH

When a health care provider, i.e. a physician, nurse, dentist or pharmacist, meets with a smoking patient, he or she has a responsibility to interfere and discourage tobacco use.[4,5] The first thing is to ask whether or not the patient is a smoker. Already, by asking, one shows to the patient that one cares about smoking and that smoking might be of importance in relation to health. It is important that the patient's smoking be handled in a neutral way without anger or condemnation. The smoker should be informed about the risks of smoking, and the information should be individualized for the particular patient. The patient's motivation should then be assessed.

STAGES OF MOTIVATION

Some smokers are contented smokers: they do not consider quitting and do not think about the dangers of smoking. But many smokers would like to quit. Motivation to do so can be regarded as a cyclic process of changes, as described by

Table 6.1 Prochaska's and Goldstein's modified stages of motivation to quit smoking[6]

1. Do you plan to quit smoking in the next six months?
Answer 'No': Precontemplation stage

2. Do you plan to quit smoking in the next month?
Answer 'No' and 'Yes' to 1: Contemplation stage

3. Have you tried to quit in the last year?
Answer: 'Yes' and 'Yes' to 2: Preparation stage

Subjects who have already quitted:
Did you quit less than six months ago?
Answer 'Yes': Action stage

Did you quit more than six months ago?
Answer 'Yes': Maintenance stage

Prochaska and Goldstein.[6] They proposed five stages of motivation to quit: precontemplation, contemplation, preparation, action and maintenance. From three questions, it is possible to determine at which stage the individual smoker is (Table 6.1). Some smokers may move through all stages, while some may skip one or more stages. The therapist's approach to the smoker depends on the stage: in the preparation stage, support and advice about NRT and golden rules of smoking cessation are relevant, while relapse prevention strategies and support are adequate in the action stage. The use of the questions in Table 6.1 is an easy and quick way to classify the motivational stage of the individual smoker and then to apply the right treatment approach.

It might also be relevant to ask if the smoker has decided to quit completely or just to cut down. If the smoker is only interested in cutting down, the stage can be considered as the precontemplation stage.

Depending on the stage of motivation, smokers should receive brochures and other self-help material about smoking or smoking cessation. Smokers who are ready to quit tobacco use should receive minimal smoking cessation treatment, consisting of NRT, clinician-provided assistance and skills training.[7] More detailed guidelines for smoking cessation have recently been published by the Agency for Health Care Policy and Research in the USA.[8,9] However, there are some basic principles related to successful smoking cessation that are important for the therapist to consider: smokers must stop smoking completely at quit day (even one or two cigarettes per day during the first one or two weeks of cessation are usually followed by relapse):

- the use of NRT lessens withdrawal symptoms and improves cessation outcomes;
- follow-up should be arranged to prevent relapse (which is highest during the first three to six weeks, then gradually declines, similarly to other addictions);
- if the patient relapses, he or she should be encouraged to make another attempt to quit later on.

CARBON MONOXIDE IN EXPIRED AIR

In most smoking cessation studies, sustained abstinence is used as the outcome measure. It consists of the smoker's statement of not smoking now and not having smoked since the last visit, together with biochemical verification by carbon monoxide (CO) in expired air. CO measurement is an easy and inexpensive way to verify abstinence biochemically. The half-life of CO varies between four and six hours, and the cut-off value between non-smokers and smokers is usually 10 parts per million (ppm). Most non-smokers attain CO values of 1–4 ppm, and some use a cut-off value of 6 ppm. Subjects exposed to extensive passive smoking might attain values of 6–9 ppm.

CO levels are most often measured with a portable CO monitor (Bedfont Monitor, Sittingbourne, UK) in expired air after a 15 s breath-hold, with a CO value of less than 10 ppm verifying abstinence.[10] The result is displayed immediately. Calibrations have to be performed at least every six months using a 50 ppm CO test gas. False-positive values might be observed in subjects with lactose malabsorption. Although an ethanol filter is present, high ethanol concentrations in the breath might interfere with measurements. Drifting of the zero-point might be observed if many smokers are tested consecutively. Without CO monitoring, up to 10% of failures might state that they do not smoke.

NICOTINE REPLACEMENT THERAPY

The rationale for nicotine substitution is as follows. When quitting smoking, the administration of nicotine decreases withdrawal symptoms in the first months, thus allowing the subject to cope with the behavioural and psychological aspects of smoking (Table 6.2).

Withdrawal symptoms (craving for cigarettes, irritability, anxiety, depression, drowsiness, difficulty in concentrating, restlessness, headache, hunger, sleep disturbances) are usually assessed on a four-point scale (0 = not at all; 1 = mild; 2= moderate; 3 = severe).[11,12] Withdrawal symptoms often appear four to eight hours after quitting, peak during the first week (days 3–5), and then gradually decline over the next two to four weeks. Nicotine dependence is measured by the Fagerström Test of Nicotine Dependence (FTND) with a possible scoring of 0–10 (most dependent)[13] (Table 6.3).

Table 6.2 The principle of nicotine replacement therapy (NRT)

- Principle: quit cigarettes
- Use NRT to reduce withdrawal
- Break the psychological addiction
- After two to four months, stop NRT

With the nicotine replacement products used today, lower nicotine levels are attained compared with smoking (i.e. the high peak plasma levels of nicotine reached during smoking are not achieved) (Figure 6.1). Patients are weaned off nicotine replacement products

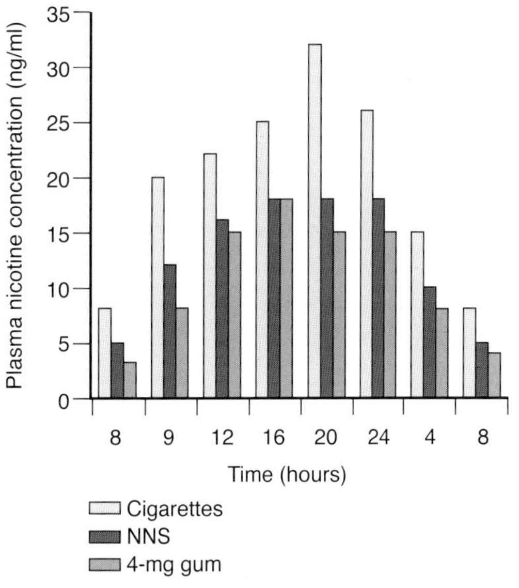

Figure 6.1
Plasma nicotine levels during cigarette smoking, nicotine nasal spray (NNS) use and 4-mg nicotine chewing gum use.

Table 6.3 Fagerström Test for Nicotine Dependence (FTND)

Item		Answer	Score
1.	How soon after you wake up do you smoke your first cigarette?	Within 5 min	3
		6–30 min	2
		31–60 min	1
		61 min or more	0
2.	Do you find it difficult to refrain from smoking in places where it is forbidden, e.g. in church, at the library, in the cinema, etc.?	Yes	1
		No	0
3.	Which cigarette would you most hate to give up?	The first one in the morning	1
		All others	0
4.	How many cigarettes per day do you smoke?	1–10	0
		11–20	1
		21–30	2
		31 or more	3
5.	Do you smoke more frequently during the first hours after waking than during the rest of the day?	Yes	1
		No	0
6.	Do you smoke if you are so ill that you are in bed most of the day (or absent from work)?	Yes	1
		No	0
		Total score	0–10

(usually over two to six weeks) when withdrawal symptoms are lessened owing to decreased dependence. The average 12-month success rate reported in most studies is about 15–25%.[8,9]

Nicotine is the drug of choice to assist smoking cessation. Results reported in a recent meta-analysis of 53 trials with 17 703 subjects, who received various forms of NRT (gum, patch, nasal spray and inhaler), indicated that NRT doubled long-term (6–12 months) quit rates.[14] The odds ratio for success of NRT compared with controls was 1.73 (95% confidence interval, CI, 1.60–1.86). The odds ratio for the different nicotine replacement products were 1.63 for gum, 1.84 for patch, 2.27 for nasal spray and 2.08 for inhaler (Table 6.4).

No studies yet have directly compared the efficacy of different forms of nicotine administration.

The nicotine replacement products described above are self-dosing systems to be used ad libi-

Table 6.4 Efficacy of NRT

- Meta-analysis controlled trials
- Success rates sustained for one year
- Odds ratio 1.73 (95% CI 1.60–1.86)
- Gum: 1.63
- Patch: 1.84
- Nasal spray: 2.27
- Inhaler: 2.08

Table 6.5 NRT formulations

Gum
2 and 4 mg content: 0.8–1.2 mg and 1.2–1.5 mg absorbed

Patch
15 mg/16 h; 21 mg/24 h

Inhaler
10 mg in one container: 4–5 mg released (2–3 mg in clinical use)

Nasal spray
0.5 mg/dose in each nostril

tum, in contrast to the patch, which 'infuses' about 1 mg of nicotine per hour at a constant rate.

Nicotine chewing gum

Gum users should only chew a piece five to ten times until they can taste the nicotine, then let the gum rest in the cheek for a few minutes, and then chew again to expose a new surface of the gum. Free nicotine can then be absorbed and reduce side-effects due to swallowed nicotine. The gum can be chewed for about 20–30 minutes. About 0.8–1.2-mg of nicotine is absorbed from a piece of 2-mg nicotine gum, and 1.2–1.5 mg of nicotine from a 4-mg piece[15] (Table 6.5). With use of nicotine gum throughout the day, blood levels of one-third (for 2-mg gum) and two-thirds (for 4-mg gum) of the nicotine obtained through smoking are achieved.[16,17]

A basic advantage of gum is the possibility of self-titrating the dose, in contrast to the patch, which delivers a fixed dose. Thus it is possible to use a piece of gum whenever it is wanted or needed during the day. The principal disadvantage of gum use is potential underdosing, which might explain the lack of effect in several trials. The approximate dose equivalent for most nicotine patches is approximately 20 pieces of the 2-mg gum, whereas the mean number of pieces of gum consumed daily is only around five or six in most studies. Thus underdosing is a plausible explanation for the lack of efficacy in several studies.[18,19]

From these observations, it would be logical to attempt to raise the consumed dose either by increasing the number of pieces of gum chewed or by using the higher-dose (4-mg) gum. In four studies comparing the 4- and 2-mg gums, the 4-mg gum was superior to the 2-mg gum for short-term outcome. Another way to increase the amount of consumed gum might be to administer it in fixed-dosage schedules as shown by Killen et al.[20]

Side-effects of gum consist mainly of mild, transient, local symptoms in the mouth, throat and stomach due to swallowed nicotine (i.e. nausea, vomiting, indigestion and hiccups). After adequate instruction, most smokers can learn to use the gum properly. However, without instructions many will discontinue use or underdose themselves.

In the Lung Health Study, among 3094 smokers who were followed for five years, the use of the 2-mg gum appeared safe and did not produce cardiovascular problems or other adverse events, even in subjects who continued to smoke and still used nicotine gum.[21]

It is suggested that smokers be instructed to stop smoking completely, use the nicotine gum on a fixed schedule (i.e. every hour, from early morning, for at least 8–10 hours) and to use extra pieces of gum whenever needed.

The optimal duration of treatment is not known; however, in most studies, the gum has been used for at least 6–12 weeks and up to one year. Individualization of treatment duration is recommended.

Nicotine transdermal patch

The nicotine patch is a fixed nicotine delivery system that releases about 1 mg of nicotine per hour for 16 hours (daytime patch) or for 24 hours (24-hour patch). Nicotine substitution is about 50% of the smoking level (21-mg patch/24 h and 15-mg patch/16 h) (Table 6.5). The nicotine curve attained in plasma with patches is flat, without the high peaks attained by cigarette smoking. It is much easier to administer the patch and to use it compared with gum, but it is not possible to self-titrate.[22] The recommended treatment duration is 8–12 weeks.

In a multicentre smoking cessation trial from the USA, examining the effect of 0, 7-mg, 14-mg and 21-mg nicotine patches, a dose–response effect of increasing nicotine dosages was reported.[23] Two large placebo-controlled trials with 600 and 1686 smokers have recently been published.[24,25] The one-year success rate was 9.3% in the active patch group versus 5.0% in the placebo patch group in the first study,[24] and 9.0% versus 6.3% in the other study.[25] Among 19 studies examining long-term (i.e. 6–12 months) smoking cessation success, 10 showed a significant outcome in favour of the nicotine patch.[22] The pooled success rate was 15.8% for active patches versus 8.8% for placebos (odds ratio 1.98; 95% CI 1.70–2.30).

Side-effects are mainly mild local skin irritation, occurring in 10–20% of subjects. In only 1.5–2% of subjects was the patch terminated owing to more persistent and severe skin irritation at the patch location.[22]

Because of its ease of use, the patch may be the first choice of nicotine delivery system today. Transdermal nicotine replacement does increase success in smoking cessation with minimal adjunctive support.

Nicotine inhaler

An inhaler consists of a mouthpiece and a plastic tube with a porous plug impregnated with nicotine, which releases nicotine vapour when air is drawn through the plug. Most of the nicotine is absorbed through the mouth and throat. Each inhaler contains 10 mg of nicotine and can release approximately 4–5 mg nicotine (Table 6.5). In clinical use, each inhaler releases approximately 2–3 mg of nicotine, and the number of inhalers used daily averages five or six. Thus, nicotine levels comparable to those found during use of the 2-mg nicotine gum are attainable (i.e. relatively low concentrations).

Few controlled trials have been conducted with nicotine inhalers. The efficacy and safety of the nicotine inhaler were examined in a double-blind, clinical, smoking cessation trial.[26] The first published study was a one-year, randomized, double-blind, placebo-controlled trial that enrolled 286 smokers. The success rates for smoking cessation were 15% and 5% at 12 months ($p < 0.001$) for active and placebo respectively. The mean nicotine substitution based on determinations after one to two weeks of therapy was 38–43% of smoking levels. The treatment was well accepted, and no serious adverse events were reported. Three other studies have confirmed the above finding, with odds ratios in favour of active treatment of 1.6, 2.2 and 1.6.[27] The inhaler may replace some of the habit patterns associated with smoking (e.g. oral and handling reinforcement), along with providing nicotine replacement. At least four inhalers should be used per day, the optimal number being 4–10 per day and the duration of use three months, with another three months of down-titration if needed. With rapid and frequent puffing, it is possible to increase the dose.

Nicotine nasal spray

The nicotine nasal spray (NNS) consists of a multidose, hand-driven, pump spray with nicotine solution. Each puff contains 0.5 mg nicotine; thus a 1 mg dose is delivered if both nostrils are sprayed as recommended (see Table 6.5). The NNS is a strong and rapid means of delivering nicotine into the body with a pharmacokinetic profile closer to cigarettes. After a single dose of 1 mg nicotine, the peak level is reached within 5–10 minutes, with average plasma trough levels of 16 ng/ml. Three published studies with the NNS indicate that the one-year success rates for active NNS versus placebo respectively were 26% and 10%, 27% and 15%, and 27% and 17%.[28,29]

This strong spray induces localized side-effects, such as sneezing, nasal secretion and irritation, and congestion, watery eyes and coughing. Up to 5% of subjects rate these side-effects as unacceptable; however, most symptoms decrease within a few days after the spray is initiated. Highly nicotine-dependent smokers might be the target group for this delivery mode of nicotine.

The NNS should be used for three months, but has been used for up to one year in some studies. The dose is from 10 to 40 puffs in each nostril per day.

PREDICTORS OF OUTCOME

In the CEASE study comprising 3575 subjects, initial cessation was a very strong predictor of long-term success, since 25% of the first-week abstainers attained 12 months' success, versus only 3% of the subjects still smoking in the first week.[30]

In a smoking cessation study comprising 259 subjects, we reported a quit rate of 0.7% after 12 months for primary failures in the study.[31] Although we offered active nicotine patches to the failures, only 57% could be persuaded to return for a 12-month follow-up visit.

In a multicentre study comprising 1686 smokers using nicotine patches, early abstinence from smoking was the strongest predictor of sustained abstinence.[32] Of first-week abstainers, 25% of 277 in the active group and 28% of 182 in the placebo group achieved long-term success, as opposed to first-week smokers (4% of 565 in the active group and 2% of 662 in the placebo group). In a similar study comprising 1200 subjects, all but one of the 96 subjects achieving long-term abstinence quit during the first week of cessation.[33]

Observations in the above four studies emphasize that the first weeks after quit-day are the most important regarding long-term outcome, which should be underlined to smokers when they have decided to quit. A week's trial of the patch, proceeding to longer use if abstinence is achieved, may be an effective policy, and might be a more cost-effective way to administer NRT.

COMBINATION OF TWO DIFFERENT NRTs

Laboratory studies have shown that the combination of nicotine gum and patch might relieve withdrawal symptoms to the same degree as when smoking.[34] A few studies have been published about combinations of two NRT products. A short-term increase in success has been observed in some, but no statistically significant 12-month increases have been found.

A dose–response effect has been observed with both the nicotine gum and patch. Even 22- and 44-mg patches have been tested with promising results after four weeks of treatment, namely success rates of 45% and 68%. In two studies, the degree of nicotine substitution was compared with outcome, and in both higher success rates were found with increasing degree of substitution. In the CEASE study comprising 3575 subjects, a higher success rate was achieved with 25-mg 16-hour patches compared with 15-mg patches.[30]

WEIGHT GAIN

Weight gain can be regarded as a withdrawal symptom due to increased hunger and increased caloric intake. However, the low and flat nicotine levels produced by NRT are not able to prevent a decrease in metabolic rate after cessation of cigarette use. A weight gain of 4–5 kg for abstainers after one year is found in most studies. About half of the participants are afraid of gaining weight, and this may be a more prominent problem for females.

Weight-gain prevention using caffeine plus ephedrine or the serotonergic anorexic drug dexfenfluramine did not increase the success rate, in contrast to what might have been expected.

OTHER DRUGS

Clonidine, an α_2-noradrenergic agonist, has been used as a smoking cessation agent in 15 controlled trials.[35] Only five studies met inclusion criteria in a recent meta-analysis comprising 722 subjects, and the odds ratio of success with clonidine versus placebo was 1.87 (95% CI 1.27–2.77). However, a high incidence of adverse effects (median 71%) occurred (i.e. dry mouth, sedation, dizziness and symptomatic postural hypotension).

The most promising drug today is bupropion (Zyban), an antidepressive agent, which has recently been approved in the USA as an anti-smoking agent.[36] It increased outcome in smoking cessation compared with placebo, and had an additive effect in combination with nicotine therapy.[37] The study comprised 893 subjects, and the 12-month success rates were 5.5% for placebo, 9.8% for 21-mg nicotine patch, 18.4% for 300 mg bupropion, and 25.5% for 300 mg bupropion plus 21-mg nicotine patch. Both groups with bupropion were more effective compared with the nicotine patch alone. However, the combination of bupropion and patch was not statistically different from bupropion alone.

Other antidepressants have been tested in smoking cessation, but no promising results have been reported. Since depression has a higher incidence among smokers and occurs as a withdrawal symptom during smoking cessation, this area will probably attract pharmaceutical companies to test newer antidepressants as possible smoking cessation agents in the near future.

HARM REDUCTION

This is a new concept, which has to be investigated further over the next few years. It could be applied to smokers who are unable to quit or who are not motivated to quit completely (i.e. recalcitrant smokers). The concept is that a reduction in the number of daily cigarettes maintained by sustained use of NRT will reduce the harm of smoking.[38] Many questions arise from this concept: Is it possible to maintain a 50% reduction in the daily number of smoked cigarettes for more than two or three months? How much

Table 6.6 NRT use: 1

1–9 cigarettes/day (not evidence-based) • 2-mg gum • Inhaler 7–9 cigarettes/day • As above, or • Patch: 10-mg/16 h or 7-mg/24 h

Table 6.7 NRT use: 2

10–20 cigarettes/day • Patch: 15-mg/16 h or 14-mg/24 h • Gum: 2- or 4-mg • Inhaler 15–20 cigarettes/day • As above, or • NNS

Table 6.8 NRT use: 3

21+ cigarettes/day • Patch: 25-mg/16 h or 21-mg/24 h • Gum: 4-mg • NNS • Inhaler • Gum as rescue in relapse situations • NRT as long-term use if needed

Table 6.9 NRT use: 4

• Use of NRT in smokers as withdrawal suppressor • Meetings, workplaces, travel • Few hours: gum, inhaler • 6 or more hours: gum, inhaler, patch • Instruct smokers to try a piece of gum/inhaler before travel starts

compensation will occur over time (i.e. will there be greater inhalation of toxic substances per cigarette smoked)? Could the motivation to quit be increased by this approach? Will the concept interfere with ordinary smoking cessation and confuse the important message about complete cessation in the first week to attain long-term success? And is this a cost-effective approach, i.e. would the cost per saved life be much higher compared with ordinary smoking cessation?

CONCLUSIONS

A pragmatic treatment schedule is shown in Tables 6.6–6.9. Since it is not possible to present a treatment approach that is evidence-based in all aspects, revisions have to be made as evidence appears from new controlled studies.

In summary, nicotine replacement therapy greatly enhances cessation outcomes; however, cessation counselling and behavioural strategies are important adjuncts for maintaining long-term cessation of smoking.

The relative effect of NRT is a doubling of the long-term success rate. Nicotine gum, patches and inhalers are first-line drugs, while nicotine nasal sprays are for more heavily dependent smokers. The patch might not be the first choice for heavily dependent smokers – at least, higher-dose patches should be used. The duration of NRT is approximately three months, with individual variations.

NRT is a very cost-effective treatment compared with several other medical treatments, and should be implemented much more widely in the future.

Particular focus on the first week after quitting might lead to a more effective use of NRT: in first-week smokers, NRT should be stopped after one to two weeks; in first-week abstainers treatment should be continued for two to three months.

Physicians and other health care providers have an obligation to discourage tobacco use in their patients and to deliver up-to-date assistance in smoking cessation.

REFERENCES

1. USDHHS, *The Health Benefits of Smoking Cessation: A Report of the Surgeon General*. DHHS CDC 90-8416, US Department of Health and Human Services, Public Health Service, Centers for Disease Control, Center for Chronic Disease Prevention and Health Promotion, Office on Smoking and Health: Rockville, MD, 1990.
2. Fiscella K, Frank P, Are nicotine patches cost effective. *JAMA* 1996; **275**: 1247–51.
3. Peto R, Lopez AD, Boreham J et al, *Mortality from Tobacco in Developed Countries 1950–2000*. Oxford University Press: Oxford, 1994.
4. WHO, Guidelines for controlling and monitoring the tobacco epidemic. Pre-publication draft. WHO: Geneva, 1995.
5. Tønnesen P, Gritz ER, Gray N, Nielsen IR, Smoking prevention and cessation. In: *Clinical and Biological Basis of Lung Cancer Prevention* (Martinet Y, Hirsch FR, Martinet N et al, eds). Birkhäuser Verlag: Basel, 1998: 15–29.
6. Prochaska JO, Goldstein MG, Process of smoking cessation. Implications for clinicians. *Clin Chest Med* 1991; **12**: 727–35.
7. American College of Chest Physicians, American Thoracic Society, Asia Pacific Society of Respirology, Canadian Thoracic Society, European Respiratory Society International Union against Tuberculosis and Lung Diseases. Smoking and Health: a physician's responsibility. A statement of the Joint Committee on Smoking and Health. *Eur Respir J* 1995; **8**: 1808–11.
8. USDHHS, *Tobacco and the Clinician: Interventions for Medical and Dental Practice*. NCI 94-3693. US Department of Health and Human Services, Public Health Service, National Institutes of Health: Rockville, MD, 1994.
9. Fiore MC, Bailey WC, Cohen SJ et al, *Smoking Cessation*. Clinical Practice Guideline 18, AHCPR 96-0692, US Department of Health and Human Services, Public Health Service, Agency for Health Care Policy and Research: Rockville, 1996.
10. Jarvis MJ, Russell MA, Saloojee Y, Expired air carbon monoxide: a simple breath test of tobacco smoke intake. *BMJ* 1980; **281**: 484–5.
11. APA, *Diagnostic and Statistical Manual of Mental Disorders – IV*. American Psychiatric Association: Washington, DC, 1994.
12. Hughes JR, Gust SW, Skoog K et al, Symptoms of tobacco withdrawal. A replication and extension. *Arch Gen Psychiatry* 1991; **48**: 52–9.
13. Fagerström KO, Heatherton TF, Kozlowski LT. Nicotine addiction and its assessment. *Ear Nose Throat J* 1991; **69**: 763–8.
14. Silagy C, Mant D, Fowler G, Lancaster T, Nicotine replacement therapy for smoking cessation. *Cochrane Library*. Update Software: Oxford, 1998; 2.
15. McNabb ME, Ebert RV, McCusker K, Plasma nicotine levels produced by chewing nicotine gum. *JAMA* 1982; **248**: 865–8.
16. McNabb ME, Chewing nicotine gum for 3 months: What happens to plasma nicotine levels? *Can Med Assoc J* 1984; **131**: 589–92
17. Tønnesen P, Fryd V, Hansen M et al, Two and four mg nicotine chewing gum and group counseling in smoking cessation: an open, randomized, controlled trial with a 22 month follow-up. *Addict Behav* 1988; **13**: 17–27.
18. Tønnesen P, Fryd V, Hansen M et al, Effect of nicotine chewing gum in combination with group counseling on the cessation of smoking. *N Engl J Med* 1988; **318**: 15–8.
19. Puska P, Bjorkqvist S, Koskela K. Nicotine

containing chewing gum in smoking cessation: a double-blind trial with half year follow-up. *Addict Behav* 1979; **4**: 141–6.

20. Killen JD, Fortmann SP, Newman B, Varady A, Evaluation of a treatment approach combining nicotine gum with self-guided behavioural treatments for smoking relapse prevention. *J Consult Clin Psychol* 1990; **58**: 85–92.
21. Murray RP, Bailey WC, Daniels K et al, Safety of nicotine polacrilex gum used by 3094 participants in the Lung Health Study. *Chest* 1996; **109**: 438–45.
22. Fagerstrøm KO, Säwe U, Tønnesen P, Therapeutic use of nicotine patches: efficacy and safety. *J Smoking-Related Dis* 1992; **3**: 247–61.
23. Transdermal Nicotine Study Group, Transdermal nicotine for smoking cessation. *JAMA* 1991; **22**: 3133–8.
24. Russell MAH, Stableton JA, Feyerabend C et al, Targeting heavy smokers in general practice: randomized controlled trial of transdermal nicotine patches. *BMJ* 1993; **306**: 1308–12.
25. Imperial Cancer Research Fund General Practice Research Group, Effectiveness of a nicotine patch in helping people to stop smoking: results of a randomized trial in general practice. *BMJ* 1993; **306**: 1304–8.
26. Tønnesen P, Nørregaard J, Mikkelsen K et al, A double-blind trial of a nicotine inhaler for smoking cessation. *JAMA* 1993; **269**: 1268–71.
27. Schneider NG, Olmstead R, Nilsson F et al, Efficacy of a nicotine inhaler in smoking cessation: a double-blind, placebo-controlled trial. *Addiction* 1996; **91**: 1293–306.
28. Sutherland G, Stapleton JA, Russell MAH et al, Randomised controlled trial of a nasal nicotine spray in smoking cessation. *Lancet* 1992; **340**: 324–9.
29. Blondal T, Franzon M, Westin A et al, Controlled trial of nicotine nasal spray with long term follow-up. *Am Rev Respir Dis* 1993; **147**: A806.
30. Tønnesen P, Paoletti P, Gustavsson G et al, Higher dosage nicotine patches increase one-year smoking cessation rates: results from the European CEASE trial. *Eur Respir J* 1999; **13**: 238–46.
31. Nørregaard J, Tønnesen P, Simonsen K et al, Smoking habits in relapsed subjects from a smoking cessation trial after one year. *Br J Addiction* 1992; **87**: 1189–94.
32. Yudkin PL, Jones L, Lancaster T, Fowler GH, Which smokers are helped to give up smoking using transdermal nicotine patches? Results from a randomized, double-blind, placebo-controlled trial. *Br J Gen Pract* 1996; **46**: 145–8.
33. Stapleton JA, Russell MAH, Feyerabend C et al, Dose effects and predictors of outcome in a randomised trial of nicotine patches in general practice. *Addiction* 1995; **90**: 31–42.
34. Fagerström KO, Schneider NG, Lunnel E, Effectiveness of nicotine patch and nicotine gum as individual versus combined treatment for tobacco withdrawal symptoms. *Psychopharmacology* 1993; **110**: 251–7.
35. Glourlay SG, Stead LF, Benowitz NL, A meta-analysis of clonidine for smoking cessation. *Cochrane Library*. Update Software: Oxford, 1997; 1.
36. Gawin F, Comptom M, Byck R, Buspirone reduces smoking. *Arch Gen Psychiatry* 1989; **46**: 288.
37. Hurt RD, Sachs DP, Glover ED et al, A comparison of sustained-release bupropion and placebo for smoking cessation. *N Engl J Med* 1997; **337**: 1195–202.
38. Fagerström KO, Tejding R, Westin Å, Lunell E, Aiding reduction of smoking with nicotine replacement medications: hope for the recalcitrant smoker? *Tobacco Control* 1997; **6**: 311–16.

Transition to early lung cancer management: Is the molecular diagnostic revolution going to change lung cancer care?

James L Mulshine, Melvyn S Tockman

Contents

INTRODUCTION

Lung cancer is the leading cause of cancer death in the USA. The 160 000 deaths from this disease in 1997 will exceed the combined mortality of breast, colon, ovarian, cervix and prostate cancer.[1] Similar trends exist for most other developed nations. Tobacco-derived carcinogens cause about 90% of lung cancer deaths, and represent the single most preventable cause of excess mortality.[2] Lung cancer remains a major public health problem, despite enormous public education efforts. According to the US Centers for Disease Control and Prevention, primary prevention of youth smoking is a priority, since only about 3% of smokers are successful each year in discontinuing the habit.[3] Nevertheless, since the publication of the first Surgeon General's report on smoking, more than three decades ago, over 40 million smokers in the USA have responded to the public health message by stopping their smoking. Yet, as a result of accrued bronchial epithelial cell injury, former smokers maintain a persistently elevated risk for lung cancer. For the first time, major thoracic oncology centers have diagnosed more new cases of lung cancer in former smokers than in current smokers.[4] Even if all smoking were to abruptly stop, lung cancer would remain a major source of mortality for decades, both because of the insidious, persistent nature of the carcinogenic injury and because of the modest success of treatment approaches for this cancer.[5] This chapter reviews the development and the prospects for early lung cancer detection. To complement the important public health benefits of smoking cessation, new efforts of comparable intensity are required to improve the health prospects for the former smokers who still face a high probability of premature death from lung cancer. Improving the outcome with this disease by defining early lung cancer management approaches could result in considerable societal benefit.

HISTORICAL SUMMARY

With chest X-ray detection, most new lung cancers are found with at least regionally metastatic disease. Evaluations initiated after clinical presentation of symptoms or signs of lung cancer are associated with an even higher occurrence of regional or distant metastases. Over the last 30 years, aggressive treatment of advanced lung cancer has not resulted in major reductions in disease-related mortality. Delayed awareness of lung cancer combined with the limited curative potential of existing systemic treatments accounts for the five-year survival rate of only 13%.[1] A key to improving outcomes for this disease is to develop technology that routinely identifies preinvasive lung cancer. The nature of lung cancer while it is still confined to the airway has emerged as a major focus for molecular biologists. The concept of regional airway injury due to chronic tobacco exposure was termed 'field cancerization' back in the 1950s by Slaughter.[6] 'Field cancerization' was an abstract concept that was useful at a theoretical level to convey the broad nature of the epithelial injury from exposure to tobacco combustion products. With today's molecular tools, a more concrete assessment of bronchial epithelial injury can be achieved.

The pioneering work of Saccomanno and Auerbach extrapolated to the lung compartment the cytomorphological progression model developed by Papanicolaou for the early detection of cervical cancer.[7,8] With the possible exception of modern helical CT imaging, chest X-ray detection of lung cancer has not substantially changed over the last 30 years. In the 1950s and 1960s, numerous trials of radiographic screening had failed to reduce lung cancer mortality. Refractory to treatment, the outcome of metastatic disease with median survivals measured in months is a known problem. These factors drove the interest of Saccomanno and others in the 1960s to propose better early lung cancer detection.[7] Saccomanno worked with a large population of uranium miners who were exposed to high doses of radioactivity prior to the implementation of industrial exposure guidelines. Beginning with the cytological criteria that had been established for cervical cancer detection, Saccomanno defined criteria for the progression of epidermoid lung cancer. In addition, he devised a technique to recover intact bronchial epithelial cells from the viscous, mucoid sputum specimen. Further, he defined fixation conditions to preserve cytomorphological features of the bronchial epithelial cells which allowed for excellent preservation of nuclear detail. Preliminary trials using these techniques in the early 1970s suggested that sputum cytology analysis was highly specific, especially for early squamous lung cancer – the most common lung cancer cell type at that time. These promising findings led to the large NCI-sponsored randomized trials conducted at Johns Hopkins, Memorial–Sloan Kettering and the Mayo Clinic. The focus of these trials was to determine if screening with two clinical diagnostic tests (sputum cytology and chest X-ray screening) resulted in a favorable reduction in lung cancer mortality compared with radiographic screening alone. As is well known, the outcome of that trial showed a favorable effect on the detection rate for many clinical parameters. For the most important outcome, namely deaths from lung cancer, there was no significant long-term effect on reducing lung cancer-related mortality. The conclusion from those trials was that lung cancer screening using standard clinical chest X-ray and sputum cytology did not work.[8–10] The yield from adding sputum cytology to chest X-ray screening was an increase in diagnostic sensitivity of only 10–15%.

This negative trial result dampened interest in the area of early lung cancer detection for many years. As we have recently reviewed, although a number of international studies have subsequently addressed this issue, none resulted in a conclusion different from that of the NCI-cooperative trial.[11,12] The difference in successful cytomorphological screening for cervical cancer and failure in lung cancer merits consideration. An obvious explanation is that the morphological progression seen in squamous cancers of the lung, as in those of the cervix, is not shared by other histologies. In lung cancer, the cytomorphological progression for cell types other than squamous cancer has still not been defined. Since the large majority of lung cancers are no longer squamous cancers, the benefit of detection of the squamous subset is diluted by the large number of non-squamous lung cancer cases.

CURRENT STANDARD CLINICAL LUNG CANCER MANAGEMENT

To this day, with only the rarest exception, the fortunate individuals who are cured of lung cancer were diagnosed with early stage disease. Surgical resection is employed when the full extent of the cancer can be safely removed. The majority of lung cancer patients are diagnosed with more advanced disease than can be managed with surgery. The non-surgical management of patients with lung cancer involves a significant professional challenge, since the outcome is likely to involve the death of the patient. In this instance, the clinical course is measured only in months, despite the skill and attentiveness of the practitioner. The virulence of this most commonly lethal cancer has been a constant since the lung cancer epidemic emerged at the beginning of this century. Lack of progress in treating advanced lung cancer was shown by a recent study. To evaluate the survival outcome, a careful balance of the prognostic features for a cohort of patients, treated for lung cancer in the Intramural Program of the NCI in the decade after the mid-1970s, was compared with a cohort of patients for a decade beyond 1985.[13] The survival curves from the two eras were nearly identical. As reflected in the sobering historical analysis of the NCI Intramural Group, progress in the treatment of this disease has been difficult.

Clinical research in lung cancer management has clearly produced refinements in surgical, radiotherapeutic and medical management. Current lung cancer treatments can be delivered to appropriate patient groups with a more favorable therapeutic index than in the past. The ability to deliver lung cancer therapy with less morbidity is a significant research accomplishment. To build on this modest progress, we must understand the reasons for the failure of current lung cancer clinical management. From this perspective, both the failure of treatment for advanced (metastatic) cancer and the vast number of former smokers still at risk for lung cancer mandate a reconsideration of how to achieve meaningful early lung cancer detection.

FUTURE DEVELOPMENTS: FOCUS ON MANAGING EARLY LUNG CANCER

The natural history of epithelial cancer is that the transformed genome of a single initiated cell provides a local growth advantage that, over the course of years, gradually expands and evolves to a critical tumor burden. In general, the larger the existing tumor burden, the easier it is to make a diagnosis of lung cancer. Unfortunately, the likelihood of a favorable outcome also deteriorates with increasing tumor burden. To provide the greatest probability of arresting early lung cancer (before metastatic spread), an early diagnosis should be made while the premalignant cells are confined to the epithelium.

Lung cancer is the result of the chronic carcinogen exposure to a large surface area with a range of normal respiratory epithelial cell populations. The many histologies of lung cancer probably reflect this complicated biology.

Currently, the precise sequence of genetic events leading to the development of an invasive cancer remains speculative. We know that a variety of carcinogens can interact with any of the normal cell populations found in the bronchial epithelium. Depending on the carcinogen exposure and the host's ability to handle xenobiotic injury, the natural history of the cancer will be variable. Effective strategies for early lung cancer detection must reconcile these alternative pathways to carcinogenesis.

MANAGING THE COSTS OF SCREENING

Beyond the issue of cost per assay, the direct and indirect costs of the clinical management associated with false-negative and false-positive assay determinations are significant. Achieving a balance between increasing the sensitivity of detection for early lung cancer, responsibly consuming health care resources as well as minimizing the misdiagnosis of screening subjects are major challenges for population-based cancer management approaches. In developing population screening approaches for cancer detection, it is critical to educate both the medical community and the general public about the goals and nature of this type of research. During the early stage in the development of early cancer detection technology, there will be problems with overly sensitive, insufficiently specific assays. Examples of this problem are currently evident with prostate-specific antigen (PSA) screening for prostate cancer, where the risk-to-benefit aspects of this early detection effort are controversial.[14] The ultimate benefit to society from comprehensive early cancer detection will only be achieved by strategic management through successively more specific testing, rather than doing nothing while awaiting an elusive 'holy grail' – a single test with perfect sensitivity and perfect specificity.

Table 7.1 Issues with population-based lung cancer screening

- Identify molecular marker indicative of altered gene expression (protein, RNA, DNA)
- Select specimen collection, preparation and preservation method to optimize marker preservation
- Define economical, high-throughput diagnostic assay
- Validate utility with prospective study
- Integrate diagnostic approach with appropriate clinical intervention
- Validate the integrated management approach for evidence of lung cancer-related mortality

Fortunately, with improving molecular biology, the question of translating laboratory discovery to lung cancer screening has reemerged. The previously disappointing results from conducting screening with highly specific diagnostic tests (sputum cytology and chest X-ray) illustrates how one negative collaborative trial could arrest research interest for over a decade. A thoughtful developmental approach is essential to prevent this field from again losing support. In anticipating sources of problems with sputum immunocytochemical analysis as a screening tool, incorporating the lessons from the long experience with the refinement of cervical cancer screening may be instructive.

Fundamental to translating laboratory techniques to population lung cancer screening, there are a variety of practical issues that need to be addressed. Some examples of such issues are listed in Table 7.1. Automated imaging of cervical cytology smears has led to accurate, high-throughput screening for cervical cancer. Since detection of lung cancer biomarkers by evaluation of airway epithelial cells requires preservation of cellular integrity, early detection of lung cancer also may require the incorporation of an automated, computer-assisted microscopy platform. Only with recent breakthroughs in computer technology has this task become a realistic goal. Cytometric image processing is a complex computational task, and success in this application is in large part due to the exponential reduction in the cost of computing over the last decade. The clinical opportunity now is to try to exploit computer capabilities to conduct routine cytological image analysis that defines the cells in a sputum specimen of bronchial epithelial origin. Assay of these cells of interest must be completed rapidly enough to enable analysis of the requisite number of samples for population-based screening. While automated image analysis of cervical cytology has contributed greatly to this technology, cervical cancer differs from lung cancer, since squamous cell is the single dominant histological type of cervical cancer. A cytomorphological technique comparable to the approaches used in cervical cancer screening has already been reported with sputum analysis.[15] At this time, though, the benefit of this purely cytomorphometric approach is restricted to detecting squamous lung cancer. Since the dominant histology of lung cancer in the USA is now adenocarcinoma, and the preinvasive morphological changes of adenocarcinoma are not known, lung cancer is a much greater challenge for image analysis techniques than is squamous cancer of the cervix. A clinician using a cytomorphological technique could reassure a patient only about the likelihood of a squamous cancer, but no statement could be made about small cell cancer or adenocarcinomas. Given the vexing issues that could arise in that circumstance, improving the approach to detect all forms of lung cancer seems essential. A useful lesson from the NCI-sponsored clinical trial is that, in order for a lung cancer screening test to be ultimately successful in significantly reducing lung cancer-related mortality, the detection tool must be capable of detecting all lung cancer cell types.[16] From a reproducibility, speed and cost perspective, it will be critical to employ a computer-driven image analysis system, but, to achieve a more sensitive detection capability, additional aspects of the biology of early lung cancer will have to be incorporated into the image analysis approach.

The status of lung cancer biomarker targets has recently been reviewed,[17] and there are a number of promising directions to consider. Along with a number of co-workers, we have reported the result of a prospective, non-concurrent trial using an immunocytochemical approach to early detection of lung cancer.[18] We have worked together with a group of talented investigators for the last decade to improve this approach.[19–24] The immunocytochemical analysis for the overexpression of the antigen heterogeneous nuclear ribonucleoprotein (hnRNP) A2/B1 by computerized image analysis, described by Tockman, is being commercialized under a Collaborative Research and Development Agreement between the National Cancer Institute, Johns Hopkins University, the Moffitt Cancer Center at the University of South Florida, the institutions of the Lung Cancer Early Detection Working Group and Chiron Diagnostics. This dedicated effort to develop an automated, sputum-based, immunocytological image analysis system for population screening for lung cancer has created the infrastructure required to routinely identify preinvasive lung cancer. In the three independent cohorts studied with this cellular-based diagnostic approach, the accuracy for detecting lung cancer is between 70% and 90%, with a diagnostic sensitivity of between 80% and 90%.[18,19] We have performed a series of studies to try to understand the biological basis for this assay success.

To achieve early lung cancer detection, the goal is to find differentially expressed determinants that reveal the presence of the early clonal populations of lung cancer cells. We have detected differential expression of hnRNP in the epithelial lining cells of the tracheobronchial tree of individuals who later developed lung cancer. Our successful early detection experience has been with analysis of bronchial epithelial cells recovered from the sputum. The sputum-based immunocytochemical assay is done in a precise, standardized fashion. Washed cells from a sputum specimen are spun down on a slide. In the original assay configuration, a cytotechnologist surveys each slide and marks the location of the morphologically recognizable, bronchial epithelial 'sentinel cells' that demonstrate 'regular metaplasia.' Using an image analysis algorithm that was optimized for the staining reagents used in this assay, the hnRNP content (immunoreactivity) in these 'sentinel cells' is quantitated at two wavelengths.[23] Using a discriminant function, values combined from the two-wavelength analysis that exceed a predefined cutoff are called positive and the cases with lesser values are considered negative. This approach was employed in the prospective analyses of the three independent cohorts evaluated to date with the sputum immunocytochemical approach.[18,19] The difference between this approach and the conventional cytomorphological approaches is that the endpoint in the sputum immunocytochemical assay is the relative level of antigen expression in a defined population of sentinel cells. In conventional cytomorphological analysis, done either by a cytologist or by a computer, the endpoint is a distribution of cell measurements. The experience at Johns Hopkins showed that the atypical cells found on cytology spontaneously reverted back to normal in over 80% of the cases. In contrast, the status of hnRNP-expressing cells measured by the immunohistochemical technique rarely changed spontaneously.[25]

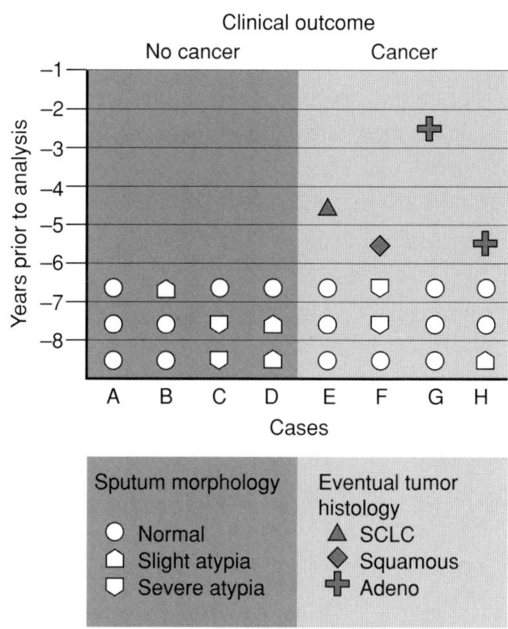

Figure 7.1
Schematic representation of the selection process used to identify a monoclonal antibody that detects early cancer cells.[7] Sputa specimens containing exfoliated bronchial epithelial prospectively acquired in a high-risk population were kept until clinical follow-up could establish what sputum came from individuals who did and did not go on to develop cancer. In a non-concurrent, prospective study, 22 positive cancer cases and 40 negative never-cancer cases showed a highly significant correlation of marker expression with actual cancer outcome; the odds ratio is 70, with a 95% confidence interval of 10.5–297.8.[7]

In Figure 7.1, we show a cartoon of the matrix for selecting the monoclonal antibody used for the early lung cancer detection approach that we have previously reported.[18,19] To select informative early detection markers, we assayed marker expression prospectively in an archive of annual sputum samples obtained over several years from a population of heavy smokers studied at Johns Hopkins during the early lung cancer detection trial. The long- term cancer status information for the study participants was determined during a total subsequent follow-up up of eight years.[18,19] From that study, we learned that in the natural history of sputum atypia the majority of atypical sputum cells revert back to a normal appearance without evolving to cancer.[8] As shown schematically in Figure 7.1, cytological progression was found rarely to be an informative marker of early lung cancer. Sputum morphology was unsuccessful as an early cancer biomarker owing to non-specific morphological changes that bore little relation to ultimate cancer outcome. For detection of early cancer, as morphology is waning as an informative tool, biomarkers are waxing in their clinical utility. Many genetic lesions reported with established lung cancer are now commonly reported in preneoplastic settings.

Applying ever more sensitive molecular diagnostics, a variety of genetic lesions are being found in normal appearing bronchial epithelium, including trisomy of chromosome 7, allelic deletions and microsatellite alterations.[26–29] In the preliminary analysis of our sputum-based early detection trial using the marker selected with the matrix outlined in Figure 7.1, most of the cancer cases were early stage, detected by overexpression of the cellular protein hnRNP A2/B1 without any evidence of morphological atypia.[19] Many lines of recent evidence suggest that the early clonal changes in the carcinogen-exposed airway may be accurately reflected by molecular markers in exfoliated sputum cells. New molecular approaches to early lung cancer detection are poised to take advantage of new diagnostic technologies that have the potential for rapid, accurate, low-cost screening.

Another aspect of this challenge is that, in the general population, the probability of developing a lung cancer is typically less than 0.001%. From a statistical perspective, using clinical features to define populations with higher risks of developing lung cancer improves the prospects for assay success and reduces the clinical trial size required to validate the effectiveness of early detection tools. Conversely, using a higher-risk cohort for clinical investigation means that the performance characteristics of an early detection assay are likely to be better then would be expected for assay precision in screening a general-risk population. The pragmatic decision to concentrate on high-risk populations for lung cancer screening also implies accepting that the cancers occurring in low-risk populations may not be detected. Consideration of the pre-test probability of a positive diagnostic assay is a critical issue to be defined in the evaluation of the utility of a particular test in a particular clinical setting. Using clinical features to define populations at high risk for developing lung cancer can increase the a priori chance of detecting a cancer by only an order of magnitude compared with other heavy smokers. When starting with such a vast at-risk population (every other adult in America is an ever-smoker, including both current and former smokers), reducing the size of a target screening population involves massive economic consequences. So, as with any other public health effort, the strategy for defining the optimal population for lung cancer screening has to be defined and validated carefully.

A priority for screening approaches is to ensure that the sensitivity of the process is high, while performing the screening procedure at a reasonable cost. The calibration issue of where to set a level of detection is a critical but unresolved question. The conclusion from the previous sputum plus chest X-ray screening study was that these diagnostic tests were highly specific, but insufficiently sensitive – frequently not detecting cancer until it was advanced and metastatic. High sensitivity for neoplastic changes prior to metastatic spread is a requirement for a successful lung cancer screening test. Since the precise time at which a tumor evolves from localized to metastatic cannot be established with certainty, one can only speculate about how to routinely handle this situation. Screening measures will have to be applied in a 'healthy', non-patient cohort before the probability of developing has occurred for the average person. As this research matures, the dynamic nature of population-based management will become evident. Depending on the risk profile of the cohort, the cost and side-effects of the interventions, and the specifics of the management will evolve as the performance characteristics of the components improve.

IMPACT OF MICROPROCESSOR INTEGRATED BIOCHIP TECHNOLOGY

A revolution in diagnostic technology is being spawned by the integration of improved computer capability with the ability to conduct biological assays on silicon dioxide microchips.[30,31] The lower cost of computer technology makes both the complex computational challenge of image analysis and the possibility of full assay automation feasible. Assay techniques are evolving with remarkable speed and with the potential to be more efficient, comprehensive and economical. This prospect is moving beyond the medical and scientific community, and is capturing the attention of the investment community, as reflected in a recent issue of *Fortune*.[32] 'Biochip technology' is emerging as a practical tool with the capability of performing large numbers of hybridization or binding reactions on a single clinical specimen, with the potential for enormous throughput in a timely and economical fashion. The first clinical application of biochip instrumentation was reported recently in the evaluation of polymorphisms of the HIV-1 protease gene. Many competing biochip approaches are simultaneously being developed. Although formidable technical and societal obstacles remain, the refinement of this technology is proceeding at a rate reminiscent of the early computer industry. We now have the opportunity to evaluate whether such technology could enable significant improvements in speed and accuracy for cancer detection and management.

This feasibility of moving to routine detection of lung cancer while it is in its early cellular phase is enhanced by the ongoing revolution in molecular diagnostics. In addition, the ability to diagnose truly early lung cancer also provides a situation in which local therapies are relevant, since the full extent of early cancerous involvement is limited to the epithelium. In most cancer settings, control of localized disease has been possible. As a result, for a particular organ site, long-term cancer survival strongly reflects the frequency of success in detecting early stage cancer. Conversely, diseases such as lung and pancreatic cancer that are seldom found in the early stages have high mortality rates. To complement the long-term benefit of primary lung cancer prevention, especially for the large cohort of former smokers, developing more effective clinical lung cancer management strategies is essential for nearer-term mortality reduction.

IS LUNG CHEMOPREVENTION WITH A FAVORABLE THERAPEUTIC INDEX POSSIBLE?

The introduction of serum-based screening for early prostate cancer was problematic owing to the morbidity of the downstream clinical management options for the PSA-detected cases.[14] To avoid this scenario with early lung cancer detection approaches, specific interventions with modest morbidity appropriate for the stage at which early lung cancer is detected must be developed.

With the developing capability of routinely detecting early lung cancer as it arises on the respiratory epithelial surface, new possibilities evolve for epithelium-directed interventions as well. A leading candidate for upper aerodigestive chemoprevention, based on the positive clinical trial results from the MD Anderson Hospital, is the use of orally administered 13-*cis*-retinoic acid.[33–35] While large clinical trials are evaluating the benefit of this strategy, it is apparent that the side-effects of headache, itchiness and chelitis compromise the utility of this drug for chemoprevention. In collaborations with collaborators at NIH, including Dedrick and DeLuca, we have reviewed the salient issues involved in developing an aerosolized chemoprevention approach to lung cancer.[36] The pharmacology of oral delivery of retinoids to the bronchial epithelium is undermined both by high enterohepatic clearance (> 75% first pass) and by extensive serum binding by albumin (which rapidly binds 99.9% of the free retinoids).[36] Albumin greatly reduces the in vitro antiproliferative effect of retinoids,[37] so we have speculated that alternative drug delivery approaches may greatly improve the prospects for controlling early lung cancer. Aerosol delivery technology has greatly improved over the last decade, so that uniform delivery to the entire pulmonary epithelium is more achievable. There is an intuitive logic in exploiting the same route of delivery for the chemoprevention agent as followed by the offending carcinogen.

The dynamics of regional drug delivery have been modeled, which is relevant since aerosolized drug delivery represents a specialized example. The critical feature of the aerosol approach is that a high first-pass concentration of aerosolized drug is delivered to the clonal populations of early cancer cells on the bronchial epithelium. At the same time the drug formulation must insure that a relatively low drug exposure of normal tissues occurs via spillover of the drug into the systemic circulation. The predictions from this model may guide aspects of candidate drug selection. From a tumor biology perspective, the selection of fenretinide is attractive because it is more potent in stimulating apoptosis.[38] The concept of programmed cell death or apoptosis has been catapulted to critical attention in the cancer biology community in recognition of the central importance of this regulatory mechanism to the pathogenesis of cancer.[39] The ability to actively eliminate clonal populations of malignant cells from the respiratory epithelium by apoptosis, which we call 'clonal clearance', may be the fundamental goal for the long-term success of lung cancer chemoprevention. Apoptosis in lung cancer cells can be modulated by many other drugs, so the clinician may need a wide array of clinical intervention tools for direct epithelial delivery in managing individuals who live long term with dynamic field cancerization changes in their airway epithelium. The formal clinical evaluation of these issues will help define the most important variables to predict successful pharmacological intervention with lung cancer confined to the airway.

The initial retinoid experience may guide the subsequent development of additional epithelium-directed chemoprevention approaches. The ability to compare the effect of one retinoid with that of another is dependent on the availability of sensitive tools to establish the actual effect of the retinoids on the target bronchial epithelial cells. In refining the best agent, dose, formulation and delivery system for aerosolized delivery, biomarkers developed for early lung cancer detection may also be adapted to allow precise yet economical monitoring of the response by the bronchial epithelium, using the new diagnostic instrumentation. Aerosolized chemotherapy delivery has already demonstrated an improved therapeutic index in Japanese clinical trials using 5-fluorouracil in the treatment of local and regionally advanced lung cancer.[40] The clinical precedent from the infectious disease literature with aerosolized drug delivery suggests a cautious basis for optimism for this type of approach.[36]

For lung cancer prevention cohorts identified either with new-generation diagnostics or by traditional clinical risk profiles, long-term compliance with a chemoprevention program will be sustainable only if the morbidity is modest. Clinical trials with aerosolized chemoprevention agents will be starting soon to evaluate the actual benefit of these approaches. Achieving improvement with the therapeutic index is the goal, so that the low morbidity of aerosolized delivery of chemoprevention agents for early lung cancer can increase the benefit of the rapidly evolving molecular diagnostics.

In closing, achieving more effective lung cancer outcomes will require the integrated and simultaneous development of both diagnostic and intervention capabilities, but promising candidate tools are rapidly evolving. While redoubled efforts at primary lung cancer prevention are appropriate with children and current smokers, improved management options for former smokers to reduce their lung cancer mortality would be an important step forward.

REFERENCES

1. Parker SL, Tong T, Bolden S, Wingo PA, Cancer statistics, 1997. *CA Cancer J Clin* 1997; **47**: 5–25.
2. Peto R, Lopez AD, Boreham J et al, Mortality from tobacco in developed countries: indirect estimation from national vital statistics. *Lancet* 1992; **339**: 1268–88.
3. United States Centers for Disease Control and Prevention, Cigarette smoking among adults – United States, 1993. *MMWR* 1994; **43**: 925–30.
4. Papadimitrakopoulou VA, Hong WK, Biomarkers as intermediate endpoints in chemoprevention trials. In: *Clinical and Biological Basis of Lung Cancer Prevention* (Martinet Y, Vignaud JM, Martinet N et al, eds). Birkhäuser: Basel, 1998: 305–12.
5. Gaffney M, Altshuler B, Examination of the role of cigarette smoke in lung carcinogenesis. *J Natl Cancer Inst* 1988; **80**: 925–31.
6. Slaughter DP, Southwick HW, Smejkal W, 'Field cancerization' in oral stratified squamous epithelium. *Cancer* 1953; **6**: 963–8.
7. Saccomanno G, Archer VE, Auerbach O, Development of carcinoma of the lung or reflected in exfoliated cells. *Cancer* 1974; **33**: 256–70.
8. Bailar JC, Early lung cancer cooperative study group: early lung cancer detection. Summary and conclusion. *Am Rev Respir Dis* 1984; **130**: 565.
9. Bailar JC, Editorial. Screening for lung cancer – Where are we now? *Am Rev Respir Dis* 1984; **130**: 541.
10. Tockman MS, Levin ML Frost JK et al, Screening and detection of lung cancer. In: *Lung Cancer* (Aisner J, ed). Churchill Livingstone: New York, 1985: 25–40.
11. Tockman MS, Mulshine JL, Early lung cancer detection: status and new strategies. *Prim Care Cancer* 1998; **18**: 22–5.
12. Mulshine JL, Zhou J, Treston AM et al, New approaches to the integrated management of early lung cancer. *Hematol Oncol Clin North Am* 1997; **11**: 235–52.
13. Chute JP, Venzon DJ, Hankins L et al, Outcomes of patients with small cell lung cancer during 20 years of clinical research at the US National Cancer Institute. *Mayo Clin Proc* 1997; **72**: 901–12.
14. Woolf SH, Screening for prostate cancer with prostate-specific antigen. *N Engl J Med* 1995; **333**: 1401–6.
15. Payne PW, Sebo TJ, Doudkine A et al, Sputum screening by quantitative microscopy: a re examination of a portion of the national cancer insti-

tute cooperative early lung cancer study. *Mayo Clin Proc* 1997; **72**: 697–704.

16. Tockman MS, Mulshine JL, Sputum screening by quantitative microscopy: a new dawn for lung cancer detection. Editorial. *Mayo Clin Proc* 1997; **72**: 788–90.
17. Hirsch FR, Brambilla E, Gray N et al, Prevention and early detection of lung cancer – clinical aspects. *Lung Cancer* 1997; **17**: 163–74.
18. Tockman, MS, Gupta PK, Myers JD et al, Sensitive and specific monoclonal antibody recognition of human lung cancer antigen on preserved sputum cells: a new approach to early lung cancer detection. *J Clin Oncol* 1988; **6**: 1685–93.
19. Tockman MS, Mulshine JL, Piantadosi S et al, LCEWDG Investigators, YTC Investigators, Prospective detection of preclinical lung cancer: results from two studies of hnRNP overexpression. *Clin Cancer Res* 1997; **3**: 2237–46.
20. Zhou J, Jensen SM, Steinberg SM et al, Expression of early lung cancer detection marker p31 in neoplastic and non-neoplastic respiratory epithelium. *Lung Cancer* 1996; **14**: 85–97.
21. Zhou J, Mulshine JL, Unsworth EJ et al, Purification and characterization of a protein that permits early detection of lung cancer. *J Biol Chem* 1996; **271**: 10 760–6.
22. Montuenga L, Zhou J, Avis I et al, The early lung cancer marker, heterogeneous nuclear ribonucleoprotein (hnRNP) A2/B1 is an oncofetal antigen. *J Respir Cell Mol Biol* 1998; **19**: 554–62.
23. Tockman MS, Gupta PK, Pressman NJ, Mulshine JL, Cytometric validation of immunocytochemical observations in developing lung cancer. *Diagn Cytopathol* 1994; **9**: 615–22.
24. Scott FM, Modali R, Lehman TA et al, High frequency of K-ras codon 12 mutations in bronchoalveolar lavage fluid of patients at high risk for second primary lung cancer. *Clin Cancer Res* 1997; **3**: 479–82.
25. Zhou J, Mulshine JL, Ro JY et al, Expression of heterogeneous nuclear ribonucleoprotein A2/B1 in bronchial epitihelium of chronic smokers. *Clin Cancer Res* 1998; **4**: 1631–40.
26. Brambilla E, Early detection of lung cancer. In: *Clinical and Biological Basis of Lung Cancer Prevention* (Martinet Y, Vignaud JM, Martinet N et al, eds). Birkhäuser: Basel, 1998: 39–56.
27. Sozzi G, Miozzo M, Donghi R et al, Deletions of 17p and p53 mutations in pre neoplastic lesions of the lung. *Cancer Res* 1992; **52**: 6097–82.
28. Sozzi G, Miozzo M, Pastorino U et al, Genetic evidence for an independent origin of multiple pre neoplastic and neoplastic lung lesion. *Cancer Res* 1995; **55**: 135–40.
29. Crowell RE, Gilliland FD, Temes RT et al, Detection of trisomy 7 in nonmalignant bronchial epithelium from lung cancer patients and individuals at risk for lung cancer. *Cancer Epidemiol Biomarkers Prev* 1996; **5**: 631–7.
30. Eggers M, Hogan M, Reich RK et al, A microchip for quantitative detection of molecules utilizing luminescent and radioisotope reporter groups. *BioTechniques* 1994; **17**: 516.
31. Kozal MJ, Shah N, Shien N et al, Extensive polymorphisms observed in HIV-1 clade B protease gene using high-density oligonucleotide array. *Nature Med* 1996; **2**: 753–9.
32. Stipp D, Gene chip breakthrough. *Fortune* 1997; **135**: 56–73.
33. Lippman S, Benner S, Hong W, Cancer Chemoprevention. *J Clin Oncol* 1994; **12**: 851–73.
34. Hong W, Lippman S, Itri L et al, Prevention of second primary tumours with isotretinoin in squamous-cell carcinoma of the head and neck. *N Engl J Med* 1990; **323**: 825–7.
35. Benner SE, Pajak TF, Lippman SM, Hong WK, Prevention of second primary tumours with isotretinoin is squamous cell carcinoma of the head and neck: long term follow-up. *J Natl Cancer Inst* 1994; **86**: 140–1.
36. Mulshine JL, De Luca LM, Dedrick RL, Regional delivery of retinoids: a new approach to early lung cancer intervention. In: *Clinical and Biological Basis of Lung Cancer Prevention* (Martinet Y, Vignaud JM, Martinet N et al, eds). Birkhäuser: Basel, 1998: 273–84.
37. Avis I, Mathias A, Unsworth EJ et al, Analysis of small cell cancer growth inhibition by 13-*cis*-

retinoic acid: importance of bioavailability. *Cell Growth Diff* 1995; **6**: 485–92.

38. Oridate N, Lotan D, Xu X-C et al, Differential induction of apoptosis by all-*trans*-retinoic acid and *N*-(4-hydroxyphenyl)retinamide in head and neck squamous cell carcinoma cell lines. *Clin Cancer Res* 1996; **2**: 855–63.
39. Thompson C, Apoptosis in the pathogenesis and treatment of disease. *Science* 1995; **267**: 1456–9.
40. Tatsumura T, Koyama S, Miyazaki, The usefulness of the nebulization of chemotheraphy in the treatment of lung cancer. *Jpn J Chest Dis* 1995; **54**: 631–7.

Pathology: Revised classification of epithelial tumours of the lung (WHO/IASLC*)

Yukio Shimosato

Contents Introduction • Benign epithelial tumours (papillomas and adenomas) • Preinvasive lesions • Malignant epithelial tumours

INTRODUCTION

Almost two decades have passed since the second edition of the World Health Organization's (WHO) *Histological Typing of Lung Tumours*[1] was published in 1981. In 1985, the Pathology Panel of the International Association for the Study of Lung Cancer (IASLC) recommended a revision of the subtyping of small cell carcinoma, uniting oat cell and intermediate cell types in one 'small cell' category, since microscopic distinction between these two subtypes is often difficult and the therapeutic response and outcome are similar, with the addition of small cell/large cell type as a separate category because of possible differences in biological behaviour from pure small cell carcinoma.[2,3] Since then, considerable progress has been made in the understanding of the morphology and biology of lung tumours, such as atypical (bronchioloalveolar) adenomatous hyperplasia and neuroendocrine carcinoma. Therefore, after the 7th World Conference of the IASLC held in Colorado, with the official recommendation of the IASLC and the WHO, the Pathology Panel of the IASLC and the Core Group of the WHO Classification of Lung and Pleural Tumours met for the first time in 1995 to consider revision of lung and pleural tumour classification, and had several discussions before reaching a consensus in July 1998. The revised classification was presented at the Congress Meeting of the International Academy of Pathology in October 1998.

This chapter deals with the outline of the revised classification for epithelial tumours of the lung. For soft tissue tumours, mesothelial tumours, miscellaneous tumours, lymphoproliferative diseases, tumour-like lesions, etc., readers should refer to the third edition of the WHO's *Histological Typing of Lung and Pleural Tumours*.[4]

Table 8.1 lists epithelial tumours of the bronchi and lung, which consist of benign, preinvasive and invasive malignant tumours.

**Participants:* WD Travis* (Chair); TV Colby,* B Corrin,* Y Shimosato,* E Brambilla* (Coordinators); E Alvarez-Fernandez,* SP Hammer,* PS Hasleton,* FR Hirsch,* B Mackay,* H Popper,* RH Steele* (Core Panel Members); S Aisner,* A Churg, LP Dehner, AF Gazdar,* DW Henderson, NA Jambhekar, MN Koss, KM Muller, N Petrovitchev, P Saldiva, M Sheppard, S Wagenaar, W-H Li (Extended Panel of Reviewers) (*IASLC Pathology Panel Members).

Table 8.1 WHO histological classification of epithelial tumours of the lung (revised 10 October 1998)

EPITHELIAL TUMOURS

Benign

- Papillomas
    - Squamous cell papilloma
        - Exophytic
        - Inverted
    - Glandular papilloma
    - Mixed squamous and glandular papilloma
- Adenomas
    - Alveolar adenoma
    - Papillary adenoma
    - Adenomas of salivary gland type
        - Mucous gland adenoma
        - Pleomorphic adenoma
        - Other
    - Mucinous cystadenoma
    - Others

Preinvasive lesions

- Squamous dysplasia/carcinoma in situ
- Atypical adenomatous hyperplasia
- Diffuse idiopathic pulmonary neuroendocrine cell hyperplasia

Invasive malignant

- Squamous cell carcinoma
    - Variants:
        - Papillary
        - Clear cell
        - Small cell
        - Basaloid
- Small cell carcinoma
    - Variant:
        - Combined small cell carcinoma
- Adenocarcinoma
    - Acinar
    - Papillary
    - Bronchioloalveolar carcinoma
        - Non-mucinous (Clara cell/type II pneumocyte) type
        - Mucinous (goblet cell) type
        - Mixed mucinous and non-mucinous (Clara cell/type II pneumocyte and goblet cell) type, or indeterminate cell type

Table 8.1 Continued
Solid adenocarcinoma with mucin formation
Adenocarcinoma with mixed subtypes
Variants:
Well-differentiated fetal adenocarcinoma
Mucinous ('colloid') adenocarcinoma
Mucinous cystadenocarcinoma
Signet ring adenocarcinoma
Clear cell adenocarcinoma
Large cell carcinoma
Variants:
Large cell neuroendocrine carcinoma
Combined large cell neuroendocrine carcinoma
Basaloid carcinoma
Lymphoepithelioma-like carcinoma
Clear cell carcinoma
Large cell carcinoma with rhabdoid phenotype
Adenosquamous carcinoma
Carcinomas with pleomorphic, sarcomatoid or sarcomatous elements
Carcinomas with spindle and/or giant cells
Pleomorphic carcinoma
Spindle cell carcinoma
Giant cell carcinoma
Carcinosarcoma
Pulmonary blastoma
Carcinoid tumours
Typical carcinoid
Atypical carcinoid
Carcinomas of salivary gland type
Mucoepidermoid carcinoma
Adenoid cystic carcinoma
Others
Unclassified carcinomas

BENIGN EPITHELIAL TUMOURS (PAPILLOMAS AND ADENOMAS)

In squamous papillomas, 'inverted papilloma' similar to those seen in the upper respiratory tract has been added, although it is very rare and the present author has yet to experience a case.

A variety of tumours are listed under adenomas, among which alveolar adenoma, papillary adenoma and mucinous cystadenoma are rare.

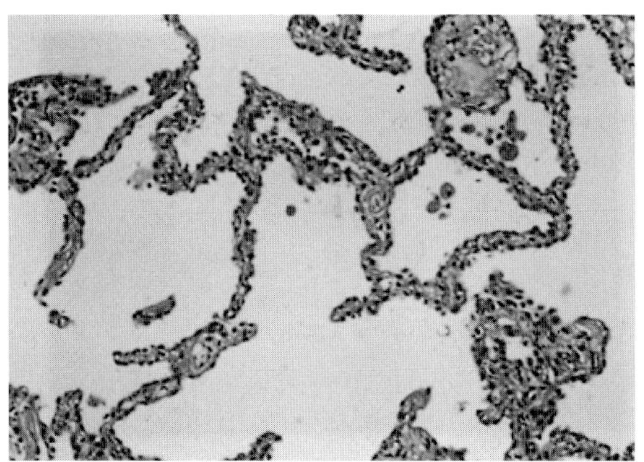

Figure 8.1
Atypical adenomatous hyperplasia (AAH) of mild degree. Alveolar lining is replaced by slightly atypical dome-shaped type II pneumocytes.

The distinction between mucinous cystadenoma and mucinous cystadenocarcinoma can be difficult. Pleomorphic adenoma is histologically identical to the salivary gland tumour of the same name and often detected as an endobronchial polypoid tumour. Mucous gland adenoma consists of mucus-filled cysts, tubules and glands, but lacks squamous and intermediate cells seen in low-grade mucoepidermoid carcinoma.

PREINVASIVE LESIONS

Squamous dysplasia and squamous cell carcinoma in situ were described in the previous edition of the classification. They represent a continuum of cytological changes, and distinction between severe dysplasia and carcinoma in situ may at times be difficult or impossible. Therefore diagnosis of such lesions should be confirmed by other pathologists before treatment.

Atypical adenomatous hyperplasia (AHH) is a dysplastic lesion of bronchioloalveoli, in which alveolar epithelial cells are replaced by atypical cuboidal to low columnar, non-mucinous cells with dense nuclei, inconspicuous nucleoli and scanty cytoplasm (Figure 8.1).[5,6] The alveolar septa are slightly thickened, and may be infil-

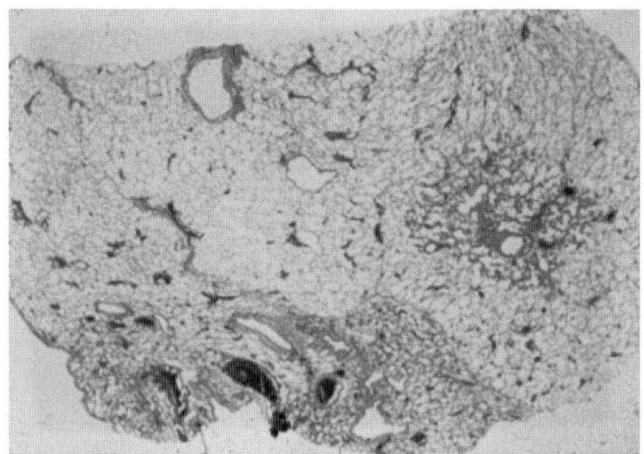

(a)

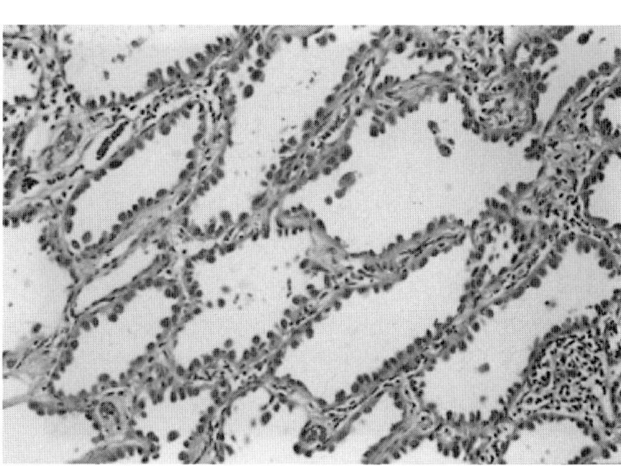

(b)

Figure 8.2
Atypical adenomatous hyperplasia (AAH) of moderate-to-severe degree. (a) A low-power view discloses a lesion with accentuated alveolar structures on the right. (b) High-power magnification reveals dome- or peg-shaped atypical epithelial cells with hyperchromatic nuclei and scanty eosinophilic cytoplasm.

trated by lymphocytes. They are often 5 mm or less in diameter, and may be detected by thinly sliced or helical computed tomography (helical-CT). The degree of cellular atypia varies from mild to severe, and the criteria for severe-degree AAH resemble, but fall short of, criteria for bronchioloalveolar carcinoma of the non-mucinous (Clara cell/type II pneumocyte) type (Figure 8.2). Intranuclear eosinophilic inclusions may be present, mitotic figures are hardly ever seen, and stromal invasion is absent. AAH is considered to be preneoplastic, since it is often seen at the periphery of adenocarcinoma and bronchioloalveolar carcinoma of the non-mucinous type.[7,8] However, the prognosis of resected lung carcinoma was found to be unaffected by association with AAH,[9] and the risk of progression to adenocarcinoma appears to be low, judging from the incidence of AAH and bronchioloalveolar carcinoma, as in the case of adenomatous polyp of the colon. AAH was designated by some as bronchioloalveolar (cell) adenoma,[10,11] but use of the term adenoma is not recommended, since it has been used for other lesions.

Diffuse idiopathic pulmonary neuroendocrine cell hyperplasia

Neuroendocrine cell hyperplasia observed as an increased number of scattered neuroendocrine cells in a limited area, or linear proliferations, or small nodules of neuroendocrine cells in bronchioli may be seen as a non-specific reaction secondary to airway or interstitial inflammation and/or fibrosis. However, rare cases of diffuse idiopathic pulmonary neuroendocrine cell hyperplasia are seen without airway inflammation or diffuse interstitial fibrosis, and they are often associated with multiple tumourlets or one or more carcinoid tumours.[12,13] In this setting, this lesion appears to be preneoplastic – but how often it becomes neoplastic is not known.

MALIGNANT EPITHELIAL TUMOURS

Malignant epithelial tumours comprise:

- squamous cell carcinoma;
- small cell carcinoma;
- adenocarcinoma;
- large cell carcinoma;
- adenosquamous carcinoma;
- carcinoma with pleomorphic, sarcomatoid or sarcomatous elements;
- carcinoid tumours;
- carcinoma of the salivary gland type;
- unclassified carcinomas.

Each subtype will be briefly explained, with emphasis placed on the changes in definition and terminology in the third edition of the classification.

Squamous cell carcinoma

In the revised edition, four variants are included, which may be the predominant feature of the tumour but more often may be focal. Spindle cell (squamous) carcinoma of the second edition is classified in the third edition as pleomorphic carcinoma under carcinomas with pleomorphic, sarcomatoid or sarcomatous elements.

Variants of squamous cell carcinoma

Papillary variant[12]

This arises in large bronchi, grows endobronchially, and may branch at the bronchial bifurcation, extending along bronchial lumina with minimally invasive growth. A verrucous growth pattern may be noted.

Clear cell variant

Clear cell changes may be seen in squamous cell carcinoma.

Small cell variant[12,14]

This is composed of small cells lacking the characteristic nuclear features of small cell carcinoma,

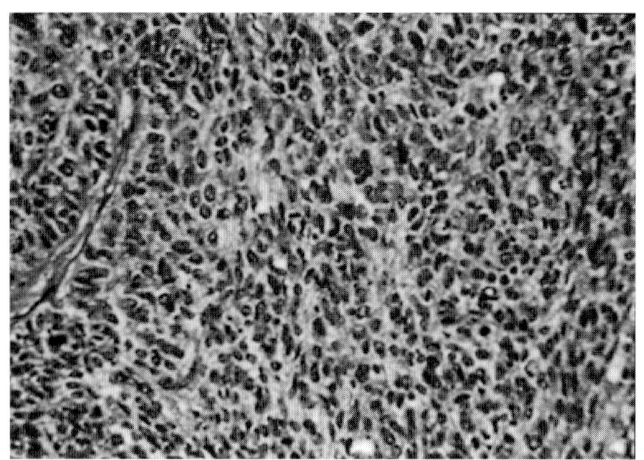

Figure 8.3
Squamous cell carcinoma, small cell variant. There is diffuse growth of small cells with oval to irregular hyperchromatic nuclei and faintly stained cytoplasm, which lack the characteristic nuclear features of small cell carcinoma. Mitotic figures are frequent. Elsewhere, squamous cell differentiation was evident.

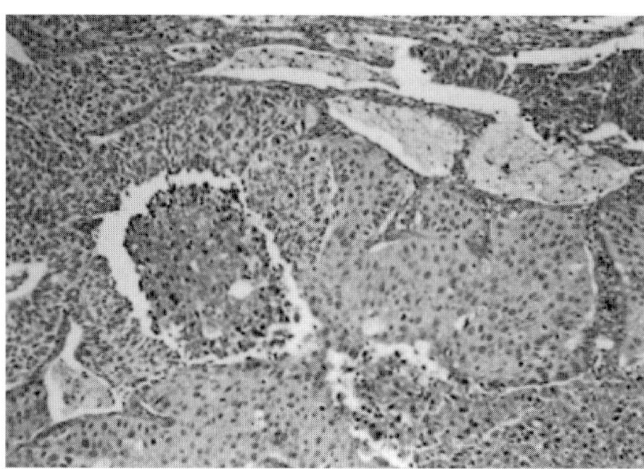

Figure 8.4
Combined small cell carcinoma. Features of small cell carcinoma are seen on the left, and large cell carcinoma suggestive of squamous cell differentiation on the right.

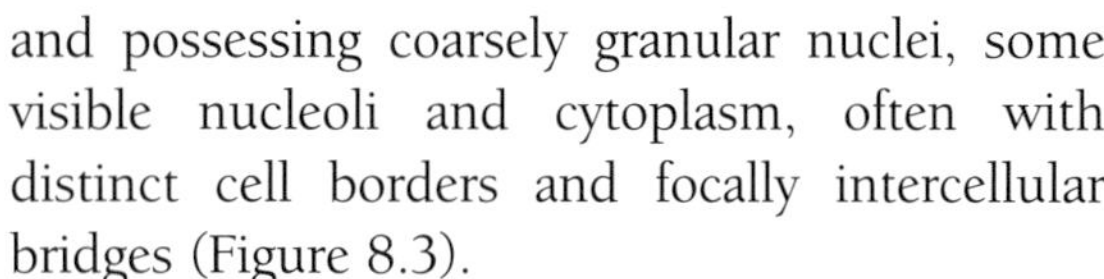

and possessing coarsely granular nuclei, some visible nucleoli and cytoplasm, often with distinct cell borders and focally intercellular bridges (Figure 8.3).

Basaloid variant[12]
This is characterized by prominent palisading of cells at the periphery of the tumour cell nests and by the presence of squamous cell differentiation in some parts.

Squamous cell carcinomas are graded as well, moderately well and poorly differentiated according to the degree of differentiation or to the amount of large cell component.

Small cell carcinoma

As already mentioned, on the recommendation of the IASLC Pathology Panel, oat cell carcinoma and small cell carcinoma of intermediate cell type were put together as small cell carcinoma (pure). Small cell carcinoma is characterized by diffuse growth or solid nests of small cells with oval to spindle nuclei, finely granular nuclei, inconspicuous nucleoli, thin nuclear membrane, scanty faintly stained or very finely granular cytoplasm, and ill-defined cell borders. Cancer cells are smaller than three resting lymphocytes. Mitotic figures are frequently seen, often 60–70 per 10 high-power fields.

A variant, *combined small cell carcinoma* (Figure 8.4), is defined as small cell carcinoma combined with non-small cell elements – usually adenocarcinoma, squamous cell carcinoma or large cell carcinoma (small cell/large cell carcinoma of the previous IASLC classification[2,3]) – but rarely with a spindle cell or giant cell component, which should be specified at diagnosis.

Small cell carcinomas arise from and destroy both hilar large bronchi and peripheral small bronchi, and grow subepithelially, very rarely replacing bronchial surface epithelium when tumours extend along bronchi. Small cell carcinoma in situ has not been experienced. Frequent association of squamous cell carcinoma in situ or dysplasia with small cell carcinoma is probably due to common carcinogenic agents in both types of carcinoma. Coagulation necrosis with basophilic staining of vascular walls (DNA incrustation) is occasionally seen.

Bronchial biopsy is often accompanied by a crushing effect of the forceps, which is also seen in cellular lesions including inflammation. Even when entire tissue fragments are crushed, free tumour cells attached to the tissue fragments may be sufficiently preserved for cytodiagnosis of small cell carcinoma.

Immunohistochemistry reveals neuroendocrine markers such as chromogranin and synaptophysin. Leu 7 and neuron-specific enolase are less specific. One-third to one-quarter of cases may not reveal neuroendocrine markers immunohistochemically or neurosecretory granules by electron microscopy.

Peripheral small cell carcinoma in stages I and II (T1–2N0–1M0) can be successfully treated by surgery and chemotherapy, the five-year survival rate being about 30–40%.[15]

Adenocarcinoma

Adenocarcinomas have been subdivided in more detail than in the previous edition, i.e. mixed type and five variants were added, and bronchioloalveolar carcinomas were subdivided by cell type. Many primary adenocarcinomas of the lung display differentiation towards peripheral airway epithelial cells such as Clara cells and type II pneumocytes, either entirely or in some parts of the tumour, which can be easily distinguished from metastatic adenocarcinomas to the lung from other organs. However, some pulmonary adenocarcinomas resemble carcinomas of the breast and salivary gland, while others may simulate signet ring carcinoma of the stomach and well-differentiated colorectal adenocarcinoma.

Small adenocarcinomas (i.e. those < 2 cm in diameter) frequently display a uniform histological pattern, but adenocarcinomas of larger size are frequently of mixed histology, with a combination of acinar (or tubular), papillary and bronchioloalveolar patterns, or solid nests of large cells with or without mucin formation.[7,8] These findings indicate that adenocarcinomas probably arise as a single cell type, and show cellular anaplasia and metaplasia as they grow to become tumours of mixed histology and increased anaplasia or atypia. Acinar and papillary adenocarcinomas, and solid adenocarcinomas with mucin formation, may arise anywhere from bronchi to bronchioloalveoli, either growing endobronchially or as nodular peripheral tumours, but bronchioloalveolar carcinomas of Clara cell type or type II pneumocyte type always arise from the bronchioloalveolar region.

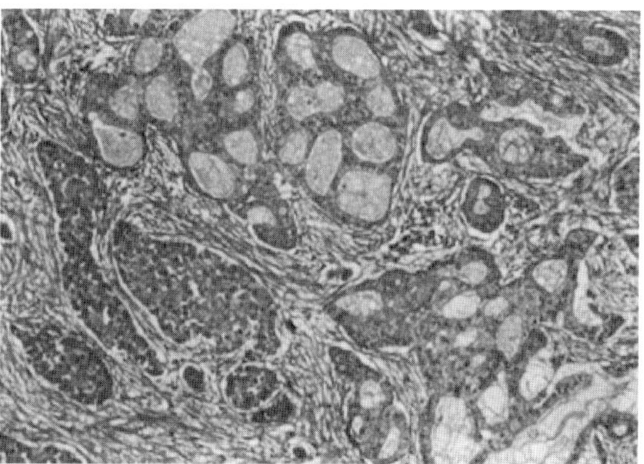

Figure 8.5
Acinar adenocarcinoma. Tubular and cribriform patterns are made up of mucinous cells. Solid nests of mucin-forming cells are present in the left lower corner.

Acinar adenocarcinoma

Acinar adenocarcinoma is composed of acini or tubules, often lined by mucin-producing cells, which may resemble bronchial glands and ducts (Figure 8.5). The individual cells, however, may simulate bronchial surface epithelial cells at

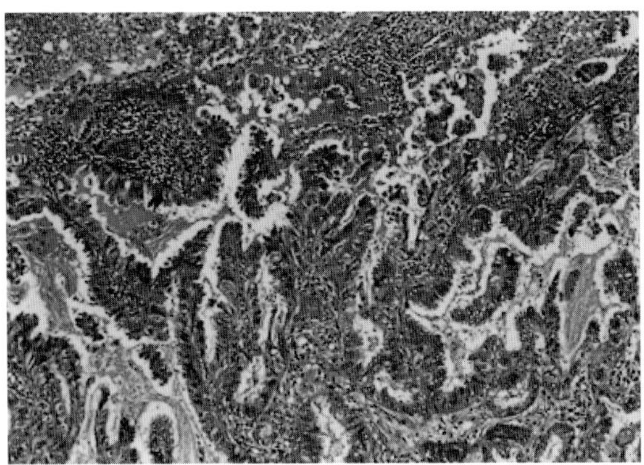

Figure 8.6
Papillary adenocarcinoma with its own fibrovascular stroma. Irregular papillary structures with a moderate amount of fibrovascular stroma destroy the lung parenchyma, and lepidic growth is noted only in minute areas.

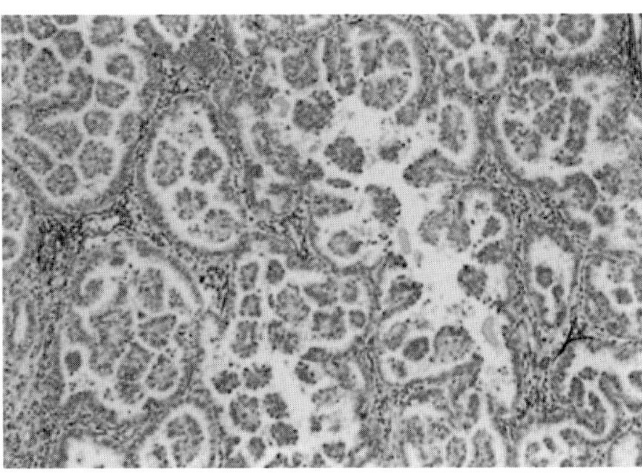

Figure 8.7
Papillary adenocarcinoma with secondary and tertiary papillary branching in bronchiolo-alveolar growth. Elastic fibres remaining in alveolar septa on the left of the photograph are lost on the right. (Elastica stain.)

times. In predominantly bronchioloalveolar adenocarcinomas made up of non-mucinous (Clara cell or type II pneumocyte) type, tubules, which are often found in the central portion of the tumour, may also be called acini, and the tumour is diagnosed as mixed adenocarcinoma of bronchioloalveolar and acinar patterns.

Papillary adenocarcinoma

Tumours predominantly composed of papillary pattern are classified as papillary adenocarcinoma. There are two types of papillary pattern: one is a 'true' papillary structure, in which columnar or cuboidal cells produce their own fibrovascular stroma and grow in papillary fashion and invade the lung parenchyma (Figure 8.6); the other is seen in the bronchioloalveolar pattern, in which cuboidal to low columnar Clara cells/type II pneumocytes replacing alveolar lining display complicated secondary and tertiary papillary branches (Figure 8.7). The latter is designated as papillary instead of bronchioloalveolar, because it is often associated with invasive growth and poorer prognosis than pure bronchioloalveolar carcinoma.

Bronchioloalveolar carcinoma

Tumours consisting of cuboidal to columnar cells that replace bronchioloalveolar lining cells without stromal, vascular or pleural invasion, are designated as bronchioloalveolar carcinoma, i.e. tumours of pure bronchioloalveolar pattern. There are three subtypes, according to constitutive cells.

Bronchioloalveolar carcinoma: non-mucinous (Clara cell/type II pneumocyte) type

'Clara cells' are either columnar or peg-shaped, with cytoplasmic snouts and eosinophilic cytoplasm. Nuclei may be situated apically, and the

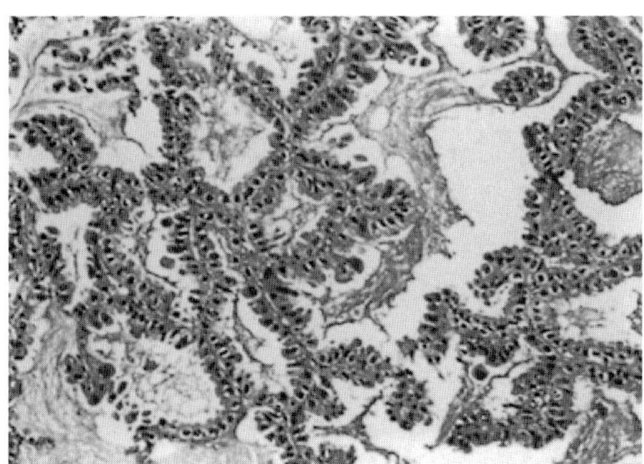

Figure 8.8
Bronchioloalveolar carcinoma of non-mucinous (Clara cell/type II pneumocyte) type. Columnar to peg-shaped tumour cells with some cytoplasmic snouts replace the alveolar lining.

degree of atypia and nucleolar size vary in areas and from case to case (Figure 8.8). 'Type II pneumocyte type' cells are dome-shaped or cuboidal, with finely vesicular cytoplasm and often small nuclei with or without nucleoli. The presence of tumours showing a combination of these two cell types indicates a close relationship between these cells. Eosinophilic nuclear inclusions are seen in both cell types. Immunohistochemically, surfactant apoprotein was initially thought to be specific to these cell types, but was later found to be positive in some pulmonary adenocarcinomas of other subtypes, such as acinar and papillary adenocarcinomas. Carcinoembryonic antigen (CEA) was positive in about 70% of cases.

This type of tumour is often nodular and associated with central or subpleural alveolar collapse with condensation of elastic fibres ('fibrosis or sclerosis'), and has been erroneously interpreted as 'scar cancer'. If stromal, vascular or pleural invasion is evident, the tumour is classified as mixed adenocarcinoma with predominant bronchioloalveolar pattern. Invasive growth is suggested when tumour cell nests show increased cell atypia or mucin production and are

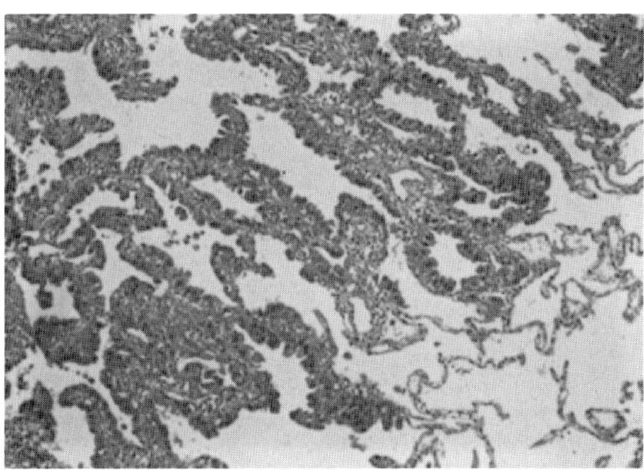

(a)

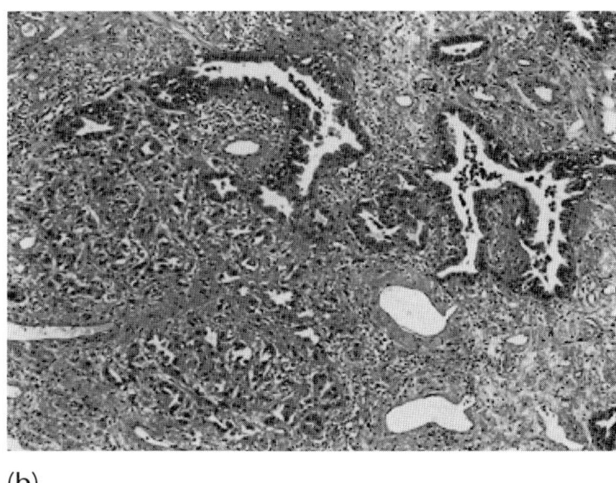

(b)

Figure 8.9
Mixed adenocarcinoma with predominant bronchioloalveolar pattern. (a) The bulk of the tumour is made up of non-mucinous-type tumour cells arranged in a bronchioloalveolar pattern. (b) In small areas at the site of alveolar collapse ('fibrosis') near the centre of the tumour, more atypical tumour cells are arranged in irregular tubules and small acini, accompanied by small amounts of collagen.

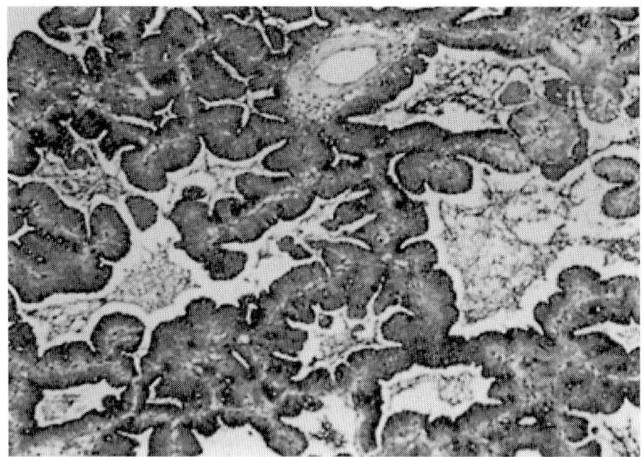

Figure 8.10
Bronchioloalveolar carcinoma of mucinous (goblet cell) type. Tumour cells arranged in a bronchioloalveolar pattern contain apical cytoplasmic mucus. (Alcian blue–PAS stain.)

associated with proliferation of fibroblasts and collagenization (Figure 8.9). Intra-alveolar complicated secondary and tertiary papillary branches also suggest areas of invasive growth elsewhere. Aerogenous spread may be seen in the surrounding lung, but is rare in unrelated segments or lobes.

Differentiation from AAH may be difficult at times, since these two categories are part of a continuous spectrum. At present, there is no distinct line dividing the two, although degree of cell atypia and cell density, nuclear accumulation of p53 products, and CEA immunoreactivity may be indicators,[5,6,8] and the diagnosis may be arbitrary.

Bronchioloalveolar carcinoma: mucinous (goblet cell) type
The tumour is composed of tall columnar cells with varying amounts of cytoplasmic mucus, frequently displacing small to medium-sized nuclei with small nucleoli to the base of the cells, and distending alveoli with mucin (Figure 8.10). This subtype may take the form of growth as a peripheral solitary nodule, disseminated multiple nodules or diffuse involvement of the lung such as lobar pneumonia, and frequently displays aerogenous spread. Lymphatic and haematogenous metastases are rare and late phenomena. A growth pattern identical to that of bronchioloalveolar carcinoma is seen in metastases from other organs such as the pancreas and uterine cervix. However, coagulation necrosis of the tumour is seen only exceptionally in the primary but often in metastatic tumours.

Bronchioloalveolar carcinoma: mixed mucinous and non-mucinous (Clara cell/type II pneumocyte and goblet cell) type, or indeterminate cell type
The mixed mucinous and non-mucinous subtype is very rare. The indeterminate cell type includes a probable bronchial surface epithelial cell type producing no or little mucin.[14]

Solid adenocarcinoma with mucin formation

This tumour consists of solid nests of frequent mucin-containing cells without acinar or papillary structures. If a few acini are seen, the tumour is classified as poorly differentiated acinar adenocarcinoma. A few mucin-containing cells may be seen in squamous cell carcinoma and large cell carcinoma. Since the presence of many mucin-containing cells is required for diagnosis, H&E sections are sufficient for diagnosis in most cases, but mucin stain may be needed for confirmation in some.

Adenocarcinoma with mixed subtypes

The majority of adenocarcinomas seen in routine practice are mixtures of acinar, papillary and/or bronchioloalveolar patterns. Adenocarcinoma with predominantly bronchioloalveolar pattern and minute areas of invasive growth, which often show an acinar pattern, is also subtyped as mixed adenocarcinoma (Figure 8.9). In adenocarcin-

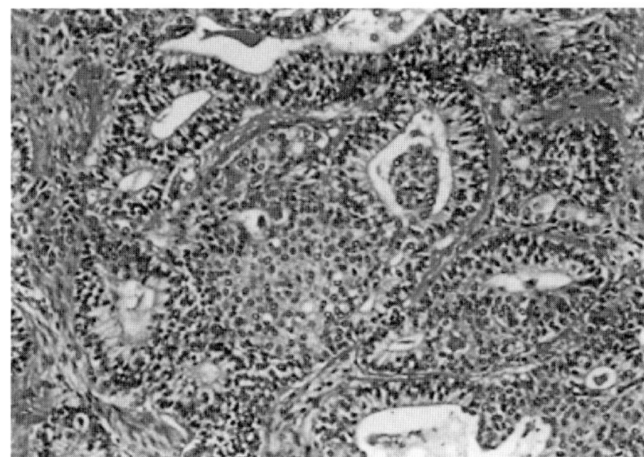

Figure 8.11
Well-differentiated fetal adenocarcinoma. Tubules are composed of tall columnar cells with clear cytoplasm, resembling fetal lung tubules. A morule, which is in continuity with tubular epithelial cells, is seen in the centre, and consists of polygonal cells with finely granular cytoplasm and some optically clear nuclei. The cytoplasm contained immunoreactive synaptophysin and chromogranin A.

oma with mixed subtypes, each element and its amount should be mentioned.

Variants of adenocarcinoma

Well-differentiated fetal adenocarcinoma[12]
This was initially reported as a pulmonary endodermal tumour resembling fetal lung,[16] and is composed of papillotubular structures, made up of tall columnar cells with clear cytoplasm resembling fetal lung tubules or the epithelial component of pulmonary blastoma. It is also characterized by the presence of morules in continuity with clear columnar cells (Figure 8.11). They are composed of polygonal cells with finely granular cytoplasm, some possessing neuroendocrine markers. Optically clear nuclei are frequent, and contain biotin.[17] In contrast to pulmonary blastoma, the prognosis is favourable when the tumour is resectable. It should be differentiated from the histologically similar 'highly malignant fetal lung-type adenocarcinoma', which lacks morules and displays more nuclear atypia.[18]

Mucinous ('colloid') carcinoma[11,12,14]
This rare tumour is similar to the gastrointestinal adenocarcinoma that used to be called by the same name; it is grossly gelatinous, and mucin-producing neoplastic epthelial cells float in pools of mucin.

Mucinous cystadenocarcinoma[11,12,14]
Another rare tumour, this is similar to the tumour of the same name in ovary and pancreas. It is cystic, and at times difficult to differentiate from mucinous cystadenoma. Such a tumour can be diagnosed as low-grade mucinous cystadenocarcinoma.

Signet ring adenocarcinoma[11,12,14]
Signet ring carcinoma of the stomach metastasizes to the lung via the lymphatics, and can be differentiated from the primary lung cancer by the location of the tumour.

Clear cell adenocarcinoma
Clear cell changes are also seen in adenocarcinoma, either focally or entirely.

Adenocarcinoma combined with a spindle cell or giant cell component is designated as pleomorphic carcinoma (see under 'Carcinoma with pleomorphic, sarcomatoid or sarcomatous elements').

Large cell carcinoma

This is a poorly differentiated carcinoma, which does not show cytological or histological features of squamous cell carcinoma, small cell carcinoma or adenocarcinoma. Individual tumour cells are large and polygonal, with vesicular nuclei, and

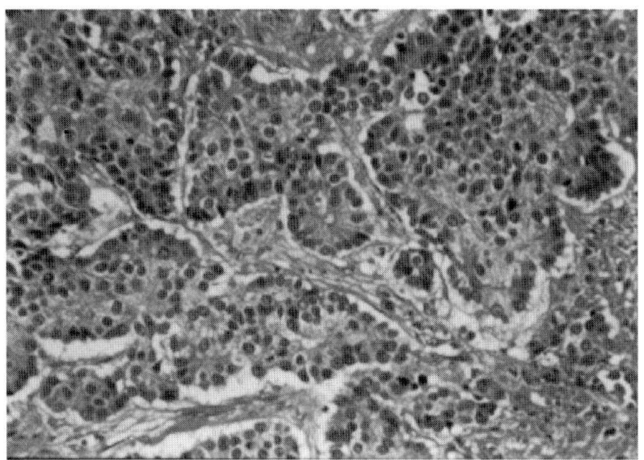

Figure 8.12
Large cell neuroendocrine carcinoma (LCNEC). Solid nests and rosette-like structures are made up of polygonal cells with finely granular nuclei. The tumour was positive for N-CAM.

often with prominent nucleoli and a moderate amount of cytoplasm. The presence of a few cells with cytoplasmic mucus does not exclude a diagnosis of large cell carcinoma. Ultrastructurally and also immunohistochemically, the tumour cells often display features characteristic of squamous or glandular cells, and, in a few instances, neuroendocrine cells.

Variants of large cell carcinoma

Large cell neuroendocrine carcinoma
Large cell carcinoma with histological features suggesting neuroendocrine differentiation, such as organoid nesting, trabeculae, rosette-like structure and palisading at the periphery of nests, is designated as large cell neuroendocrine carcinoma (LCNEC) (Figure 8.12) . It can be verified by electron microscopy and/or immunohistochemistry.[12,13,19,20]

Nuclei are either granular hyperchromatic or vesicular, often with prominent nucleoli. Cytoplasm is abundant and finely granular. Mitotic figures are frequent (11 or more), averaging 75 per 10 high power fields. Immunohistochemically, chromogranin A, synaptophysin and N-CAM can be stained positively. The latter shows positive staining on cell membrane focally, while small cell carcinoma displays positive membrane staining in toto.

Some adenocarcinomas and squamous cell carcinomas, which do not show features suggestive of neuroendocrine cells, may reveal neuroendocrine markers immunohistochemically or electron-microscopically. These tumours are simply classified as either adenocarcinoma or squamous cell carcinoma with notes on the presence of neuroendocrine features, although some prefer to place them under the category of non-small cell neuroendocrine carcinoma.

Basaloid carcinoma
This uncommon tumour consists of lobular and trabecular nests of small monomorphic cuboidal to fusiform cells with a palisading pattern at the periphery of the nests.[12] Nuclei are moderately hyperchromatic, with a few perhaps inconspicuous nucleoli, and cytoplasm is scanty. Mitotic figures are frequent. There are no intercellular bridges or keratinization. Comedo-type necrosis is often seen. Rosettes may be present, but lack neuroendocrine markers. This tumour arises in proximal bronchi, and often displays endobronchial growth. If it is combined with either squamous or glandular components, it is classified as squamous cell carcinoma and adenocarcinoma, with basaloid features, respectively.

Lymphoepithelioma-like carcinoma
This is also a rare tumour, but is said to be seen in southeast Asia, where it has been claimed to be frequently associated with Epstein–Barr virus (EBV). The present author has seen a case that showed a combination of lymphoepithelioma-

like features and adenocarcinoma but was not associated with EBV. Histologically, it is similar to nasopharyngeal carcinoma of the same name, and is composed of nests of large polygonal cells with vesicular nuclei and distinct nucleoli infiltrated by lymphoid cells.

Clear cell carcinoma
Large cell carcinomas composed of polygonal cells with clear or foamy cytoplasm are called clear cell carcinoma. Clear cytoplasm may or may not contain glycogen. The tumour should be differentiated from clear cell carcinoma metastatic from other organs.

Large cell carcinoma with rhabdoid phenotype
This is characterized by cytoplasmic eosinophilic globules consisting of intermediate filaments, which are positive for vimentin or cytokeratin. Rhabdoid cells are noted focally or extensively in the large cell component of poorly differentiated carcinoma or in large cell carcinoma. This subtype is also rare.

Adenosquamous carcinoma
Adenosquamous carcinoma consists of a mixture of a squamous cell component and an adenocarcinoma component, each occupying at least 10% of the entire tumour area. This value has been set arbitrarily. The adenocarcinoma component should be acinar, papillary or abundant mucin-producing large cells. The presence of occasional mucin-producing cells should be disregarded.

Carcinomas with pleomorphic, sarcomatoid or sarcomatous elements
This is a group of poorly differentiated carcinomas partly consisting of a sarcoma or sarcoma-like component, which may represent a continuum of epithelial and mesenchymal differentiation. It is divided into three subtypes: carcinomas with spindle and/or giant cells, carcinosarcoma, and pulmonary blastoma.

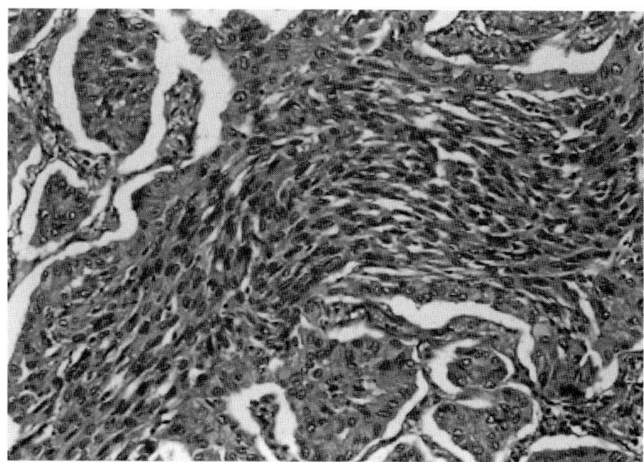

Figure 8.13
Pleomorphic adenocarcinoma. The tumour consists of nests of poorly differentiated adenocarcinoma cells and a closely associated bundle of spindle cells. A non-mucinous bronchioloalveolar pattern was noted elsewhere.

Carcinomas with spindle and/or giant cells
These include three different subtypes: pleomorphic, spindle cell and giant cell carcinomas.

Pleomorphic carcinomas
These consist of a mixture of areas displaying features of adenocarcinoma, squamous cell carcinoma or large cell carcinoma, and areas with spindle cell or giant cell components occupying at least 10% of the tumour (Figure 8.13).

Spindle cell and giant cell carcinomas
Pure spindle cell carcinoma and giant cell carcinoma are rare. Epithelial markers may be demonstrated in the spindle cell component, the giant cell component or both. If not, separation from sarcoma is difficult. 'Giant cells' are mono- or

multinucleated, polygonal and often dyscohesive, with emperipolesis by polymorphonuclear leukocytes or lymphocytes.

Carcinosarcoma

This is a carcinoma consisting of carcinoma and sarcoma with heterologous elements such as neoplastic cartilage, bone or striated muscle. If heterologous elements are absent, the tumour is classified as pleomorphic carcinoma.

Pulmonary blastoma

This is a biphasic tumour consisting of an immature epithelial component, which may simulate tubules of the fetal lung, and an immature mesenchymal component, which may differentiate towards bone, cartilage and striated muscle. Morular structures are not found.

Carcinoid tumours

The histology of carcinoid tumours of the lung is similar to that of tumours of the same name in other organs, consisting of organoid, trabecular, insular, palisading, ribbon-like or rosette-like arrangements, which are closely associated with fine vasculature. Tumour cells characteristically possess finely granular cytoplasm and nuclei with a finely granular chromatin pattern. Nucleoli may be present. Spindle cells, oxyphilic (oncocytoid) cells and clear cells may be found, as are glandular structures. Ossification, sclerosis and amyloid deposits may be seen in stroma.

Carcinoid tumours are subclassified into typical and atypical carcinoid tumours.[12,13] In the former, foci of coagulation necrosis are absent, and mitotic figures are 1 or less per 10 high power fields. They may show some cell atypia, increase in cellularity and lymphatic invasion, but their prognosis is excellent. In the atypical tumours, the mitotic count is 2–10 per 10 high power fields, and foci of coagulation necrosis, often punctate, may be present. The most important factor separating atypical from typical carcinoid tumour is the mitotic activity of the tumour. Therefore distinction between the two may be impossible on small biopsy specimens.

Carcinoid tumours are found in both major bronchi and peripheral lung. The tumour may be associated with neuroendocrine cell hyperplasia, particularly with peripheral carcinoid tumours. Immunohistochemically, neuroendocrine markers, such as chromogranin A, synaptophysin, N-CAM, neuron-specific enolase and Leu 7 are often positive, and the tumour may also contain immunoreactive serotonin, pancreatic polypeptide, adrenocorticotrophic hormone, etc. Carcinoid syndrome may be noted when metastasis to the liver is present. The outcome of atypical carcinoid tumours is much poorer than that of typical carcinoid tumours, and the five-year survival rate is 50–70%.[12,13]

Carcinoma of the salivary gland type

Some low-grade bronchial carcinomas are histologically identical to the salivary gland tumours of the same name, such as mucoepidermoid carcinoma and adenoid cystic carcinoma.[11,12,14] There are also histologically similar high-grade carcinomas in both organs, which in the lung are probably of bronchial gland origin and are arbitrarily included under the heading of acinar adenocarcinoma.

Mucoepidermoid carcinoma

Mucoepidermoid carcinoma of low-grade malignancy arises usually from segmental and subsegmental bronchi, and often displays endobronchial growth. It is composed of squamous cells, mucous cells and intermediate cells. Acinar or tubular structures are frequent, and cystic changes may be prominent, but keratinization is absent or inconspicuous.

Mucoepidermoid carcinoma of high-grade malignancy should be differentiated from adenosquamous carcinoma, in which the characteristic admixture of squamous cells and mucin-containing cells within a single nest is not noted.

Adenoid cystic carcinoma

This has a characteristic cribriform pattern consisting of small tumour cells, in which microcystic spaces and stroma contain connective tissue mucin and may become hyalinized. Tubular or ductal structures lined by double layers of cuboidal cells containing secretion may be present. Cells of myoepithelial nature can be demonstrated by immunostaining for smooth muscle actin and vimentin. This tumour arises from the trachea and main bronchi. Because of the infiltrative nature of this tumour, the surgical resection line should be checked carefully for the presence of invading tumour. This tumour should be differentiated from high-grade malignant acinar adenocarcinoma showing a cribriform pattern.

Other carcinomas of salivary gland type

Acinic cell carcinoma, epimyoepithelial carcinoma and malignant mixed tumour of the bronchus are very rare.

Unclassified carcinomas

These are carcinomas that cannot be placed in any of the above categories.

REFERENCES

1. World Health Organization, *Histological Typing of Lung Tumours. International Classification of Tumours, No. 1*, 2nd edn. World Health Organization: Geneva, 1981.
2. Yesner R, Classification of lung cancer histology. *N Engl J Med* 1985; **312**: 652–3.
3. Hirsch FR, Matthews MJ, Aisner S et al, Histological classification of small cell lung cancer: Changing concepts and terminology. *Cancer* 1988; **62**: 973–7.
4. Travis WD, Colby TV, Corrin B et al, *Histological Typing of Lung and Pleural Tumours. International Classification of Tumours, No. 1*, 3rd edn. World Health Organization: Geneva, 1999.
5. Nakayama H, Noguchi M, Tsuchiya R et al, Clonal growth of atypical adenomatous hyperplasia of the lung: cytofluorometric analysis of nuclear DNA content. *Mod Pathol* 1990; **3**: 314–20.
6. Kitamura H, Kameda Y, Nakamura N et al, Atypical adenomatous hyperplasia and bronchioloalveolar lung carcinoma. Analysis by morphometry and the expression of p53 and carcinoembryonic antigen. *Am J Surg Pathol* 1996; **20**: 553–62.
7. Kurokawa T, Matsuno Y, Noguchi M et al, Surgically curable 'early' adenocarcinoma in the periphery of the lung. *Am J Surg Pathol* 1994; **18**: 431–8.
8. Shimosato Y, Noguchi M, Matsuno Y, Adenocarcinoma of the lung: its development and malignant progression. *Lung Cancer* 1993; **9**: 99–108.
9. Suzuki K, Nagai K, Yoshida J et al, The prognosis of resected lung carcinoma associated with atypical adenomatous hyperplasia: a comparison of prognosis of well-differentiated adenocarcinoma associated with atypical adenomatuos hyperplasia and intrapulmonary metastasis. *Cancer* 1997; **79**: 1521–6.
10. Miller RR, Bronchioloalveolar cell adenoma. *Am J Surg Pathol* 1990; **14**: 904–12.
11. Shimosato Y, Part II, Lung tumors. In: *Biopsy Interpretation of the Lung* (Shimosato Y, Miller RR). Raven Press: New York, 1994: 199–394.
12. Colby TV, Koss MN, Travis WD, *Tumors of the Lower Respiratory Tract*. Third series, Fascicle 13, *Atlas of Tumor Pathology*. Armed Forces Institute of Pathology: Washington, DC, 1995.
13. Corrin B, Neuroendocrine neoplasms of the lung. *Curr Diagn Pathol* 1997; **4**: 239–50.
14. Shimosato Y, Pulmonary neoplasms. In: *Diagnostic Surgical Pathology*, 3rd edn (Sternberg SS, ed). Raven Press: New York, 1999.
15. Naruke T, Goya T, Tsuchiya R, Suemasu K, Prognosis and survival in resected lung carcinoma based on the new international staging system. *J Thorac Cardiovasc Surg* 1988; **96**: 440–7.
16. Kradin RL, Kirkham SE, Young RH et al,

Pulmonary blastoma with argyrophil cells and lacking sarcomatous feature (pulmonary endodermal tumor resembling fetal lung). *Am J Surg Pathol* 1982; **6**: 165–72.
17. Nakatani Y, Kitamura H, Inayama Y et al, Pulmonary endodermal tumor resembling fetal lung: the optically clear nucleus is rich in biotin. *Am J Surg Pathol* 1994; **18**: 637–42.
18. Kodama T, Shimosato Y, Watanabe S et al, Six cases of well differentiated adenocarcinoma simulating fetal lung tubules in pseudoglandular stage. *Am J Surg Pathol* 1984; **8**: 735–44.
19. Travis WD, Linnoila RI, Tsokos MG et al, Neuroendocrine tumour of the lung with proposed criteria for large cell neuroendocrine carcinoma: an ultrastructural, immunohistochemical, and flow cytometric study of 35 cases. *Am J Surg Pathol* 1991; **15**: 529–33.
20. Jiang S-X, Kameya T, Shoji M et al, Large cell neuroendocrine carcinoma of the lung: a histologic and immunohistochemical study of 22 cases. *Am J Surg Pathol* 1998; **22**: 526–37.

9 Clinical diagnosis and basic evaluation

Eric J Olson, James R Jett

Contents Introduction • History • Physical examination • Imaging • Diagnostic techniques • Overview of basic evaluation • Future developments

INTRODUCTION

Lung cancer is among the most common and lethal forms of cancer. In the USA and many other countries, it is the leading cause of cancer-related mortality. Global lung cancer incidence and mortality rates should continue to increase as a result of the ongoing use of tobacco products. Remarkable increases in lung cancer death rates have been documented in central and eastern European countries in parallel with rising cigarette consumption.[1] Five-year survival rates for all stages of lung cancer are disappointingly less than 15%. Three- to five-year disease-free rates for resected stage I lung cancer as high as 60–90% have been reported, but less than 20% of all lung cancers are stage I at the time of diagnosis. It is imperative that clinicians be familiar with the evaluation of lung cancer, given its tremendous worldwide public health impact and the prognostic importance of early cancer detection.

Lung cancer outcome depends on the cell type and stage of disease at presentation based on the tumor, node, metastasis (TNM) classification. Accordingly, the essential aspects of lung cancer evaluation are the histological distinction of small cell (SCLC) and non-small cell (NSCLC) types and accurate determination of the extent of disease so that appropriate treatment can be initiated. The evaluation of lung cancer begins with a careful history and physical examination, followed by testing to obtain a tissue diagnosis and stage the extent of disease. This chapter will review aspects of clinical presentation, imaging and diagnostic testing for bronchogenic carcinoma. Details regarding staging are covered in Chapter 10.

HISTORY

Lung cancers are clinically silent for the majority of the time, since, theoretically, they grow from a single malignant cell to a potentially detectable lesion. Occasionally, lung cancer is discovered incidentally in an asymptomatic patient, for instance as a solitary pulmonary nodule on a routine chest radiograph. Smoking history,[2] concurrent chronic obstructive pulmonary disease (COPD)[3] and previous exposures to certain occupational carcinogens[4] predict a higher risk for bronchogenic carcinoma. The majority of lung cancer patients are symptomatic at the time of diagnosis. Local tumor growth, regional extension, metastases, paraneoplastic phenomena or a combination of mechanisms may cause tumor-associated symptoms (Table 9.1). There are no characteristics of clinical presentation that absolutely distinguish between NSCLC and SCLC.

Local effects

The most common initial symptom of lung cancer is cough, which occurs in 45–75% of patients.

Table 9.1 Aspects of lung cancer presentation

Asymptomatic
Symptomatic
Effects of local tumor growth
Cough
Bronchorrhea
Fever, chills, purulent sputum production (postobstructive pneumonitis)
Dyspnea
Hemoptysis
Wheeze
Stridor
Chest pain
Effects of regional tumor extension
Hemidiaphragm paralysis
Hoarseness
Dysphagia
Bronchoesophageal fistula
Pericardial effusion/tamponade/ tachyarrhythmias
Lymphangitic carcinomatosis
Pulmonary nodules
Tumor microembolism
Pleural effusion
Superior vena cava syndrome
Pancoast's syndrome
Metastatic effects
Adrenal
Liver
Central nervous system
Bone
Paraneoplastic effects
See Table 9.2

Causes include bronchial mucosa tumor invasion, postobstructive pneumonitis/atelectasis, tumor cavitation or pleural effusion. Although cough is a nonspecific symptom, a change in the character of the cough, such as new hemoptysis or coexistent fever and chills, may signal a cause other than smoking-related bronchitis. Bronchorrhea, the expectoration of large-volume thin mucoid secretions, may be seen with advanced bronchioloalveolar carcinoma, but is rare. Lung cancer is an unusual cause of chronic cough in patients with a normal chest radiograph.[5] One-third to one-half of patients initially report dyspnea that may arise from large airway obstruction, postobstructive pneumonitis/atelectasis, pleural effusion, lymphangitic metastases, pericardial effusion, or concurrent illnesses such as COPD. Dyspnea in a lung cancer patient with a normal chest radiograph may be due to pulmonary thromboembolism or, less commonly, tumor microembolism. Lung cancer presents with hemoptysis in many patients as a result of tumor necrosis, mucosal ulceration, tumor erosion into pulmonary vasculature, postobstructive pneumonia and pulmonary thromboembolism. Retrospective studies reveal that bronchogenic carcinoma accounts for 19–29% of cases of hemoptysis. In patients with a normal chest radiograph and hemoptysis, only 2–9% are subsequently found to have lung cancer.[6] Hemoptysis is commonly blood-streaked sputum, although large central tumors may lead to massive hemoptysis that can result in death by asphyxiation. Tumor involvement of the parietal pleura, chest wall, and mediastinum leads to chest pain as an initial complaint in 25–50% of patients. Other causes of pain include rib cage metastases, pulmonary embolism and postobstructive pneumonitis. Pneumothorax is a rare cause of chest pain and dyspnea in lung cancer patients.

Regional extension effects

Direct mediastinal extension by lung cancer or metastases to mediastinal lymph nodes can lead to a variety of presentations due to the diversity of adjacent structures. Phrenic nerve involvement by tumor may cause ipsilateral diaphragmatic paralysis, demonstrated on chest radiography by hemidiaphragm elevation often in the setting of a centrally located mass. If lung cancer is not initially identified as the etiology of diaphragm paralysis, it is unlikely to become the explanation over time.[7] Hoarseness – a finding at presentation in 2–18% of lung cancer patients – is usually attributable to unilateral left vocal paralysis resulting from damage to the left recurrent laryngeal nerve anywhere along its intrathoracic course. Extrinsic esophageal compression by tumor or metastatic lymph nodes may cause dysphagia. Postprandial coughing raises the possibility of broncho-esophageal fistula. Pericardial involvement by hematogenous, lymphatic or direct extension routes may cause asymptomatic pericardial fluid/thickening detected radiographically, tachyarrhythmias or pericardial tamponade. Autopsy series suggest that as many as 30% of patients may have cardiac involvement by lung cancer, but not nearly as many are suspected ante mortem.

In addition to its characteristic tendency to spread to hilar and mediastinal lymph nodes, lung cancer may metastasize within the lung in several patterns. One type is lymphangitic carcinomatosis, which usually appears on chest radiograph as focal or diffuse reticular or reticulonodular interstitial infiltrates and Kerley B lines, possibly combined with central adenopathy and pleural effusions. By high-resolution chest computed tomography (CT), this process characteristically appears as irregular nodular thickening along bronchovascular bundles and interlobular septa, consistent with the role of lymphatics in this form of dissemination.[8] Intrapulmonary metastases may also appear as single or multiple nodules/masses in one or both hemithoraces. A management dilemma occurs in patients with otherwise resectable lung cancer who have one or more radiographically indeterminate lung nodules. The differential diagnosis is broad, but includes synchronous lung cancers, granulomatous processes, silicotic nodules, metastatic extrapulmonary malignancies, Wegener's granulomatosis, and others. An individualized approach to these situations is generally recommended. Lung cancer microembolism to the pulmonary arterial system, a rare form of intrathoracic metastasis, produces dyspnea and is very difficult to diagnose ante mortem. Diagnosis has been occasionally accomplished by cytological examination of blood drawn through a wedged pulmonary artery catheter.

Pleural effusion

Lung cancer and breast cancer are the most common causes of malignant pleural effusion. Malignant pleural effusions due to lung cancer are generally on the same side as the main tumor. They may be moderate to large in size, bloody, and recurrent following thoracentesis. Pleural effusions develop in the setting of malignancy from local effects of the tumor (pleural metastases, lymphatic obstruction, bronchial obstruction with pneumonia or atelectasis, and chylothorax), systemic effects (pulmonary thromboembolism and hypoalbuminemia), or as complications of therapy.[9] The main mechanism for malignant pleural effusion formation is altered lymphatic drainage. Metastatic tumor implants on the pleural surface may alter capillary permeability and further increase pleural fluid formation. In most cases, metastatic involvement of the pleura is thought to begin with hematogenous seeding of the visceral pleura, followed by subsequent movement and attachment of tumor cells to the parietal pleural surface.

Malignant effusions are usually exudative (effusion meets at least one of the following criteria: pleural fluid/serum total protein ratio >0.5, pleural fluid/serum lactate dehydrogenase (LDH) ratio >0.6, or pleural fluid LDH $>$two-thirds of the upper limits of normal of the serum) and lymphocytic (>50%) predominant. The fluid may appear serous, serosanguineous or frankly bloody. The initial thoracentesis of a malignant effusion reveals malignant cells 50% of the time. The cytological yield increases to 65% and 70% on the second and third attempts respectively. Pleural fluid cytology is more sensitive than pleural biopsy primarily because pleural metastases tend to be focal and percutaneous biopsy is performed blindly. Pleural biopsy adds very little to the overall diagnostic yield when combined with cytology.[10] Therefore a second thoracentesis is usually performed rather than closed pleural biopsy if malignant effusion is suspected.[11] Low pleural fluid pH (<7.30) and glucose (<60 mg/dl) values predict higher pleural fluid cytology yields, but also predict poor response to pleurodesis and short survival time.[9]

Malignant cells in pleural fluid indicate T4 or stage IIIB disease in NSCLC, and this eliminates further consideration of surgical resection. It is important to remember, however, that the mere presence of a pleural effusion does not categorically preclude surgery for NSCLC (see Chapter 10). Other conditions that can cause pleural fluid without direct tumor involvement of the pleura include postobstructive pneumonitis/atelectasis, pulmonary embolism, or illnesses unrelated to the tumor, such as congestive heart failure, nonobstructive pneumonia and cirrhosis. Therefore the physician must thoroughly evaluate pleural effusion in NSCLC patients with otherwise potentially resectable disease. Unfortunately, series have demonstrated that only 5–10% of lung cancer patients with cytologically negative pleural effusions are ultimately found to have operable disease.[12]

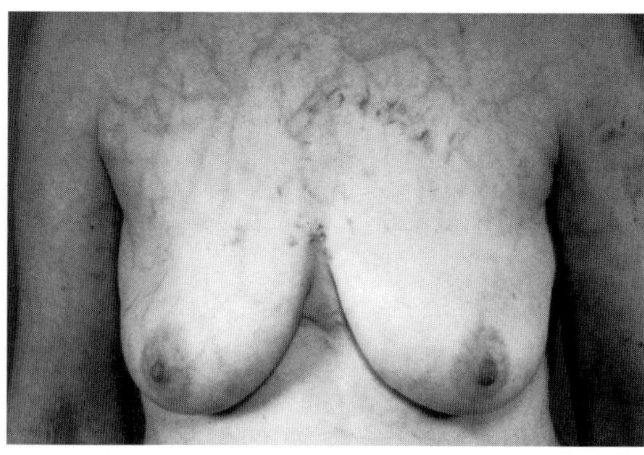

Figure 9.1
Tortuous, prominent, collateral venous drainage over the upper torso in superior vena cava syndrome. (Courtesy of JH Ryu, MD, Mayo Clinic, Rochester, MN.)

Superior vena cava syndrome

Several well-known syndromes result from regional growth of lung cancer. Obstructed venous flow due to extrinsic compression of the superior vena cava by adjacent bronchogenic carcinoma causes the superior vena cava syndrome.[13] Clinical manifestations result from venous hypertension above the level of the obstruction. Symptoms and signs typically include headache and facial fullness (which may be worse in the recumbent position), swelling and ruddiness of the face, neck and upper extremities, distended neck veins, and prominent/tortuous collateral venous drainage over the upper torso (Figure 9.1). Chest radiography may reveal mediastinal widening or a right perihilar mass. Bronchogenic carcinoma is the leading cause, but only 4% of lung cancers present in this manner. The differential diagnosis also includes lymphoma, metastatic extrathoracic malignancies, granulomatous mediastinal inflammation/fibrosis, postirradiation fibrosis and aortic aneurysms. Although the treatment goal remains prompt initiation of palliative chemotherapy or radiation, superior vena cava syndrome is no longer regarded as a medical emergency.[14] Diagnostic studies can be safely executed, and a tissue diagnosis should be obtained before starting therapy. Chemotherapy

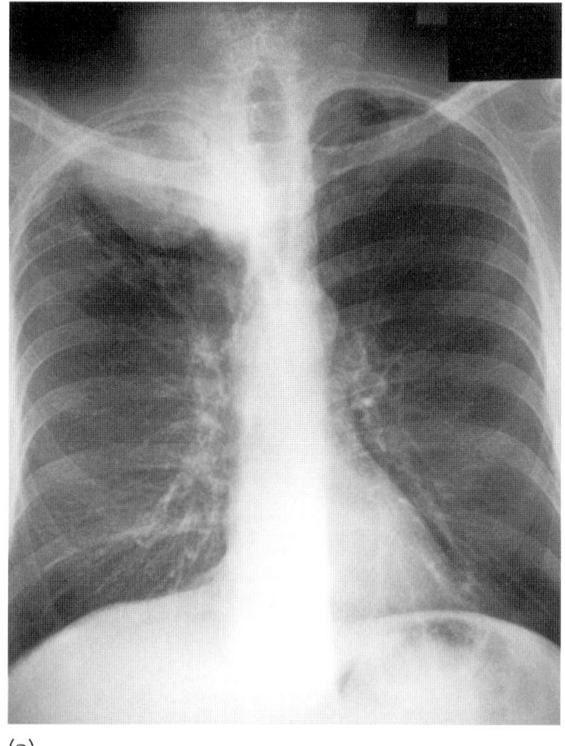

(a)

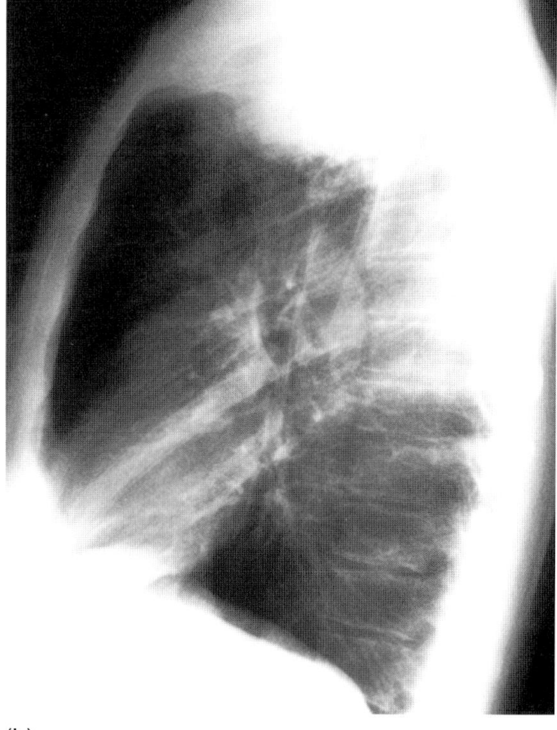

(b)

(c)

Figure 9.2
(a) Posteroanterior and (b) lateral chest radiographs and (c) CT appearance of a large right superior sulcus tumor in a 52-year-old smoker who presented with right shoulder pain. Transthoracic needle aspiration revealed squamous cell carcinoma.

or radiotherapy will relieve the obstruction symptoms in most lung cancer patients with superior vena cava syndrome.

Pancoast's syndrome

Pancoast's syndrome is characterized by a tumor situated in the extreme apical region of the hemithorax called the superior sulcus, in conjunction with ipsilateral shoulder and medial scapular discomfort. Patients may also have pain, with or without muscle wasting in the ulnar nerve (C8, T1) distribution, and Horner's syndrome (ptosis, miosis and ipsilateral facial anhidrosis). Most patients do not have all of these signs and symptoms until late in the course of the disease. Tumor invasion of the adjacent chest wall, brachial plexus and sympathetic ganglion is the cause of the clinical manifestations. The clinical findings vary depending on the extent to which the adjacent structures are involved. Superior sulcus tumors may manifest on chest radiograph as unilateral apical thickening (>5 mm), apical mass (Figure 9.2) or bony destruction.[15] Magnetic resonance imaging (MRI) has been shown to more accurately define the local magnitude of superior sulcus tumors than CT. The majority of cases of Pancoast's syndromes are due to NSCLC, but SCLC, metastatic extrapulmonary cancer and infectious conditions (bacterial, mycobacterial and fungal) have also been implicated. Tissue diagnosis is recommended, and transthoracic needle aspiration is frequently and successfully employed in this regard. Pancoast's tumors are generally defined as stage IIB, IIIA or IIIB lesions (see Chapter 10).

Metastatic effects

Approximately 40–50% of NSCLC patients present with metastatic disease that precludes surgical resection. SCLC has an even greater propensity to metastasize earlier in its course. Consequently, SCLC is considered a systemic disease at the time of diagnosis, even if it appears to be limited to the chest. Lung cancer dissemination may occur via lymphatic, hematogenous or interalveolar routes.[16] Metastases to nearly every organ have been described, but the most common sites of involvement are the lung, adrenals, liver, central nervous system and bone. Clinical manifestations depend upon the extent of specific organ dysfunction induced by metastases. Quoted frequencies of metastases differ depending upon whether initial presentation or autopsy series are cited.

Adrenal

Adrenal metastases are common in lung cancer, and are reported in 25–45% of autopsy series. They are usually asymptomatic, and are initially detected as unilateral adrenal gland enlargement on staging chest CT extended to the upper abdomen. In two series totalling 576 NSCLC patients, 4–7.5% were found to have an isolated unilateral adrenal mass with approximately 30–40% of the adrenal lesions found to be malignant.[17,18] Adrenal adenomas occur in 2–10% of the general population, and typically appear on CT as homogeneous, low-attenuation (due to fat content), well-circumscribed lesions less than 3 cm in diameter.[11] A suspicious adrenal enlargement must be pursued with CT-guided needle biopsy in NSCLC patients before a curative thoracic surgical attempt is undertaken. More recently, chemical shift MRI has been shown to be 96% sensitive and 100% specific for distinguishing adenomas, and may ultimately eliminate the need for percutaneous biopsies in selected patients.[19] The differential diagnosis for benign adrenal enlargement includes adrenal adenomas, nodular hyperplasia and hemorrhagic cysts.

Liver

Metastatic involvement of the liver is common and usually clinically silent early in the course of disease. Liver metastases are particularly common with SCLC. They are found in 25% of SCLC patients at the time of presentation and in 60% at autopsy. History and physical examination do not dependably detect liver metastases. Liver involvement may be suggested by abnormalities on the initial staging CT or by elevated liver test values. Advanced liver involvement may be associated with systemic symptoms, such as anorexia, weight loss and jaundice.

Central nervous system

Lung cancer is the most common cause of brain metastases. Clinical and autopsy data indicate that approximately 40% of lung cancer patients will develop brain metastases. Small cell and adenocarcinoma are the most common histological types of lung cancer to cause brain metastases. Although occasionally asymptomatic, brain metastases usually cause either nonfocal symptoms, such as headache (most common), nausea and vomiting, or focal abnormalities, including seizures, hemi-sensorimotor changes and cranial nerve deficits. Neurological symptoms precede lung cancer symptoms in most patients with concurrent disease. Metastases develop more commonly in the cerebral hemispheres, particularly in the parietal and frontal lobes, than in the cerebellum. Metastatic lesions are detected by CT or MRI. Central nervous system metastases signal stage IV disease and generally herald an ominous prognosis, but neurosurgical advances have resulted in successful resection of solitary brain metastases, leading to improvements in neurological status and survival.[20] Surgery is considered in medically appropriate patients with potentially resectable intrathoracic primaries whose solitary metastatic lesions are large, superficial, causing symptoms requiring immediate relief, or associated with significant edema or hemorrhage.[21]

Other forms of central nervous system involvement by metastatic lung cancer include spinal cord metastases and leptomeningeal carcinomatosis. Intraspinal lesions usually cause back pain that is worsened by movement, straining and supine positioning. Neurological deficits from spinal cord compression, such as sensory defects at or below the level of the lesion, paraparesis or paraplegia, and bowel/bladder incontinence tend to develop quickly, progress rapidly and be irreversible. In this event, spinal metastases become a medical emergency, for which steroids should be started pending definitive therapy. Leptomeningeal carcinomatosis is uncommon, and uniformly predicts a short survival time. Neurological symptoms may also result from a number of paraneoplastic syndromes which are discussed below.

Bone

Skeletal metastases occur in approximately 25–30% of lung cancer patients, and are typically found as osteolytic lesions in the vertebral bodies, ribs, and the long bones of the arms and legs. These lesions usually produce pain or elevations of calcium or alkaline phosphatase.[11] Twenty percent of SCLC patients may also have bone marrow involvement, which may not initially be accompanied by clinical or laboratory abnormalities. Bony metastases may be detectable on plain radiographs. If these are negative, a bone scan should be obtained. If the diagnosis remains in doubt, MRI of the specific bony structure is the most sensitive test for the detection of bony metastases.

Paraneoplastic effects

Bronchogenic carcinomas are associated with paraneoplastic syndromes more than any other tumor. Ten to twenty percent of lung cancer patients will develop paraneoplastic syndromes. These diverse phenomena, most of which are more common with SCLC, result from effects of lung cancer on other organ systems beyond those related to the physical presence of the primary or metastatic lesions. The clinical manifestations are frequently nonspecific, and are mediated by the ectopic production of biologically active peptides, cytokines and antibodies.[22] An awareness of the paraneoplastic syndromes is important, since they may be the presenting feature of an otherwise difficult to detect lung cancer in its earlier or recurrent stages. With the clinically frustrating exception of the neurological syndromes, the course of most paraneoplastic syndromes is analogous to that of the underlying lung cancer. Table 9.2 lists the paraneoplastic syndromes associated with lung cancer. The most

Table 9.2 Paraneoplastic syndromes associated with lung cancer (modified from the literature[11,22])

Endocrine/metabolic	Musculoskeletal
Hypercalcemia	Polymyositis
Syndrome of inappropriate antidiuretic hormone (SIADH) (hyponatremia)	Myopathy
Cushing's syndrome	Neurological
Gynecomastia	Lambert–Eaton myasthenic syndrome
Galactorrhea	Peripheral neuropathy
Acromegaly	Cerebellar degeneration
Carcinoid syndrome	Limbic encephalitis
Hyperthyroidism	Polyradiculopathy
Hypercalcitoninemia	Myelopathy
Hyperglycemia	Opsoclonus/myoclonus
Hypoglycemia	Dysautonomia
Hypouricemia	Retinopathy
Cachexia/anorexia	Hematological
Cutaneous	Anemia
Clubbing/hypertrophic osteoarthropathy	Polycythemia
Dermatomyositis	Hypercoagulable state
Acanthosis nigricans	Migratory thrombophlebitis
Erythema gyratum repens	Disseminated intravascular coagulation
Hyperpigmentation	Nonbacterial thrombotic endocarditis
Urticaria	Leukocytosis/leukemoid reaction
Vasculitis	Dysproteinemia
Pruritis	Eosinophilia
Basex's syndrome (acrokeratosis)	Thrombocytopenic purpura
Tylosis	Renal
Erythroderma	Glomerulonephritis
Acquired ichthyosis	Tubulointerstitial disorders
Erythema annulare centrifugum	Nephrotic syndrome
Sign of Leser–Trelat	

common paraneoplastic syndromes are discussed below.

Hypercalcemia

Hypercalcemia is the most frequently encountered paraneoplastic syndrome. Lung cancer is the most commonly responsible malignancy, with squamous cell the usual histological type. Hypercalcemia generally results from tumor production of parathyroid hormone-related peptide (PTHrP).[23] Rarely, hypercalcemia is due to osteolytic bony metastases or aberrant elaboration of other cytokines. PTHrP mimics the actions of endogenous parathyroid hormone

(PTH), so hypercalcemia results from heightened osteoclastic bone breakdown, decreased bone formation and decreased renal calcium excretion. The manifestations of hypercalcemia are malaise, weakness, fatigue, abdominal pain, constipation, anorexia, polydipsia, polyuria, confusion, hyporeflexia and shortened QT interval on ECG. Coma and death are late manifestations. Diagnosis is made by demonstrating a combination of increased serum ionized calcium level (or disproportionate increase in total serum calcium relative to the serum albumin), normal or low PTH level by immunoassay (to rule out primary hyperparathyroidism), and exclusion of other causes of hypercalcemia (granulomatous disorders such as sarcoidosis, hyperthyroidism, adrenal insufficiency, acute renal failure, Paget's disease, and medications such as thiazide diuretics and vitamin D). It is also very important to rule out bony metastases. PTHrP is detectable by radioimmunoassay, but problems remain with test sensitivity. Treatment strategies are volume repletion with normal saline, increased urinary calcium excretion with a loop diuretic such as furosemide, decreased bony resorption with bisphosphonates, calcitonin or gallium, and treatment of the underlying malignancy.[24] The last may be difficult, since hypercalcemia usually occurs with advanced disease. The median survival with hypercalcemia is two to three months.

Syndrome of inappropriate antidiuretic hormone

The cardinal manifestation of the syndrome of inappropriate antidiuretic hormone (SIADH) is hyponatremia due to the inappropriately sustained ectopic production of arginine vasopressin (AVP; antidiuretic hormone), which acts on the distal renal tubule to promote free-water conservation. Small cell is almost always the underlying lung cancer histological type.[25] SIADH can occur with equal frequency in limited and extensive SCLC. Clinical manifestations of hyponatremia are due to cerebral edema, and occur more in relation to the rate of fall of the serum sodium than to the absolute serum sodium level. Because the hyponatremia usually develops slowly in SIADH, many patients are asymptomatic at presentation. Early symptoms include fatigue, weakness, nausea and anorexia. The diagnostic criteria for SIADH are: hyponatremia, serum, hypoosmolality (<275 mosmol/kg), inappropriately increased urine osmolality (>200 mosmol/kg), natriuresis (urine sodium >20 mmol/l), clinical euvolemia, and the absence of renal, adrenal and thyroid dysfunction. Central nervous system disorders, other pulmonary lesions (notably pneumonia) and drugs (including cyclophosphamide, tricyclic antidepressants, thiazide diuretics, morphine and vincristine) can also cause SIADH. Asymptomatic or mildly symptomatic patients may be treated with restriction of water intake to less than 1 liter per day (although sustained compliance is difficult) and demeclocycline (which gradually blocks the action of AVP on the kidney). More serious symptoms, such as seizures, cognitive decline and mental status changes, or more profound hyponatremia (serum sodium <120 mmol/l) should be treated with normal (0.9%) saline and a loop diuretic. The use of hypertonic (3%) saline is rarely indicated. Use of normal saline alone may actually decrease the serum sodium concentration, so a loop diuretic must be added. The goal should be to raise the serum sodium at a maximum rate of 2 mmol/l/h (maximum 20 mmol/l/day) to a target of 120–125 mmol/l. More aggressive sodium correction may theoretically result in central pontine myelinolysis – a devastating central neurological insult usually resulting in death.

Ectopic adrenocorticotropic hormone syndrome

Cushing's syndrome describes a constellation of findings due to excess glucocorticoid production.

Approximately 80% of adrenocorticotropic hormone (ACTH)-dependent cases of Cushing's syndrome are due to Cushing's *disease* – an ACTH-secreting tumor of pituitary origin. The remaining cases are due primarily to ectopic ACTH or corticotropin-releasing hormone (CRH) production, usually by SCLC (most common) or bronchial carcinoid tumors. Ectopically produced ACTH directly stimulates adrenal glucocorticoid release, while CRH triggers ACTH release from the pituitary. Slowly growing carcinoid tumors may be accompanied by the classic features of Cushing's syndrome, including truncal weight gain, moon facies, hypertension, purplish cutaneous striae, hirsutism, glucose intolerance and proximal muscle weakness. Cushing's manifestations in more rapidly growing SCLC are usually limited to weight loss, hypertension, edema, weakness, poor skin integrity, hypokalemic alkalosis and glucose intolerance. Overall, less than 5% of SCLC patients develop Cushing's syndrome, and its occurrence predicts a shorter survival time, perhaps because of the co-morbidities induced by glucocorticoid excess. An elevated 24–hour urinary free-cortisol level (typically >275 nmol/day) and failure to suppress cortisol during low-dose dexamethasone challenge confirm the presence of Cushing's syndrome.[26] An ectopic source of ACTH is suggested by lack of suppression with high-dose dexamethasone and serum ACTH levels greater than 40 pmol/l, yet exceptions exist such as the tendency of some carcinoids to be suppressed by high-dose dexamethasone. Treatment options include resection (carcinoid tumors), chemotherapy (SCLC), bilateral adrenalectomy, or medical suppression of adrenal glucocorticoid production with ketoconazole, aminoglutethimide or metyrapone.

Neurological syndromes

There are several stereotypical neurodegenerative syndromes that occur primarily in SCLC patients.[27] These paraneoplastic syndromes are distinct from the nonfocal neurological dysfunction induced by the systemic effects of cancer. They are felt to be sequelae of autoimmune phenomena that can involve any level(s) of the nervous sytem (brain, cranial nerves, spinal cord, peripheral nerves, neuromuscular junction and muscle). The proposed pathogenic sequence begins with the ectopic expression by tumor cells of antigens similar to those normally expressed in the nervous system. The shared antigen is sensed as foreign, and an immune response ensues causing nervous system injury and clinical deficits.[28] In support of this mechanism are the observations that these syndromes are associated with specific detectable antibodies, nervous system injuries are strikingly limited to specific cell types, deposits of immunoglobulin have been demonstrated in areas of neuronal cell loss, and the characteristic antibodies are made in the central nervous system by autoreactive lymphocytes. The prototypical process of the autoantibody pathogenic mechanism is the Lambert–Eaton myasthenic syndrome. However, not all patients with clinically similar syndromes have detectable autoantibodies; attempts to induce similar syndromes in animals with passive immunoglobulin transfer or immunization with the culprit antigen have been largely unsuccessful, and immunosuppressants are not usually effective treatments. Our understanding of these syndromes continues to evolve.

Lambert–Eaton myasthenic syndrome

Proximal muscle weakness, hyporeflexia and autonomic dysfunction (dry mouth, erectile dysfunction, constipation, blurred vision) characterize Lambert–Eaton myasthenic syndrome (LEMS). The pathognomonic electromyographic finding is a marked increase of the compound muscle action potential following high rates of nerve stimulation.

Similarly, augmented strength and reflexes can be demonstrated on physical examination after maximal contraction of the involved muscle groups. Clinical manifestations are due to antibodies to P/Q-type voltage-gated calcium channels expressed on the presynaptic cholinergic synapses of peripheral nerves that interfere with the release of acetylcholine.[29] These voltage-gated calcium channels also appear on SCLC cells. Treatments of potential benefit include 3,4-diaminopyridine (which increases presynaptic calcium influx), plasma exchange, intravenous immunoglobulin and treatment of the underlying tumor. Approximately one-third to one-half of LEMS patients will improve with treatment of the underlying SCLC. However, not all patients with LEMS have an underlying malignancy.

Antineuronal nuclear autoantibodies-1-associated (ANNA-1) syndromes

ANNA-1, also known as anti-Hu antibodies, are IgG antibodies that recognize a family of nuclear mRNA-binding proteins expressed in SCLC cells and neurons of the central and peripheral nervous systems. These antibodies are distinct from the autoantibodies of systemic lupus erythematosus, and whether ANNA-1 antibodies have a pathogenic role in the neurological manifestations remains unclear. Seropositivity for ANNA-1 is associated with a diverse set of neurological disorders that can occur in varying combinations. Lucchinetti and colleagues[30] reported on the wide spectrum of neurological and oncological findings in 162 ANNA-1 seropositive patients. Twice as many women were afflicted as men. By the end of follow-up, a malignancy had been detected in 142 patients (88%), with 81% having SCLC. Seventeen of the SCLC patients developed at least one other malignancy. Neurological signs associated with ANNA-1, in decreasing frequency, were neuropathy (sensory > mixed somatic > autonomic > motor), cerebellar ataxia, limbic encephalitis (neurocognitive and neurobehavioral deficits), polyradiculopathy, LEMS, myopathy, myelopathy, opsoclonus/myoclonus, motor neuronopathy, brachial plexopathy and aphasia. Gastrointestinal dysmotility occurred in 38 (28%) patients, as manifested primarily by gastroparesis and intestinal pseudoobstruction due to involvement of the myenteric plexus. The neurological manifestations preceded the cancer diagnosis in 96% of patients, and usually progressed in a subacute manner. None of the 49 patients who received immunosuppressant therapy (steroids, plasma exchange, intravenous immunoglobulin or cyclophosphamide) experienced neurological improvement. Somewhat ironically, ANNA-1 seropositivity is associated with more limited stage SCLC at presentation, higher complete tumor response to chemotherapy and longer survival.[31] Patients with unexplained neurological findings, ANNA-1 positivity and a history of smoking should undergo a thorough search for SCLC, including a chest CT with contrast. Five to fifteen percent of SCLC patients may be ANNA-1 seropositive without neurological findings.

Other neurological paraneoplastic syndromes

Type 2 antineuronal nuclear autoantibodies (ANNA-2), also known as anti-Ri antibodies, are linked with opsoclonus/myoclonus (opsoclonus are involuntary, conjugate, arrhythmic high-amplitude, saccadic eye movements) in the setting of breast cancer. Paraneoplastic cerebellar degeneration is associated with a specific anti-Purkinje cell antibody called anti-Yo (PCA 1) in females with breast and gynecological malignancies. Similar syndromes can occur in SCLC and NSCLC, but lung cancer patients are typically ANNA-2 or anti-Yo seronegative. Cancer-associated retinopathy is a rare complication of SCLC, and is felt to be due to detectable antibodies directed at the retinal photoreceptor layer or ganglion cells.

Other paraneoplastic syndromes

Clubbing of the fingers and toes is characterized by loss of the angle between the base of the nail bed and cuticle, rounded nails and enlargement of the digit tips.[32] Hypertrophic osteoarthropathy (HPO) is a painful proliferative periostitis that classically involves the long bones of the arms and legs.[32] The affected bones reveal periosteal new bone formation on plain radiographs, and increased, symmetric uptake on radionuclide studies. Clubbing and HPO are rare entities that can occur together or as isolated findings. The cause(s) remains unknown, but they can occur in conjunction with bronchogenic carcinoma, as well as a variety of cardiopulmonary suppurative processes (bronchiectasis, cystic fibrosis, empyema and subacute bacterial endocarditis), usual interstitial pneumonitis/idiopathic pulmonary fibrosis, pulmonary arteriovenous malformations, congenital cyanotic heart disease inflammatory bowel disease and cirrhosis. The potential association between polymyositis and lung cancer remains controversial. Similarly, it is unclear how thoroughly the physician should search for malignancy in patients with unexplained venous thromboembolism. A prudent strategy may be to maintain a low threshold of suspicion for malignancy when venous thromboembolism develops without conventional risk factors, and to proceed with additional testing as directed by history, physical examination and routine initial investigations.[33]

PHYSICAL EXAMINATION

A careful physical examination is a vital component of lung cancer evaluation, since it may provide important diagnostic, prognostic and staging clues. General appearance may be normal or may reveal debilitation, cachexia, lethargy, pallor, jaundice, fever or significant co-morbidities. Blood pressure irregularities can be seen in conjunction with neurological or adrenal paraneoplastic phenomena. Hoarseness suggests recurrent laryngeal nerve compromise.

Respiratory system examination should be conducted in an orderly manner. On inspection, tachypnea may signal painful rib metastases, pleural effusions or postobstructive pneumonia, while expiratory prolongation is consistent with underlying COPD. Signs of venous hypertension limited to the head, neck and arms are seen with superior vena cava syndrome, while jugular venous hypertension and pulsus paradoxus are signs of pericardial tamponade from metastatic disease. Pain may cause the patient to favor the upper extremity ipsilateral to a superior sulcus tumor. Neck palpation may yield evidence of spread to supraclavicular lymph nodes. Focal rib tenderness implies metastases. Direct extension of lung cancer to the chest wall is rarely palpable. The combination of percussible dullness, diminished breath sounds and reduced fremitus suggests pleural effusion, hemidiaphragm dysfunction due to phrenic nerve entrapment, or postobstructive pneumonitis/atelectasis. Bronchial breath sounds and increased fremitus indicate consolidation with patent proximal airways. Focal wheezing is detected with central airway compromise by an endobronchial tumor or extrinsic compression, generalized wheezing with COPD. Concurrent interstitial lung diseases, such as asbestosis, may be heralded by characteristic Velcro-type inspiratory crackles. Depending on their distribution, rubs may be due to venous thromboembolic events or metastatic pericardial or pleural involvement.

The remainder of the examination is equally important. Pertinent skin findings include cutaneous metastases, typically over the torso and scalp, and Basex's syndrome, which is hyperkeratosis of the acral regions. Acanthosis nigricans, brown velvety plaques of the groin, back of neck

Table 9.3 Karnofsky Performance Scale (from Margolis[45])

Definition	Percentage	Criteria
Able to carry on normal activity and to work; no special care needed	100	Normal; no complaints; no evidence of disease
	90	Able to carry on normal activity; minor signs or symptoms of disease
	80	Normal activity with effort; some signs or symptoms of disease
Unable to work; able to live at home; cares for most personal needs; a varying amount of assistance is needed	70	Cares for self; unable to carry on normal activity or to do active work
	60	Requires occasional assistance, but is able to care for most needs
	50	Requires considerable assistance and frequent medical care
Unable to care for self; requires equivalent of institutional or hospital care; disease may be progressing rapidly	40	Disabled; requires special care and assistance
	30	Severely disabled; hospitalization is indicated, although death may not be imminent
	20	Very sick; hospitalization necessary; active supportive treatment necessary
	10	Moribund; fatal processes progressing rapidly

and axillae, may be paraneoplastic phenomena, but are more commonly seen with obesity and diabetes. The differential diagnosis for bony pain in the cancer setting includes skeletal metastases and HPO. Liver metastases may be palpable. A thorough nervous system examination is crucial, especially in patients with headache, sensorimotor complaints and back pain. Unilateral lower extremity swelling, tenderness and erythema may accompany deep venous thromboses.

The history and physical examination findings can be combined to estimate general health status, such as by the Karnofsky Performance Scale (Table 9.3). This clinical index provides a convenient framework to rate the impact of the lung cancer and co-morbidities on the patient. Performance status has been shown reproducibly to be an important prognostic variable in NSCLC and SCLC, and usually influences treatment decision-making.

IMAGING

Standard chest radiograph

The standard posteroanterior and lateral chest radiograph is usually the first test to suggest bronchogenic carcinoma, and it helps to assess the intrathoracic extent of cancer, guides subsequent work-up, and identifies simultaneous thoracic disease.[34] The spectrum of possible findings is broad, but the most common are a localized opacity (nodule or mass), pleural effusion, infiltrate, atelectasis and adenopathy. Certain radiographic appearances may suggest histological types of lung cancer, but these generalizations are not absolute. Squamous cell carcinoma usually presents as a large mass, centered at or near the hilum, that may cavitate. SCLC may also present as a rapidly enlarging central mass with contiguous hilar and mediastinal involvement. Only 5–10% of SCLCs present as peripheral lung lesions. Adenocarcinoma typically arises peripherally as a solitary nodule or mass. Large cell carcinoma is characteristically a large peripheral mass. Brochioloalveolar carcinoma may appear as a nodule or an alveolar infiltrate that can be diffuse. The drawbacks of plain chest radiography include lack of specificity and resolution limitations. Lesions smaller than 2–3 mm are not reliably detectable, and the regions behind the heart and clavicle may be difficult to interpret. Estimates are that chest radiography is 70–80% accurate in the overall detection of lung cancer, 50–60% sensitive in the detection of hilar adenopathy, and less than 50% sensitive in the detection of mediastinal adenopathy.[35]

Computed tomography

CT greatly enhances the imaging of bronchogenic carcinoma by providing further definition of the primary lesion's appearance, detecting concurrent parenchymal or pleural disease missed by plain chest radiograph, demonstrating lymphangitic spread of malignancy, guiding diagnostic maneuvers, and evaluating hilar and mediastinal lymph node metastases. CT also helps in the evaluation of distant metastases by the routine practice of extending the examination to include the liver and adrenals. The delineation by CT of the relation of bronchogenic carcinoma to surrounding structures is particularly important, since these findings significantly influence prognosis and, in the case of NSCLC, surgical options. However, the resolution limitations of CT in this regard must be acknowledged. Consensus calls for intrathoracic lymph nodes larger than 1 cm in diameter to be considered abnormal by CT. The sensitivity and specificity of CT to detect hilar and mediastinal lymph node metastases range from 50% to 90%.[36] The sensitivity of CT suffers from microscopic lymph node metastases, while its specificity is influenced by benign causes of lymphadenopathy, such as reactive hyperplasia, granulomatous inflammation and anthracosis. CT also has difficulties in accurately diagnosing chest wall or mediastinal structure invasion, detecting endobronchial lesions, and differentiating tumor from adjacent atelectasis or pneumonia. Hence CT is not a substitute for histological information, and patients must not be denied surgery for NSCLC based simply on CT findings without tissue confirmation.

Solitary pulmonary nodule

A solitary pulmonary nodule (SPN) is a common clinical radiological dilemma. Defined as a singular rounded lesion entirely surrounded by lung normal parenchyma and without associated lymphadenopathy, an SPN may be due to malignant and benign causes (Table 9.4).[37] The majority of SPNs are benign. Most malignant SPNs are clinical stage I bronchogenic carcinomas. SPNs are usually incidental findings on plain chest radiographs obtained for other purposes. The ques-

Table 9.4 Causes of solitary pulmonary nodules (from Midthun et al[37])

Infectious granuloma
Tuberculosis
Histoplasmosis
Coccidioidomycosis
Bronchogenic carcinoma
Metastatic cancer
Breast
Head and neck
Colon
Renal cell
Sarcoma
Germ cell
Bronchial carcinoid
Hamartoma
Organizing pneumonia/abscess
Wegener's granulomatosis
Rheumatoid nodule
Arteriovenous malformation
Pulmonary infarction
Bronchogenic cyst
Lipoma
Amyloidoma

tions become whether the SPN is benign or malignant, and whether it should be observed, biopsied or removed. The evaluation begins, if possible, with review of previous chest radiographs. A nodule that has been radiographically stable for at least two years is, by definition, benign, and no further maneuvers are necessary. A steadily growing nodule is considered malignant, and should be resected immediately. When comparison studies are insufficient, the next step is to assess for calcification in the nodule with plain or computed tomography. Central, concentric or popcorn calcification patterns are reliable indicators of their benign nature. Eccentric calcification does not rule out malignancy. Thin-section CT images may also detect fat within the nodule; this indicates hamartoma, which is always benign. Taking advantage of the differences in vascular supply between benign and malignant nodules, Swenson and colleagues demonstrated that the level of nodule enhancement detected by thin-section CT after injection of intravenous contrast reliably differentiated benign from malignant lesions (Figure 9.3). Using 15 Hounsfield units as the threshold for enhancement, sensitivity of this technique was 98% and specificity 58%.[38] If a nodule does not enhance, it is almost always benign (98% sensitivity). If radiological studies are inconclusive, clinical factors predicting a higher risk of malignancy include advanced age of the patient, smoking history, prior malignancies and larger nodule size. The patient's wishes must be considered in the decision-making process. Lesions 3 cm or more in size are malignant in over 90% of cases, and should not be observed. If a lesion is not removed and is indeterminate then it must be observed. Observation typically involves obtaining serial chest CT scans every three months for the first year and every six months during the second year.[37] Serial plain chest radiographs do not reliably detect enlargement of small nodules. If the nodule grows, it must be resected. If the nodule is stable for two years, it is safe to assume that it is benign. The potential for metastases during observation of malignant nodules over three to six months is unknown, but there is no proof that this brief period of observation is detrimental to survival.

Magnetic resonance imaging

MRI does not have a routine role in the evaluation of lung cancer. However, its superiority over CT in distinguishing tumor abutment versus invasion of chest wall, vertebral and mediastinal structures makes it a useful adjunct in situations such as superior sulcus tumors and possible

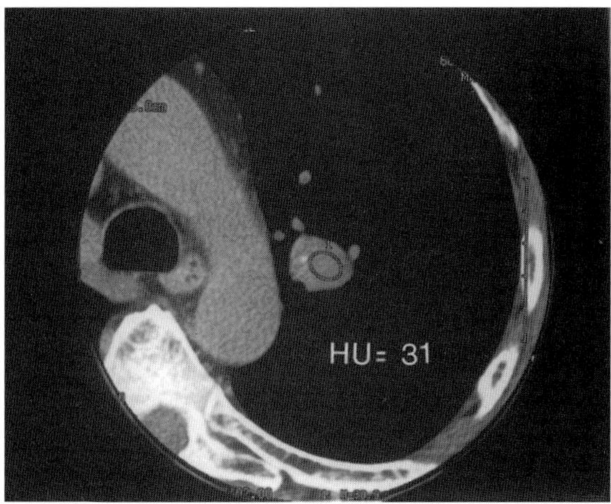

(a)

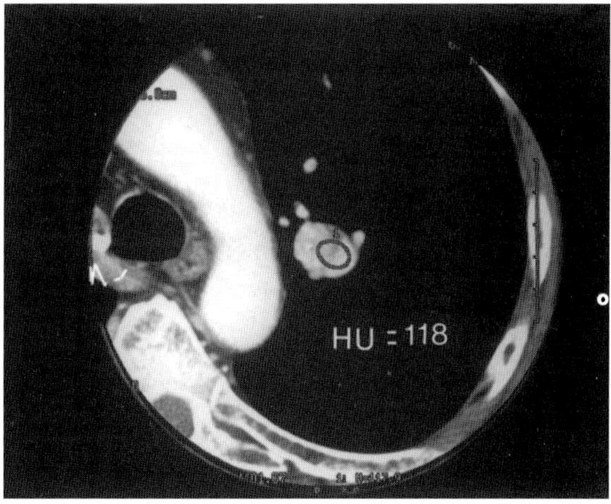

(b)

Figure 9.3
CT images demonstrating enhancement of 87 Hounsfield units (HU) of a left lung nodule after injection of iodinated contrast (31 HU on the precontrast image versus 118 HU on the postcontrast image). The circle within the nodule circumscribes the region used to measure enhancement.

neuroforaminal encroachment.[39] MRI is limited by cardiac and respiratory motion artifact, lack of widespread availability and expense.

Nuclear medicine studies

In NSCLC patients with marginal pulmonary function, quantitative ventilation–perfusion ($\dot{V}/\dot{Q}$) lung scans can be used to assess candidacy for lung resection. The fraction of total ventilation or perfusion from the contralateral lung is multiplied by the preoperative forced expiratory volume in 1 second (FEV_1) to predict postoperative FEV_1 for patients undergoing pneumonectomy. An FEV_1 of 40% of predicted suggests that the patient should tolerate resection from a pulmonary perspective.[40] Bone scanning is not routinely recommended to rule out occult bony metastases in early stage bronchogenic carcinoma, but is indicated in lung cancer patients with bone pain, hypercalcemia, increased alkaline phosphatase and/or pathological fractures.[11] The technique suffers from reduced specificity, since old fractures and degenerative changes may cause lesions indistinguishable from metastases. Indeterminate abnormalities, especially over the spine and weight-bearing bones, require further plain radiographic evaluation and, in appropriate clinical circumstances, biopsy.

DIAGNOSTIC TECHNIQUES

An accurate tissue diagnosis is an essential early step in the management of lung cancer because of its therapeutic and prognostic import. Biopsy procedures are not always required before surgical therapy, but are conducted in most patients suspected of lung cancer since clinical and radiographic findings are not uniquely assigned to SCLC or NSCLC. Various techniques are available to obtain tissue for cytological and histopathological analysis.

Sputum cytology

Sputum cytology is a noninvasive method to obtain a diagnosis in appropriate situations.[41]

The yield depends on the ability of the patient to produce acceptable sputum, tumor size, location of tumor in relation to major central airways, and the cytopathologist's skills. Sensitivities of nearly 80% for detection of proximal tumors have been reported. The yield is below 20% for small (<3 cm) peripheral malignancies. The appropriate number of specimens to collect remains unclear, but one to three consecutive early morning samples or a three-day pooled sputum specimen are generally recommended. Abnormal findings may also result from concurrent pulmonary infections (false positives) or unsuspected head and neck cancers.

Flexible fiberoptic bronchoscopy

Flexible fiberoptic bronchoscopy is commonly used for diagnostic and staging purposes. Endoscopically visible abnormalities are approached with traditional biopsy forceps, brushings and washings. Transbronchial needle aspirations (TBNA) may also be performed on submucosal tumors or those causing extrinsic bronchial compression. The yield from an endoscopically visible lesion should be in excess of 80%. Peripheral lesions are sampled with fluoroscopically guided transbronchial biopsies, brushings and washings. Lesion size is the primary determinant of outcome, with yields of 25% reported for malignant lesions under 2 cm, 60–70% for lesions over 2 cm, and 80% for lesions over 4 cm.[42] Transbronchial lung biopsies should detect lymphangitic spread of malignancy. For staging purposes, bronchoscopy may occasionally detect synchronous lesions, assess proximal extent of tumor, and facilitate sampling of paratracheal, subcarinal and hilar lymph nodes by TBNA. Although technically challenging, TBNA has a sensitivity of 50% and a specificity of 90% for mediastinal staging.[43] Chest CT should be obtained before TBNA to help guide the attempts. Use of 19-gauge needles improves sensitivity by allowing procurement of cytological and histological specimens. TBNA should be obtained before sampling other endoscopically visible lesions to avoid false-positive results. Bleeding is a very infrequent complication of TBNA. Bronchoscopy in COPD patients confers only a slightly increased risk if obstruction is severe.[44]

Transthoracic needle aspiration

Peripheral lesions or those with extension to the mediastinum, chest wall or pleura may also be sampled by fluoroscopically or CT-guided transthoracic needle aspiration (TTNA). Suspicious peripheral lesions are sometimes directly resected for diagnosis and treatment if surgery would be the anticipated maneuver regardless of TTNA results. However, TTNA may be applied when a tissue diagnosis is needed but the patient cannot or will not undergo surgery, the patient is undecided about surgery pending tissue confirmation of cancer, or fiberoptic bronchoscopy was nondiagnostic.[45] Yields above 90% have been reported.[46] Pneumothorax is the main complication, occurring in up to 30% of cases, yet less than 15% will require a chest tube. Tumor seeding of the biopsy tract is a very rare complication. Increased-risk situations for TTNA include bullous emphysema in the region to be biopsied, lesions located away from the pleural surface, a poorly cooperative patient, and underlying lung disease whose impact would significantly increase if pneumothorax developed.[47] There is a substantial false-negative rate (20–30% of patients with a negative TTNA may have a malignant lesion),[11] so indeterminate or negative TTNA results must not be interpreted as a diagnostic endpoint. A repeat TTNA is diagnostic in 35–65% of cases.[11] Percutaneous radiologically guided needle aspiration is used to confirm metastases to liver, bone and adrenals.

Thoracic surgery techniques

Cervical mediastinoscopy or anterior mediastinotomy have been the traditional routes by which histological verification of mediastinal metastases has been obtained. These are safe procedures whose findings may obviate the need for further surgery in NSCLC patients. Cervical mediastinoscopy allows sampling of the right paratracheal and subcarinal nodes, while anterior mediastinotomy accesses the left paratracheal, supraaortic and aortopulmonary window nodes.[11] It remains controversial whether mediastinal sampling should be routinely performed before all surgery for NSCLC, but it should be performed in any patient felt to be a surgical candidate whose chest CT reveals mediastinal lymph nodes over 1 cm in diameter. Video-assisted thoracoscopic surgery (VATS) is a more recent, less-invasive technique for sampling of indeterminate peripheral nodules, pleural thickening and effusions, and mediastinal/hilar lymph nodes. Scalene or supraclavicular lymph node biopsy is an appropriate diagnostic and staging procedure in the setting of clinically significant enlargement. The patient with a suspicious lesion (enlarging or spiculated nodule) without evidence of metastatic disease may go directly to thoracotomy for definitive diagnosis and treatment.

OVERVIEW OF BASIC EVALUATION

The purpose of the basic evaluation is to efficiently and accurately establish the diagnosis and initial extent of lung cancer. Aspects of this process are influenced by local practice biases. The core elements include a careful history and physical examination, posteroanterior and lateral chest radiographs and basic blood tests, including complete blood count and chemistry profile (especially electrolytes, serum calcium, alkaline phosphatase, aspartate aminotransferase, albumin, total bilirubin and creatinine).[11] While the cost-effectiveness of the blood tests can be debated, they may suggest metastatic disease, paraneoplastic phenomena or co-morbidities. Chest CT with extension to upper abdominal CT is routinely obtained to define the primary lesion and locoregional extent of disease. Testing for extrapulmonary metastases is pursued as directed by the initial information. Biopsy of suspected metastases may allow simultaneous diagnosis and staging. Head CT and bone scanning are not routinely performed on asymptomatic patients with NSCLC and clinically early stage disease, although this remains controversial.[48] For peripheral chest lesions, the diagnostic options are TTNA, bronchoscopy, VATS and thoracotomy. It is unclear whether TTNA or bronchoscopy is the better initial choice. TTNA may enjoy a higher yield for smaller lesions, but also a higher complication rate. Bronchoscopy allows for endobronchial visualization, and would still be performed at the time of thoracotomy if TTNA were positive. For central lesions or hemoptysis with negative chest film, sputum cytology is also an option, and bronchoscopy is usually favored over TTNA.

Additional pulmonary testing may be necessary if surgical resection is considered. Given the common etiological thread of smoking, it is not surprising that 80–90% of lung cancer patients also have COPD, 20–30% of them with severe disease.[44] Lung resection, incisional pain, medical appliances, and postoperative use of sedatives and analgesics impact negatively on lung function and defense. Preoperative spirometry and diffusing capacity D_{LCO} should be obtained. Patients with $FEV_1 > 1.5$–2 l, maximal voluntary ventilation (MVV) > 50% of predicted and $D_{LCO} > 60\%$ of predicted can proceed to thoracotomy. Patients with values below these may need to undergo a more thorough examination that includes quantitative $\dot{V}/\dot{Q}$ lung scanning and/or exercise testing with evaluation of maximum oxygen uptake. Although no value categorically precludes surgery, predicted postoperative $FEV_1 < 40\%$ of predicted, hypercapnia ($P_{CO_2} > 45$), or maximal oxygen consumption <10 ml/kg/min during exercise testing predict significant postoperative problems.[40] The use of VATS and limited resections has dramatically changed the definition of inoperability due to pulmonary limitations.

FUTURE DEVELOPMENTS

Given the dramatic differences in overall lung cancer survival versus those enjoyed with resectable stage I disease, interest will continue to focus on methods of earlier lung cancer detection and more accurate staging.[49] The recent use of spiral CT scanners allows for extremely rapid thoracic imaging at a reduced radiation dose, thereby imparting the benefits of CT sensitivity with the speed and radiation levels of more traditional radiographic imaging. Spiral CT scanning may become the screening tool of the future.[50] Autofluorescence bronchoscopy exploits differences in light energy emission between normal and dysplastic/malignant tissue to facilitate detection of mucosal abnormalities at a theoretically earlier stage. Positron emission tomography (PET) scanning is an emerging and promising nuclear medicine application that may more accurately separate malignant from benign lung nodules, assess regional spread and detect visceral metastases.[39] It is hoped that these new techniques, combined with greater participation of patients in prospective clinical trials (currently only 1% of lung cancer patients in the USA are enrolled), will result in improved lung cancer survival rates.

REFERENCES

1. Kubik AK, Parkin DM, Plesko I et al, Patterns of cigarette sales and lung cancer mortality in some Central and Eastern European countries, 1960–1989. *Cancer* 1995; **75**: 2452–60.
2. American Thoracic Society, Cigarette smoking and health. *Am J Respir Crit Care Med* 1996; **153**: 861–5.
3. Tockman MS, Anthonisen NR, Wright EC et al, Airways obstruction and the risk for lung cancer. *Ann Intern Med* 1987; **106**: 512–18.
4. Yesner R, Pathogenesis and pathology. *Clin Chest Med* 1993; **14**: 17–30.
5. Irwin RS, Curley FJ, French CL, Chronic cough: the spectrum and frequency of causes, key components of the diagnostic evaluation, and outcome of specific therapy. *Am Rev Respir Dis* 1990; **141**: 640–7.
6. Poe RH, Israel RH, Marin MG et al, Utility of fiberoptic bronchoscopy in patients with hemoptysis and a non localizing chest roentgenogram. *Chest* 1988; **93**: 70–5.
7. Piehler JM, Pairolero PC, Gracey DR, Bernatz PE, Unexplained diaphragmatic paralysis: a harbinger of malignant disease? *J Thorac Cardiovasc Surg* 1982; **84**: 861–4.
8. Munk PL, Muller NL, Miller RR, Ostrow DN, Pulmonary lymphangitic carcinomatosis: CT and pathologic findings. *Radiology* 1988; **166**: 705–9.
9. Sahn SA, Pleural diseases related to metastatic malignancies. *Eur Respir J* 1997; **10**: 1907–13.
10. Prakash UBS, Reiman HM, Comparison of needle biopsy with cytologic analysis for the evaluation of pleural effusion: analysis of 414 cases. *Mayo Clin Proc* 1985; **60**: 158–64.
11. American Thoracic Society, European Respiratory Society, Pretreatment evaluation of non-small-cell lung cancer. *Am J Respir Crit Care Med* 1997; **156**: 320–32.
12. Decker DA, Dines DE, Payne WS et al, The significance of a cytologically negative pleural effusion in bronchogenic carcinoma. *Chest* 1978; **74**: 640–2.

13. Parish JM, Marschke RF, Dines DE, Lee RE, Etiologic considerations in superior vena cava syndrome. *Mayo Clin Proc* 1981; **56**: 407–13.
14. Ahmann FR, A reassessment of the clinical implications of the superior vena cava syndrome. *J Clin Oncol* 1984; **2**: 961–9.
15. Arcasoy SM, Jett JR, Superior pulmonary sulcus tumours and Pancoast's syndrome. *N Engl J Med* 1997; **337**: 1370–6.
16. Patel AM, Peters SG, Clinical manifestations of lung cancer. *Mayo Clin Proc* 1993; **68**: 273–7.
17. Oliver TW, Bernardino ME, Miller JI et al, Isolated adrenal masses in non-small cell bronchogenic carcinoma. *Radiology* 1984; **153**: 217–18.
18. Ettinghausen SE, Burt ME, Prospective evaluation of unilateral adrenal masses in patients with operable non-small cell lung cancer. *J Clin Oncol* 1991; **9**: 1462–6.
19. Schwartz LH, Ginsberg MS, Burt ME et al, MRI as an alternative to CT-guided biopsy of adrenal masses in patients with lung cancer. *Ann Thorac Surg* 1998; **65**: 193–7.
20. Patchell RA, Tibbs PA, Walsh JW et al, A randomized trial of surgery in the treatment of single metastases to the brain. *N Engl J Med* 1990; **322**: 494–500.
21. Black PMcL, Solitary brain metastases: radiation, resection, or radiosurgery. *Chest* 1993; **103**(4 Suppl): 367–9S.
22. Patel AM, Davila DG, Peters SG, Paraneoplastic syndromes associated with lung cancer. *Mayo Clin Proc* 1993; **68**: 278–87.
23. Burtis WJ, Parathyroid hormone-related protein: structure, function, and measurement. *Clin Chem* 1992; **38**: 2171–83.
24. Bilezikian JP, Management of acute hypercalcemia. *N Engl J Med* 1992; **326**: 1196–203.
25. List AF, Hainsworth JD, Davis BW et al, The syndrome of inappropriate secretion of antidiuretic hormone in small cell lung cancer. *J Clin Oncol* 1986; **4**: 1191–8.
26. Kaye TB, Crapo L, The Cushing's syndrome: an update on diagnostic tests. *Ann Intern Med* 1990; **112**: 434–44.
27. Hinton RC, Paraneoplastic neurologic syndromes. *Hematol Oncol Clin North Am* 1990; **10**: 909–25.
28. Dalmau J, Posner JB, Paraneoplastic syndromes affecting the nervous system. *Semin Oncol* 1997; **24**: 318–28.
29. Lennon VA, Kryzer TJ, Griesmann GE et al, Calcium-channel antibodies in the Lambert–Eaton syndrome and other paraneoplatic syndromes. *N Engl J Med* 1995; **332**: 1467–74.
30. Lucchinetti CF, Kimmel DW, Lennon VA, Paraneoplastic and oncologic profiles of patients seropositive for type I antineuronal nuclear autoantibodies. *Neurology* 1998; **50**: 652–7.
31. Graus F, Dalmau J, Rene R et al, Anti-Hu antibodies with small-cell lung cancer: association with complete response to therapy and improved survival. *J Clin Oncol* 1997; **15**: 2866–72.
32. Hansen-Flaschen J, Nordberg J, Clubbing and hypertrophic osteoarthropathy. *Clin Chest Med* 1987; **8**: 287–98.
33. Prins MH, Hettiarachchi RJ, Lensing AW, Hirsch J, Newly diagnosed malignancy in patients with venous thromboembolism. Search or wait and see? *Thromb Haemost* 1997; **78**: 121–5.
34. Karsell PR, McDougall JC, Diagnostic tests for lung cancer. *Mayo Clin Proc* 1993; **68**: 288–96.
35. Swensen SJ, Brown LR, Conventional radiology of the hilumand mediastinum in bronchogenic carcinoma. *Radiol Clin North Am* 1990; **28**: 521–38.
36. Dales RE, Stark RM, Raman S, Computed tomography to stage lung cancer: approaching a controversy using meta-analysis. *Am Rev Respir Dis* 1990; **141**: 1096–101.
37. Midthun DE, Swensen SJ, Jett JR, Approach to the solitary pulmonary nodule. *Mayo Clin Proc* 1993; **68**: 378–85.
38. Swensen SJ, Lung nodule enhancement at CT: multicenter study. Society of Thoracic Radiology Meeting, San Juan, Puerto Rico, 1998. Session 4, Paper 26.
39. Broderick LS, Tarver RD, Conces DJ, Imaging of lung cancer: old and new. *Semin Oncol* 1997; **24**: 411–18.

40. Dunn WF, Scanlon PD, Preoperative pulmonary function testing for patients with lung cancer. *Mayo Clin Proc* 1993; **68**: 371–7.
41. Mehta AC, Marty JJ, Lee FYW, Sputum cytology. *Clin Chest Med* 1993; **14**: 69–85.
42. Arroliga AC, Matthay RA, The role of bronchoscopy in lung cancer. *Clin Chest Med* 1993; **14**: 87–98.
43. Harrow EM, Wang KP, The staging of lung cancer by bronchoscopic transbronchial needle aspiration. *Chest Surg Clin North Am* 1996; **6**: 223–35.
44. American Thoracic Society, Standards for the diagnosis and care of patients with chronic obstructive pulmonary disease. *Am J Respir Crit Care Med* 1995; **152**: S77–120.
45. Margolis ML, Non-small cell lung cancer-clinical aspects, diagnosis, staging, and natural history. In: *Fishman's Pulmonary Diseases and Disorders,* 3rd edn (Fishman AP, Elias JA, Fishman JA et al, eds). McGraw-Hill: New York, 1998: 1759–81.
46. Salazar AM, Westcott JL, The role of transthoracic needle biopsy for the diagnosis and staging of lung cancer. *Clin Chest Med* 1993; **14**: 99–110.
47. American Thoracic Society, Guidelines for percutaneous transthoracic needle biopsy. *Am Rev Respir Dis* 1989; **140**: 255–6.
48. Silvestri GA, Littenberg B, Colice GL, The clinical evaluation for detecting metastatic lung cancer: a meta-analysis. *Am J Respir Crit Care Med* 1995; **152**: 225–30.
49. Midthun DE, Jett JR, Early detection of lung cancer: today's approach. *J Respir Dis* 1998; **19**: 59–69.
50. Kaneko M, Eguchi K, Ohmatsu H et al, Peripheral lung cancer: screening and detection with low-dose spiral CT versus radiography. *Radiology* 1996; **201**: 798–802.

10 Staging, classification and prognosis

Peter Goldstraw

Contents

INTRODUCTION

It is logical that this chapter should fall between the preceding one on diagnosis and evaluation and those that follow on the treatment modalities for non-small cell lung cancer (NSCLC) and small cell lung cancer (SCLC). At its most simplistic, 'staging' is the process by which the clinician decides the appropriate therapy for a patient diagnosed to have lung cancer. However, staging should not be thought of as a set of investigations that are performed between diagnosis and treatment. Many of the tests that are undertaken to establish the diagnosis (such as chest radiography, bronchoscopy and pleural aspiration cytology) provide valuable information as to stage. Often the choice of test by which to establish the diagnosis will be made on the basis of the clinician's assessment of the probable stage of the disease. Tests undertaken to decide stage proceed in parallel with those required to establish the diagnosis and others to assess patient fitness for possible treatment options, often interweaving and providing information across these categories. Tests may have to be repeated if they are undertaken without sufficient foresight to look beyond the diagnosis and consider the consequential issues of treatment. Sometimes treatment may be recommended after staging and before a firm diagnosis. A surgeon may 'stage' a patient and recommend thoracotomy with only the strong clinical–radiographic suspicion of lung cancer and without pursuing the diagnosis to a cytological or histological conclusion. In such circumstances, the surgeon will establish the diagnosis as the first step at thoracotomy using rapid, 'frozen section' histology before proceeding with treatment by pulmonary resection.

We shall consider the separate aspects of staging: the 'staging system', the 'staging process' and the 'staging tests'.

THE STAGING SYSTEM

The internationally recognized system for the staging of lung cancer is the TNM system devised by the Union Internationale Contre le Cancer (UICC).[1] This provides an internationally recognized shorthand to describe the extent of the disease, in which a T descriptor tells of the extent of the primary tumour, an N descriptor the extent of lymph node involvement, and an M descriptor the presence or absence of distant metastases. A number attached to each descriptor indicates progressively advancing disease. The latest revision of this came into use at the end of 1997.[2] The descriptors are defined in Table 10.1. Thus a tumour of 5 cm in diameter, involving the ipsilateral mediastinal glands and with an additional pulmonary nodule, believed to malignant, in the

Table 10.1 TNM descriptors[a]

Primary tumour (T)

TX Primary tumour cannot be assessed; or tumour is proven by the presence of malignant cells in sputum or bronchial washings but is not visualized by imaging or bronchoscopy

T0 No evidence of primary tumour

Tis Carcinoma in situ

T1 Tumour ≤ 3 cm in greatest dimension, surrounded by lung or visceral pleura, without bronchoscopic evidence of invasion more proximal than the lobar bronchus[b] (i.e. not in the main bronchus)

T2 Tumour with any of the following features of size or extent:

- >3 cm in greatest dimension
- involves main bronchus, ≥ 2 cm distal to the carina
- invades the visceral pleura
- associated with atelectasis or obstructive pneumonitis that extends to the hilar region but does not involve the entire lung

T3 Tumour of any size that directly invades any of the following: chest wall (including superior sulcus tumours), diaphragm, mediastinal pleura, parietal pericardium; or tumour in the main bronchus <2 cm distal to the carina, but without involvement of the carina; or associated atelectasis or obstructive pneumonitis of the entire lung

T4 Tumour of any size that invades any of the following: mediastinum, heart, great vessels, trachea, oesophagus, vertebral body, carina; or tumour with a malignant pleural or pericardial effusion,[c] or with satellite tumour nodule(s) within the ipsilateral primary-tumour lobe of the lung

Regional lymph nodes (N)

NX Regional lymph nodes cannot be assessed

N0 No regional lymph node metastasis

N1 Metastasis to ipsilateral peribronchial and/or ipsilateral hilar lymph nodes, and intrapulmonary nodes involved by direct extension of the primary tumour

N2 Metastasis to ipsilateral mediastinal and/or subcarinal lymph node(s)

N3 Metastasis to contralateral mediastinal, contralateral hilar, ipsilateral or contralateral scalene, or supraclavicular lymph node(s)

Distant metastasis (M)

MX Presence of distant metastasis cannot be assessed

M0 No distant metastasis

M1 Distant metastasis present[d]

[a]Reproduced with kind permission of Dr CF Mountain and the Editor of *Chest*.[2]

[b]The uncommon superficial tumour of any size with its invasive component limited to the bronchial wall, which may extend proximal to the main bronchus, is also classified T1.

[c]Most pleural effusions associated with lung cancer are due to tumour. However, there are a few patients in whom multiple cytopathological examinations of pleural fluid show no tumour. In these cases, the fluid is non-bloody and is not an exudate. When these elements and clinical judgement dictate that the effusion in not related to the tumour, the effusion should be excluded as a staging element and the patient's disease should be staged T1, T2 or T3. Pericardial effusion is classified according to the same rules.

[d]Separate metastatic tumour nodule(s) in the ipsilateral non-primary-tumour lobe(s) of the lung is also classified M1.

Table 10.2 Stage grouping: TNM subsets[a,b]

Stage	TNM subset
0	Carcinoma in situ
IA	T1N0M0
IB	T2N0M0
IIA	T1N1M0
IIB	T2N1M0
	T3N0M0
IIIA	T3N1M0
	T1N2M0
	T2N2M0
	T3N2M0
IIIB	T4N0M0
	T4N1M0
	T4N2M0
	T1N3M0
	T2N3M0
	T3N3M0
	T4N3M0
IV	Any T Any N M1

[a]Staging is not relevant for occult carcinoma, designated TXN0M0.
[b]Reproduced with the kind permission of Dr CF Mountain and the Editor of *Chest*.[2]

other ipsilateral lobe would be described as T2N2M1.

For convenience, TNM subsets with similar survival prospects and for which treatment options would be similar are combined into stage groups (Table 10.2); the example just given would fall into stage IV.

Many clinicians feel that such detailed staging is irrelevant for SCLC, and consider that a cruder division into 'limited' and 'extensive' disease allows clinical decisions to be made on treatment.[3] Limited disease is defined as tumour that is restricted to one hemithorax, often including the ipsilateral supraclavicular fossa, basically a single radiotherapy field, while any wider disease, including distant metastases, is considered as extensive disease. Although this distinction is certainly sufficient for the vast majority of sufferers with this cell type, the TNM stage remains relevant for the fortunate patient with unusually localized disease, for whom surgical therapy or multimodality therapy should be considered.

THE STAGING PROCESS

The clinician is confronted with a bewildering array of tests that may, when used appropriately, provide information as to the extent of disease and therefore permit staging of the patient and allow advice to be given on therapy. The value and place of each test will be discussed in the next section. The clinician may utilize any and all such tests to construct a clinical/evaluative TNM stage, designated cTNM. Such tests may include surgical exploration, such as mediastinoscopy and video-assisted thoracoscopy (VATS), undertaken prior to a decision to recommend treatment. It is as well to remember that, as one proceeds with this information-gathering exercise, the tests become increasingly costly and more invasive. Once sufficient information has been collected to permit a decision as to which treatment is appropriate for the individual patient, further tests become obtrusive and unwarranted. The difficulty for the clinician is to know where to draw the line and to decide that the evidence is sufficiently reliable as to make the case for a particular treatment.

There can be no rigid protocol for staging, and the clinician will decide the next step based upon the overall picture as it emerges as each step

Table 10.3 Pretreatment minimal staging 3

Step 1

Investigation		Patient group	Confirmatory tests
Clinical history	Weight loss and performance status	All patients	As appropriate
Clinical examination		All patients	As appropriate
Chest radiographs	PA Lateral	All patients	Aspiration of effusion (considered positive if cytology malignant)
Blood tests	Hb Alkaline phosphatase Transaminase Lactate dehydrogenase	All patients	As for high-risk patients in Step II

If still thought suitable for curative treatment, proceed to Step II

Step II

Investigation	Patient group	Confirmatory tests
Bronchoscopy	All patients with central tumours or those in whom central extension is suspected	The features of proximal, extrinsic compression are unreliable and require further evaluation of the mediastinum by CT and/or mediastinal exploration
Bone scan	High-risk group[a]	Skeletal radiographs ± CT/MRI of bone if dubious positive result
CT chest and upper abdomen (to lower pole of kidneys with intravenous contrast enhancement of mediastinal vessels)	All patients if available	Dubious findings confirmed (not necessarily histological)
Liver ultrasound	High-risk group[a] if CT of abdomen not available	
Brain assessment by CT or MRI	Advisable in high-risk group[a]	

Table 10.3 Continued

[a]High-risk patients are those having non-specific features identified by Hooper et al.[8]

- Unexplained anaemia (Hb <11 g%)
- Unexplained weight loss (>8 lb (3 kg) in 6/12)
- Abnormal alkaline phosphatase or transaminase
- Where any clinical suspicion of metastatic disease exists
- Patients with stage III disease

If still thought suitable for curative treatment, proceed to Step III

Step III

Investigation	Patient group
(a) Bronchoscopy if not previously undertaken	All patients
(b) Thoracoscopy (video-assisted)	If pleural effusion present and cytology negative but clinical suspicion remains, do a pleural biopsy
(c) Mediastinal exploration • It is recommended that this is performed preoperatively by:	
• Transcarinal aspiration • Cervical mediastinoscopy	Patients in whom CT suggests mediastinal invasion or if CT shows nodes >1.0 cm
• Additional evaluation of the subaortic fossa by left anterior mediastinotomy	The above groups with tumours of the left upper lobe or left main bronchus
• *This must be performed intraoperatively*	*All patients* – including those whose mediastinum has been assessed preoperatively
• Palpation insufficient	
• Careful and extensive mediastinal dissection	
• Separate labelling as per Naruke or ATS of excised nodes for subsequent histological examination (only N1 nodes on resection specimen)	
• Re-evaluation of T stage	

Proceed with definitive therapy, which will be surgical resection in all but the most unusual circumstances provides additional information. For most clinicians, the critical point in the staging process is reached once the patient's disease has been shown to be too extensive to permit surgical treatment. The oncologist or radiotherapist might still consider other staging tests to be important in defining the most appropriate regimen. If the patient comes through the assessment of the clinician and is still considered operable, the surgeon will almost certainly wish to define the stage more precisely before making a final decision to operate. As this frequently involves a decision as to the probable extent of resection, and the use of surgical investigations such as mediastinoscopy, this step should be left to the surgeon.

The issue of which tests are considered the minimum necessary to establish cTNM has been considered by the IASLC, and is one that is regularly updated at their workshops.[4] Their recommendations are shown in Table 10.3. The American Thoracic Society and the European Respiratory Society have accepted similar recommendations.[5]

Once a decision has been made as to treatment, the cTNM assigned to that patient should not be changed in the records. Additional information will accumulate if the patient proceeds to thoracotomy and pulmonary resection. This will allow an updated stage to be established, the postsurgical/pathological stage, or pTNM. This should be recorded, but does not replace the cTNM.

The manual for staging of cancer produced by the American Joint Committee for Cancer Staging and End-Results Reporting[6] allows and recommends that a record be made of the assessment of residual disease after treatment. This is most usually applied after surgical resection. The designation R is used to define this. RX indicates that it is not possible to evaluate the presence of residual disease. R0 indicates that no residual disease remains after complete resection, R1 that microscopic residual tumour remains, and R2 that macroscopic residual tumour remains after what must be considered an incomplete resection. Most workers interpret the R1 status as applying to the case where the resection margins are unexpectedly positive on subsequent histological examination of the resection specimen. This classification is not part of the staging system, but represents good practice.

As time passes, the disease may recur or progress, and additional tests may be indicated to establish a re-treatment or rTNM. Some would consider that our ultimate insight into the extent of disease is realized at autopsy, when aTNM can be created. However, time is the ultimate test, and our understanding of disease progression is curtailed by death, preventing the development of clinically relevant disease that could be overlooked at autopsy.

THE STAGING TESTS

In an age of technological progress, it is often necessary to remind oneself and one's staff of the importance of good clinical acumen. All of our elaborate scans have to be directed by clinical assessment and interpreted in the light of this.

Clinical history and examination

These remain the most basic and most cost-effective assessments of disease extent. The clinician, while enquiring as to symptoms of the primary tumour, will be looking to assess performance status and co-morbid conditions, but a few questions are relevant to assess stage. The presence of chest wall pain is more accurate at determining chest wall invasion than a computed tomographic (CT) scan. The presence of unexplained weight loss should alert the clinician to the increased possibility of disseminated disease in such patients. A patient may well dismiss weight loss as attributable to changes in diet and a deliberate attempt at weight reduction. Further enquiry may show that repeated previous attempts at weight reduction have failed without the assistance of disseminated malignancy! The patient coming to see a chest specialist will not volunteer the recent onset of bone pain, assuming it to be degenerative or traumatic in nature, and may assume that hoarseness is due to the trauma of coughing. Similarly, patients and their relatives may rationalize the change in personality as being due to anxiety after hearing the diagnosis and dismiss neurological symptoms as being due to minor nerve damage. A careful examination should focus upon any questions raised in the history, and there should also be an examination for cervical lymphadenopathy and hepatomegaly. The ability to detect enlarged neck nodes improves with practice, and this important examination should not be designated to the most junior member of the team.

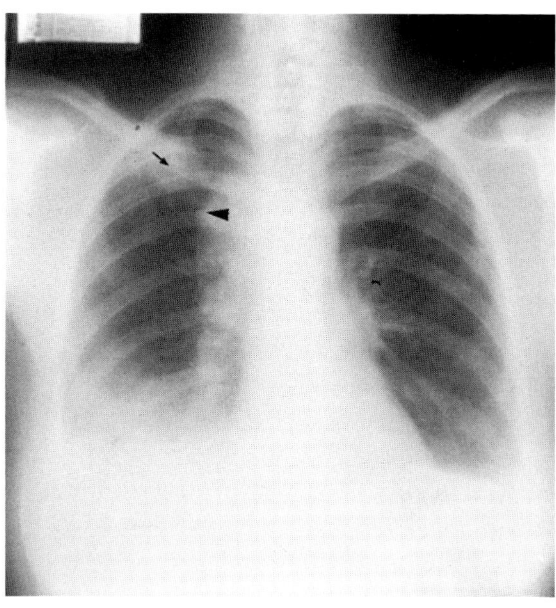

Figure 10.1
The chest radiograph of a patient with a mass in the right upper lobe (arrow). The film also shows gross widening of the superior mediastinum (arrowhead), strongly suggestive of mediastinal nodal disease, but there is, in addition, a right pleural effusion. Aspiration cytology of the effusion gave the diagnosis of adenocarcinoma, allowed staging of the disease and also showed the patient to be inoperable.

Chest radiography

This is usually the starting point in further evaluation. While it usually provides clues as to the diagnosis it also gives valuable staging information as to tumour size and possible local invasion.[7] It is as well to check the radiograph for rib erosion, elevation of the hemidiaphragm, the presence of other lung nodules or evidence of an effusion (Figure 10.1). The presence of such features may allow one to cut short the process of assessment by establishing the diagnosis and staging the patient with a single investigation, such as pleural aspiration cytology.

Haematological parameters

Parameters such as anaemia, disturbance of liver enzymes and elevation of serum alkaline phosphatase are reliable indicators, suggesting a greater probability of distant disease.[8] Such tests are inexpensive and widely available, and should be a routine part of the staging process.

Bronchoscopy

For the patient who remains operable at this point, a wide vista of additional tests may be appropriate. The diagnosis may be established by sputum cytology, an under-utilized investigation, but for all patients except those with extensive disease bronchoscopy will be undertaken. This provides an opportunity for more accurate determination of cell type by histological examination, and allows one to assess the proximal extent of the disease within the tracheobronchial tree. The fibreoptic bronchoscope is an excellent screening tool for the respiratory physician, but in borderline cases the surgeon will wish to examine the airway with respiration suspended under general anaesthesia, often using the rigid bronchoscope with its wider field of view and facility for larger biopsies.

Computed tomography

This has greatly aided the staging of lung cancer, and the proliferation of CT scanning facilities attests to the enormous value of this investigation. However, much depends upon technical aspects of the scanner, the protocol used for the study and the experience of the radiologist.[9] CT scans of the chest provide an enormous amount of three-dimensional information on disease extent. One can analyse the individual components of the scan, assessing the accuracy with which CT can detect mediastinal gland involvement, mediastinal invasion, chest wall invasion, the presence of additional pulmonary nodules, or deposits in the abdominal organs or brain.

In reality, the value of the information provided by CT scanning is far greater than the sum of its component parts. The three-dimensional construct helps the surgeon anticipate the possible extent of resection, the technical problems that may be encountered and the areas to inspect for possible tumour extension. The surgeon can use such information in evaluating the patient's fitness for such extended surgery, to guide intraoperative assessment and to plan the operative strategy to deal with likely areas of extension or concern. It does not matter to the surgeon that such areas of concern may prove to be fallacious – it is better to be prepared – but for the clinician the lack of specificity must be an ever-present concern in evaluating the true extent of disease. One would not want to deny the patient potentially curative surgery on the basis of a radiographic feature that lacks accuracy. Confirmatory tests are often necessary, particularly if the decision hinges on a single, adverse CT feature. The significance of *additional pulmonary nodules* will depend upon geographical factors such as the local prevalence of benign granulomatous disease. In one study, 67% of such nodules were shown to be definitely benign, and only 11% were definitely malignant.[10]

Mediastinal lymph nodes can be seen more easily on CT than with conventional radiology.[11] As the size of such nodes increases, so does the probability that they contain metastases. However, there is no size criterion below which deposits are excluded with certainty, nor above which deposits are certain to be present (Figure 10.2). As one increases the size limit permitted for normality, those nodes deemed 'abnormal' are more likely to contain metastases, and the evaluation gains greater specificity but at the cost of declining sensitivity. If one applies a lower cut-off, the reverse applies: sensitivity rises at the expense of falling specificity, and one is more likely to designate nodes as 'abnormal' when they do not contain metastases.[12] This is the dilemma for the radiologist. The commonest compromise is to report nodes as abnormal if their short-axis diameter is greater than 1.0 cm.[13] The accuracy of this assessment depends upon many factors: the speed of the scanner, the use of contrast to enhance the mediastinal vessels, and the rigour with which lymph node deposits are sought at thoracotomy. The reported sensitivity and specificity fall from 70–80% to 60% when the CT assessment is subjected to detailed intrathoracic staging.[14–16] Abnormal nodes larger than this should be examined by mediastinal exploration to gain histological confirmation of their involvement. Such enlarged nodes within the superior mediastinum are accessible to cervical mediastinoscopy and anterior mediastinotomy (see below). Enlarged nodes beyond the reach of these techniques can be accessible to VATS,[17] but such nodes have less impact on the results of surgical treatment, and their accurate designation can usually be left until

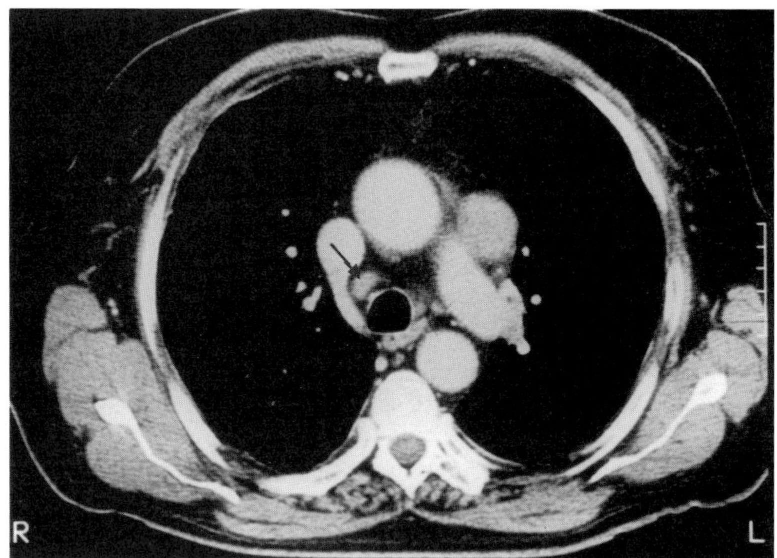

Figure 10.2
A CT scan of the chest, with contrast enhancement of the mediastinal vessels. An enlarged node is visible in the right paratracheal area (arrow). Although this node was larger than 1 cm, it was shown at mediastinoscopy to be benign, and this was confirmed at subsequent thoracotomy.

thoracotomy. If the CT scan of the chest shows that the mediastinal nodes are within this size limit, the surgeon may proceed to thoracotomy without mediastinal exploration.[18]

Mediastinal invasion may be suggested on CT, but this assessment is unreliable[19] unless there is gross involvement (Figure 10.3). More frequently the CT scan of the chest will show that the tumour, and the associated atelectasis or consolidation, are contiguous with the mediastinal outline (Figure 10.4). If CT does not demonstrate a fat line separating these two opacities, the

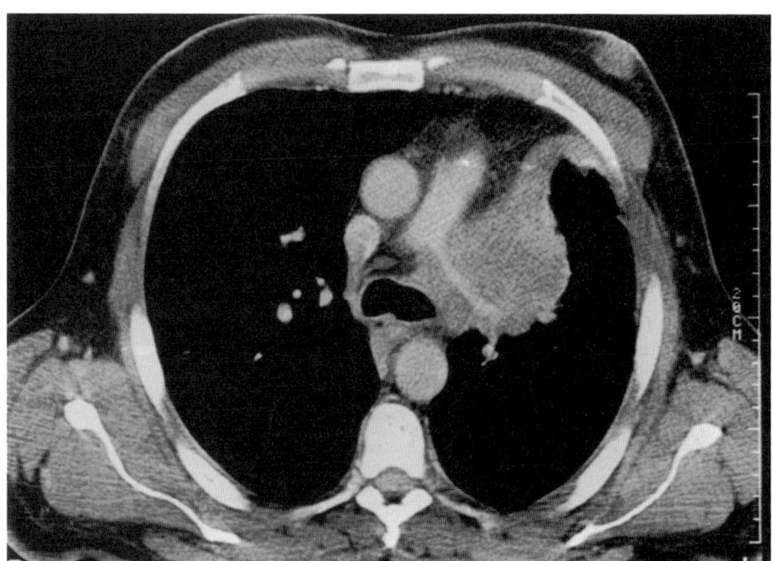

Figure 10.3
A CT scan of a patient with a left upper lobe tumour. The CT shows unequivocal evidence of irresectable involvement of the mediastinum, with tumour encircling the main pulmonary artery to its origin. A left anterior mediastinotomy would be unnecessary unless tissue diagnosis was required.

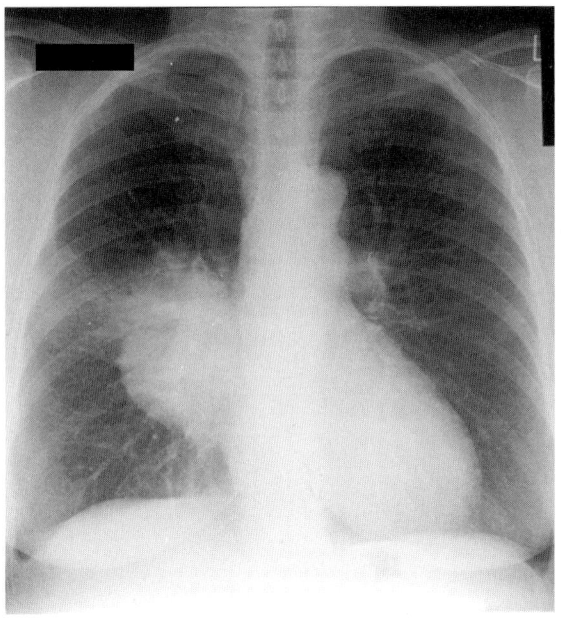
(a)

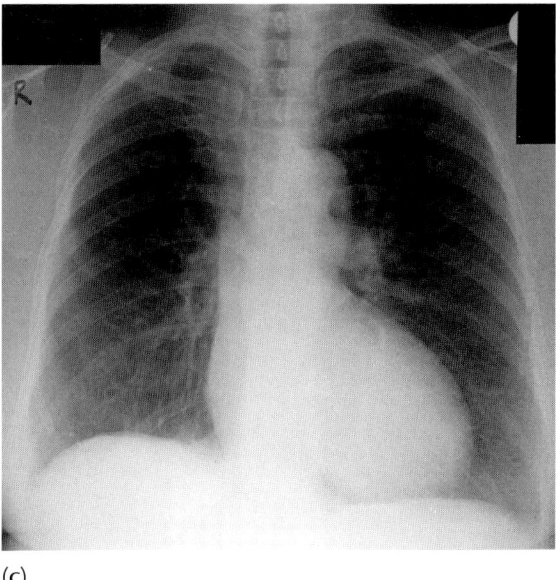

(c)

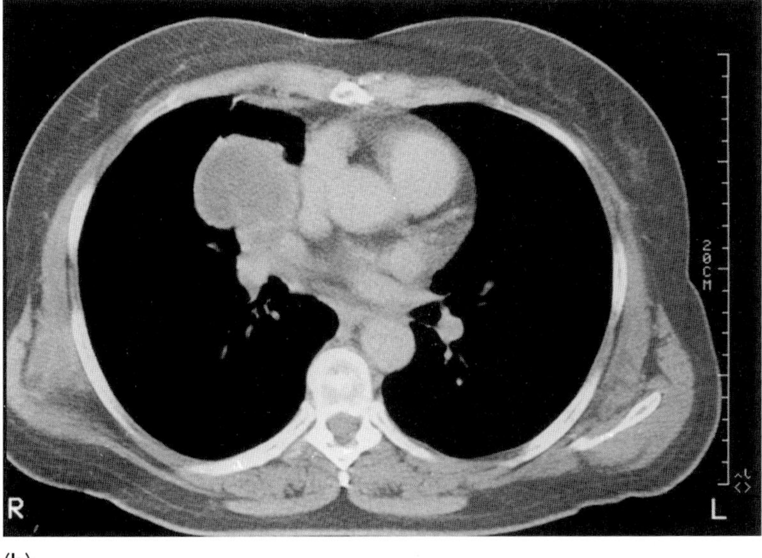

(b)

Figure 10.4
(a) A chest radiograph and (b) a CT scan of a patient with a tumour in the right middle lobe. This was pronounced inoperable by the clinician. The appearances are not unequivocal, and at thoracotomy resection of a T2N0 tumour was possible by bilobectomy. (c) This chest radiograph was taken three years later, when the patient was well and disease-free.

radiologist will warn that invasion may be present.[20] This judgement carries a sensitivity and specificity of around 60%,[21] but it is imperfect and dependent upon the experience of the radiologist. Such a worry can usually be resolved by mediastinoscopy (Figure 10.5), with the addition of mediastinotomy in appropriate cases. A suggestion of mediastinal invasion beyond the reach of

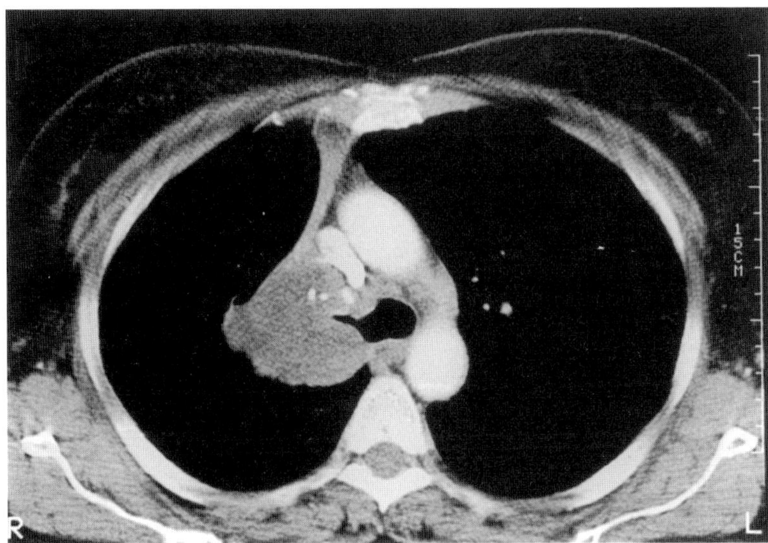

Figure 10.5
The CT scan of a patient with a tumour in the right upper lobe encroaching upon the mediastinum and the right main bronchus. This was evaluated by mediastinoscopy and was found to be resectable. The patient underwent right upper lobectomy and sleeve resection for a T2N1 tumour.

these techniques can be inspected using VATS, but is usually left until thoracotomy when a more determined assessment of resectability can be made without the danger of massive bleeding.

The CT evaluation of *chest wall invasion* is similarly imperfect unless rib erosion or extension outside the chest wall can be demonstrated.[22] Fortunately, such invasion does not preclude successful resection with good survival results.[23,24]

Most clinicians when requesting a CT scan will ask for the chest study to extend into the abdomen to the lower pole of the kidneys in a search for *distant metastases* in the liver, abdominal nodes, adrenals and kidneys. While this is a useful

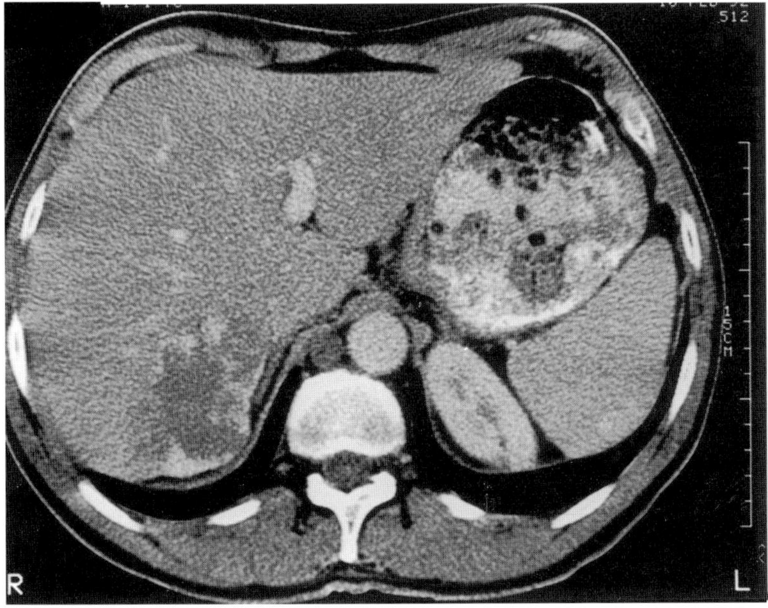

Figure 10.6
The CT of the abdomen suggested a liver metastasis. The appearances were not clarified by ultrasound, and a needle biopsy showed a benign haemangioma.

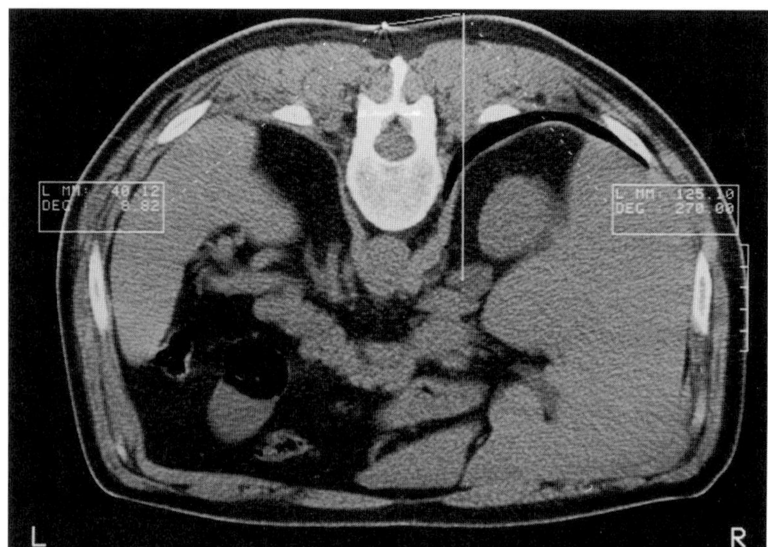

Figure 10.7
A CT-guided needle biopsy of an indeterminate mass in the right adrenal gland. It showed the presence of an adenoma.

addition to the CT protocol, an isolated abnormality should not be taken as proof unless there is confirmatory evidence that such an abnormality is metastatic (Figure 10.6).[25] This may require CT-guided needle biopsy (Figure 10.7). We have found this to be a useful role for positron emission tomography (PET), if this is available (see below). The addition of CT of the brain is debated. Undoubtedly, the number of unsuspected metastases discovered is small (around 5%),[26] but, since this has a profound effect on the advisability of thoracotomy, we routinely undertake CT of the brain, chest and abdomen prior to surgery.[27]

Scintigraphic scans

These are largely obsolete, with the exception of bone scintigraphy.[28] This has retained a place in staging, not because of its accuracy but because no other technique has emerged to image the whole skeleton readily. Most clinicians use bone scans selectively in 'high-risk' individuals, in whom distant metastases have been suggested clinically by symptoms or the presence of non-specific features such as weight loss or disturbed blood parameters.[29,30] Since false-positive bone scans can occur with trauma and degenerative conditions, it is as well to follow-up any abnormality with skeletal radiology, and in doubtful cases a local CT or magnetic resonance image (MRI) of the area.[31]

Abdominal ultrasound

This is widely available, and in experienced hands is as good as CT at detecting metastases in the liver[32] or adrenals.[33] If CT is not available, ultrasound should be performed in high-risk cases. Ultrasound is helpful to obtain additional information to characterize any abdominal abnormality on CT, and may obviate the need for needle biopsy.

Mediastinal exploration

This is a very valuable surgical assessment, which may be used in all cases prior to surgery but in most centres is now used selectively to evaluate the mediastinum when CT has suggested the presence of enlarged mediastinal nodes or mediastinal invasion.[34] *Cervical mediastinoscopy*[35] is undertaken under general anaesthesia through a short cervical

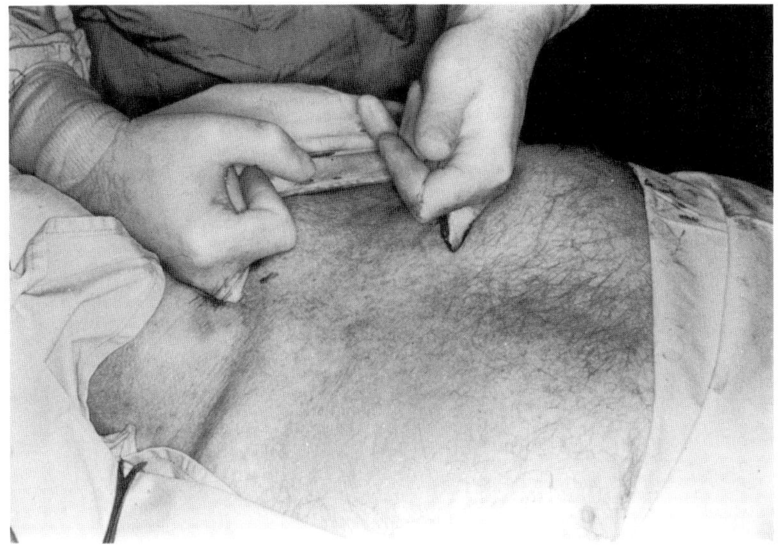

Figure 10.8
This patient has a tumour in the left upper lobe, and the surgeon is undertaking evaluation by cervical mediastinoscopy and left anterior mediastinotomy. After all biopsies have been taken, bi-digital palpation of the subaortic fossa will exclude invasion or gross mediastinal gland enlargement in this critical area.

incision. It allows inspection and biopsy in the paratracheal region to both sides of the trachea and at the carina, excluding gross, often irresectable, nodal metastases and assuring resectability. When wishing to inspect the area around the aortic arch and subaortic fossa, as in patients with tumours arising in the left upper lobe or reaching the left main bronchus, cervical mediastinoscopy should be supplemented by *left anterior mediastinotomy.*[35] This allows digital examination and, if necessary, cautious biopsy of disease in this area (Figure 10.8). It is applied selectively, depending upon the CT appearances in this area of the mediastinum.[36] Such techniques do not exclude more subtle mediastinal disease, but, with experience, ensure that complete resection is possible in 95% of negative cases.[37,38] The surgeon will often be encouraged to proceed with thoracotomy and resection when other, less accurate, techniques such as CT have raised doubts.

Mediastinal needle biopsy

This can be undertaken through the bronchoscope.[39] Suitable target nodes should be identified in the main carina or the paratracheal area, usually on CT. This technique may obtain tissue diagnosis and confirm irresectability, but there is a small risk of false-positive samples.[40] It is not a reliable alternative to staging the mediastinum by surgical exploration prior to thoracotomy.

Transoesophageal ultrasound

This has been used to assess the presence of mediastinal node enlargement, but is limited by the same size criteria as CT.[41] The transoesophageal route is attractive as a conduit to examine the mediastinum below the carina, beyond the reach of the mediastinoscope, checking areas where CT has suggested mediastinal invasion. The results have proven unreliable.[42]

Positron emission tomography

PET using the ^{18}F-labelled glucose analogue fluoro-2-deoxy-D-glucose (FDG–PET) has emerged as an exciting addition to the staging tests. It is expensive and not widely available, and we are still assessing its cost-effectiveness. It provides an alternative, metabolic search for malignant disease that is independent of the anatomical features of the deposits.[43] It can characterize the lung lesion reliably in most cases,[44] failing only to detect very small deposits and indolent cases such as bronchoalveolar carcinoma.[45] False-positive cases can occur with chronic inflammatory conditions, most notably tuberculosis. PET may thus have a role in diagnosis, and its place relative to bronchoscopy or needle aspiration is under discussion.[46] Interest, however, has focused on the possibility that PET could aid the non-invasive search for metastatic disease in the mediastinum and at distant sites.[47] PET is more accurate in the detection of mediastinal nodal disease than CT and even mediastinal exploration, with a reported sensitivity of 80–100% and a specificity of 70–100%.[48] The images produced at present by FDG–PET scanners are indistinct and lack anatomical precision. It is difficult to accurately define the margins of the hilum and mediastinum. Most centres having access to PET continue to rely upon CT and confirm positive PET findings by mediastinal exploration, thus adding to the expense of staging.[49] There is also the philosophical problem as to whether one wishes to detect all mediastinal nodal deposits. There are many reports of five-year survival rates of 20–30% after complete resection in the presence of N2 disease.[38,50–52] Mediastinal exploration will miss such subtle N2 disease, perhaps to the patient's benefit, encouraging one to proceed with surgery with complete resection in 85% of cases.[38] PET will detect otherwise-unsuspected distant metastases in 11–29% of patients otherwise thought suitable for thoracotomy.[53–55] The specificity of this evaluation is 100%. We have utilized PET selectively in an attempt to characterize the additional abnormalities found on our routine CT survey of patients coming to thoracotomy in whom the mediastinum has been evaluated by CT and mediastinal exploration.[56] When such lesions showed high uptake on PET, they were all shown to be malignant by biopsy or radiological follow-up (Figure 10.9). When PET uptake was absent at this site, all but one of the 13 lesions were shown to be benign (specificity 100%, sensitivity 93%). To our surprise, despite these patients having a greater prospect of metastatic disease than most, we found only one lesion not shown on CT that subsequently proved to be metastatic. Such a role for PET seems to be a reasonable alternative to invasive evaluation of the CT abnormalities.

Magnetic resonance imaging

This is little or no more accurate than CT in routine staging. Some authorities consider that the ability to visualize in planes other than the axial gives MRI an advantage in difficult areas such as the lung apex and lower mediastinum.[57] Most would recommend MRI when evaluating Pancoast's tumour (Figure 10.10).[58] The special value of this investigation is as a problem-solving tool looking at the central nervous system. MRI is more accurate than CT at detecting and characterizing brain lesions.[59] We would recommend its use if CT of the brain shows an abnormality or when clinical suspicion remains after a negative CT. The routine use of MRI as a screening tool for asymptomatic brain metastases has not been shown to be of value. Similarly, if the CT raises doubts as to tumour extension around the spine and into the spinal canal, MRI will give clearer definition and valuable information.

Intrathoracic staging

The tests described above should allow one to determine cTNM and in appropriate cases recommend thoracotomy. For the surgeon, however, the staging process does not end there. We have come to appreciate that a detailed re-evaluation at thoracotomy is a valuable step prior to proceeding with resection. *Intrathoracic staging* will evaluate areas of concern remaining after CT

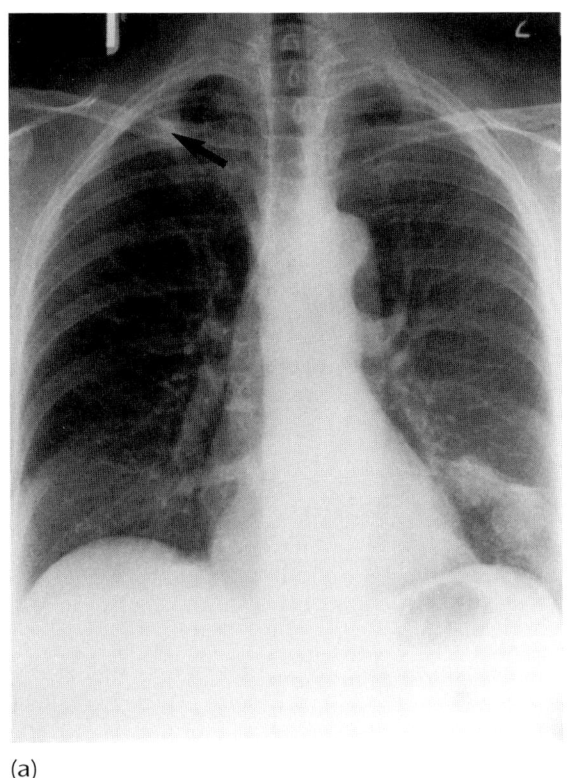

(a)

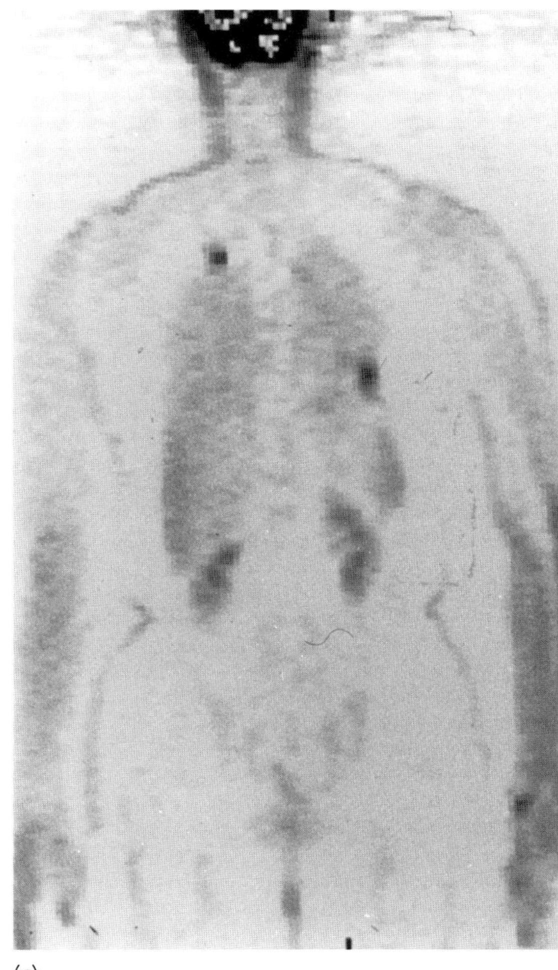

(b)

(c)

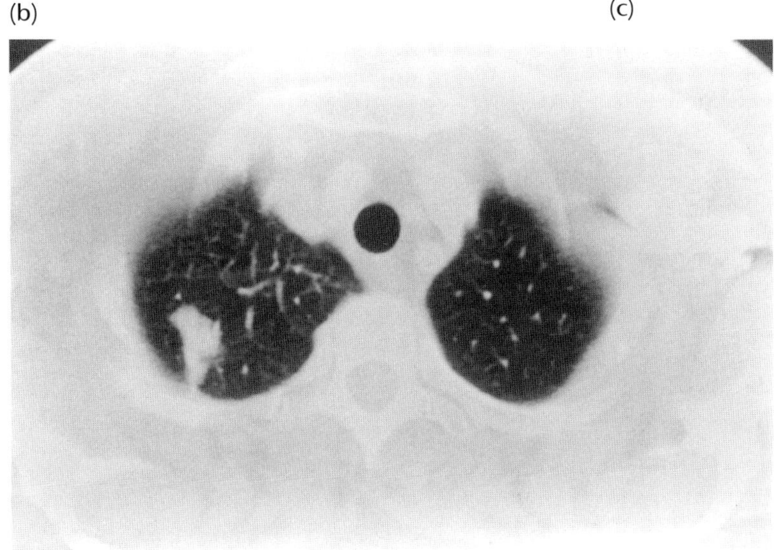

Figure 10.9
(a) The chest radiograph of a patient who presented with a tumour in the left lower lobe; there is an additional lesion at the right apex (arrow). (b) The CT scan did not suggest that this additional lesion was a tumour. (c) An FDG–PET study showed high uptake in both lesions, and the right-sided lesion was confirmed histologically to be malignant.

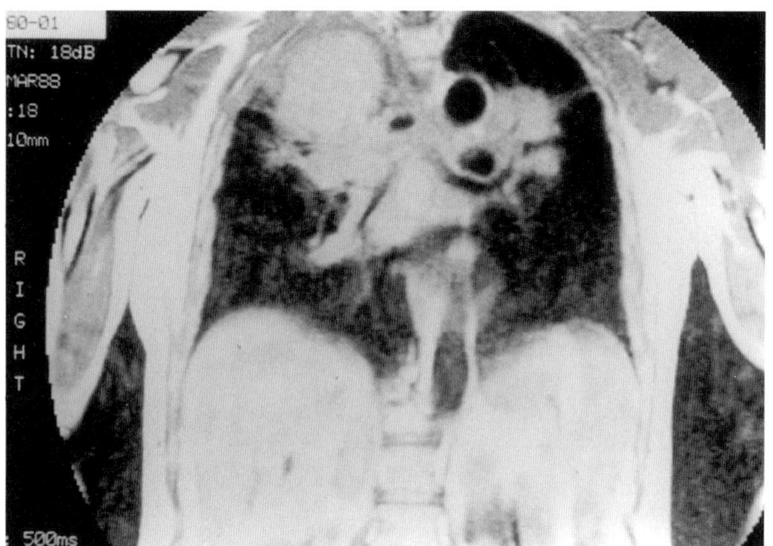

Figure 10.10
An MRI scan of a patient with a right-sided Pancoast's tumour. The scan gives a coronal reconstruction of this difficult area, but also suggested nodes at the main carina, which were confirmed to contain metastatic disease at mediastinoscopy.

and subsequent mediastinal evaluation, search for additional lesions in the lung and pleura not seen on CT, examine for satellite nodules[60] and permit a thorough evaluation of nodal extent by *systematic nodal dissection*.[61] There is debate as to the value of pleural lavage cytology as a routine step immediately after opening the chest. Kondo and his colleagues found positive pleural cytology in 9% of cases, and showed it to have a strong negative impact on prognosis.[62] Other workers have confirmed the incidence of positive cytology, but did not find a statistically significant influence on prognosis after resection.[63]

Despite rigorous preoperative staging with CT and, where appropriate, mediastinal exploration, cTNM will be shown to be inaccurate in over half of the patients coming to thoracotomy.[64] While occasionally cTNM will overestimate the extent of disease, in most cases the disease will be shown to be more extensive. It is clearly important that the surgeon obtains such valuable insight into the extent of disease before making a decision about whether to proceed with resection and when judging the extent of pulmonary resection necessary to achieve complete resection. Systematic nodal dissection (SND) begins with the excision of all mediastinal fat and the lymph nodes contained therein (Figure 10.11). It is recommended that the nodes be labelled in accordance with an internationally recognized chart, such as that devised by Naruke (Figure 10.12).[65] It is our routine procedure to slice these nodes at the operating table and examine the internal architecture before deciding whether rapid histological confirmation is necessary by frozen section analysis. If resection is deemed possible, we proceed to examine the N1 nodes similarly, in a centrifugal fashion until the extent of resection has been determined. The only nodes remaining in the resection specimen can be assumed to be N1. In such a way, the surgeon will ensure complete resection with the minimum resection of lung parenchyma. We have shown that SND will disclose N2 disease in 18% of patients coming to thoracotomy without histological evidence preoperatively, and only 60% of patients will be shown to be node-negative.[66] This study confirmed that SND could not be omitted

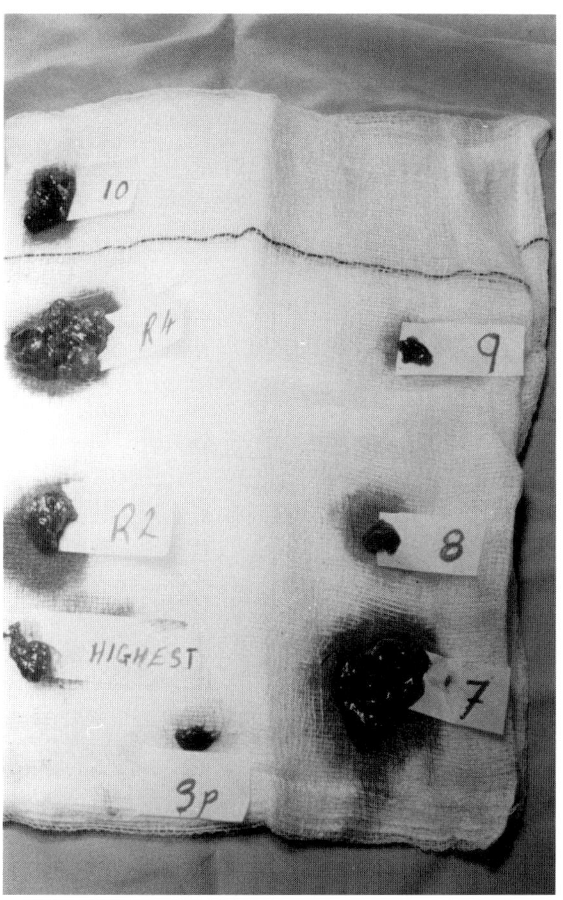

Figure 10.11
An operative specimen showing fat and lymph node stations removed during the first step in systematic nodal dissection (SND). These can be correlated with the Naruke chart (Figure 10.12; and see also Appendix 1, pages 363–79) to show that a complete circumnavigation of the right side of the mediastinum has been accomplished.

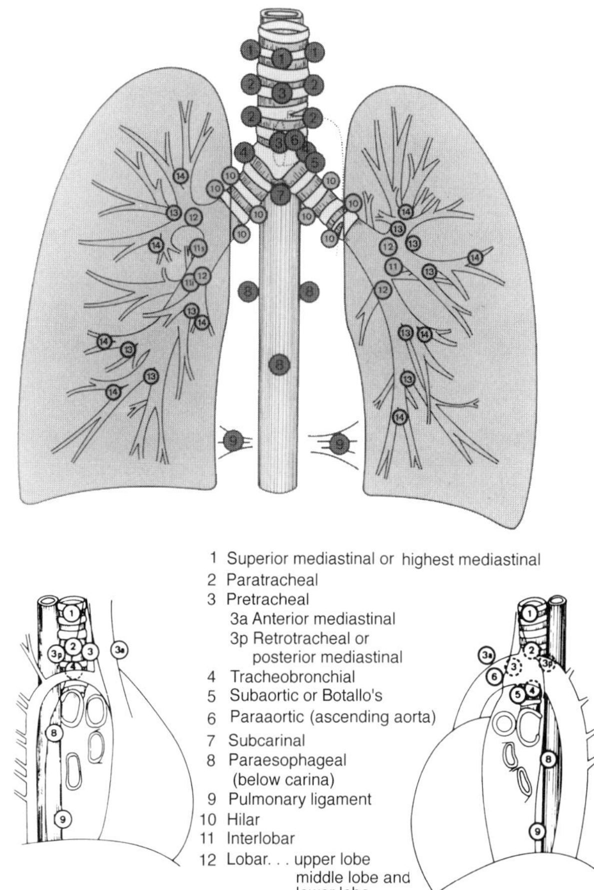

Figure 10.12
The nodal chart devised by Naruke. The lymph node stations are numbered: 1–9 indicate mediastinal nodal stations. (Reproduced with permission of Dr T Naruke and Mosby Inc from J Thorac Cardiovasc Surg 1978; **76**: 832–9.[65])

on the basis of cell type, tumour size, tumour origin, lobe of origin or by preoperative mediastinal exploration.

Since 'skip' lesions to the mediastinal nodes without hilar node involvement were found in 6% of cases, the assessment of the mediastinum is important irrespective of the findings in the hilum. If mediastinal node deposits are discovered at thoracotomy and yet complete resection has been confirmed to be feasible, the surgeon must decide whether to proceed with resection, balancing the reduced prospects of survival after complete resection and the added morbidity and mortality of pulmonary resection. The surgeon will be aware that the patient has already necessarily incurred the morbidity and mortality of thoracotomy,[67] and will base the decision to resect upon the patient's fitness, the extent of resection necessary, the cell type, and the number and position of positive nodes. Complete resection will be deemed appropriate in 85% of cases, although the perioperative mortality is higher and the five-year survival rate reduced to around 20%.[38]

Subsequent histological examination of lymph node stations removed at surgery will show metastases that the surgeon had not appreciated in up to 9% of cases.[68] The pathologist will also study the specimen and attached lymph nodes, looking for the presence of pleural invasion and satellite lesions that may have eluded the surgeon. Some authors have suggested that the use of *monoclonal antibody stains* will detect nodal deposits not seen with conventional stains in up to 6% of lymph nodes in 22% of patients.[69] Others have suggested that this is the result of taking additional slices of the nodes and that the majority of such micrometastases will be found with conventional stains by more thorough histological examination.[70]

To establish the pTNM, the clinician will thus have to scrutinize the operative findings and study the detailed pathology report. The accuracy of pTNM will depend heavily on the detailed nature of such reports.

OTHER PROGNOSTIC INDICATORS

Only *performance status* equals stage in its impact on survival after all treatment modalities. Other factors such as *weight loss* and the presence of *systemic symptoms* are accepted as important. *Gender*, *cell type*, *degree of differentiation* and *vascular invasion* may be significant, but reports vary depending upon stage and whether surgery was possible.[71] Age has an impact on treatment, but is not an independent variable. Certainly, information on these factors should be recorded and data presented in any report of results. There is great interest in *biological markers* in lung cancer, and the hope that a panel of markers, including oncogenes and tumour suppressor genes, can provide an independent, biological method of anticipating outcome. At present, our knowledge of these markers is imperfect.[71] It is recommended that, where possible, cryopreserved tissue from well-staged, surgical specimens should be stored for future studies.

PROGNOSIS

The survival of patients with each stage of disease is discussed in detail in the chapters on treatment in this book, but a few comments are pertinent when considering staging. When reading the literature on the results of treatment of lung cancer, especially surgical series, the reader is reminded of two phenomena: what Shields has termed 'the diminishing denominator',[72] and the impact of 'stage migration' or the 'Will Rogers effect'.[73]

The diminishing denominator can give a false impression of the value of surgery in an advanced stage of lung cancer by reporting only the results on patients found to be within this stage at thoracotomy and surviving complete resection. Other patients are 'censored' from the analysis if found at thoracotomy not to fall into the study population, if resection is not possible, if incomplete resection has been performed and even if dying after operation. The reported survival of patients in this stage who survive complete resection gives little guidance to the clinician armed only with cTNM, and results are further inflated by the use of actuarial survival statistics. Thus 400 patients with a presumptive stage may proceed to thoracotomy. One hundred patients will be found to be ineligible at thoracotomy, 85 will be irresectable, 100 undergo incomplete resection, 15 die after surgery, and the actuarial survival of the 10 who survive to five years after complete resection is computed to be 20%. While this may impress the unwary, closer study reveals that more patients will die of such unwarranted surgery than those in whom the prognosis is improved, at a cost of 400 major operations and much morbidity.

Stage migration is an inevitable consequence of more detailed staging. As one refines the group under study, those eliminated cascade into the more advanced stages, swelling their numbers. These new recruits have a better prognosis than the original patients do in that group, defined by cruder staging techniques, and the prognosis of the group is thus improved. The shifting populations are evident in any study giving details of the results of surgery based upon cTNM and pTNM. In one study,[74] the number of patients who fell into the T1N0 category fell from 349 to 264 when shifting from cTNM to pTNM, and conversely the number of patients with T3N0 disease rose from 109 to 147. This demonstrates the improved staging achieved by thoracotomy. The five-year survival of patients based upon pTNM will always be superior to that based upon cTNM, and this effect is more pronounced in higher stage groups. In another study,[2] the five-year survival rate of T1N0 patients rose from 61% to 67%, a 10% improvement, when moving from cTNM to pTNM, while the survival rate of T3N0 patients rose from 22% to 38%, an improvement of 87% in the survival of this group. These statistical realities are legitimate, but one must resist the temptation to attribute the improved survival to the staging evaluation itself.

When evaluating the benefits of any treatment for lung cancer, it is important to study the report carefully, to determine the true denominator and to note the tests used to define the population under study. Thus the reader may be better able to place into context the results reported in the following chapters of this book.

REFERENCES

1. International Union against Cancer (UICC), The birth of the TNM. *UICC Magazine* 1988; **9**: 1–3.
2. Mountain CF, Revisions in the International System for Staging Lung Cancer *Chest* 1997; **111**: 1710–17.
3. Ihde D, Makuch RW, Carney DN et al, Prognostic implications of stage of disease and sites of metastases in patients with small cell carcinoma treated with intensive combination chemotherapy. *Am Rev Respir Dis* 1981; **123**: 500–7.
4. Feld R, Abratt RP, Graziano SL et al, Pretreatment minimal staging and prognostic factors for non-small cell lung cancer. *Lung Cancer* 1997; **17**(Suppl 1): s3–10.
5. Anonymous, Pretreatment evaluation of non-small-cell lung cancer. *Am J Respir Crit Care Med* 1997; **156**: 320–32.
6. American Joint Committee on Cancer Staging and End Results Reporting, *AJCC Cancer Staging Manual*, 5th edn. Lippincott-Raven: Philadelphia, 1997.
7. Romney BM, Austin JH, Plain film evaluation of carcinoma of the lung. *Semin Roentgenol* 1990; **25**: 45–63.
8. Hooper RG, Beechler CR, Johnson MC, Radioisotope scanning in the initial staging of bronchogenic carcinoma. *Am Rev Respir Dis* 1978; **118**: 279–86.
9. Bollen ECM, Goei R, Hof-Grootenboer BEv et al, Interobserver variability and accuracy of computed tomographic assessment of nodal status in lung cancer. *Ann Thorac Surg* 1994; **58**: 158–62.
10. Keogan MT, Tung KT, Kaplan DK et al, The significance of pulmonary nodules detected on CT staging for lung cancer. *Clin Radiol* 1993; **48**: 94–6.
11. Osborne DR, Korobkin M, Ravin CE et al, Comparison of plain radiography, conventional tomography, and computed tomography in detecting intrathoracic lymph node metastases from lung carcinoma. *Radiology* 1982; **142**: 157–61.

12. Dales RE, Stark RM, Raman S, Computed tomography to stage lung cancer. Approaching a controversy using meta-analysis. *Am Rev Respir Dis* 1990; **141**: 1096–101.
13. Kayser K, Bach S, Bulzebruck H et al, Site, size, and tumour involvement of resected extrapulmonary lymph nodes in lung cancer. *J Surg Oncol* 1990; **43**: 45–9.
14. Lewis JWJ, Pearlberg JL, Beute GH et al, Can computed tomography of the chest stage lung cancer? Yes and no. *Ann Thorac Surg* 1990; **49**: 591–5.
15. Dillemans B, Deneffe G, Verschakelen J, Decramer M. Value of computed tomography and mediastinoscopy in preoperative evaluation of mediastinal nodes in non-small cell lung cancer. A study of 569 patients. *Eur J Cardiothorac Surg* 1994; **8**: 37–42.
16. McLeod TC, Bourgouin PM, Greenberg RW et al, Bronchogenic carcinoma: analysis of staging in the mediastinum with CT by correlative lymph node mapping and sampling. *Radiology* 1992; **182**: 319–23.
17. Landreneau RJ, Hazelrigg SR, Mack MJ et al, Thoracoscopic mediastinal lymph node sampling: useful for mediastinal lymph node stations inaccessible by cervical mediastinoscopy. *J Thorac Cardiovasc Surg* 1993; **106**: 554–8.
18. Goldstraw P, Kurzer M, Edwards D, Pre-operative staging of lung cancer: accuracy of computed tomography versus mediastinoscopy. *Thorax* 1983; **38**: 10–5.
19. Glazer HS, Kaiser LR, Anderson DJ et al, Indeterminate mediastinal invasion in bronchogenic carcinoma: CT evaluation. *Radiology* 1989; **173**: 37–42.
20. Armstrong P, Preoperative computed tomographic scanning for staging lung cancer. *Thorax* 1994; **49**: 941–3.
21. Wursten HU, Vock P, Mediastinal infiltration of lung carcinoma (T4N0–1): the positive predictive value of computed tomography. *Thorac Cardiovasc Surg* 1987; **35**: 355–60.
22. Ratto GB, Piacenza G, Frola C et al, Chest wall involvement by lung cancer: computed tomographic detection and results of operation. *Ann Thorac Surg* 1991; **51**: 182–8.
23. Pairolero PC, Trastek VF, Payne WS, Treatment of bronchogenic carcinoma with chest wall invasion. *Surg Clin North Am* 1987; **67**: 959–64.
24. Shah SS, Goldstraw P, Combined pulmonary and thoracic wall resection for stage III lung cancer. *Thorax* 1995; **50**: 782–4.
25. Gillams A, Roberts CM, Shaw P et al, The value of CT scanning and percutaneous fine needle aspiration of adrenal masses in biopsy-proven lung cancer. *Clin Radiol* 1992; **46**: 18–22.
26. Mintz BJ, Tuhrim S, Alexander S et al, Intracranial metastases in the initial staging of bronchogenic carcinoma. *Chest* 1984; **86**: 850–3.
27. Grant D, Edwards D, Goldstraw P, Computed tomography of the brain, chest, and abdomen in the preoperative assessment of non-small cell lung cancer. *Thorax* 1988; **43**: 883–6.
28. Quinn DL, Ostrow LB, Porter DK et al, Staging of non-small cell bronchogenic carcinoma. Relationship of the clinical evaluation to organ scans. *Chest* 1986; **89**: 270–5.
29. Ramsdell JW, Peters RM, Taylor AT Jr et al, Multiorgan scans for staging lung cancer: correlation with clinical evaluation. *J Thorac Cardiovasc Surg* 1977; **73**: 653–9.
30. Salvatierra A, Baamonde C, Llamas JM et al, Extrathoracic staging of bronchogenic carcinoma. *Chest* 1990; **97**: 1052–8.
31. Gold RI, Seeger LL, Bassett LW, Steckel RJ, An integrated approach to the evaluation of metastatic bone disease. *Radiol Clin North Am* 1990; **28**: 471–83.
32. Snow JH Jr, Goldstein HM, Wallace S, Comparison of scintigraphy, sonography, and computed tomography in the evaluation of hepatic neoplasms. *Am Roentgen Ray Soc* 1979; **132**: 915–18.
33. Abrams HL, Siegelman SS, Adams DF et al, Computed tomography versus ultrasound of the adrenal gland: a prospective study. *Radiology* 1982; **143**: 121–8.
34. Goldstraw P, CT Scanning in the pre-operative

assessment of non-small cell lung cancer. In: *Lung Cancer: Basic and Clinical Aspects* (Goldstraw P, Hansen HH, eds). Martinus Nijhoff: Boston, 1986: 183–99.

35. Goldstraw P, Mediastinal exploration by mediastinoscopy and mediastinotomy. *Br J Dis Chest* 1988; **82**: 111–20.
36. Jiao X, Magistraelli P, Goldstraw P, The value of cervical mediastinoscopy combined with anterior mediastinotomy in bronchogenic carcinoma of the left upper lobe. *Eur J Cardio-thorac Surg* 1997; **11**: 450–4.
37. Pearson FG, Delarue NC, Ilves R et al, Significance of positive superior mediastinal nodes identified at mediastinoscopy in patients with resectable cancer of the lung. *J Thorac Cardiovasc Surg* 1982; **83**: 1–11.
38. Goldstraw P, Mannam GC, Kaplan DK, Michail P, Surgical management of non-small-cell lung cancer with ipsilateral mediastinal node metastasis (N2 disease). *J Thorac Cardiovasc Surg* 1994; **107**: 19–27.
39. Brynitz S, Struve-Christensen E, Borgeskov S, Bertelsen S, Transcarinal mediastinal needle biopsy compared with mediastinoscopy. *J Thorac Cardiovasc Surg* 1985; **90**: 21–4.
40. Cropp AJ, DiMarco AF, Lankerani M, False-positive transbronchial needle aspiration in bronchogenic carcinoma. *Chest* 1984; **85**: 696–7.
41. Kondo D, Imaizumi M, Abe T et al, Endoscopic ultrasound examination for mediastinal lymph node metastases of lung cancer. *Chest* 1990; **98**: 586–93.
42. Muller LC, Glaser K, Salzer GM, Aufschnaiter M, Transesophageal sonography in central bronchial carcinoma. *Eur J Cardio-thorac Surg* 1990; **4**: 226–8.
43. Hughes JM, ^{18}F-Fluorodeoxyglucose PET scans in lung cancer. *Thorax* 1996; **51**(Suppl 2): s16–22.
44. Duhaylongsod FG, Lowe VJ, Patz EF Jr et al, Detection of primary and recurrent lung cancer by means of F-18 fluorodeoxyglucose positron emission tomography (FDG PET). *J Thorac Cardiovasc Surg* 1995; **110**: 130–9.
45. Scott WJ, Schwabe JL, Gupta NC et al, PET–Lung tumour study group. Positron emission tomography of lung tumours and mediastinal lymph nodes using (^{18}F) fluorodeoxyglucose. *Ann Thorac Surg* 1994; **58**: 698–703.
46. Gould MK, Lillington GA, Strategy and cost in investigating solitary pulmonary nodules. *Thorax* 1998; **53**(Suppl 2): s32–7.
47. Obers VJ, Leiman G, Girdwood RW, Spiro FI, Primary malignant pleural tumours (mesotheliomas) presenting as localized masses. Fine needle aspiration cytologic findings, clinical and radiologic features and review of the literature. *Acta Cytol* 1988; **32**: 567–75.
48. Schiepers C, Role of positron emission tomography in the staging of lung cancer. *Lung Cancer* 1997; **17**(Suppl 1): s29–35.
49. Vansteenkiste J, Stroobants SG, De Leyn P et al, Lymph node staging in non-small-cell lung cancer with FDG–PET scan: a prospective study on 690 lymph node stations from 68 patients. *J Clin Oncol* 1998; **16**: 42–9.
50. Martini N, Flehinger BJ, The role of surgery in N2 lung cancer. *Surg Clin North Am* 1987; **67**: 1037–49.
51. Naruke T, Goya T, Tsuchiya R, Suemasu K, The importance of surgery to non-small cell carcinoma of lung with mediastinal lymph node metastasis. *Ann Thorac Surg* 1988; **46**: 603–10.
52. Vansteenkiste J, De Leyn P, Deneffe G et al, Survival and prognostic factors in resected N2 non-small cell lung cancer: a study of 140 cases. *Ann Thorac Surg* 1997; **63**: 1441–50.
53. Valk PE, Pounds TR, Hopkins DM et al, Staging non-small cell lung cancer by whole body positron emission tomographic imaging. *Ann Thorac Surg* 1995; **60**: 1573–82.
54. Weder W, Schmid RA, Bruchhaus H et al, Detection of extrathoracic metastases by positron emission tomography in lung cancer. *Ann Thorac Surg* 1998; **66**: 886–93.
55. Lewis P, Griffin S, Marsden P et al, Whole-body ^{18}F-fluorodeoxyglucose positron emission tomography in preoperative evaluation of lung cancer. *Lancet* 1994; **344**: 1265–6.
56. Kutlu CA, Pastorino U, Maisey M, Goldstraw P,

Selective use of PET scan in the preoperative staging of NSCLC. *Lung Cancer* 1998; **21**: 177–84.
57. Gefter WB, Magnetic resonance imaging in the evaluation of lung cancer. *Semin Roentgenol* 1990; **25**: 73–84.
58. Heelan RT, Demas BE, Caravelli JF et al, Superior sulcus tumours: CT and MR imaging. *Radiology* 1989; **170**: 637–41.
59. Webb WR, MR imaging in the evaluation and staging of lung cancer. *Semin Ultrasound CT MR* 1988; **9**: 53–66.
60. Deslauriers J, Brisson J, Cartier R et al, Carcinoma of the lung. Evaluation of satellite nodules as a factor influencing prognosis after resection. *J Thorac Cardiovasc Surg* 1989; **97**: 504–12.
61. Goldstraw P, Report on the International Workshop on Intrathoracic Staging. London, October 1996. *Lung Cancer* 1997; **18**: 107–11.
62. Kondo H, Asamura H, Suemasu K et al, Prognostic significance of pleural lavage cytology immediately after thoracotomy in patients with lung cancer. *J Thorac Cardiovasc Surg* 1993; **106**: 1092–7.
63. Hillerdal G, Dernevik L, Almgren S-O et al, Prognostic value of malignant cells in pleural lavage at thoracotomy for bronchial carcinoma. *Lung Cancer* 1998; **21**: 47–52.
64. Fernando HC, Goldstraw P, The accuracy of clinical evaluative intrathoracic staging in lung cancer as assessed by postsurgical pathologic staging. *Cancer* 1990; **65**: 2503–6.
65. Naruke T, Suemasu K, Ishikawa S, Lymph node mapping and curability at various levels of metastasis in resected lung cancer. *J Thorac Cardiovasc Surg* 1978; **76**: 832–9.
66. Graham ANJ, Chan KJM, Pastorino U, Goldstraw P, Systematic nodal dissection in the intrathoracic staging of patients with non-small cell lung cancer. *J Thorac Cardiovasc Surg* 1999; **117**: 264–51.
67. Annual Returns, The Society of Cardiothoracic Surgeons of Great Britain and Ireland. Unpublished data (available from the Society).
68. Gaer JA, Goldstraw P, Intraoperative assessment of nodal staging at thoracotomy for carcinoma of the bronchus. *Eur J Cardio-thorac Surg* 1990; **4**: 207–10.
69. Passlick B, Izbicki JR, Kubuschok B et al, Detection of disseminated lung cancer cells in lymph nodes: Impact on staging and prognosis. *Ann Thorac Surg* 1996; **61**: 177–83.
70. Nicholson AG, Graham ANJ, Pezzella F et al, Does the use of immunohistochemistry to identify micrometastases provide useful information in the staging of node-negative non-small cell lung carcinomas? *Lung Cancer* 1997; **18**: 231–40.
71. Graziano SL, Non-small cell lung cancer: clinical value of new biological predictors. *Lung Cancer* 1997; **17**(Suppl 1): s37–58.
72. Shields TW, The significance of ipsilateral mediastinal lymph node metastasis (N2 disease) in non-small cell carcinoma of the lung. A commentary. *J Thorac Cardiovasc Surg* 1990; **99**: 48–53.
73. Feinstein AR, Sosin DM, Wells CK, The Will Rogers Phenomenon: stage migration and new diagnostic techniques as a source of misleading statistics for survival in cancer. *N Engl J Med* 1985; **312**: 1604–8.
74. Naruke T, Goya T, Tsuchiya R, Suemasu K, Prognosis and survival in resected lung carcinoma based on the new international staging system. *J Thorac Cardiovasc Surg* 1988; **96**: 440–7.

11 Treatment of non-small cell lung cancer

11.1 Treatment of NSCLC: Surgery

Robert J Korst, Ryosuke Tsuchiya

Contents

INTRODUCTION

Lung cancer is one of the leading causes of cancer death worldwide. Approximately 80% of cases of newly diagnosed lung cancer are of the non-small cell type (NSCLC). Unfortunately, a large percentage of these patients will have inoperable disease on the basis of distant metastases (stage IV) or locally advanced disease (stage IIIb). For the remaining patients with early stage disease (stages I and II), as well as selected patients with locally advanced disease (stage IIIa), complete surgical resection remains the best hope for cure, provided that the operative risk is tolerable.

Over the past four decades, several points regarding the conduct of resection have become accepted as the surgical management of NCSLC has evolved:

- Incomplete resections leaving either gross or microscopic disease behind will fail to cure the disease, and are rarely indicated in a palliative setting. Intraoperative frozen section analysis should be employed frequently to ensure negative margins.
- General oncologic principles should be followed, including resection of the tumor and surrounding normal lung (lobectomy or pneumonectomy) with draining lymphatics and lymph nodes.
- The mediastinal lymph nodes should be dissected to accurately stage the patient.
- En bloc resection of the tumor and surrounding structures is desirable whenever technically possible.

Survival after surgical resection for NSCLC is stage-dependent (Table 11.1.1). Despite the development of the principles mentioned above, only 13% of all patients can presently be expected to be cured of their disease. This dismal figure underscores the need for prevention as well as continued investigation into better treatment options for patients with NSCLC.

HISTORICAL SUMMARY

Although non-anatomic pulmonary resection for lung cancer had been reported in 1895, the first anatomic lobectomy was performed by Davies in 1912. It was not until the advent of an effective underwater drainage system, however, that pulmonary resection could safely be performed

Table 11.1.1 Survival following resection of NSCLC by stage (see text for references)

Stage	Five-year survival rate (%)
Stage I	
Overall	76
T1N0M0	84
T2N0M0	68
Stage II	
T1–2N1M0	47
T3N0M0:	
Chest wall invasion	56
Mediastinal invasion	29
Proximal bronchus	36
Stage III	
N2:	
Clinically negative mediastinum	34
Clinically positive mediastinum	9

on more of a routine basis. Following a report by Graham of the first pneumonectomy in 1933, surgical resection became the treatment of choice for lung cancer. Over the next several decades, various types of anatomic lung resections continued to be described, including segmentectomy, sleeve lobectomy and pneumonectomy, as well as resection for superior sulcus tumors.

Through the 1970s and 1980s, it became recognized that, despite radical resection with negative margins, many patients with resected NSCLC ultimately died of their disease, with the majority of recurrences being distant metastases. This was especially true for patients found to have disease metastatic to the lymph nodes (locally advanced disease) at the time of resection. As a result of this observation, combined with the disappointing results obtained with postoperative chemotherapy and radiation therapy, investigators began to report improved survival in selected patients with ipsilateral mediastinal node metastases (N2) detected preoperatively who received preoperative 'induction' chemotherapy. It is hoped that this improved survival may translate to patients with lesser-stage, poor-prognosis disease (T2N0–1) as well as those with limited distant metastases (M1) – strategies currently under investigation.

STAGE I DISEASE (T1–2N0)

Patients with this early stage of NSCLC typically present without symptoms, and most are cured with primary surgical excision. These tumors are usually peripheral in location, and are discovered on a routine chest radiograph. These peripheral 'coin lesions' are mainly adenocarcinomas, including bronchioloalveolar carcinomas. Uncommonly, a radiographically 'occult' tumor may be discovered. Unlike the peripheral lesions, occult tumors are mainly squamous in histology, and patients may present with hemoptysis. Not infrequently, occult tumors are detected during screening bronchoscopy after a previous lung resection,[1] or in patients who have undergone bronchoscopy as part of the workup for another process, such as head and neck or esophageal cancer. In areas where lung cancer screening of high-risk populations using sputum cytology is utilized, occult NSCLC is detected more readily than in areas where screening is not routinely practiced.

When evaluating a patient with a stage I NSCLC, a CT scan of the chest and upper abdomen should be obtained with intravenous contrast to assess the mediastinum, lungs, liver and adrenal glands for metastatic disease. Other tests, such as bone and brain scans, are not routinely indicated in asymptomatic patients, since the yield is very low. If enlarged mediastinal lymph nodes are detected on CT scan, cervical mediastinoscopy is indicated to obtain histologic confirmation, since a significant number of these nodes will be inflammatory in nature. The use of routine mediastinal lymph node biopsy in the presence of normal sized nodes on CT scan remains controversial, and is not routinely practiced.

Complete surgical excision is the treatment of choice for stage I NSCLC, provided that the operative risk is acceptable. Patients should undergo preoperative pulmonary function testing to assess lung reserve, as well as cardiac evaluation if indicated from the patient's history. The operation of choice is anatomic lobectomy, which can be performed through a variety of incisions, the most common being a posterolateral thoracotomy. Limited resections (wedge resection or segmentectomy) should be avoided whenever possible because of the higher rate of local recurrence and worse long-term survival when these lesser resections are performed.[2] Limited resections remain an option, however, for patients with poor pulmonary reserve. Occasionally, a more extensive resection needs to be performed when the location of the tumor is such that removal of a single lobe is not adequate. When the tumor protrudes into the mainstem bronchus, sleeve lobectomy is the procedure of choice to obtain negative bronchial margins; however, a tumor involving the bronchus intermedius requires a bilobectomy, while a lesion more extensively involving the mainstem bronchus requires pneumonectomy. Pneumonectomy may also be indicated in the rare circumstances when the tumor is closely associated with the proximal, extrapericardial, pulmonary artery. For upper lobe lesions that invade the pulmonary artery to the lower lobe, a vascular sleeve resection can be performed, sparing the lower lobe.

Although it has been suggested that mediastinal lymph node dissection is unnecessary in patients with very small T1 tumors, the vast majority of patients undergoing resection for NSCLC should have this procedure routinely performed. Although this approach has never been demonstrated to improve survival, it is the only way to accurately stage a patient's disease, and adds very little time and morbidity to the operation. In addition, approximately 16% of patients with peripheral T1N0 tumors where the primary tumor is less than 3 cm in size will have mediastinal node metastases.[3] When resecting a right-sided tumor, the right paratracheal, pretracheal, subcarinal and inferior pulmonary ligament nodes should be dissected. On the left, the preaortic, aortopulmonary window, subcarinal and inferior pulmonary ligament nodes are accessible.

The operative mortality rate following pulmonary lobectomy for all stages of disease should not surpass 2%, but should be considerably less for patients with stage I disease. Morbidity and mortality increase with higher stages of disease and extended resections. The operative mortality rate following pneumonectomy is near 6% in most series, with some being even lower.[4] The five-year survival rate for patients with completely resected T1N0 lesions surpasses 80% in some reports, while this figure is reduced to approximately 65% for T2N0 tumors. The overall five-year survival rate for patients with completely resected stage I NSCLC is approximately 75%.[5]

No form of adjuvant therapy is currently recommended after resection of stage I disease. Current research efforts are geared toward determining which patients with stage I disease are at a higher risk for relapse, with the focus being on molecular markers. Recurrences following complete resection for stage I NSCLC are mainly in the form of

Table 11.1.2 Sites of first distant recurrence following resection in 159 patients with stage I NSCLC[6]

Site	Number
Brain	51
Lung	20
Liver	14
Bone	11
Other	8
Disseminated	5

distant metastases, as displayed in Table 11.1.2. Patients should be followed with serial chest radiographs and physical examinations after resection for NSCLC, with the intent of detecting both recurrent disease and new primary tumors.

STAGE II DISEASE (T1–2N1 AND T3N0)

N1 disease

Patients with T1–2N1 NSCLC represent a small subset in the spectrum of this disease, usually comprising less than 10% of patients coming to surgery. As with stage I, the majority of patients can be effectively treated with lobectomy, although about a third will require pneumonectomy, mainly because of involved hilar lymph nodes adherent to the pulmonary artery or major bronchi. In addition, it is increasingly more important to perform a thorough mediastinal lymph node dissection in this group of patients because of the higher incidence of occult N2 disease.

One controversial issue that arises when operating on patients with N1 disease is the meaning of an involved 'sump' node. The sump nodes are defined as interlobar nodes lying on the bronchus or pulmonary artery in the major fissure. When these nodes are involved by tumor, the implication is that tumor cells have entered the lymphatic channels of the adjacent lobe, and serious consideration should be given to performing a pneumonectomy to obtain a complete resection. This approach, however, has never been demonstrated to improve survival – in part because of the small number of patients with this problem.

Recurrence following complete resection for T1–2N1 NSCLC is common, with five-year survival rates approaching only 45%.[7] As with stage I, the most common form of recurrence is distant metastatic disease, especially if the tumor is an adenocarcinoma or large cell carcinoma. Patients enjoying a better prognosis tend to be those with small primary tumors, squamous histology and only one involved lymph node. Although postoperative radiation therapy has been shown to decrease the local recurrence rate, this has not translated into improved survival.[8] In addition, there is no consistent benefit from the use of adjuvant chemotherapy in this group, either.

T3N0 disease

Chest wall involvement

T3 tumors invading the chest wall are readily amenable to surgical resection. As a general guideline, one rib above and one below the gross margin of the tumor should be taken to ensure negative margins. Although en bloc resection is desirable and should be achieved whenever possible, discontinuous resection can be done when absolutely necessary, as long as meticulous attention is paid toward documenting margins. It currently remains controversial whether a complete chest wall resection, including ribs, is necessary for tumors invading only the parietal pleura. A parietal pleurectomy with negative deep margins may be sufficient, but should be used with extreme caution.

Following resection, the issue of chest wall reconstruction needs to be addressed. The first question regarding this is whether the chest wall reconstruction is really necessary, and this usually depends on the assessment of chest wall stability. After resection of short segments of one or two ribs, or up to three posterior segments under the paraspinous muscles or scapula, reconstruction is not usually necessary. When reconstruction is undertaken, the Marlex/methyl methacrylate sandwich technique readily restores stability and prevents the flail chest phenomenon during breathing. A Gore-Tex patch, stretched tightly, has also been used with acceptable results. Mortality following chest wall resection is low, but is related to the size and location of the defect in the chest wall, the amount of lung resected and the technique of reconstruction.

Factors that affect long-term survival following resection of these tumors are the extent of chest wall involvement, the ability to completely resect the tumor, and the presence or absence of lymph node involvement. The overall five-year survival rate of patients with T3N0M0 tumors invading the chest wall undergoing complete en bloc surgical resection is approximately 50–60%.[9] Patients with a T3N0M0 tumor that involves only the parietal pleura have a better prognosis than those where the tumor invades muscle and ribs (62% and 35% five-year survival rates respectively).[9]

T3 tumors invading the chest wall are peripheral, and therefore less likely to spread to mediastinal lymph nodes. However, when present, N1 or N2 nodal disease negatively impacts long-term survival following resection of these tumors. Most surgeons believe that patients with T3N2M0 tumors have a negligible five-year survival, and should not be offered primary surgical therapy. It is therefore important in patients with tumors invading the chest wall to perform cervical mediastinoscopy to rule out N2 or N3 disease prior to undertaking a pulmonary and chest wall resection.

The role of adjuvant therapy for tumors invading the chest wall remains undefined, but results have not been encouraging. Although no clear survival benefit has been noted, patients with incompletely resected tumors or those with hilar or mediastinal nodal metastases should receive postoperative radiation therapy to decrease the incidence of local recurrence.[8] Intraoperative implantation of radioisotopes may be of some benefit for those patients who undergo an incomplete resection. The role of induction chemoradiotherapy in poor-prognosis tumors (N2 disease, full-thickness chest wall invasion) is now being investigated.

Tumors invading the mediastinum

Tumors invading the mediastinal pleura, fat, nerves and pericardium but not the major mediastinal vessels or organs represent another subset of the T3 classification. These patients have a notoriously poor five-year survival following surgical resection alone. In part, this poor survival is due to the high likelihood of mediastinal node metastases and the low rate of complete resection attained when the mediastinum is invaded. Additionally, even when these tumors are completely resected and the mediastinal nodes are negative, patients with T3 disease invading the mediastinum have a worse prognosis when compared with other types of T3 tumors.[10]

Owing to the high frequency of N2 disease, patients with evidence of mediastinal invasion on CT scan should undergo cervical mediastinoscopy to rule out nodal involvement or T4 disease. If N2 disease is detected, induction (neoadjuvant) therapy may offer these patients a better chance of long-term survival, if surgical resection is being considered. If there is no N2, N3 or T4 disease found at mediastinoscopy, these patients can undergo primary surgical resection with five-year survival rates of 30% if complete resection can be performed.[10]

Tumors in proximity to the carina

Tumors within 2 cm but not involving the main carina comprise another subset of T3 tumors. As with the other T3 tumors, patients with these proximal bronchial lesions are candidates for surgical resection. Technical considerations when resecting tumors involving the main bronchi pertain to the extent of resection, intraoperative airway management and techniques of sleeve resection. Small, solitary, squamous cell lesions confined to the left main bronchus with no invasion through the bronchial wall can very occasionally be handled with excision of the main bronchus alone, with total lung preservation and primary anastomosis. However, frequently these lesions are multiple, and are best treated with endobronchial laser or radiation (brachytherapy). If resection is being considered for a solitary proximal lesion on the right, however, usually a pneumonectomy or right upper lobe sleeve resection is required because of the close proximity of the right upper lobe orifice to the main bronchus. Sleeve lobectomy (versus pneumonectomy) is the preferable resection when possible for tumors extending into the orifice of the lobar or mainstem bronchus with no peribronchial or hilar nodal involvement.

When there is invasion of peribronchial tissues or N1 disease is present, sleeve lobectomy can be attempted if the disease is limited, but pneumonectomy is usually required for extranodal spread. If the tumor extends very close to the carina, resection of the main bronchus flush with the trachea may be required to encompass the tumor with negative margins. In this case, stapling of the bronchial stump may not be possible, and a hand-sewn closure may be required. If not, tracheal sleeve pneumonectomy is the procedure of choice.

Airway management and ventilation are of paramount importance when the proximal bronchi are resected. Standard double-lumen endobronchial tubes or endobronchial blockers with single-lung ventilation can be utilized for sleeve resections of the main bronchi. Tracheal sleeve pneumonectomy requires ventilation of the distal remaining lung. This problem can be handled in several ways, including passage of a thin single-lumen endotracheal tube past the anastomotic site, jet ventilation into the distal lung, or in-field ventilation through the open bronchus using sterile ventilator tubing.

Factors that adversely affect long-term survival following resection include peribronchial extension of the tumor and the presence of N2 nodal metastases. The overall five-year survival rate following complete resection for tumors within 2 cm of the carina is currently reported to be 36%;[11] however, patients with tumor confined to the main bronchi with no invasion of peribronchial tissues or associated N2 disease have been reported to have a five-year survival rate of 80% in one series.[12] Patients with T3 tumors approaching the carina associated with N2 nodal metastases separate from the primary tumor ('true' N2) have a negligible five-year survival. Patients with N2 disease that is present by virtue of direct spread from the primary tumor, however, remain surgical candidates. Therefore we feel it is mandatory to perform cervical mediastinoscopy prior to an attempted resection to identify those patients with 'true' mediastinal nodal disease who would receive no benefit from primary surgical resection. If N2 nodes are identified at cervical mediastinoscopy, induction radio- and/or chemotherapy may be of value, but this awaits clinical trials.

STAGE III DISEASE

Stage IIIa (T3N1) disease

T3 tumors with associated ipsilateral bronchopulmonary or hilar lymph node involvement comprise the first category of stage IIIa disease. The preferred treatment is again complete resection via lobectomy with mediastinal lymph node dissection. The previously mentioned issues concerning N1 disease apply in this setting as well.

Stage IIIa (N2) disease

The decision to perform primary surgical resection for patients with N2 disease requires careful preoperative selection, since the overall five-year survival rate for patients with N2 disease undergoing surgical resection alone is a mere 5–15%. Those with only single-station intracapsular nodal disease, T1 primary tumors, and 'clinically' negative mediastinums by mediastinoscopy or CT scanning are reported to enjoy a five-year survival rate of approximately 30% following complete surgical resection, compared with less than 10% for those with 'bulky' N2 disease identified preoperatively and those with associated T3 primary tumors.[13] Patients with left upper lobe tumors and N2 disease confined to level 5 or 6 have the best prognosis of all, with five-year survival rates as high as 42% when completely resected.[14] Unfortunately, patients with 'minimal' N2 involvement for whom primary surgery is beneficial represent a small fraction of all patients with N2 disease, and further therapeutic advances clearly need to be made for those patients with bulky, 'clinical', N2 disease.

As a result of these survival figures, when performing thoracotomy for NSCLC, it is advisable to biopsy the mediastinal lymph nodes prior to completing the pulmonary resection. If intraoperative frozen section analysis reveals unsuspected multistation N2 disease, or total nodal replacement with tumor, careful consideration should be given to closing the wound without performing the pulmonary resection to administer 'preoperative' chemo(radio)therapy. If no nodal metastases or only microscopic nodal metastases are discovered at one station, the pulmonary resection should commence.

Postoperative adjuvant chemotherapy and/or radiation therapy have been used in an attempt to improve survival for patients with resected stage IIIA (N2) NSCLC. Neither modality has been shown to be of significant benefit compared with surgery alone; however, a reduction in local recurrence is seen.[8] Unfortunately, 80% of patients undergoing surgical resection for NSCLC with N2 nodal disease have recurrences at distant metastatic sites (especially brain), suggesting that further systemic therapy is needed to improve survival.

Most adjuvant chemotherapy trials have not shown prolonged survival following resection for patients with N2 disease. A recent meta-analysis of 52 randomized trials of adjuvant chemotherapy for completely resected NSCLC suggested only a small advantage (3% at two years) of cisplatin-based chemotherapeutic regimens given in the adjuvant setting.[15] Recently, a Japanese study of 323 patients suggested a significant survival advantage for patients receiving oral tegafur plus uracil (UFT) following complete surgical resection of NSCLC compared with surgery alone.[16] Since only 55 of these patients were stage IIIA, however, the extrapolation of these data to patients with N2 disease is, at most, limited. The role of adjuvant chemotherapy has yet to be defined in patients with stage IIIA NSCLC, and is continuing to be studied in clinical trials as newer, more active and less toxic agents become available.

Induction (neoadjuvant) chemotherapy

Induction chemotherapy emerged as an option for patients with N2 disease after it became clear that only a minority of these patients benefit from surgical resection alone and that preoperative radiation therapy has no effect on survival. To date, many phase II trials of induction chemotherapy or chemoradiation therapy both

Table 11.1.3 Three phase III trials of induction chemotherapy for NSCLC with ipsilateral mediastinal lymph node metastases

Author	Number of patients[a]	Chemotherapy agents	Percent resectable[a]	Median survival[a,b]
Pass[19]	13/14	Cisplatin Etoposide	85/86	29/16
Roth[20]	26/32	Cisplatin Etoposide Cyclophosphamide	61/66	64/11
Rosell[21]	30/30	Mitomycin Ifosfamide Cisplatin	85/90	26/8

[a]Induction chemotherapy followed by surgery group/surgery alone group.
[b]Overall median survival in months.

with or without postoperative adjuvant therapy have been reported. Preoperative chemotherapy, such as the MVP (mitomycin, vindesine and cisplatin) regimen utilized at the Memorial Sloan–Kettering Cancer Center in New York and the University of Toronto have shown survival benefit in this group of patients when compared with historical controls.[17,18] The majority of reports, however, deal with preoperative chemoradiation, and essentially mirror the results of the previously mentioned induction chemotherapy trials. Although hundreds of patients have been enrolled in such phase II studies, no real effect of the treatment can be assessed for two reasons. First, the chemotherapy and radiotherapy protocols have varied widely from one trial to the next, as did the extent of preoperative staging, making the results difficult to interpret. Second, patients in these phase II trials are not randomized, and therefore no control groups exist other than historical data.

There have been three small phase III trials comparing induction chemotherapy and surgical resection to surgical resection alone in the treatment of patients with N2 disease (Table 11.1.3). Although different chemotherapy protocols were utilized and the numbers were small, the survival rates reported were significantly higher than in the control arms. Surprisingly, in all three studies, the rate of complete resection was no different in the treatment arms compared with the control arms. These three small phase III trials and the phase II trials that have been matched to historical controls seem to suggest an improvement in survival for these patients, at least with induction chemotherapy.

Treatment-related mortality in the induction trials has resulted from the chemotherapy, radiation therapy and surgery, or a combination of these modalities. Most trials report a treatment-related death rate in the range of 5–15%. Chemotherapy-related deaths are dependent on the specific agent and dose, as well as the immunosuppressive effects of these drugs. Morbidity following induction chemotherapy can be manifested in several organ systems.

Pulmonary function studies should be repeated after induction chemotherapy to assess the pulmonary effects of such drugs as mitomycin and cyclophosphamide, which appear to be toxic to both the pulmonary endothelium and the epithelium, resulting in impaired diffusion of gases. Cardiac toxicity of doxorubicin should be assessed with a myocardial imaging study following the administration of this drug, and creatinine clearance should be measured following treatment with cisplatin if the serum creatinine level has become elevated. These chemotherapy-specific toxicities demand that the induction chemotherapy patient be monitored more closely in the perioperative period to prevent failure of an already-compromised organ system.

Bronchial obstruction needs to be relieved prior to the administration of cytotoxic drugs to avoid postobstructive pneumonia and death during leukopenic events. This can be handled either with radiation therapy or endobronchial laser resection. Radiation therapy is also associated with toxicity that, when given in combination with chemotherapy and surgery, can result in the patient's demise. Examples include the enhanced pulmonary toxicity when radiation therapy is used with mitomycin, the myocardial damage when it is used with doxorubicin, and the higher incidence of bronchopleural fistula in irradiated patients following pulmonary resection.

Morbidity and mortality from the surgical procedure itself can be minimized by careful anesthetic management, close perioperative monitoring of cardiac, pulmonary and fluid status, as well as some specific interventions to treat certain toxicities. For example, mitomycin pulmonary toxicity appears to be exacerbated by high inspired oxygen fractions. Therefore the lowest possible oxygen concentration in the inspired gases should be used, while maintaining adequate oxygenation of the blood. Perioperative corticosteroids can effectively treat both mitomycin- and radiation-induced pulmonary toxicity as well. Tight control over fluid administration should be realized, thereby avoiding pulmonary edema as a result of impaired cardiac and renal function, but still maintaining enough volume for adequate end-organ perfusion.

Stage IIIb (T4 or N3) disease

Patients with this stage of locally advanced NSCLC are considered inoperable. Rare exceptions do exist, however, and generally apply to selected patients with T4 disease. Tracheal sleeve pneumonectomy can be considered for the occasional patient with endobronchial tumor involving the main carina; however, involvement of peribronchial tissue or lymph nodes should preclude this procedure. The five-year survival rate for patients with T4 (carina) N0 tumors undergoing tracheal sleeve pneumonectomy has been reported to approach 20%; however, the operative mortality rate from this procedure can be as high as 15–30%.[22,23]

It is presently debated whether subclavian artery invasion represents T3 or T4 disease, but apical tumors invading this vessel should be resected if a complete resection can be performed. This vessel can be reconstructed either primarily or with a synthetic graft. Again, for patients to benefit from such an extended resection, node-negative status should be confirmed prior to resection using cervical mediastinoscopy.

Sporadic reports exist concerning aortic resection for T4 tumors with an occasional long-term survivor,[24] but no significant survival benefit has been demonstrated in these patients. Similarly, although technically possible, resection of tumors involving the vertebral body has not been shown to provide a survival advantage.[25] These last two scenarios should be considered for clinical protocols involving induction chemo-(radio)therapy, followed by reassessment. If a significant response is seen, resection can be considered in the protocol setting.

If, at thoracotomy for presumed T3 disease, an incomplete resection is all that can be done, owing to involvement of mediastinal organs or vessels (T4), then partial resection with implantation of radioisotopes combined with postoperative external-beam radiation may provide some benefit, with a salvage rate of up to 10%, but this has never been compared with primary (external) radiotherapy as an alternative approach.

STAGE IV DISEASE

Surgery for stage IV disease is limited to young, healthy patients with a solitary site of metastatic disease, and an easily resectable primary tumor contained within the chest. An exhaustive search should be carried out prior to consideration of resection of stage IV disease, looking for other sites of metastatic disease not clearly evident by history and physical examination. Positron emission tomography (PET) may emerge as a useful test for this purpose, and all suspicious lesions should be biopsied to obtain a histologic diagnosis. Solitary bone, liver and skin metastases are rare, but the following sites warrant mentioning because of their more frequent occurrence.

Brain metastases

Approximately one-third of patients with NSCLC and brain metastases present initially with neurologic symptoms, with the lung cancer being found only after a search for the primary tumor has been carried out. In addition to the patients with stage IV disease at presentation, recurrences following resection of NSCLC are most commonly distant metastases and, of these, nearly 30% are located in the brain. It is now accepted that patients with solitary brain metastases from NSCLC are best treated by resection of the brain lesion followed by postoperative whole-brain radiation therapy. Using this strategy, the five-year survival rate in these patients should approach 20%. Even if a cure is not obtained, survival is prolonged and quality of life improved when compared with a non-surgical approach.[26]

When patients present with NSCLC and a single, synchronous brain metastasis, and both lesions are resectable, the brain tumor should be resected prior to the primary tumor, provided that no urgent intrathoracic process is occurring (e.g. massive hemoptysis). This strategy is based on the observation that recovery from intracranial surgery is less intensive than that from thoracotomy. If the resectability of either lesion is in question prior to surgery, one should approach the questionable lesion first to ensure that both lesions can be completely resected prior to undertaking a potentially unnecessary operation. If a brain metastasis is found but a search for the primary tumor is negative, one should proceed with resection of the intracranial tumor.

Adrenal metastases

Solitary metastases to the adrenal glands are being diagnosed with greater frequency owing to routine scanning of the upper abdomen with newer-generation, spiral CT scanners. The utility of adrenalectomy for a solitary NSCLC metastasis, however, has not yet been demonstrated, and is currently under investigation in clinical protocols. Certainly, patients with solitary adrenal metastases should be referred to participate in such protocols.

Lung metastases

Not uncommonly, patients will present with what appears to be a solitary pulmonary metastasis. This should be resected whenever possible owing to the significant survival benefit obtained by a surgical strategy. Obviously, the patient's pulmonary function must be able to permit more than one lung resection.

SPECIAL CONSIDERATIONS

Superior sulcus tumors

Superior sulcus tumors are apical lung cancers that are at least T3 by definition, since they invade the chest wall. In addition to chest wall invasion, these tumors also invade neighboring vital structures, including the brachial plexus, vertebral body and subclavian vessels.[27] Presenting symptoms almost always include pain in the shoulder radiating down the upper, inner aspect of the arm (T1 nerve root) as well as into the ulnar distribution in the hand (C8 nerve root). Patients may also have Horner's syndrome, resulting from invasion of the stellate ganglion in the sympathetic chain – a condition that implies advanced local invasion.

Treatment of these lesions is by surgical resection. Prior to resection, mediastinal node metastases must be ruled out using cervical medastinoscopy owing to the poor prognosis of these patients after resection when N2 disease is present. Several different operative approaches have been described, depending on whether the tumor invades the anterior or posterior aspect of the first rib. It is agreed that posterior lesions should be approached through a posterolateral thoracotomy extending up to the neck, as described by Paulson. This enables the scapula to be lifted off the chest wall and allows access to the apex of the hemithorax from outside the chest wall. Tumors that appear to invade more anteriorly can be approached through any number of anterior approaches, the most common being an L-shaped transcervical incision[28] and the hemiclamshell approach.[29] The advantage of the hemiclamshell incision is easy access to the pulmonary hilum for the performance of lobectomy with mediastinal lymph node dissection. In addition to lobectomy, the standard operation for superior sulcus tumors includes the resection of at least the first rib, the transverse processes of the vertebral bodies associated with each resected rib, and the T1 nerve root.

Following complete resection, the five-year survival rate of patients with superior sulcus tumors is approximately 30%.[28] Unfortunately, many patients do not have a complete resection because of invasion of the previously mentioned vital structures. It has therefore become standard therapy to give patients preoperative external-beam radiation therapy in an attempt to shrink the tumor prior to an attempt at resection, with the hope of increasing the likelihood of a complete resection. The validity of this approach, however, has never been proven, and many patients still undergo incomplete resections. An option currently available is preoperative chemoradiation in a protocol setting, but no data from these studies are yet available.

Multiple primary tumors

It is not uncommon for patients to present with more than one lung malignancy. Either these tumors represent synchronous primaries or one lesion is a metastasis from the other. When the tumors are of different histologies, the diagnosis of synchronous primary lung cancers is made. If the lesions are of the same histology, cervical mediastinoscopy should be routinely performed, because if positive mediastinal nodes are discovered then the chance of one lesion being metastatic rises. Pathologic evidence of two separate primary tumors is the presence of carcinoma in situ in both lesions; however, this information is rarely present at the time of surgery.[30] In many equivocal instances, the 'benefit of the doubt' is given to the patient, and the tumors are labelled as synchronous primaries.

Optimal oncologic treatment for patients with synchronous primary NSCLC is two staged lobectomies for contralateral tumors, and bilobectomy or pneumonectomy for ipsilateral tumors. In cases where the resectability of one lesion is questioned, the questionable tumor should be resected first.

If the patient's lung function permits only one lobectomy, a decision must be made as to which lesion will be resected via lobectomy and which will be approached with a limited resection. Generally, the limited resection should be reserved for the smaller, squamous cell cancers, since these are less likely to spread via lymphatics than adenocarcinomas. Limited resection should consist of segmentectomy instead of wedge resection whenever possible. A third option is to perform multiple segmentectomies in patients with limited pulmonary reserve.

Bronchioloalveolar carcinoma

Bronchioloalveolar carcinoma (BAC) represents a unique subtype of NSCLC that appears to be increasing in incidence. This increase may be real, or may represent heightened recognition of this variant by pathologists. This disease seems to occur mainly in elderly women with a negligible smoking history. Three distinct clinical scenarios seem to be able to arise with BAC.

First, and most commonly, patients may present with a solitary pulmonary nodule. These lesions are usually picked up by routine chest radiograph, and are asymptomatic. Mediastinal lymph nodes are uncommonly involved. Treatment is lobectomy, and long-term survival seems to be excellent.

Second, some patients with BAC will present with small lesions on CT scan that resemble infiltrates. These lesions tend to be multiple, and also tend to recur frequently following resection, especially in areas of lung distant from the primary tumor (multifocal BAC). This implies that this form of BAC may be spread throughout the airway by means of aerosol. Standard treatment is presently resection, but care must be given to the conservation of lung, since these tumors tend to recur with great frequency. Whether or not these patients benefit from repeated attempts at resection is currently unknown.

Third, a minority of patients will present with a lobar infiltrate representing lobar replacement with BAC. Radiologic studies give the appearance of dense consolidation that has arisen over a period of weeks to months. This presentation of BAC carries a poor prognosis, with many patients recurring with widespread infiltrative disease and respiratory failure following resection. For this reason, it is unknown if these benefit at all from resection.

Prognosis in patients with BAC seems to correlate most with the radiographic appearance of the lesion(s).[31] Other factors that have been implicated as poor prognosticators in some studies, but not in others, are a mucinous histology and the presence of vascular invasion. The effect of chemotherapy remains unknown in patients with BAC. Isolated reports of successful double-lung transplantation for recurrent BAC with long-term survivors have been described, but this procedure remains investigational in the treatment of BAC.[32]

Positive resection margins

Every attempt should be made intraoperatively to resect with negative margins. Frozen section analysis should be used to confirm negative margins, and, when positive, further tissue should be resected. A positive bronchial resection margin can be treated by resection of the bronchus and performance of a bronchoplastic procedure, or even pneumonectomy if necessary. Carcinoma in situ remaining at the bronchial stump may not adversely effect prognosis,[33] but this has not conclusively been proven and even this early disease should currently be resected.

Minimally invasive resections

Video-assisted (VATS) pulmonary resections, including lobectomy, are currently being investigated as primary therapy for NSCLC. Although VATS lobectomy is technically possible to perform, its theoretical advantage of decreased postoperative pain is not yet proven. In addition, a thoracotomy still needs to be performed to remove the specimen, and there have been reports of tumor seeding and increased local recurrence following minimally invasive resections.[34] As a result, minimally invasive pulmonary resections for NSCLC cannot yet be routinely advocated, but may be applicable in highly selected cases.

Completion pneumonectomy

Patients with locally recurrent NSCLC or second primary tumors following resection should be evaluated in a similar fashion to those who present with their first cancer. If there is no evidence of distant disease and the remaining pulmonary function is adequate, these patients should be considered for completion pneumonectomy.

Completion pneumonectomy is a technically challenging operation, requiring that the surgeon review the previous operative notes to learn about the anatomy and potential hazards of the reoperation. Mobilization of the lung should be performed intrapleurally whenever possible to avoid excessive bleeding and damage to neighboring structures. Intrapericardial ligation of the vessels also serves to reduce the chance of hemorrhage. Intraoperative use of topical hemostatic agents as well as efficient coagulating devices is helpful.

The operative mortality rate following completion pneumonectomy is in the region of 10%, slightly higher than that seen with standard pneumonectomy.[35] Postoperative morbidity is in the region of 20%, with a significant proportion of complications related to bleeding. Long-term survival rate in patients with NSCLC who undergo this operation is approximately 30%, indicating that completion pneumonectomy is a worthwhile procedure in selected patients.[35]

PALLIATIVE SURGERY

Pleural disease

Patients with diffuse pleural disease (T4) typically present with dyspnea and a pleural effusion. The diagnosis should be confirmed, and is most easily obtained by placement of a chest tube and examination of the fluid for malignant cells. Once the diagnosis of a malignant pleural effusion is confirmed, pleurodesis with sterile talc or other pleural irritant is warranted to prevent recurrence.

If a patient presents with obvious end-stage metastatic disease and a new pleural effusion, a simple thoracentesis may relieve some of the dyspnea and allow the patient to be discharged home to their family. This strategy should be reserved for patients who are anticipated to expire within the next few weeks.

Thoracoscopic exploration is warranted in the following selected instances:

- if the fluid is negative for malignant cells and a malignant diagnosis will affect the treatment plan;
- if the lung fails to re-expand after drainage of fluid, in which case thoracoscopic intervention may be necessary just for the strategic placement of chest tubes to facilitate expansion;
- after a poor result from a bedside pleurodesis as manifested by the rapid reaccumulation of fluid.

The role of formal decortication is very limited in these patients because of their extremely short life expectancy.

Endobronchial disease

Unresectable endobronchial tumor is a not-infrequent occurrence in patients with NSCLC. Typically, these patients may present with airway occlusion with distal pulmonary collapse and pneumonia, dyspnea and hemoptysis. The endobronchial disease may be the manifestation either of the primary tumor extending proximally in the airway or of nodal disease eroding into the proximal tracheobronchial tree. Frequently, the patient has had a previous pulmonary resection and has a recurrence at the bronchial stump.

Adequate palliation can be obtained using either laser or stenting techniques. For bleeding lesions, therapy with the Nd:YAG laser and electrocoagulation are the preferred approaches. Obstructing lesions can be treated using either approach. A combination of débridement through a rigid bronchoscope and laser treatment to obtain hemostasis is often an effective technique. Care must be taken not to blindly laser tumor in the proximal segmental bronchi, since perforation can occur. Recently, photodynamic therapy (PDT) has been used in cases of endobronchial NSCLC. This technique needs further evaluation before it can be routinely used for this disease.

Endobronchial stents are typically of the silicone rubber or self-expanding wire variety. The type of disease most amenable to stenting is that associated with a patent airway both proximal and distal to the obstructing lesion. Silicone stents are deployed using a rigid bronchoscope, while self-expanding wire stents are typically deployed over a guidewire using fluoroscopy as a guide. Silicone stents are removable, while wire stents are not; however, the indications for stent removal in patients with inoperable NSCLC are few.

SUMMARY

Surgery for NSCLC has evolved considerably over the past 50 years. Resection is currently indicated for patients with early stage (I, II, selected IIIA) disease, while chemotherapy and radiotherapy are used for more advanced disease. The mainstay of surgical therapy remains anatomic lobectomy with complete mediastinal lymph node dissection, provided the patient can physically tolerate this procedure. Care must be taken to ensure a complete resection, since incomplete resections do not cure.

New strategies for different stages of disease are constantly being evaluated in the randomized, controlled setting. Strategies currently under investigation include the use of preoperative 'induction' chemotherapy for poor-outcome, lesser-stage disease (T2 > 5 cm), induction chemoradiotherapy for superior sulcus tumors, as well as a randomized trial designed to determine if the best mode of local disease control is surgical resection or radiotherapy. It is through carefully controlled trials such as these that new inroads will be established in the care of patients with NSCLC.

REFERENCES

1. Saito Y, Sato M, Sagawa M et al, Multicentricity in resected occult bronchogenic squamous cell carcinoma. *Ann Thorac Surg* 1994; **57**: 1200–5.
2. Ginsberg RJ, Rubinstein L, for The Lung Cancer Study Group, Randomized trial of lobectomy versus limited resection for patients with T1N0 non-small cell lung cancer. *Ann Thorac Surg* 1995; **60**: 615–23.
3. Asamura H, Nakayama H, Kondo H et al, Lymph node involvement, recurrence and prognosis in resected small peripheral, non-small cell lung carcinomas: Are these carcinomas candidates for video-assisted lobectomy? *J Thorac Cardiovasc Surg* 1996; **111**: 1125–34.
4. Ginsberg RJ, Hill LD, Eagan RT et al, Modern 30-day operative mortality for surgical resections in lung cancer. *J Thorac Cardiovasc Surg* 1983; **86**: 654–8.
5. McCormack P, Martini N, Primary lung cancer. *NY State J Med* 1980; **80**: 618.

6. Martini N, Bains MS, Burt ME et al, Incidence of local recurrence and second primary tumours in resected stage I lung cancer. *J Thorac Cardiovasc Surg* 1995; **109**: 120–9.
7. Martini N, Burt ME, Bains MS et al, Survival after resection of stage II non-small cell lung cancer. *Ann Thorac Surg* 1992; **54**: 460–6.
8. Lung Cancer Study Group, Effects of postoperative mediastinal radiation in completely resected stage II and stage III epidermoid cancer of the lung. *N Engl J Med* 1986; **315**: 1377–81.
9. McCaughan BC, Martini N, Bains MS, McCormack PM, Chest wall invasion in carcinoma of the lung. Therapeutic and prognostic implications. *J Thorac Cardiovasc Surg* 1985; **89**: 836–84.
10. Martini N, Yellin A, Ginsberg RJ et al, Management of non-small cell lung cancer with direct mediastinal involvement. *Ann Thorac Surg* 1994; **58**: 1447–51.
11. Faber LP, Jensik RJ, Kittle CF, Results of sleeve lobectomy for bronchogenic carcinoma in 101 patients. *Ann Thorac Surg* 1984; **37**: 279–85.
12. Nakahashi H, Yasumoto K, Ishida T et al, Results of surgical treatment of patients with T3 non-small cell lung cancer. *Ann Thorac Surg* 1988; **46**: 178–81.
13. Martini N, Flehinger BJ, The role of surgery in N2 lung cancer. *Surg Clin North Am* 1987; **67**: 1037–49.
14. Patterson GA, Piazza D, Pearson FG et al, Significance of metastatic disease in subaortic lymph nodes. *Ann Thorac Surg* 1987; **43**: 155–9.
15. Non-Small Cell Lung Cancer Collaborative Group, Chemotherapy in non-small cell lung cancer: a meta-analysis using updated data on individual patients from 52 randomized, clinical trials. *BMJ* 1995; **311**: 899–909.
16. Wada H, Hitomi S, Teramatsu T, Adjuvant chemotherapy after complete resection in non-small cell lung cancer. *J Clin Oncol* 1996; **14**: 1048–54.
17. Martini N, Kris MM, Flehinger BJ et al, Preoperative chemotherapy of stage IIIa (N2) non-small cell lung cancer: the Memorial Sloan–Kettering experience with 136 patients. *Ann Thorac Surg* 1993; **55**: 1365–74.
18. Burkes RL, Ginsberg RJ, Shepherd FA et al, Induction chemotherapy with mitomycin, vindesine and cisplatin for stage III unresectable non-small cell lung cancer: results of the Toronto phase II trial. *J Clin Oncol* 1992; **10**: 580–6.
19. Pass HI, Pogrebniak HW, Steinberg SM et al, Randomized trial of neoadjuvant therapy for lung cancer: Interim analysis. *Ann Thorac Surg* 1992; **53**: 992–8.
20. Roth JA, Fossella F, Komaki M et al, A randomized trial comparing perioperative chemotherapy and surgery with surgery alone in resectable stage IIIA non-small cell lung cancer. *J Natl Cancer Inst* 1994; **86**: 673–80.
21. Rosell R, Gomez-Codina J, Camps C et al, A randomized trial comparing preoperative chemotherapy plus surgery with surgery alone in patients with non-small cell lung cancer. *N Engl J Med* 1994; **330**: 153–8.
22. Dartevelle PG, Khalife J, Chapelier A et al, Tracheal sleeve pneumonectomy for bronchogenic carcinoma: a report of 55 cases. *Ann Thorac Surg* 1988; **46**: 68–72.
23. Tsuchiya R, Goya T, Naruke T, Suemasu K, Resection of tracheal carina for lung cancer. Procedures, complications and mortality. *J Thorac Cardiovasc Surg* 1990; **99**: 779–87.
24. Tsuchiya R, Asamura H, Kondo H et al, Extended resection of the left atrium, great vessels, or both for lung cancer. *Ann Thorac Surg* 1994; **57**: 960–5.
25. Grunenwald D, Mazel C, Girard P et al, Total vertebrectomy for en bloc resection of lung cancer invading the spine. *Ann Thorac Surg* 1996; **61**: 723–6.
26. Burt M, Wronski M, Arbit E et al, Resection of brain metastases from non-small cell lung carcinoma. Results of therapy. *J Thorac Cardiovasc Surg* 1992; **103**: 399–411.
27. Pancoast HK, Importance of careful roentgen-ray investigation of apical chest tumours. *JAMA* 1924; **82**: 1407.
28. Dartevelle P, Chapelier AR, Macchiarini P et al, Anterior transcervical–thoracic approach for radical resection of lung tumors invading the thoracic inlet. *J Thorac Cardiovasc Surg* 1993; **105**: 1025–34.

29. Korst RJ, Burt ME, Cervicothoracic tumours: results of resection by the 'hemiclamshell' approach. *J Thorac Cardiovasc Surg* 1998; **115**: 286–95.
30. Martini N, Melamed MR, Multiple primary lung cancers. *J Thorac Cardiovasc Surg* 1975; **70**: 606–12.
31. Dumont P, Gasser B, Rouge C et al, Bronchoalveolar carcinoma. Histopathologic study of evolution in a series of 105 surgically treated patients. *Chest* 1998; **113**: 391–5.
32. Etienne B, Vertocchi M, Gamondes J-P et al, Successful double-lung transplantation for bronchioloalveolar carcinoma. *Chest* 1997; **112**: 1423–4.
33. Snijder RJ, de la Riviere AB, Elbers HJJ, van den Bosch JMM, Survival in resected stage I lung cancer with residual tumor at the resection margin. *Ann Thorac Surg* 1998; **65**: 212–16.
34. Downey RJ, McCormack P, LoCicero III J, The Video-Assisted Thoracic Surgery Study Group. Dissemination of malignant tumors after video-assisted thoracic surgery: a report of twenty-one cases. *J Thorac Cardiovasc Surg* 1996; **111**: 954–60.
35. Gregoire J, Deslauriers J, Guojin L, Rouleau J, Indications, risks and results of completion pneumonectomy. *J Thorac Cardiovasc Surg* 1993; **105**: 91.

11.2 Treatment of NSCLC: Radiotherapy

William T Sause, Anna Gregor

Contents Introduction • Where are we now? • Current recommendations • Future directions

INTRODUCTION

Radiation is capable of sterilizing up to 25% of all lung tumors.[1–5] Table 11.2.1 contains data from autopsies and surgical specimens following preoperative radiation, and reflects the percentage of tumors that are sterilized with radiation alone. Unfortunately, these figures are for surgically resectable lung cancer, and reflect only local control, which does not account for the biology of the tumor.

Surgery, radiation and chemotherapy are all used in the treatment of lung cancer. Surgical resection remains the primary curative modality, and may be the only treatment required in early stage disease if all cancer is removed. Unfortunately, the majority of patients present with unresectable or marginally resectable disease. The addition of radiation and chemotherapy attempts to decrease the unacceptably high incidence of local and distant failures that occur with surgery alone. Progress has been slow, however, and the overall survival of patients has remained essentially unchanged for the past 20 years. The indications for external-beam radiation include medically inoperable lung cancer, regionally advanced lung cancer where surgical resection is not feasible, and as a palliative tool in patients with advanced disease.

Table 11.2.1 Tumor sterilization by radiation alone

Series	Percentage sterilized at surgical pathology
Bromley[1]	44
Bloedorn[2]	30
Manfredi[3]	20
Klingerman[4]	23
Coy[5]	19

WHERE ARE WE NOW?

Radiation is an acceptable treatment in patients who are medically inoperable. Although not as impressive as surgical results for stage I patients, radiation is capable of curing a subset of early stage non-small cell lung cancer (NSCLC)

patients. Many studies have shown a correlation between the size of the primary tumor and survival. Sandler et al[6] reported a three-year actuarial survival rate of 30% for tumors less than 3 cm in diameter, 17% for tumors treated at 3–6 cm, and 0% for tumors greater than 6 cm in diameter. Dorosetz et al[7] also suggested that local control has less effect on survival as the size of the primary tumor increases. In 150 patients with technically resectable but medically inoperable NSCLC, the median survival was 20 months for T2 and T3 lesions, irrespective of local control. For T1 lesions, however, the median survival was 30 months if the primary was controlled, and 17 months if it was not controlled.

The dose–response relationship can be documented in T1 lesions, and a dose equivalence of greater than 65 Gy at 200 cGy per fraction should be the goal of treatment. Most patients with medically inoperable lung cancer have poor pulmonary function. Radiation therapy fields should be designed to encompass the index lesion but be limited in nodal coverage. Retrospective analysis suggests that little survival benefit is achieved with large-field design, but large fields definitely add toxicity.

In summary, radiation therapy is of benefit to patients with medically inoperable but resectable lung cancer, with a proportion of early stage patients being cured of their disease. Aggressive therapy is indicated in patients with small lesions, but as the size of the primary tumor and the extent of disease increase, the necessity for aggressive thoracic irradiation is less well defined.

Patients with stage II or IIIa disease are considered marginally resectable because of the high incidence of local failure with surgery alone. The Ludwig Cancer Study Group[8] showed an intrathoracic failure rate of 31% for stage II patients treated with surgery alone. Many investigations have retrospectively reported a decrease in local failure with postoperative irradiation.[9,10] Several prospective trials have attempted to confirm the benefit of postoperative radiation therapy. The largest North American trial was conducted by the Lung Cancer Study Group,[11] and was a prospective randomized trial comparing surgery alone with surgery plus postoperative radiotherapy in 210 patients with completely resected, stage II and stage III epidermoid lung cancer. There was one local failure in the 102 patients treated with postoperative radiation therapy, and 21 local-only failures in the 108 patients treated with surgery. This confirmed a benefit to local control with external-beam irradiation, but failed to confirm a survival benefit of postoperative radiation therapy.[12] It remains controversial whether or not postoperative radiation therapy has any impact on survival. Arguments against postoperative radiation therapy are based on the fact that most patients fail with distant disease, and that postoperative radiation does incur toxicity. Other investigators believe that the quality of the prospective trials has been poor and that increasing local control, at a minimum, can improve the disease-free survival, and perhaps the overall survival in these patients.[13]

There is currently enthusiasm for the use of chemotherapy with or without radiation as a preoperative tool in marginally resectable lung cancer.[14] Many patients have been treated in phase II trials evaluating the use of preoperative chemotherapy plus or minus radiation. Again, there appears to be an improvement in local regional control with this aggressive management approach in patients utilizing chemotherapy, radiation and surgery.[15–19] Unfortunately, the long-term survival benefit continues to remain questionable, and to date there is no good phase III evidence that preoperative treatment in these marginally resectable patients is of substantial survival benefit.[20–22] There is little doubt that these aggressive preoperative regimens increase surgical morbidity and mortality, and must be conducted with caution and preferably on study.

Patients with chest wall invasion are an unusual set of patients with stage IIB disease, and are potentially curable with surgical resection. Patterson et al[23] reported on 35 patients with chest wall invasion treated with either surgery alone or surgery plus radiation. Chest wall recurrences developed in 6 of the 22 patients who were not irradiated, compared with none of the 13 patients who were irradiated. In contrast, Allen et al[24] reported a decreased five-year survival in patients with chest wall invasion who received postoperative radiation therapy, compared with patients treated with surgery alone. This trial is difficult to interpret, because 33% of the patients treated with postoperative radiation therapy had positive lymph nodes, compared with only 6% of the patients treated surgically.

In summary, marginally resectable cases are those with locally advanced tumors or who have microscopically positive local regional lymph nodes. Local control is definitely improved with the addition of pre- or postoperative radiation therapy, but improvement in survival is controversial.

As a general rule, patients with T4 and/or N2 disease are considered surgically inoperable.[25] With supportive care consisting of antibiotics, expectorants and oxygen, it has been shown that only 4% are alive at two years. Thoracic irradiation, although rarely curative, occasionally produces a long-term survivor (disease-free for more than five years), and at least represents a useful palliative tool.[26,27] Aggressively applied non-surgical treatment can improve the median and two-year survival of some patients with unresectable locally advanced NSCLC, but the treatment can be toxic and complicated. Conversely, palliative schedules can be delivered simply and conveniently with little toxicity. Assignment of patients into aggressive treatment schedules when realistically most patients are cases for palliative treatment is an extremely important and sometimes difficult endeavor.

Many authors have attempted to place patients into good and bad prognostic categories. An early analysis by Aristizabel and Caldwell[28] suggested that patients without palpable supraclavicular nodes, superior vena cava syndrome or invasion into adjacent structures exhibited an improved five-year survival over those patients who did have these poor prognostic features.

Statistical analyses of large groups of treated patients have defined clinical variables that may predict an improved survival.[29] A Cox regression analysis of patients treated on Radiation Therapy Oncology Group (RTOG) protocols suggested that Karnofsky performance status (KPS), weight loss and age are important predictors of poor survival. In this analysis, race, histology and gender did not predict for poor survival in surgically unresectable disease. Most recently, a sophisticated recursive partitioning analysis of over 1500 patients treated on several RTOG protocols has suggested that weight loss, KPS and age are extremely important clinical variables.[30] Nodal stage is also important, but only as a yes/no variable. These clinical parameters can be extremely useful when assigning patients into aggressive versus non-aggressive treatment schedules.

Assigning patients to aggressive treatment schedules versus a more limited palliative schedule not only is important for survival but also predicts toxicity. RTOG 90-15[31] was designed to deliver concurrent chemotherapy with multiple daily fractionated radiation. More than 50% of the patients in this trial had a weight loss of greater than 5%, and the treatment-associated mortality rate was 7%, attesting to the fact that ill patients will not tolerate this type of aggressive treatment. Patients for whom one elects aggressive non-surgical treatment with radiation therapy, or with radiation therapy and chemotherapy, should be that select group with high performance status, low weight loss and age less than 70 years. If these selection criteria are met, aggressive non-surgical treatment can improve short- and long-term survival.

Historically, radiation therapy with doses of at least 60 Gy has produced a short-term survival benefit over less intensive schedules.[29] Long-term survival with 60 Gy continues to be infrequent, and local failure is still high (greater than 80%). More recently, this dose of radiation has been compared with even more aggressive radiation therapy schedules. Phase II data from the RTOG,[32] delivering 1.2 Gy twice daily to 69.6 Gy, suggests that a modest improvement in survival will occur in selected patients with regionally advanced disease. Most recently, a UK trial[33] randomized patients to 1.5 Gy, three times daily to 54.0 Gy, versus 60 Gy. In this trial, there was a statistical improvement in survival with the more aggressive treatment: an improvement in the two-year survival rate from 20% to 33%. A phase II dose-escalation trial is in progress in the USA, evaluating doses up to 80 Gy utilizing sophisticated three-dimensional treatment planning.[34]

Combination chemotherapy and radiation therapy has been utilized as a method to increase aggressive non-surgical treatment in regionally advanced lung cancer. Again, selection criteria are extremely important and, in general, are similar to those utilized for aggressive radiation therapy. Several phase III trials have been conducted analyzing the results of radiation therapy alone, versus radiation therapy with chemotherapy.[35–38] The majority of these trials suggest a modest but definitely improved median survival with combined therapy. A meta-analysis[39] also suggests a reproducible survival benefit of approximately 4% when cisplatin is incorporated into the treatment schedule. It remains unclear as to which chemotherapeutic agents are best and as to the most appropriate timing of irradiation and chemotherapy. Some of the most convincing phase III data come from a Cancer and Acute Leukemia Group B (CALGB) trial in the USA and a US intergroup trial:an improvement in the two-year survival rate from 20% to 31%.[37,38] In both of these trials, vinblastine was given 5 mg weekly five times, and cisplatin was given at 100 Gy/m^2 every three weeks two times prior to 60 Gy of external-beam radiation. In both of these large trials, there was a survival benefit to combined therapy. The development of new chemotherapeutic agents may make these schedules obsolete. Utilization of the newer combinations is probably effective and safe if they are given prior to radiation. Concurrent chemotherapy and radiation is probably more experimental when newer combinations are utilized and toxicity of combined therapy may be prohibitive.

Unfortunately, most patients are not candidates for these aggressive treatment schedules. Not only are these schedules unduly toxic, but they are also expensive and socially inconvenient. Brief, effective palliative treatment schedules should be used on most patients. These schedules incur little toxicity, and can result in useful palliation and improvement in quality of life. An adequate dose of radiation should be delivered to provide symptomatic relief, but need not cause undue medical and social hardship to the patient. Virtually every conceivable mathematical treatment schedule has been reported in the literature. Table 11.2.2[28,40–42] reflects some of the common schedules used in this situation. Often, split-course treatment or large infrequent fractions of radiation are utilized. There is an advantage to such schedules, in that one can omit subsequent treatment courses if disease progresses and makes treatment unnecessary. At our institution,[40] we utilize 12 fractions of 400 cGy for one month in the majority of these patients, and limit the spinal cord dose to seven fractions of 400 cGy. These treatments can occasionally

Table 11.2.2 Palliative schedule for advanced NSCLC

Series	Dose per fraction (cGy)	Number of fractions	Total time (days)
Aristizabal[28]	300	10	12
Sause[40]	400	12	31
Slawson[41]	500	12	84
Bleehan[42]	850 1000	2 1	8

provide a long disease-free survival, and are adequate enough to provide palliation for the majority of patients. For treatment techniques, see the Appendix to this chapter (pages 210–12).

Radiation therapy represents an extremely useful palliative tool in the management of patients with metastatic lung cancer. The more common sites of involvement include the brain, spinal cord and bone. Brain metastases will occur in approximately 35% of patients with bronchogenic carcinoma. Patients can present with severe headaches, focal weakness and, rarely, seizure activity. Prompt intervention with steroids and external-beam radiation therapy can often improve the quality of these patients' lives. Brief, high-dose per fraction radiation schedules are most appropriate in this group of patients. Between 20 and 30 Gy, delivered over five to ten fractions in one to two weeks, offers the most efficient form of palliation in these patients.[43–45] Rarely, extremely good-performance patients, with systemic disease controlled, may benefit from more aggressive radiation therapy, or even surgical resection of isolated central nervous system metastases. These aggressive forms of radiation can include cone-down fields to 40–50 Gy or specialized stereotactic radiosurgical techniques. Symptomatic improvement occurs in approximately 70% of patients.[46,47]

Bone metastases represent a common clinical problem, and painful skeletal disease can frequently be palliated with external-beam radiation therapy. Again, brief courses of high-dose per fraction treatment are more appropriate. These may include treatments of 7.0–8.0 Gy given once or twice up to 10 fractions of 3 Gy. Relief of pain and bone healing is a common phenomenon following external-beam radiation therapy.[48–50]

A relatively uncommon event in patients with bronchogenic carcinoma is spinal cord compression.[51–53] Early recognition and immediate treatment are best correlated with good results, particularly if intervention occurs prior to the patient becoming paralyzed. In these situations, the radiation dose should be somewhat more aggressive and delivered to a dose equivalent of 40–50 Gy. Approximately one-third of the patients will obtain symptomatic relief.

Bronchial symptoms, such as hemoptysis and obstructive pneumonia, can be debilitating in patients with bronchogenic carcinoma. Palliative endobronchial radiation therapy can provide relatively rapid symptomatic improvement. Endobronchial sources of radioactive material must be placed bronchoscopically, and radiation can be delivered with high-dose-rate remote after-loading sources or with low-dose-rate sources.[54] High-dose-rate catheters require several applications, delivering 600–700 cGy per fraction at 0.5 cm. Low-dose rate applications are often delivered at 100 cGy per hour to a total dose of 30 Gy. Improvement in symptoms occurs at least 50% of the time. A major complication of endobronchial irradiation is erosion of the bronchus and fatal hemoptysis. The factor most often associated with fatal hemoptysis is location of the tumor in the left upper lobe, with the pulmonary artery receiving 20–30 Gy in single 6 Gy fractions.

Toxicity associated with external-beam radiation therapy is primarily related to the critical structures located in the thorax, primarily the pulmonary parenchyma, esophagus and spinal cord. Less frequently, cardiac toxicity is a clinical problem. The most frequently encountered toxicity is related to the lung parenchyma.[55–57] As a general rule, one should not attempt to treat a patient when more than one-third of the functioning lung parenchyma is in the treatment field. No good treatment algorithms exist to correlate PFTS (pulmonary function test), volume of lung treated and radiation dose with toxicity. Acute pneumonitis, which is potentially life-threatening, can occur in up to 10% of patients treated with external-beam radiation therapy, with at least 35% of patients experiencing moderate-to-severe pulmonary symptoms. There is no question that, as field size increases, pulmonary toxicity increases. Patient selection is critical when determining the aggressiveness of treatment in an individual patient.

The esophagus has become a dose-limiting organ with modern aggressive treatment schedules. In the UK trial,[39] delivering 1.5 Gy three times a day, the incidence of esophageal stricture was 7%. In combined studies utilizing chemotherapy and twice-daily radiation, the incidence of severe esophageal toxicity approaches 30%.[58] This is related both to the intensity of therapy and to the volume of esophagus treated. One must take care to limit the volume of esophagus treated as much as possible and be aware that multiple daily fractionated radiation with concurrent chemotherapy substantially increases esophageal toxicity.

The most critical organ in the thorax is the spinal cord. In general, a dose equivalent of 45 Gy at 2.0 Gy per fraction should not be exceeded. Although the incidence of spinal cord damage is small, it represents an irreversible, severely debilitating complication of treatment, and should be avoided at all costs.

CURRENT RECOMMENDATIONS

Medically inoperable localized NSCLC can be treated with external-beam irradiation. Field sizes adequate to encompass the tumor with some margins are optimal, and a dose equivalent of at least 65 Gy at 2.0 Gy per fraction should be utilized.

In regionally advanced new metastatic NSCLC, case selection for aggressive versus palliative irradiation is important and extremely difficult. In general, only these patients with no constitutional symptoms (i.e. weight loss and KPS) should be treated aggressively. Aggressive treatment should include systemic therapy and moderately aggressive scheduling of irradiation – a minimum of 60 Gy in six weeks. Palliative patients can be treated with a variety of schedules, and probably the schedule should be tailored in some way to the extent of disease and the performance of the patient.

FUTURE DIRECTIONS

One conclusion that seems irrefutable from the multitude of randomized trials conducted over the past 20 years in NSCLC is that, in selected patients, aggressive non-surgical treatment can alter the course of the disease. Unfortunately, most patients continue to die from their cancer and much more research needs to be performed to define which patient population should be subjected to aggressive therapy. To date, our selection criteria are fairly unsophisticated, and include performance status, weight loss and perhaps age.

The recent publication of the CHART data from the UK (1.5 Gy three times a day to 54 Gy) suggests that radiation alone applied in a shortened aggressive fashion can improve survival. This aggressive treatment can increase toxicity – particularly esophageal and spinal toxicity. Modern imaging and computerized planning equipment now give us the ability to optimize irradiation.[34] Traditional radiation volumes in NSCLC have included the primary tumor and regional lymphatics, often to the thoracic inlet. Aggressive treatment schedules, which seem to have improved survival, are difficult, if not impossible, to apply to large volumes of normal tissue. One area of intense clinical research over the next 10 years will need to deal with the relationship of normal tissue tolerance and field size to tumor control with aggressively delivered, finely focused radiation.

The interaction of treatment modalities will also need focused investigation. Although surgery added to radiation and chemotherapy in stage III disease improves local control, does it improve survival? This is the topic of a current phase III trial in North America. Now do we sequence chemotherapy with irradiation? Many phase III trials suggest that sequential chemotherapy followed by irradiation creates the best therapeutic index. However, more information on NSCLC, small cell lung cancer and head and neck trials suggests that short, intense concurrent chemotherapy and irradiation may be preferred.[39,58] The question arises of how to control toxicity, particularly with the new chemotherapeutic agents, which are undoubtedly radiation sensitizers.

A better understanding of cancer biology has opened many new avenues of clinical investigation of lung cancer. Will modern biologics such as targeted antibiotics, protein inhibitors, retroviruses and a multitude of potential agents to reprogram cellular function in some way be incorporated into the management of the disease, with or without traditional treatment?

The opportunities for clinical improvement exist, utilizing the tools available to us while clinical and basic research into this virulent disease must continue. Unfortunately, NSCLC is by and large a self-inflicted neoplasm, and perhaps most of our research efforts in the future should be aimed at eradicating the distribution and promulgation of cigarettes.

REFERENCES

1. Bromley L, Szur L, Combined radiotherapy and resection for carcinoma of the bronchus. Experiences with 66 patients. *Lancet* 1955; **ii**: 937–41.
2. Bleodorn FG, Cowley RA, Cuccia CA et al, Preoperative irradiation in bronchogenic carcinoma. *Am J Roentgenol* 1964; **92**: 77–87.
3. Manfredi F, King R, Behnke R, Heimburger I, Preoperative irradiation in bronchogenic carcinoma. *Am Rev Respir Dis* 1966; **94**: 584–8.
4. Klingerman M, Order S, Integrated therapy for lung carcinoma. In: *Cancer Therapy by Integrated Radiation and Operation* (Rush B, Greenlaw R, eds). Charles C Thomas: Springfield, 1968: 67–73.
5. Coy P, Kennelly G, The role of curative radiotherapy in the treatment of lung cancer. *Cancer* 1980; **45**: 698–702.
6. Sandler HM, Curran WJ, Turrisi AT, The influence of tumor size and pretreatment staging on outcome following radiation therapy alone for stage I non-small cell lung cancer. *Int J Radiat Oncol Biol Phys* 1990; **19**: 9–13.
7. Dosoretz DE, Galmarini D, Rubenstein JH et al, Local control in medically inoperable lung

cancer: an analysis of its importance in outcome and factors determining the probability of tumor eradication. *Int J Radiat Oncol Biol Phys* 1993; **27**: 507–16.

8. The Ludwig Lung Cancer Study Group, Patterns of failure in patients with resected stage I and II non-small cell carcinoma of the lung. *Ann Surg* 1987; **205**: 67–71.
9. Choi NCH, Crillo HC, Gardiello M et al, Basis for new strategies in postoperative radiotherapy of bronchogenic carcinoma. *Int J Radiat Oncol Biol Phys* 1980; **6**: 31–5.
10. Kirsh MM, Sloan H, Mediastinal metastases in bronchogenic carcinoma: influence of postoperative irradiation, cell type, and location. *Ann Thorac Surg* 1982; **33**: 459–63.
11. The Lung Cancer Study Group, Effects of postoperative mediastinal radiation on completely resected stage I and stage II epidermoid cancer of the lung. *N Engl J Med* 1986; **315**: 1377–81.
12. The Lung Cancer Study Group, The benefit of adjuvant treatment for resected locally advanced non-small cell lung cancer. *J Clin Oncol* 1988; **6**: 9–17.
13. Van Houtte PJ, Non-small cell lung cancer: surgery and postoperative radiotherapy. In: *Lung Cancer: Principles and Practice* (Pass HI, Mitchell JB, Johnson DH, Turrisi AT, eds). Lippincott-Raven: Philadelphia, 1996: 851–61.
14. Rusch VW, Albain KS, Crowley JJ et al, Neoadjuvant therapy: a novel and effective treatment for stage IIIB non-small cell lung cancer. *Ann Thorac Surg* 1994; **58**: 290.
15. Warram J, Preoperative irradiation of cancer of the lung: final report of a therapeutic trial. A collaborative study. *Cancer* 1975; **36**: 914.
16. Burkes RL, Ginsberg RJ, Shepherd FA et al, Induction chemotherapy with mitomycin, vindesine and cisplatin for stage III unresectable non-small cell lung cancer; results of the Toronto phase II trial. *J Clin Oncol* 1992; **10**: 580.
17. Martini N, Kris M, Flehinger BJ et al, Preoperative chemotherapy for IIIa (N2) lung cancer; the Sloan–Kettering experience with 136 patients. *Ann Thorac Surg* 1993; **55**: 1365.
18. Shepherd FA, Induction chemotherapy for locally advanced non-small cell lung cancer. *Ann Thorac Surg* 1993; **55**: 1585.
19. Albain K, Rusch V, Crowley J et al, Concurrent cisplatin/etoposide + chest radiation followed by completed analysis of SWOG-8805. *Proc Am Soc Clin Oncol* 1994; **13**: 337.
20. Pass HI, Pogrebniak HW, Steinberg SM et al, Randomized trial of neoadjuvant therapy for lung cancer: interim analysis. *Ann Thorac Surg* 1992; **53**: 992.
21. Rosell R, Gomez-Codina J, Camps C et al, A randomized trial comparing preoperative chemotherapy plus surgery with surgery alone in patients with non-small cell lung cancer. *N Engl J Med* 1994; **330**: 153.
22. Roth JA, Fossella F, Komaki R et al, A randomized trial comparing perioperative chemotherapy and surgery with surgery alone in resectable stage III non-small lung cancer. *J Natl Cancer Inst* 1994; **86**: 673.
23. Patterson GA, Ilves R, Ginsberg RJ et al, The value of adjuvant radiotherapy in pulmonary and chest all resection for bronchogenic carcinoma. *Ann Thorac Surg* 1982; **34**: 692–7.
24. Allen MS, Mathisen DJ, Grillo HC et al, Bronchogenic carcinoma with chest wall invasion. *Ann Thorac Surg* 1991; **51**: 948–51.
25. Cox JD, Komaki R, Byhardt RW, Is immediate chest radiotherapy obligatory for any or all patients with limited-stage non-small cell carcinoma of the lung? Yes. *Cancer Treat Rep* 1983; **67**: 327–31.
26. Perez CA, Stanley K, Grundy G et al, Impact of irradiation technique and tumor extent in tumor control and survival of patients with unresectable non-oat cell carcinoma of the lung. *Cancer* 1982; **50**: 1091.
27. Perez CA, Bauer M, Edelstein S et al, Impact of tumor control on survival in carcinoma of the lung treated with irradiation. *Int J Radiat Oncol Biol Phys* 1986; **12**: 539.
28. Aristizabal SA, Caldwell WL, Radical irradiation with the split-course technique in carcinoma of the lung. *Cancer* 1976; **37**: 2630.

29. Stanley KE, Prognostic factors for survival in patients with inoperable lung cancer. *J Natl Cancer Inst* 1980; **65**: 25.
30. Sause W, Scott C, Byhardt R, Recursive partitioning analysis of 1592 patients on four RTOG studies in non-small cell lung cancer. *Proc Am Soc Clin Oncol* 1993; **12**: 336 (abst).
31. Byhardt RW, Scott CB, Ettinger DS et al, Concurrent hyperfractionated irradiation and chemotherapy for unresectable non-small cell lung cancer; results of Radiation Therapy Oncology Group (RTOG) 90-15. *Cancer* 1995; **75**: 2337.
32. Cox JD, Azarnia N, Byhardt RW et al, A randomized phase I/II trial of hyperfractionated radiation therapy with total doses of 60.0 Gy to 79.2 Gy; possible survival benefit with >69.6 Gy in favorable patients with Radiation Therapy Oncology Group stage III non-small cell lung carcinoma. Report of Radiation Therapy Oncology Group 83-11. *J Clin Oncol* 1990; **8**: 1543.
33. Saunders MI, on behalf of the CHART Steering Committee, A randomized multicentre trial of CHART versus conventional radiotherapy in non-small cell lung cancer. *Lung Cancer* 1997; **18**(Suppl 2): 28.
34. Emami B, Three-dimensional conformal radiation therapy in bronchogenic carcinoma. *Semin Radiat Oncol* 1996; **6**(2): 92.
35. Longeval E, Klastersky J, Combination chemotherapy with cisplatin and etoposide in bronchogenic squamous cell carcinoma and adenocarcinoma: a study by the EORTC Lung Cancer Working Party (Belgium). *Cancer* 1982; **50**: 2751.
36. LeChevalier T, Arriagada R, Quoix E et al, Radiotherapy alone versus combined chemotherapy and radiotherapy in nonresectable non-small cell lung cancer: first analysis of a randomized trial in 353 patients. *J Natl Cancer Inst* 1991; **83**: 417.
37. Dillman RO, Seagren SL, Herndon J, Green MR, Randomized trial of induction chemotherapy plus radiation therapy versus RT alone in stage III non-small cell lung cancer: five year follow-up of CALGB 84-33. *Proc Am Soc Clin Oncol* 1993; **12**: 329.
38. Sause WT, Scott C, Taylor S et al, Radiation Therapy Oncology Group (RTOG) 88-08 and Eastern Cooperative Oncology Group (EGOG) 4588: preliminary results of a phase III trial in regionally advance, unresectable non-small cell lung cancer. *J Natl Cancer Inst* 1995; **87**: 198.
39. Non-small Cell Lung Cancer Collaborative Group. Chemotherapy in non-small cell lung cancer. A meta-analysis using updated data on individual patients from 52 randomized clinical trials. *BMJ* 1995; **311**: 899–909.
40. Sause W, Sweeney RA, Plenk HP, Thomson JW, Radiotherapy of bronchogenic carcinoma. *Radiology* 1981; **140**: 209.
41. Slawson RG, Salazar OM, Poussin-Rosillo H et al, Once-a-week versus conventional daily radiation treatment for lung cancer: final report. *Int J Radiat Oncol Biol Phys* 1988; **15**: 62.
42. Bleehan N, Inoperable non-small cell lung cancer (NSCLC): a Medical Research Council randomized trial of palliative radiotherapy with two fractions or ten fractions. *Br J Cancer* 1991; **63**: 265.
43. Borgelt B, Gelber R, Kramer S et al, The palliation of brain metastases: final results of the first two studies by the Radiation Therapy Oncology Group. *Int J Radiat Oncol Biol Phys* 1980; **6**: 1.
44. Borgelt B, Gelber R, Larson M et al, Ultra rapid high dose irradiation schedules for the palliation of brain metastases: final results of the first two studies by the Radiation Therapy Oncology Group. *Int J Radiat Biol Phys* 1981; **7**: 163.
45. Kurtz JM, Gelber R, Brady LW et al, The palliation of brain metastases in a favorable patient population: a randomized clinical trial by the Radiation Therapy Oncology Group. *Int J Radiat Oncol Biol Phys* 1981; **7**: 891.
46. Lang EFJ, Slater J, Metastatic brain tumors; results of surgical and non-surgical treatment. *Surg Clin North Am* 1964; **44**: 856.
47. Levin AB, Experience in the first 100 patients undergoing computerized tomography-guided stereotactic procedures utilizing the Brown–Roberts–Wells guidance system. *Appl Neurophysiol* 1985; **48**: 45.

48. Penn CRH, Single dose and fractionated palliative irradiation for osseus metastases. *Clin Radiol* 1976; **27**: 405.
49. Arcangeli G, Micheli A, Arcangeli G et al, The responsiveness of bone metastases to radiotherapy: the effect of site, histology, and radiation dose on pain relief. *Radiother Oncol* 1989; **14**: 95.
50. Mallawar MM, Delaney TF, Treatment of metastatic cancer to bone. In: *Cancer: Principles and Practice of Oncology*, 4th edn (DeVita VT, Hellman S, Rosenberg SA, eds). JB Lippincott: Philadelphia, 1993: 2225.
51. Sorenson PS, Borgason SE, Rohde K et al, Metastatic spinal cord compression; results of treatment and survival. *Cancer* 1990; **65**: 1502.
52. Kim RY, Smith JW, Spencer SA et al, Malignant epidural spinal cord compression associated with a paravertebral mass: its radiotherapeutic outcome on radiosensitivity. *Int J Radiat Oncol Biol Phys* 1993; **27**: 1079.
53. Leviov M, Dale J, Stein M et al, The management of spinal cord compression: a radiotherapeutic success ceiling. *Int J Radiat Oncol Biol Phys* 1993; **27**: 231.
54. Mehta MP, Endobronchial radiotherapy for lung cancer. *Lung Cancer* 1996; **49**: 741–50.
55. Rubenstein JH, Richter MP, Moldofsky PJ, Solin LJ, Prospective prediction of post-radiation therapy lung function using quantitative lung scans and pulmonary function testing. *Int J Radiat Oncol Biol Phys* 1988; **15**: 83.
56. Choi NC, Kanarek DJ, Grillo HC, Effect of postoperative radiotherapy on changes in pulmonary function in patients with stage II and IIIA lung carcinoma. *Int J Radiat Oncol Biol Phys* 1990; **18**: 95.
57. Byhardt RW, Artin L, Pajak TF et al, The influence of field size and other treatment factors on pulmonary toxicity following hyperfractionated irradiation for inoperable non-small cell lung cancer – analysis of a Radiation Therapy Oncology Group protocol. *Int J Radiat Oncol Biol Phys* 1993; **27**: 537.
58. Johnson BE, Grayson J, Woods E et al, Limited stage small cell lung cancer treated with concurrent etoposide/cisplatin plus BID chest radiotherapy. *Proc Am Soc Clin Oncol* 1989; **8**: 228.

APPENDIX: EXAMPLES OF RADIOTHERAPY TECHNIQUES AND PLANNING VOLUMES

John D Stageberg, William T Sause

The following figures illustrate the radiotherapy techniques and planning volumes used in the treatment of both non-small and small cell lung cancer.

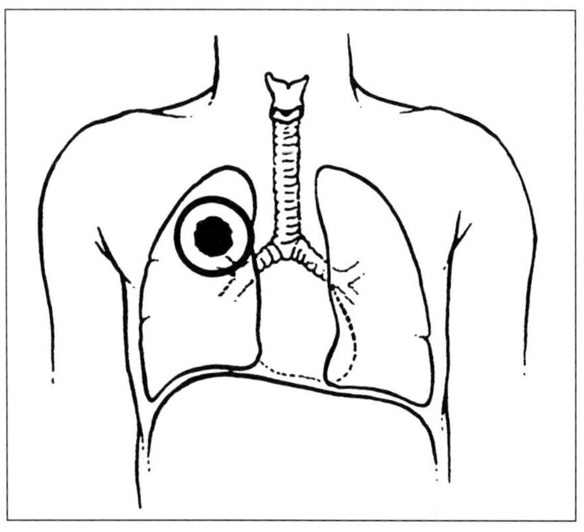

Figure A1
T1–2, N0: 2 cm margin around the primary tumor, without effective nodal irradiation.

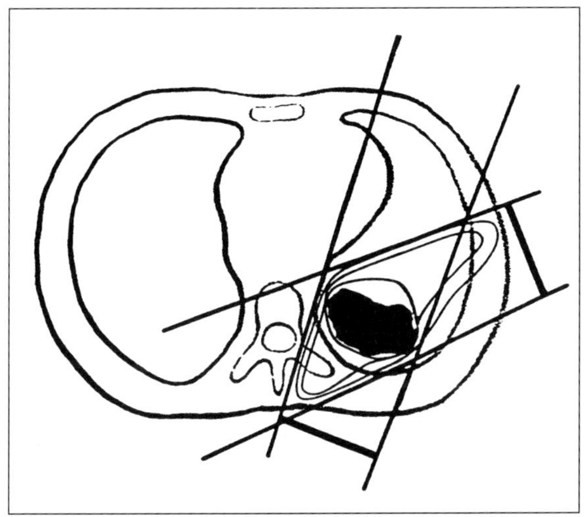

Figure A2
Computer treatment planning design: a sophisticated plan, when available, to limit the dose received by normal tissues. Note the tight idodose curve around the tumor and the limited dose to the heart and the opposite lung. Field placement is indicated by heavy straight lines.

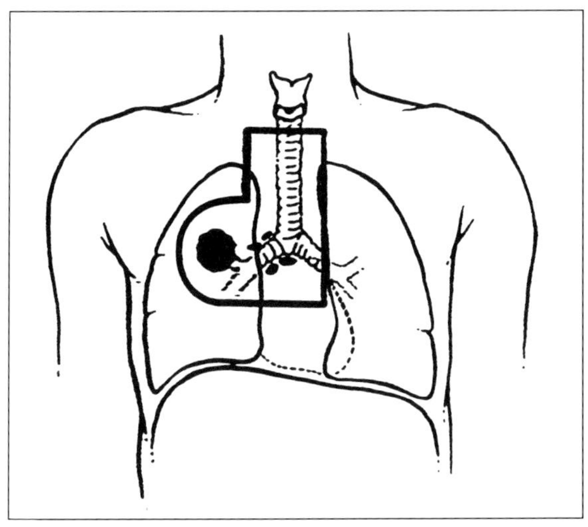

(a)

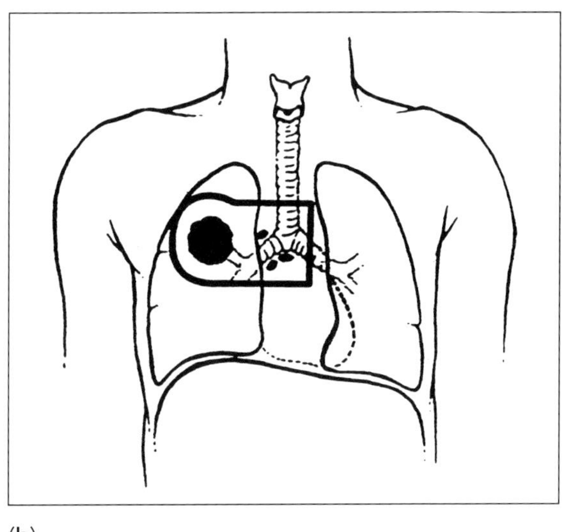

(b)

Figure A3
(a) T1–3, N1–3: 2 cm margin around the primary tumor and clinically evolved lymph nodes, including the first echelon of subclinical lymph nodes, to a dose equivalent of 50 Gy. (b) T1–3, N1–3, boost volume: boost volume should include the primary tumor and clinically involved lymph nodes with a 1 cm margin to 60–70 Gy, allowing for normal tissue tolerance. If available, sophisticated computer treatment planning may be used (see Figure A2). If treatment intent is for palliation only, treat boost field only with a variety of treatment schedules noted in the text.

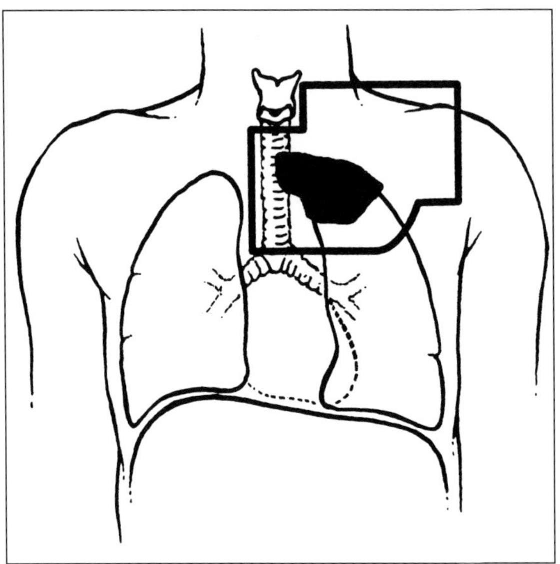

Figure A4
T4, superior sulcus tumor: treatment may include the supraclavicular nodes.

11.3 Treatment of NSCLC: Chemotherapy

Frances A Shepherd, Desmond N Carney

Contents

INTRODUCTION

Adenocarcinoma, squamous cell carcinoma and large cell anaplastic carcinoma, collectively known as non-small cell lung cancer (NSCLC), account for 75–80% of all pulmonary neoplasms. The relative proportions of these three histologic cell types have changed over the last two decades, and currently in North America adenocarcinoma is seen most frequently (in up to 35% of patients), followed by squamous (30%) and large cell (10–15%). This trend has been somewhat less pronounced in Europe, and squamous cell cancer still predominates in most Eastern countries. At the time of initial diagnosis, approximately 50% of patients with NSCLC have clinically detectable metastatic spread outside the chest, and locally advanced unresectable thoracic tumors are found in a further 10–15% of patients. Furthermore, more than 50% of the remaining patients recur either locally or at distant metastatic sites after surgery. This means that more than three-quarters of patients with NSCLC are potential candidates for systemic chemotherapy alone or with radiotherapy at some time during the course of their disease.

As we approach the end of the 20th century, we should pause to assess the contribution that chemotherapy has made to the management of this disease. The practising oncologist may be chastened to observe that only a modest improvement in survival has occurred in the last 50 years, despite the introduction of many new chemotherapeutic agents during that time. In fact, a recent review of cancer therapy in the USA has suggested that the increasing age-adjusted death rate for patients with lung cancer is having a significant *negative* effect on the rate of cancer-free survival overall.[1]

The role of systemic chemotherapy in the management of NSCLC remains one of the most controversial issues in medical oncology today.[2] The controversy applied initially only to patients with advanced, unresectable tumors, but recently, as chemotherapy has been incorporated into combined-modality treatment programs for localized resectable disease, the debate has now broadened to include virtually all stages of this cancer.

PROGNOSTIC FACTORS

When evaluating chemotherapy, it is essential to examine the prognostic factors that have the potential to affect the results of treatment. Stage is one of the most important determinants of both response and survival for virtually all cancers, and NSCLC is no exception. Several staging systems have been used over the past 30 years, but the system proposed jointly by the American Joint Committee on Cancer, the Union Internationale Contre le Cancer and the Japanese Cancer Committee[3] is the most widely accepted currently. Because stage is such an important variable, all investigators are encouraged to provide detailed documentation of stage in their reports, and to use this commonly accepted International Staging System, which has recently been revised.[4]

Twenty studies of prognostic factors were reviewed by Maki et al.[5] Some of the studies included only surgical patients, whereas others were restricted to patients with advanced inoperable disease. The variables chosen for analysis were not uniform between studies, and although all studies used univariate analysis, multivariate analyses were carried out in only 13. Furthermore, various statistical methods were applied for both univariate and multivariate analyses. Finally, four of the seven studies that involved more than 100 patients included patients with small cell histology. Despite these limitations, important observations arose from their analysis.

Prognostic factors in *operable* patients will be more important in the design of future trials if chemotherapy is applied to earlier stages of NSCLC either as adjuvant treatment after surgery, or as preoperative induction therapy in combined-modality treatment programs. An analysis of stage I (which at the time included T1N1) patients from Lung Cancer Study Group (LCSG) trials showed that pathologic subtype and TNM stage were the strongest predictors for *recurrence*, whereas performance status and postoperative infection added importantly to histologic type and tumor and nodal stage with respect to prediction of *overall survival*.[6] Some, but not all, retrospective reviews have suggested that the need for preoperative blood transfusions may have a negative effect on recurrence and survival.[7]

Most studies of prognostic factors have focused on *inoperable* patients who participated in chemotherapy trials. Usually the trials included patients with locally advanced tumors and those with hematogenous metastases. It must not be forgotten, however, that the stage IV patients in these studies represent only a select subgroup of stage IV patients overall, in that they met the eligibility requirements for the chemotherapy trials. Patients with adverse prognostic factors such as poor performance status, severe abnormalities of hepatic or renal function, brain metastases, etc. were frequently excluded from these clinical studies.

A meta-analysis of 6247 patients entered on chemotherapy trials in NSCLC identified several variables that were important for *response* to treatment.[8] Overall and complete response rates correlated strongly with stage (stage III, 39%; stage IV, 25%). Response rates were significantly higher for combination chemotherapy than for single-agent treatment, and the best results were obtained when the combination included cisplatin, a vinca alkaloid, mitomycin C or ifosfamide. This kind of analysis has yet to be done for the new chemotherapy agents that have been introduced in the last decade. A review of 699 patients with stage IV disease treated in Eastern Cooperative Oncology Group (ECOG) chemotherapy trials demonstrated lower response rates in patients with liver, bone and bone marrow involvement and a poor initial performance status.[9] A more recent meta-analysis, which focused on prognostic factors predictive of response in patients treated only with cisplatin-based chemotherapy,[10] showed that higher response rates were seen in patients with normal hemoglobin, white blood cell and platelet counts, older patients, and patients without adrenal or skin metastases. In multivariate analysis, only age and platelet count remained significant.

With respect to *survival*, almost all studies have shown that stage and performance status have the most impact. Weight loss and an elevated lactate dehydrogenase (LDH) level have also been found by some investigators to be significant, whereas age and histologic subtype do not seem to have a significant impact on survival.[5] Female gender has been associated with longer survival in several studies.[5,11] Using the statistical method of recursive partioning and amalgamation, Takigawa et al[12] showed that the best survival was seen in patients with good performance status, stage II and hemoglobin above 11 g/dl. The worst survival was seen in patients with a poor performance status and a history of weight loss irrespective of stage.[12]

Most studies of prognostic factors have focused on clinical and simple laboratory parameters. For patients undergoing surgical resection, adequate tissue is frequently available for in vitro testing, which may provide prognostic information for certain subsets of patients. Patients with diploid squamous cell carcinoma have been shown to have significantly longer survival than those with aneuploid tumors, irrespective of stage.[13] Tumor proliferative activity as measured by thymidine labelling index has been found to be prognostic in univariate analysis, although in multivariate analysis stage was found to be of greater significance.[14] In some, but not all, studies, the presence of neuroendocrine markers[15] and the ability to establish tumor cell lines in vitro have been associated with adverse prognosis.[16,17] Enhanced *ras* oncogene expression, which occurs in approximately 30% of adenocarcinomas, has also been found to correlate with shortened survival.[18] It has been reported that the survival of patients with blood type A or AB who had primary tumors negative for blood-group antigen A was significantly shorter than that of patients with antigen A-positive tumors.[19] Some authors have shown that aberrant *p53* expression predicts for resistance to cisplatin chemotherapy.[20] Increased angiogenesis is now recognized as a significant adverse prognostic variable, and this may have implications for therapy in the future, since inhibitors of angiogenesis are now being evaluated in clinical trials.[21]

It is therefore clear that many variables other than the treatment administered may influence both response and survival in patients with NSCLC. It is essential that reports of phase II trials should provide details of these important patient characteristics and that prospective randomized phase III trials should be stratified to ensure that the treatment arms achieve proper balance for the most important variables.

SINGLE-AGENT THERAPY

When chemotherapy for NSCLC was reviewed more than a decade ago by Bakowski and Crouch[22] and Joss et al,[23] they identified ifosfamide, vindesine, cisplatin and mitomycin C as the most active drugs for the treatment of this malignancy. Ten years later, these agents or their analogs still form the nucleus for most combination-chemotherapy regimens.

With the exception of one study,[9] all reviews of chemotherapy for NSCLC reported lower response rates and shorter survival for single-agent treatment compared with combination chemotherapy. Nonetheless, continued assessment of single agents is important for the identification of new active compounds that may have

Table 11.3.1 Chemotherapy agents that are active in the treatment of NSCLC

Single-agent response rate > 15%	Single-agent response rate < 15%	Investigational agents
Epirubicin (high-dose)	Cisplatin	Camptothecins:
	Carboplatin	Irinotecan (CPT-11)
		Topotecan
	Cyclophosphamide	
Ifosfamide	Anthracyclines:	Tirapazamine
	Doxorubicin	
	Epirubicin (standard-dose)	
Vinca alkaloids:	Epipodophyllotoxins:	
Vinblastine	Etoposide	
Vindesine	Teniposide	
Vinorelbine		
Gemcitabine	5-Fluorouracil	
Taxanes:	Methotrexate	

the potential to be incorporated into combination-chemotherapy regimens. Although many single agents have been evaluated over the last three decades, far fewer have demonstrated adequate activity to justify continued use in combination regimens. The most active agents in common use today are shown in Table 11.3.1.

Cisplatin and other platinum analogs

Although other chemotherapeutic drugs produce higher single-agent response rates than cisplatin, it remains an important drug in combination-chemotherapy protocols. In phase II trials, response rates from 6% to 32% (average 20%) were achieved when cisplatin was used alone in varying doses and schedules.[22] It may be administered in divided doses over three to five days or as a single large dose of up to 120 mg/m^2. The optimal dose and schedule remain controversial. Two studies suggested that a high dose (100–120 mg/m^2) was superior with respect to both response[10] and duration of response,[24] but this was not confirmed in a Southwest Oncology Group (SWOG) study that compared cisplatin 50 mg/m^2 on days 1 and 8 with 100 mg/m^2 on days 1 and 8.[25] Similar results were reported from a European Lung Cancer Working Party trial that compared cisplatin doses of 120 mg/m^2 and 30 mg/m^2 daily for two days.[26] Cisplatin is associated with only modest myelosuppression, and has demonstrated both in vivo and in vitro synergy with several other chemotherapeutic agents. For these reasons, it forms the backbone of most combination regimens. Cisplatin can also be administered concurrently with thoracic radiotherapy without undue toxicity.[27,28]

Other platinum compounds include carboplatin and iproplatin.[29,30] Both of these agents have single-agent response rates of less than 10% in previously untreated patients. Despite a response rate of only 9%, though, a prospective randomized ECOG study demonstrated significantly prolonged survival for a cohort of stage IV patients treated with carboplatin alone compared with other combination regimens.[29] Carboplatin is associated with less gastrointestinal toxicity, neurotoxicity and nephrotoxicity than cisplatin, although it is more myelosuppresive.

Ifosfamide

Cyclophosphamide has limited usefulness in the treatment of NSCLC. As a single agent it has demonstrated response rates of less than 15%, and it is seldom used in combination regimens any longer. Ifosfamide is an alkylating agent that can be used in significantly higher doses than cyclophosphamide.[31,32] It has been evaluated in varying doses and schedules, and as a single agent produces response in over 20% of patients. In lung cancer, administration of ifosfamide 1.2–2.0 g/m^2 for five consecutive days does not appear to result in response rates higher than those produced by treatment with bolus doses of 4.0–5.0 g/m^2 on day one only, despite the higher total dose delivered in the five-day schedules. Bolus therapy may, however, be associated with slightly greater toxicity.

Vinca alkaloids

Both vindesine and vinblastine are active against NSCLC. In single-arm phase II trials, vindesine, which is a semisynthetic analog of vinblastine, produced response rates that seemed to be slightly higher than those seen previously with single-agent vinblastine. However, a recent study comparing the relative usefulness of chemotherapeutic agents used in combination with cisplatin showed no added benefit for vindesine, but a significant benefit ($p > 0.001$) for vinblastine.[10] Vinorelbine is a semisynthetic vinca alkaloid that is the only vinca that is modified at the catharanthine ring rather than the vindoline ring of the molecule.[33] Like other vinca alkaloids, it acts by inhibiting microtubule assembly. Its dose-limiting toxicity is neutropenia, and it appears to be significantly less neurotoxic than other vincas. In a phase II trial of 78 untreated patients with NSCLC, partial remission was observed in 23 of 70 evaluable patients (33%). At the starting dose of 30 mg/m^2 weekly approximately one-third of cycles were delayed owing to granulocytopenia.[33] In combination with other agents, the weekly dose may need to be reduced to 25 mg/m^2.

Mitomycin C

Mitomycin C has shown reproducible single-agent activity of 15–20% when given at maximal single-agent doses. At high doses, this drug has been associated with pulmonary fibrosis, cumulative marrow suppression, prolonged thrombocytopenia, and hemolytic–uremic syndrome in a small number of patients. Pulmonary toxicity may be reduced by the administration of a steroid with mitomycin,[34] and marrow toxicity may be avoided by reducing the dose and prolonging the interval between treatments.

Epipodophyllotoxins

The epipodophyllotoxin etoposide has only modest activity against NSCLC when used as a single agent,[8] but, because of in vivo and in vitro synergy, it has been used extensively in combination with cisplatin. Etoposide is schedule-dependent, with the administration of multiple doses over several days superior to a one-day schedule of the same total dose.[35] Therefore it is usually administered intravenously over three to five days in most NSCLC protocols.

Teniposide, which differs from etoposide by only the substitution of a single thenylidine group, is also active against NSCLC. It is not available in North America, but is widely used in many European countries. Teniposide and etoposide have not been compared directly in randomized clinical trials, and so their relative activities cannot be assessed. However, it appears that teniposide in combination with cisplatin produces response rates that are similar to cisplatin–etoposide regimens.[36] Teniposide is more myelosuppressive than etoposide.

Taxanes

Paclitaxel is a novel cytotoxic agent extracted from the bark of the Pacific yew (*Taxus brevifolia*). It exerts its antitumor activity by inducing excessive polymerization of tubulin, which interferes with normal mitotic activity. In phase II trials of advanced NSCLC, paclitaxel showed consistent single-agent response rates of 20% or greater.[37] In the early trials, it was administered as a continuous infusion over 24 hours in doses up to 250 mg/m^2 every three weeks. Dose-limiting toxicities included neutropenia and peripheral neuropathy. Paclitaxel may also be administered over shorter infusion times of three hours or even one hour. Response rates appear to be similar with shorter infusion times, but the toxicity profile changes considerably. Myelosuppression is less severe, but neurotoxicity and myalgia increase substantially.

Docetaxel is a semisynthetic taxane that has the same mechanism of action and a similar spectrum of activity as paclitaxel.[38] In phase II trials, overall response rates ranging from 18% to 38% (mean 25%) were seen in previously untreated patients. The dose-limiting toxicity of docetaxel is myelosuppression. In the phase II trials, doses of 60, 75 and 100 mg/m^2 were evaluated, but no clear evidence of a dose–response effect was seen in this dosing range. Non-hematologic side-effects are usually mild. As with paclitaxel, premedication with corticosteroids is required to prevent allergic reactions. With prolonged use, docetaxel may cause edema and pleural effusions, but this toxicity may be lessened by corticosteroid administration.

Gemcitabine

Gemcitabine (2',2'-difluorodeoxycytidine, a pyrimidine antimetabolite) is a deoxycytidine analog that has shown considerable activity against NSCLC. In several phase II trials in which over 600 patients were evaluable for response, overall response rates were consistently 20% or more.[39] Gemcitabine produces only mild-to-moderate nausea and vomiting, and grade 4 myelosuppression is rare, even when very high doses of this drug are employed. It does not cause alopecia. It is usually administered weekly for three weeks at a dose of 1000–1250 mg/m^2 followed by a one-week rest period. A recent review of the phase II trials of gemcitabine showed that it was well tolerated and very effective in elderly patients,[40] and because of its favorable toxicity profile, it has been suggested as a possible alternative for the treatment of this population.

Other agents

Other agents with single-agent activity of less than 10% include lomustine, 5-fluorouracil (5-FU), methotrexate, doxorubicin and epirubicin. Response rates up to 19% may be achieved with epirubicin in high doses (135–150 mg/m^2) – but this is at the expense of greater myelosuppression and potentially greater cardiotoxicity, and these doses would not be suitable for incorporation into most combination-chemotherapy regimens.[41]

New and investigational agents

Camptothecins

The camptothecins are a new family of natural products that exert their anticancer activity through inhibition of the enzyme topoisomerase

I. These compounds form complexes with the enzyme, leading to single-strand breaks in DNA and inhibition of DNA and RNA synthesis. In a phase II trial of weekly camptothecin-11 (CPT-11, irinotecan), at a dose of 150 mg/m^2, 23 of 72 previously untreated patients with NSCLC (31.9%) achieved partial responses.[42] In a similar study of irinotecan, 100–125 mg/m^2 weekly, 31.8% of 44 patients achieved partial responses.[43] The dose-limiting toxicities observed were leukopenia and diarrhea. Unfortunately, the diarrhea caused by irinotecan may be quite severe, and may limit its usefulness in this patient population.

Topotecan has also been evaluated in patients with NSCLC. In one trial, a response rate of 15% was observed, mainly in patients with squamous histology.[44] In another trial, however, no responses were observed in the first 20 patients treated, and so the study was terminated.[45]

Tirapazamine

Tirapazamine is a benzotriazine compound that exhibits differential toxicity for hypoxic cells. Under hypoxic conditions, tirapazamine undergoes one-electron reduction by cytochrome P450 and P450 reductase to a cytotoxic free radical.[46] The free radical is believed to abstract hydrogen ions from DNA, thereby causing DNA strand cleavage and selective hypoxic cell cytotoxicity. Tirapazamine causes acute nausea and vomiting and diarrhea. Muscle cramping has been seen in some patients, as well as acute and usually rapidly reversible hearing loss. Despite the unusual but reversible ototoxicity seen with this agent, phase I and II trials have shown that it may be combined safely with cisplatin.[47]

COMBINATION CHEMOTHERAPY

Response rates in NSCLC are higher when combination chemotherapy is used compared with single-agent treatment. Although many chemotherapy regimens result in significant response, the contribution such treatment makes to prolongation of survival remains controversial. In general, survival gains have been modest in both locally advanced and disseminated disease trials. Even in the trials that have demonstrated a *statistically significant* prolongation of survival, it remains questionable to some oncologists whether the short weeks or months gained are clinically relevant in view of the potential for toxicity and the cost of the treatment involved. In advanced disease, chemotherapy is never curative, and survival curves remain exponential, with no sign of a plateau. As chemotherapy is applied to earlier stages of NSCLC, combined-modality treatment programs should not be considered successful if they result merely in a shift of the survival curve to the left with prolongation only of the median, without an accompanying increase in the level of the plateau and cure rate. In advanced disease, new regimens should be expected to produce an absolute increase in the proportion of patients who survive one year or longer.

At this time, cisplatin or a platinum analog forms the cornerstone of most combination-chemotherapy regimens that are active against NSCLC. Approximate response rates for some of the more common cisplatin-containing or carboplatin-containing regimens and other current regimens are shown in Table 11.3.2. Response rates should not be compared directly, since most reported trials are non-randomized phase II studies and contain heterogeneous patient populations with many variations in prognostic variables. Response rates and survival for individual regimens are presented in more detail in the following sections, which discuss the application of chemotherapy to various stages of NSCLC. In addition, experience with combinations using the newer agents gained from phase

Table 11.3.2 Active chemotherapeutic combinations for the treatment of NSCLC

Chemotherapeutic regimen	Range of response (%)
Cyclophosphamide, doxorubicin, cisplatin[48]	15–25
Bleomycin, etoposide, cisplatin[49]	20–40
Cisplatin and a vinca alkaloid, either vindesine or vinblastine[50]	15–30
Mitomycin C, vindesine or vinblastine, cisplatin[50]	30–60
Etoposide, cisplatin[50]	20–30
Teniposide, cisplatin[36]	22–43
Carboplatin, etoposide[29]	10–30
Ifosfamide, mitomycin C[51]	25–30
Ifosphamide, etoposide[52]	27
Ifosfamide, cisplatin[52]	18–35
Mitomycin, ifosfamide, cisplatin[53]	35–50
Ifosfamide, carboplatin, etoposide[54]	43
Ifosfamide, cisplatin, etoposide[55]	35–40
Gemcitabine, cisplatin[56]	28–54
Paclitaxel, cisplatin[57,58]	27–44
Paclitaxel, carboplatin[37]	25–62
Vinorelbine, cisplatin[59–62]	30–45
Docetaxel, cisplatin[38]	30–51

III trials will be presented in the section on the treatment of advanced disease.

ADJUVANT CHEMOTHERAPY AFTER SURGICAL RESECTION

The poor survival following surgical resection for patients with early stage tumors led to the evaluation of adjuvant chemotherapy after complete or partial resection of NSCLC. Most of the trials reported to date focused on patients with stage II (T1–2N1) or completely resected stage III (T3N0 and T1–3N1–2) tumors, but some also included stage I patients (usually T2N0). In general, to be effective in the adjuvant setting, combination-chemotherapy regimens should result in response rates of approximately 50% in patients with advanced disease, and a proportion of patients should achieve complete clinical response. The most active regimens in use today result, at best, in response in only 35–50% of patients with advanced disease, and complete clinical responses are rare. This is true even for regimens containing the newer, more active agents. It is not surprising, therefore, that a major survival advantage has not been seen in most of the prospective, randomized trials of adjuvant therapy to date.

The design and results of several prospective trials of adjuvant chemotherapy are summarized in Table 11.3.3. The trials undertaken by the

Table 11.3.3 Randomized trials of adjuvant chemotherapy after surgical resection for NSCLC

Author	Stage	Treatment[a]	Number of patients	Median survival	Survival rate (%)		
					1-year	2-year	3-year
Holmes[63]	Stage II–III, completely resected	CAP	62	23 mo	75	41	—
		BCG	68	16 mo	64	30	—
Lad[64]	Stage I–III, incompletely resected	CAP–RT	78	20 mo	60	41	24
		RT	86	13 mo	54	32	20
Feld[65]	T2N0, T1N1, completely resected	CAP	136	76 mo	89	80	60 (5-yr)
		No Rx	133	83 mo	88	73	52 (5-yr)
Ohta[69]	Stage III, completely resected	VdsP	90	31 mo	—	—	35 (5-yr)
		No Rx	91	37 mo	—	—	41 (5-yr)
Dautzenberg[67]	Stage I–III, completely resected	COPAC–RT	138	1.3/1.2 yr[b]	—	38/36[b]	17/19[b]
		RT	129	2.1/0.8 yr[b]	—	54/22[b]	34/6[b]
Wada[68]	Stage I–III, completely resected	CVUFT	115	—	—	—	61 (5-yr)
		UFT	108	—	—	—	64 (5-yr)
		No Rx	100	—	—	—	49 (5-yr)
Niiranen[66]	T1–3N0, completely resected	CAP	54	7+ yr	—	—	67 (5-yr)
		No Rx	56	5+ yr	—	—	56 (5-yr)

[a]CAP, cyclophosphamide, doxorubicin (Adriamycin), cisplatin; BCG, bacillus Calmette–Guérin; RT, radiotherapy; No Rx, no-treatment control arm; VdsP, vindesine, cisplatin; COPAC, cyclophosphamide, vincristine (Oncovin), cisplatin, doxorubicin, lomustine (CCNU); CVUFT, cisplatin, vindesine, uracil, ftorafur; UFT, uracil, ftorafur.
[b]Stage I–II/stage III.

LCSG are of particular importance, because all patients in their studies underwent careful mediastinal node sampling at surgery to ensure precise staging. The first LCSG chemotherapy trial compared postoperative cyclophosphamide, doxorubicin (Adriamycin) and cisplatin (CAP) versus immunotherapy with bacillus Calmette–Guérin (BCG) in patients with completely resected stage II or III adenocarcinoma or large-cell carcinoma.[63] Relapse-free survival was significantly better in the chemotherapy arm. However, although the median survival time was approximately seven months longer, and the two-year survival was also greater, the differences did not reach statistical significance. This trial has been criticized because it did not have a no-treatment control arm.

In another trial in patients with *incompletely resected* tumors, the LCSG also observed a benefit with postoperative CAP with radiotherapy compared with radiotherapy alone.[64] Incomplete resection was defined as a positive resection margin on microscopic examination, or the presence of metastatic cancer in the highest lymph node sampled. As in the previous study, median survival was prolonged by approximately seven months, but the three-year survival was equal in both arms. The last LCSG study evaluated the usefulness of CAP chemotherapy following complete resection of early stage tumors (T2N0 and T1N1) compared with no additional treatment. The results of this study were disappointing in that no improvement in either median or long-term survival was seen with the addition of CAP.[65]

The Finnish group also evaluated CAP chemotherapy after complete resection in patients without lymph node involvement. Although this study included patients with stage III tumors (T3N0), almost 90% of both the chemotherapy and control groups had stage I disease (T1–2N0). Disease-free survival was significantly better for patients who received chemotherapy (p=0.05), with 67% of patients alive at five years compared with only 56% of control patients.[66]

The CAP regimen was expanded to include vincristine (Oncovin) and lomustine (CCNU) (COPAC) in a multicentre French trial.[67] At a minimum follow-up time of six years, no difference in either disease-free or overall survival was seen between the group who received thoracic radiotherapy alone and those who received three courses of COPAC followed by radiation.

When these trials were designed up to 20 years ago, CAP chemotherapy was the most active regimen available for the treatment of NSCLC. However, a National Cancer Institute of Canada (NCIC) study demonstrated a higher response rate and longer survival for patients with advanced disease who received vindesine and high-dose cisplatin compared with CAP.[48] In a Japanese study, Wada et al[68] administered three cycles of vindesine and cisplatin using a low dose of cisplatin, 50 mg/m^2, followed by one year of tegafur and uracil. The control arms received either one year of uracil alone or no therapy. The five-year survival rates for the chemotherapy and uracil groups were 60.6% and 64.1% respectively, compared with 49% for the no-treatment group (p=0.053, log-rank; p=0.044, Wilcoxon). A comparison of the overall survival of the two treatment arms combined compared with that of the surgery-alone group showed a significant advantage for treatment (p=0.022). In a trial limited to patients with completely resected stage III tumors, Ohta et al also evaluated the usefulness of postoperative vindesine and cisplatin or no further treatment. Their results were similar to those of the LCSG trials in that the median survival was prolonged by approximately six months, but long-term survival was not significantly improved (five-year rates 41% and 35%).[69] Other platinum-based regimens have been evaluated by the National Kyushu Cancer Centre in Japan, but no improvement in median survival or overall survival was seen in their trial.[70] ECOG, SWOG and the Radiation Therapy Oncology Group (RTOG) have just completed a trial of postoperative etoposide and cisplatin plus radiotherapy versus radiotherapy alone in patients with completely resected stages II and IIIA NSCLC, but survival results are not yet available.

Although these studies demonstrated a definite biologic effect for adjuvant chemotherapy, the survival gains were modest at best, and frequently the benefit was reflected only in median survival, without a long-term benefit. In addition, the CAP generation of studies encountered significant problems with both patient and physician compliance, with the result that only half of the intended chemotherapy was actually administered in most of the trials. Because most of the trials were relatively small, they lacked the statistical power to show significant differences. To determine whether small but meaningful survival gains could actually be attributed to the administration of chemotherapy after surgery, a large meta-analysis was performed by the Non-Small Cell Lung Cancer Collaborative Group.[71] To evaluate the addition of chemotherapy to surgery, 14 trials including 4357 patients were studied. The results for the use of long-term alkylating agents were negative, with a combined hazard ratio of 1.15 ($p = 0.005$). However, for regimens containing cisplatin, the overall hazard ratio was 0.87 ($p=0.08$), with an absolute benefit from chemotherapy of 3% at two years and 5% at five years. When chemotherapy was added to surgery plus thoracic irradiation, the benefits were less, with an overall hazard ratio of 0.94 ($p=0.46$), and a 2% survival benefit at both two and five years.

Several groups are currently evaluating the usefulness of adjuvant chemotherapy for completely resected NSCLC and, despite the above results, this is justified for several reasons. First, since the CAP or vindesine and cisplatin studies of the 1970s and 1980s, the introduction of the serotonin (5-HT_3) antagonist class of drugs has changed the delivery of cisplatin-based chemotherapy dramatically. These new agents are much more effective at controlling chemotherapy-induced emesis, and thus may improve patient compliance in the current adjuvant chemotherapy trials. It might be expected, therefore, that, with better tolerability, and more complete treatment delivery, the cisplatin-based adjuvant trials of the future could be more effective. The second reason to continue to evaluate adjuvant chemotherapy is the availability of more active agents and chemotherapy combinations within the last decade. Some of these regimens have already been shown to be superior to previous combinations of cisplatin with either an epipodophyllotoxin[57,58] or a vinca alkaloid.[72]

At least three large randomized trials of adjuvant chemotherapy are open at this time in Europe and North America. A large European trial is being conducted by the European Organization for Research and Treatment of Cancer (EORTC) and the Adjuvant Lung Project Italy (ALPI). Patients with completely resected stage I–IIIA tumors are randomized to receive three courses of adjuvant mitomycin C, vinblastine and cisplatin or follow-up alone. Radiation is optional. The International Adjuvant Lung Cancer Trial, which was initiated by the lung cancer group at the Institut Gustave-Roussy in France, spans at least four continents, and is a trial of novel design. Patients with completely resected stages I, II and selected IIIA must receive a platinum-based regimen, but the dose of cisplatin may range from 80 to 120 mg/m^2, and the second drug may be vinblastine, vindesine, vinorelbine or etoposide according to the availability of chemotherapeutic agents in the country where the patient is being treated. Patients must receive an adequate number of treatment cycles to receive a total cisplatin dose of 300–400 mg/m^2. Radiotherapy may be administered at the discretion of the treating physicians. This trial aims to accrue 3300 patients in order to detect an absolute increase in survival of 5% at five years.

In North America, the NCIC, ECOG, SWOG and Cancer and Acute Leukemia Group B

(CALGB) are participating in a trial of adjuvant cisplatin and vinorelbine for patients with stage I (T2N0) and stage II (excluding T3N0) NSCLC. For Canadian centres, all patients have fresh frozen tumor and normal lung samples submitted to a central tumor bank. All samples are assessed by molecular methods for the presence or absence of *ras* gene mutations, and this variable serves as a stratification parameter. The determination of *ras* status for the US centers is by immunohistochemical techniques from paraffin block samples. Both this and the international trial are accruing patients, but results will not be available for several years. In the meantime, adjuvant chemotherapy is not recommended for patients with completely resected NSCLC outside a clinical trial.

CHEMOTHERAPY FOR LOCALLY ADVANCED (STAGE IIIA AND IIIB) TUMORS

Up to one-third of patients with NSCLC present with disease that remains localized to the thorax but that is thought to be too extensive for surgery. Standard management for these patients with locally advanced stages IIIA and IIIB tumors is thoracic irradiation, which results in objective tumor regression in a significant proportion of patients. This is usually accompanied by palliation of symptoms, but few patients are cured, and the five-year survival rate is usually 10% or less.

The observation that death for most patients with stage III tumors is caused by distant metastases has led to the development of combined-modality treatment programs that incorporate chemotherapy. The intent of such treatment is to eradicate the micrometastatic deposits that are obviously present at the time of initial diagnosis even though they are undetectable clinically. In addition to its systemic effects, chemotherapy may also improve local control. Chemotherapeutic agents may act as radiation sensitizers when given concurrently with radiotherapy, and radiation has the potential to be more effective when administered sequentially to smaller-bulk tumors that have responded to induction chemotherapy.

Chemotherapy and radiotherapy

Several trials were performed in the early 1980s and 1990s to determine whether the *sequential* administration of combination chemotherapy followed by thoracic radiotherapy could prolong survival for patients with locally advanced NSCLC. Most were quite small, with fewer than 50 patients per arm, but the results of some of the larger and more recent trials are summarized in Table 11.3.4. In the trial reported by Morton et al,[73] a cisplatin-based regimen was not employed, and in that of Mattson et al,[74] the CAP regimen included only low-dose cisplatin. In the studies of Dillman et al,[75,76] Le Chevalier et al,[77] Sause et al[78] and Planting et al,[79] high-dose cisplatin, 100–120 mg/m^2, was used. In the EORTC trial reported by Planting et al,[79] the radiotherapy was delivered as a split course with 30 Gy in 10 fractions followed by 25 Gy in 10 fractions. In most of the other trials, the radiotherapy was uninterrupted at a dose of 60 Gy delivered over six weeks, and in the RTOG trial reported by Sause et al,[78] there was also a hyperfractionated radiotherapy arm.

Even in the studies that employed high-dose cisplatin, the median survival in the chemotherapy arms was only in the range of one year. Furthermore, even though the prolongation of median survival achieved statistical significance in some of the studies, the actual survival gain was less than one month for two studies, approximately two months for three, and four months for the other. The two-year survival rate was similar in all studies and ranged from 12% to 15% for the radiation-alone arms and 20% to 26% for the radiation and chemotherapy arms. No or minimal

Table 11.3.4 Randomized trials of radiotherapy with or without chemotherapy in locally advanced NSCLC

Author	Radiation (Gy)	Chemo-therapy[b]	Number of patients	Median survival (months)	Survival rate (%) 1-year	2-year	3-year
Mattson[74]	55	—	119	10.3	41	15	11
	55	CAP	119	11.0	41	20	7
Morton[73]	60	—	58	9.6	43	12	7 (5-yr)
	60	MACC	56	10.4	47	23	5 (5-yr)
Dillman[75,76]	60	—	77	9.7	40	13	11
	60	PV	79	13.8	55	26	23
Le Chevalier[77]	65	—	177	10.0	41	14	4
	65	VCPC	176	12.0	51	21	12
Soresi[27]	50	—	50	11.0	48	40	?
	50	Weekly P	45	16.0	73	25	?
Schaake-Koning[28]	55	—	108	?	46	13	2
	55	Weekly P	98	?	44	19	13
	55	Daily P	102	?	54	26	16
Sause[78]	60	—	153	11.4	46		5
	60	PV	152	13.8	60		8
	60.9 HF[b]	—	156	12.2	51		6
Planting[79]	55	—	33	12.0		20	0
	55	PVds	37	12.0		20	8

[a]CAP, cyclophosphamide, doxorubicin (Adriamycin), cisplatin; MACC, methotrexate, doxorubicin, cyclophosphamide, lomustine (CCNU); PV, cisplatin, vinblastine; VCPC, vindesine, cyclophosphamide, cisplatin, lomustine; P, cisplatin; PVds, cisplatin, vindesine.
[b]HF, hyperfractionated.

survival benefit was seen at three years and five years in most of the studies, although the Dillman[75,76] and Le Chevalier[77] studies continued to show a small survival advantage beyond the two-year mark.

Concurrent chemotherapy and radiotherapy

The optimal sequence for the administration of chemotherapy and radiotherapy for locally advanced NSCLC has not yet been determined.

The *concurrent* administration of chemotherapy and radiotherapy offers all the benefits of early administration of systemic treatment, with the added potential benefit of improved local control as a result of synergy between the chemotherapeutic agents and radiation.

There have been only two randomized trials that have compared radiation therapy alone versus radiation therapy with concurrent chemotherapy.[27,28] In a study at the National Tumor Institute of Milan, patients were randomized to receive radiotherapy, 50 Gy in 28 fractions, or the same radiation with cisplatin 15 mg/m^2 weekly. Patients in the combination arm had a higher response rate (64% versus 50%), but no statistical differences were observed in disease-free or overall survival.[27] In a recent EORTC trial, patients were randomized to split-course radiotherapy, 55 Gy in 20 fractions, or to the same treatment with cisplatin either 30 mg/m^2 per week or 6 mg/m^2 daily. Response rates in the three arms were similar, but the daily cisplatin group had significantly longer survival than the no-chemotherapy group (p=0.009). The weekly cisplatin group was intermediate between the other two groups, and not significantly different from either.[28]

Studies of sequential and concurrent chemotherapy and radiotherapy are ongoing using some of the new chemotherapy agents now available. Phase I trials have shown that radiation may be combined safely with paclitaxel, docetaxel, gemcitabine and vinorelbine. The CALGB are performing a very interesting randomized phase II trial of both sequential and concurrent administration of chemotherapy. All patients receive cisplatin and are randomized to receive one of paclitaxel, vinorelbine, docetaxel or gemcitabine. The cisplatin is given on days 1 and 22, and the other drugs on days 1 and 8, then on days 22 and 29. At the beginning of the seventh week, thoracic radiotherapy starts, and the same chemotherapy drugs are continued using the same schedule of administration, but attenuated doses. Based on the results of this phase II trial, future phase III studies will be designed.[80]

Whether the concurrent administration of chemotherapy and radiotherapy is superior to sequential administration has been studied in only one randomized trial to date.[81] All patients received chemotherapy with mitomycin C, vindesine and cisplatin either before or concurrently with thoracic radiotherapy. Thoracic radiation was administered as 28 Gy in 14 fractions, followed by a 10-day rest period and another 28 Gy in 14 fractions. Three hundred and fourteen patients entered the study, and the overall response rate was higher in the concurrent arm (84% versus 66%). Median (16.5 months versus 13.3 months), two-year (37% versus 25.6%) and three-year (27% versus 12.5%) survivals were all higher for concurrent therapy (p=0.473). Marrow toxicity was higher with concurrent therapy, but this was not associated with an increased toxic death rate.

The value of adding chemotherapy to thoracic irradiation remains controversial, even today. All of the studies discussed above showed improvements in both median and two-year survivals, but this was not always accompanied by prolongation of long-term survival or increased cure rates. Because most of the trials were relatively small, they may have lacked the power to show small but meaningful differences in survival, and so several groups have undertaken meta-analyses that have now been published.[71,82,83]

The Non-Small Cell Lung Cancer Collaborative Group included trials of chemotherapy and radiotherapy for locally advanced disease in their extensive review of chemotherapy for NSCLC.[71] Using data from only seven trials (807 patients), six of which used a cisplatin-based regimen, the overall hazard ratio of 0.98 was only marginally in favor of chemotherapy. For the six cisplatin trials, the hazard ratio was 0.94, with an absolute benefit of only 2% at both two and five years. Two other analyses, which included the results from 14 trials and 1887 patients[82] and 2589 patients[83] each, had similar results. Marino et al[82] from Milan reported a reduction in mortality rates at one and two years of 5% and 18%, but no differences were detectable at the three- and five-year points. Pritchard and Anthony[83] also reported a slightly reduced risk of death with chemotherapy, with a relative risk of death of 0.87 at two years. They reported that this corresponded to a mean gain in life expectancy for the entire group of two months. Five-year data were not provided.

Induction chemotherapy and surgery

Although radiation with or without chemotherapy is standard therapy for patients with unresectable locally advanced tumors, there has been recent interest in combined-modality treatment programs of chemotherapy followed by *surgery*. Neoadjuvant or induction chemotherapy before surgery has theoretical appeal for several reasons. Response to chemotherapy may allow an otherwise-unresectable tumor to be surgically resected. However, this should not be viewed as the primary goal of treatment, since other treatment modalities can achieve local control and most patients die of distant failure. If this form of combined-modality treatment is to result in a significant prolongation of long-term survival, it will probably be as a result of eradication of micrometastatic tumor deposits. Surgical resection following chemotherapy provides a true pathologic assessment of response to induction therapy, which may be used to guide subsequent treatment. In a sense, the preoperative treatment may be viewed as an 'in vivo chemosensitivity test', and postoperative chemotherapy recommended only for those patients who demonstrate a response to their initial treatment.

There have been several phase II feasibility trials of induction chemotherapy followed by surgical resection, and the results of these studies have been reviewed by several authors.[84–87] It is impossible to draw firm conclusions from these trials, since they included mixed populations of stage IIIA and IIIB disease, and even some patients with earlier-stage tumors. Chemotherapeutic regimens were not standardized, and some patients had both combination chemotherapy and radiation before surgical resection. However, important observations may be made from these studies. Response rates achieved by these early stage, good-performance-status patients are significantly higher than those seen with the same combinations administered to patients with advanced stage IV tumors. Response ranged from 39% to as high as 76%, and complete pathologic response was documented in up to 15% of patients (predominantly with squamous pathology). Median survival ranged from 9 months to 30+ months, with an average of approximately 18 months. This, on the surface, might appear to be better than the median survival of approximately one year that is achieved with radiotherapy alone, but it should be emphasized that all of these studies represent a select subgroup of stage III patients, and that most patients with poor prognostic findings such as superior vena cava obstruction, involvement of mediastinal structures, etc., were excluded from these trials. Long-term survival and cure rate are much more difficult to interpret from the literature. The most optimistic interpretation would be approximately 25–35% survival rates at three to five years.

It is not possible to draw firm conclusions with respect to the optimal chemotherapeutic regimen to be employed as induction treatment before surgery. No single combination-chemotherapy regimen, nor any of the trials that administered both chemotherapy and radiotherapy, demonstrated apparent superiority with respect

Table 11.3.5 Randomized trials of induction chemotherapy and surgery for NSCLC

Author	Treatment[a]	Number of patients	Survival: Median (months)	Survival: Long-term (%)	p
Pass[88]	EP and surgery	13	28.7	42 (3-yr)	0.095
	versus				
	Surgery and radiation	14	15.6	18 (3-yr)	
Rosell[89]	MIC, surgery and radiation	30	26	30 (3-yr)	<0.001
	versus				
	Surgery and radiation	30	8	0	
Roth[90]	CEP and surgery	28	21	36 (5-yr)	0.056
	versus				
	Surgery alone	32	14	15 (5-yr)	
Shepherd[91]	PV and surgery	16	—	40 (2-yr)	ns[b]
	versus				
	Radiation alone	15	—	40 (2-yr)	
Elias[92]	EP, surgery and radiation	23	19	?	0.64
	versus				
	Surgery and radiation	24	23	?	

[a]EP, etoposide, cisplatin; MIC, mitomycin C, ifosfamide, cisplatin; CEP, cyclophosphamide, etoposide, cisplatin; PV, cisplatin, vinblastine.
[b]ns, not significant.

to response rate, complete resection rate, median or long-term survival.

These studies all showed that induction chemotherapy before surgical resection is feasible, but the absence of standards with respect to patient selection, induction regimens and reporting of results makes it impossible to compare these studies with historical data. The results of five prospectively randomized trials of induction chemotherapy and surgery have been published to date; they are summarized in Table 11.3.5. All of the studies were small, with 60 patients each in two,[88,90] 57 in one,[92] and only 31[91] and 27[88] in the others.

Although different chemotherapy regimens were used in the trials reported by Roth et al,[90] Rosell et al,[89] and Pass et al,[88] they all had similar results. Both median and three-year survival rates were superior in the treatment arms that included chemotherapy, and the differences were statistically significant in the trials reported by Rosell et al[89] and Roth et al.[90] In fact, the differences were so great that a decision was made to close these two studies prematurely. Despite the similarity of results, these studies are not felt to be definitive for several reasons. In part, because of the small sample sizes, both studies suffered from major imbalances in critical prognostic variables between the two arms. In the surgery-alone arm of the Roth study,[90] 10 patients (31%) had stage IIIB tumors, and a further 3 (9%) had stage IV tumors. This means that 40% of patients in that arm were not truly eligible for the trial, compared with 11% in the combined-modality chemotherapy arm, which had three patients with stage IIIB tumors and none with stage IV. In view of the small sample size, this serious stage imbalance alone could have accounted for some of the difference in outcome. In the Rosell trial,[89] all patients had stage IIIA tumors, and both arms were well balanced for clinical prognostic factors. However, in the surgery-alone group, 42% of patients were found to have mutations of the K-*ras* gene, which is known to be a significant adverse prognostic factor, compared with only 15% of the patients in the combined-modality arm. In addition, the survival in the surgery-alone arm was particularly poor, with no patient surviving to two years. Based on many historical surgical series, this survival is very much less than would be expected in a population of potentially resectable patients with stage IIIA tumors, especially since several patients had T3N0 tumors without mediastinal node involvement.

The results of a small study from the CALGB have been reported.[92] In this trial, patients received thoracic irradiation and surgical resection, with or without chemotherapy with cisplatin and high-dose etoposide with growth factor support. Median survival for the chemotherapy arm was actually *lower* than that of the control arm (19 versus 23 months respectively), although the differences were not significant ($p=0.64$).

A small Canadian trial, which was closed early in order to join the North American Intergroup study, had a slightly different design. In this study, patients in the control arm received thoracic irradiation *alone*, and the study arm consisted of induction chemotherapy with high-dose cisplatin and vinblastine followed by surgery and postoperative chemotherapy. Although the median and progression-free survival rates showed a slight trend in favor of chemotherapy and surgery, the two-year survival rate was identical at 40% in each arm.[91]

The results of a large French trial have been presented only in preliminary form.[93] In this trial, patients were randomized to proceed to immediate surgery, or to receive two courses of chemotherapy consisting of mitomycin, ifosfamide and cisplatin followed by surgical resection and postoperative chemotherapy for responding patients only. At the time of reporting, 111 patients had entered the trial, and they were well balanced for the known prognostic factors. It should be noted that patients with stage I (T2N0) and stage II were eligible for this study, and constituted more than 50% of the patients in the surgery-alone arm.

These trials certainly suggest that surgery alone may be inferior treatment for patients with potentially resectable stage IIIA tumors. They do not, however, tell us that induction chemotherapy followed by surgery is *the best* treatment for these patients. Several investigators have questioned whether surgery is necessary at all, and whether thoracic irradiation, either alone or combined with chemotherapy, might be equivalent to induction chemotherapy and surgery. Three large trials designed to answer this question are currently ongoing in Europe and North America. In the EORTC trial 08941, all patients receive three courses of induction chemotherapy, which must contain either cisplatin 100mg/m^2 or carboplatin 350mg/m^2. Other drugs in the regimen may be chosen by the institution, and two phase II trials of gemcitabine–cisplatin and carboplatin–cisplatin are ongoing within the induction portion of this study. Responding and stable patients are then randomized to receive thoracic irradiation or to undergo surgical resection. In the North American Intergroup high-priority trial, all patients receive etoposide and cisplatin administered concurrently with thoracic radiotherapy. Randomization, which takes place at the time of study entry, is to surgical resection or to a boost of radiotherapy. Two further courses of chemotherapy are given after the surgery or boost radiation. Finally, the British Medical Research Council trial is very similar to the Canadian trial. In this study, patients receive either thoracic irradiation alone or induction chemotherapy followed by surgery. It will be several years before the results of any of these trials are available.

CHEMOTHERAPY FOR ADVANCED DISEASE

The role of chemotherapy in advanced (stage IV) disease remains controversial to this day. Since patients are not curable at this stage, the primary goals of therapy must be palliation of symptoms and prolongation of survival. Response rate alone is an inadequate measure of the usefulness of combination chemotherapy. Response must be accompanied by meaningful prolongation of survival without unacceptable toxicity. Recently it has been suggested that prolongation of median survival for only a few weeks is also not adequate justification for treatment, and that the success of chemotherapy for advanced disease should be based on the proportion of patients who achieve long-term survival of one year or more. With the new agents and combinations that are now available, at least 35–40% of patients should achieve one-year survival. However, it is recognized that a major proportion of patients may experience improvement in symptoms even in the absence of a 50% reduction in tumor mass.[94] Despite response rates as low as 25–30%, improvement in major lung cancer-related symptoms such as cough, chest pain and shortness of breath may be seen in as many as two-thirds of patients.

There seems to be little doubt that response to chemotherapy is associated with prolongation of survival. Despite this, the overall contribution that chemotherapy makes to survival remains modest. There have been seven prospectively randomized trials of chemotherapy versus best supportive care for patients with advanced NSCLC, the results of which are summarized in Table 11.3.6. Only in the studies of Quoix et al,[100] Rapp et al[48] and Cormier et al[95] were statistically significant prolongations of survival achieved with chemotherapy. However, it should be noted that in the Cormier trial,[95] the patients in the best-supportive-care arm had a very short median survival of only 8.5 weeks. Furthermore, in the Rapp study,[48] survival for patients in the high-dose cisplatin and vindesine arm was less than four months longer than that of patients in the control arm.

The Non-Small Cell Lung Cancer Collaborative Group also assessed the benefit of chemotherapy for advanced disease in their meta-analysis.[71] Data were available from 11 trials and a total of 1190 patients. Eight of the studies used cisplatin in doses ranging from 40 to 120 mg/m^2 and either a vinca alkaloid or etoposide. The analysis showed a benefit from chemotherapy, with a hazard ratio of 0.73 (p=0.095). Although the overall increase in median survival was only one and a half months, there was an absolute increase in one-year survival rate of 10%. This

Table 11.3.6 Randomized trials of chemotherapy versus supportive care for patients with advanced NSCLC

Author	Chemotherapy[a]	Number of patients	Median survival (weeks)	p
Cormier[95]	MACC	20	30.5	0.0005
	BSC	19	8.5	
Rapp[48]	VdsP	44	32.6	0.01 (VdsP vs BSC)
	CAP	43	24.7	0.05 (CAP vs BSC)
	BSC	50	17.0	
Ganz[96]	Vb1P	22	18.6	0.26
	BSC	26	14.4	
Woods[97]	VdsP	97	27.0	0.33
	BSC	91	17.0	
Cellerino[98]	CEP/MEC	58	34.3	0.135
	BSC	57	21.1	
Kaasa[99]	VdsP	44	22.0	0.29
	BSC	43	16.5	
Quoix[100]	VdsP	24	28	<0.0013
	BSC	22	10	

[a]MACC, methotrexate, doxorubicin (Adriamycin), cyclophosphamide, lomustine (CCNU); BSC, best supportive care; VdsP, vindesine, cisplatin; CAP, cyclophosphamide, doxorubicin, cisplatin; VblP, vinblastine, cisplatin; CEP, cyclophosphamide, epirubicin, cisplatin; MEC, methotrexate, etoposide, lomustine.

long-term survival benefit has not been confirmed by all authors. In a slightly smaller meta-analysis of seven studies and 700 patients, Souquet et al[101] reported that chemotherapy caused a significant reduction in mortality at six months, but no benefit at 12 and 18 months.

Because of concerns that the small survival benefit seen in the combination-chemotherapy arms of the Canadian trial might be associated with unacceptable financial cost, a formal economic evaluation of this study was undertaken.[102] It is interesting, and perhaps surprising, that this evaluation demonstrated that the use of combination chemotherapy *was* cost-effective. This was due to the high costs of supporting patients on the supportive-care arm, who actually spent *more* time in hospital than patients on either of the chemotherapy arms. Economic analyses of other clinical trials have also been reported.[103] The European trial that compared vinorelbine alone to cisplatin in combination with either vinorelbine or vindesine showed a

Table 11.3.7 Randomized trials of new chemotherapy combinations versus single-agent cisplatin

Author	Cisplatin dose (mg/m^2)	Dose of study drugs	Number of patients	Response rate (%)	Survival	
					Median	1-year (%)
Wozniak[59]	100	None	218	10	6.0 mo	16
	100	Vinorelbine 25 mg/m^2/wk	214	25	7.0 mo	35
Sandler[104]	100	None	154	10	32 wk	28
	100	Gemcitabine 1000 mg/m^2/wk × 3	155	32	39 wk	39
von Pawel[105]	75	None	219	14	28 wk	22
	75	Tirapazamine 390 mg/m^2	218	28	35 wk	33
Gatzemeier[106]	100	None	205	17	37 wk	32
	30	Paclitaxel 175 mg/m^2 (3 h)	202	26	35 wk	35

significant survival advantage for the cisplatin–vinorelbine arm over the other two arms at a cost of only US$17 700 per year of life gained. The cost for vindesine–cisplatin was US$22 100 per year of life gained. These two studies thus suggest that chemotherapy should not be withheld from NSCLC patients for financial reasons.

Combinations incorporating some of the new chemotherapeutic agents have now been evaluated in randomized trials, some of which have been summarized in Tables 11.3.7–11.3.9.

The results of four trials of new-drug combinations versus single-agent cisplatin are summarized in Table 11.3.7. In a SWOG study, vinorelbine 25 mg/m^2 per week in combination with cisplatin 100 mg/m^2 was compared with the same dose of cisplatin alone.[59] The overall response rate for the combination was 26%, compared with only 10% for cisplatin alone. Median and one-year survival rates were also longer for the combination, at seven months and 35%, compared with only six months and 16% for single-agent treatment ($p=0.0005$). Not unexpectedly, toxicity was higher in the combination arm. There were 20 episodes of neutropenic fever (12%) compared with none in the cisplatin-alone arm, and four treatment-related deaths compared with only one.

The Hoosier Oncology Group compared a combination of gemcitabine 1000 mg/m^2 per week × 3 with cisplatin 100 mg/m^2 versus cisplatin alone,[104] and had similar response and survival results to those in the SWOG trial. In the CATAPULT 1 study,[105] cisplatin at a dose of only 75 mg/m^2 was compared against cisplatin with tirapazamine. Once again, response and survival rates were superior for the combination arm.

Unlike these three trials, the trial reported by Gatzemeier et al,[106] which compared single-agent cisplatin 100 mg/m^2 versus a combination of cisplatin 80 mg/m^2 and paclitaxel 175 mg/m^2

Table 11.3.8 Randomized trials of new single agents versus standard or new chemotherapy combinations

Author	Cisplatin dose (mg/m²)	Dose of study drugs	Number of patients	Response rate (%)	Survival	
					Median	1-year (%)
Depierre[60]	None	Vinorelbine 30 mg/m²/wk	119	16	32 wk	23
	80	Vinorelbine 30 mg/m²/wk	121	43	33 wk	30
Gil Deza[61]	None	Vinorelbine 30 mg/m²/wk	73	42	32 wk	NR[a]
	100	Vinorelbine 30 mg/m²/wk	89	42	41 wk	NR
Le Chevalier[62]	None	Vinorelbine 30 mg/m²/wk	188	14	31 wk	30
	120	Vinorelbine 30 mg/m²/wk	182	30	40 wk	35
	120	Vindesine 3 mg/m²/wk	179	19	32 wk	30
Manegold[107]	None	Gemcitabine 1000 mg/m²/wk × 3	72	18	6.6 mo	26
	100	Etoposide 100 mg/m² × 3	75	15	7.6 mo	24
Perng[108]	None	Gemcitabine 1250 mg/m²/wk × 3	27	19	37 wk	40
	80	Etoposide 80 mg/m² × 3	25	21	48 wk	33

[a]NR, not reported.

administered over three hours, did not have positive results.[106] Although the response rate was higher for the combination-chemotherapy arm (26% versus 17%; $p=0.028$), there were no differences in either median or one-year survival rates. The authors suggested that this might have been due to taxane treatment given to patients in the cisplatin-alone arm at the time of disease progression. Neutropenia, peripheral neuropathy, and arthralgias and myalgias were reported more frequently in the paclitaxel–cisplatin arm, although better quality-of-life scores were also reported in that arm. This was probably due to a higher rate of nausea and vomiting, anorexia and constipation reported by patients treated with the higher dose of cisplatin in the single-agent arm.

Although it may no longer be appropriate to study single-agent cisplatin, the new drugs have shown high enough response and survival rates in phase II trials to justify their evaluation as single agents in randomized trials. The results of five such studies are shown in Table 11.3.8.

In three studies, single-agent vinorelbine 30 mg/m^2 per week was compared with a combination of vinorelbine and cisplatin.[60–62] Despite variable cisplatin doses, the results of the three trials were remarkably similar. With the exception of the study reported by Gil Deza et al,[61] response rates were significantly higher in the combination arm, and ranged from 30%[62] to 43%.[60] Median and one-year survival rates were also superior for the combination arms, although it should be noted that single-agent vinorelbine resulted in median survivals of greater than 30 weeks in all of the studies and a one-year survival rate of 30% in one French trial.[62] As might be expected, nausea and vomiting were seen more frequently in patients treated with cisplatin, and myelosuppression and neurotoxicity were also greater in the combination arms.

There have been two trials of single-agent gemcitabine compared with etoposide and cisplatin.[107,108] Single-agent gemcitabine had been shown in phase II studies to produce response in approximately 20% of patients,[39] and this was confirmed in these two randomized trials. The response rates were similar in both trials, with gemcitabine demonstrating activity that was equal to or better than the combination in each study. Although the median survival was slightly less for patients treated with single-agent gemcitabine, the one-year survival was actually better in the gemcitabine-alone arm in one small Taiwanese trial.[108] Both studies demonstrated significantly lower toxicity for patients treated with single-agent gemcitabine. In the German trial,[107] only 2% of gemcitabine patients had grade 4 neutropenia, compared with 12% of those treated with cisplatin and etoposide, and only 11% of patients had grade 3 nausea and vomiting, compared with 29% treated with the combination. Perng et al[108] reported only 3.7% grade 3/4 leukopenia for gemcitabine alone, compared with 30.7% for patients treated with etoposide and cisplatin. Only 3.7% of patients on gemcitabine had grade 3 nausea and vomiting, compared with 34.6% on the combination arm.

Virtually all of the new agents underwent phase I and II trials, which showed that they could be administered safely in combination with cisplatin or carboplatin. These new combinations were then compared in randomized studies with regimens that were hitherto considered standard treatment for patients with advanced NSCLC. The results of seven such trials are summarized in Table 11.3.9.

Paclitaxel was compared with standard therapy with cisplatin and an epipodophylloxin in two large randomized trials.[57,58] In an ECOG study, cisplatin 75 mg/m^2 was given to all patients, and paclitaxel was administered over 24 hours at doses of 135 or 250 mg/m^2, and compared with standard therapy with etoposide 100 mg/m^2 for three days. Higher response rates were seen in the paclitaxel arm, with no significant difference in response or survival rates seen between the low- and high-dose paclitaxel arms. Both paclitaxel arms had survival that was significantly longer than that of the etoposide–cisplatin arm ($p=0.03$). The paclitaxel arms were associated with higher rates of grade 4 granulocytopenia, neurotoxicity and myalgias, which were clearly dose-related.

The EORTC undertook a similar study[58] in which cisplatin 80 mg/m^2 was administered with either paclitaxel 175 mg/m^2 over three hours or teniposide 100 mg/m^2 daily for three days. This study showed that, while paclitaxel yielded a

Table 11.3.9 Randomized trials of standard chemotherapy combinations versus new chemotherapy combinations

Author	Cisplatin dose (mg/m²)	Dose of study drugs	Number of patients	Response rate (%)	Survival Median	Survival 1-year (%)
Bonomi[57]	75	Paclitaxel 135 mg/m² (24 h)	189	27	9.6 mo	37
	75	Paclitaxel 250 mg/m² (24 h)	191	32	10 mo	39
	75	Etoposide 100 mg/m² × 3	194	12	7.7 mo	32
Giaccone[58]	80	Paclitaxel 175 mg/m² (3 h)	155	44	9.4 mo	41
	80	Teniposide 100 mg/m² × 3	157	30	9.7 mo	43
Belani[109]	75	Etoposide 100 mg/m² × 3	179	15	39 wk	37
	None	Carboplatin AUC 6[a] Paclitaxel 223 mg/m² (3 h)	190	23	33 wk	32
Le Chevalier[62]	None	Vinorelbine 30 mg/m²/wk	188	14	31 wk	30
	120	Vinorelbine 30 mg/m²/wk	182	30	40 wk	35
	120	Vindesine 3 mg/m²/wk	179	19	32 wk	30
Cardenal[110] (phase II trial)	100	Gemcitabine 1250 mg/m²/wk × 3	69	41	8.7 mo	32
	100	Etoposide 100 mg/m² × 3	62	22	7.2 mo	26
Crino[111]	100	Gemcitabine 1000 mg/m²/wk × 3	155	38	37 wk	33
	100	Mitomycin C 6 mg/m² Ifosfamide 3 g/m²	152	26	39 wk	34
Comella[112] (phase II trial)	50 mg/m² /wk × 2	Gemcitabine 1000 mg/m²/wk × 2 Vinorelbine 25 mg/m²/wk × 2	55	62	NR[b]	NR
	60 × 1	Epirubicin 60 mg/m² × 1 Vindesine 3 mg/m² × 1 Lonidamine 75 mg p.o. daily	50	35	NR	NR

[a]AUC 6, 'area under the curve' dosing of 6.
[b]NR, not reported.

higher overall response rate (44% versus 30%; $p=0.03$), this did not result in either a median or one-year survival advantage. However, the toxicity profile in this study was considerably different from that of the ECOG trial. The paclitaxel arm had only 24% grade 3/4 neutropenia and only 3% febrile neutropenia, compared with 63% and 27% respectively for the teniposide arm. Grade 3/4 neurotoxicity was higher in the paclitaxel arm (12% versus 4%).

Belani et al[109] reported the results of a trial that compared cisplatin and etoposide against high-dose paclitaxel 225 mg/m^2 over three hours and carboplatin using 'area under the curve' dosing of 6. Despite the high dose of paclitaxel used in this study, the overall response rate was a disappointing 23%, although this was significantly better than the 15% achieved with cisplatin–etoposide ($p=0.059$). However, both the median and one-year survival rates were lower for the paclitaxel arm than for the etoposide–cisplatin arm.

Vinorelbine in combination with high-dose cisplatin has been compared with vindesine and cisplatin.[62] Vinorelbine was associated with significantly higher response rates as well as median and one-year survival rates. Neutropenia was higher in the vinorelbine–cisplatin arm ($p < 0.001$), but neurotoxicity was significantly greater in the vindesine–cisplatin arm ($p < 0.004$).

Gemcitabine combinations have also been evaluated in randomized clinical trials.[110–112] A small Spanish study[110] compared gemcitabine 1250 mg/m^2 weekly for three weeks with cisplatin 100 mg/m^2 versus etoposide 100 mg/m^2 daily × 3 plus cisplatin. Preliminary results have been published only in abstract form. The response rate was twice as high in the gemcitabine arm, and median and one-year survivals also favored gemcitabine. Neutropenia was similar in both arms, although thrombocytopenia was greater in the gemcitabine arm (20% versus 3.5%), and all other toxicities were similar.

Crino et al[111] reported the results of an Italian trial of gemcitabine and cisplatin compared with mitomycin C, ifosfomide and cisplatin (MIC). Although the MIC regimen is not used commonly in North America, it is considered one of the standard regimens for the treatment of advanced NSCLC in the UK and Europe. This study showed an overall response rate of 38% for gemcitabine and cisplatin compared with only 26% for MIC ($p=0.03$). However, despite the response advantage for the gemcitabine arm, median and one-year survival rates were similar, with 37 weeks and 33% for gemcitabine and 39 weeks and 34% for MIC. Hematologic toxicity was slightly higher in the gemcitabine arm for both absolute neutrophil count and platelet count, and more patients in the gemcitabine arm required red blood cell and platelet transfusions.

The group of the National Tumor Institute of Naples have also shown that gemcitabine may be combined with cisplatin and vinorelbine.[112,113] A small randomized trial that compared this combination with a combination of vindesine, cisplatin and lonidamine has been published only in abstract form. The overall response rate of 62% favored the gemcitabine arm, but survival data have not yet been published.

Although it is clear that chemotherapy exerts a biological effect in patients with advanced NSCLC, broad generalizations cannot be made for the treatment of this group of patients as a whole. Whenever possible, patients should be treated on clinical trials of either new agents or new combinations of drugs. Continued research in patients with advanced disease is essential to identify regimens that may have sufficient activity to justify their future use in patients with earlier stages of disease. At this time, chemotherapy is sufficiently active to justify its use in patients who want treatment and who understand its limitations. Treatment must be individualized, and should be offered to good-performance-status patients who have the greatest chance to benefit from therapy and the least potential to develop toxicity. It seems that combinations incorporating the new agents are modestly superior to the standard regimens used until the early 1990s. Improvements have been seen in response rates, although, on the whole, survival gains have been small. Some agents have resulted in response and survival rates equivalent to those of combination chemotherapy, but with significantly less toxicity. In a patient population in which the aim of treatment is mainly palliation, this could be viewed as an important improvement over current standard therapy.

REFERENCES

1. Bailor JC, Smith EM, Progress against cancer! *N Engl J Med* 1986; **314**: 1226–32.
2. Vokes EE, Bitran JD, Vogelzang NJ, Chemotherapy for non-small cell lung cancer. The continuing challenge. *Chest* 1991; **99**: 1326–8.
3. Mountain C, A new international staging system for lung cancer. *Chest* 1986; **89**: 225S.
4. American Joint Committee on Cancer, Thorax: lung. In: *AJCC Cancer Staging Manual*. Lippincott-Raven: Philadelphia. 1997: 127–41.
5. Maki E, Feld R, Prognostic factors in patients with non-small cell lung cancer. A critique of the world literature. *Lung Cancer* 1991; **7**: 27–35.
6. Gail MH, Eagan RT, Feld R et al, Prognostic factors in patients with resected stage 1 non-small cell lung cancer: a report from the Lung Cancer Study Group. *Cancer* 1984; **54**: 1802–13.
7. Keller S, Groshen S, Martini N, Kaiser L, Blood transfusion and lung cancer recurrence. *Cancer* 1983; **62**: 606–10.
8. Donnadieu N, Paesmans M, Sculier J-P, Chemotherapy of non-small cell lung cancer according to disease extent: a meta-analysis of the literature. *Lung Cancer* 1991; **7**: 243–52.
9. Bonomi PD, Finkelstein DM, Ruckdeschel JD et al, Combination chemotherapy versus single agents followed by combination chemotherapy in stage IV non-small cell lung cancer: a study of the Eastern Cooperative Oncology Group. *J Clin Oncol* 1989; **17**: 1602–13.
10. Borges M, Sculier JP, Paesmans M et al, Prognostic factors for response to chemotherapy containing platinum derivatives in patients with unresectable non-small cell lung cancer. *Lung Cancer* 1996; **16**: 21–33.
11. Ferguson MK, Skosey C, Hoffman PC, Golomb HM, Sex-associated differences in presentation and survival in patients with lung cancer. *J Clin Oncol* 1990; **8**: 1402–7.
12. Takigawa N, Segawa Y, Okahara M et al, Prognostic factors for patients with advanced non-small cell lung cancer: univariate and multivariate analyses including recursive partitioning and amalgamation. *Lung Cancer* 1996; **15**: 66–7.
13. Sahin AA, Ro JY, el-Naggar AK et al, Flow cytometric analysis of the DNA content of non-small cell lung cancer. Ploidy as a significant prognostic indicator in squamous cell carcinoma of the lung. *Cancer* 1990; **65**: 530–7.
14. Alama A, Constantini M, Repetto L et al, Thymidine labelling index as prognostic factor in resected non-small cell lung cancer. *Eur J Cancer* 1990; **26**: 622–5.
15. Berendsen HH, de-Leij L, Popperma S et al, Clinical characterization of non-small cell lung cancer tumours showing neuroendocrine differentiation features. *J Clin Oncol* 1989; **11**: 1614–20.
16. Stevenson H, Gazdar A, Phelps R et al, Tumor cell lines established in vitro, an independent prognostic factor for survival in non-small cell lung cancer. *Ann Intern Med* 1990; **113**: 764–70.
17. Carney DN, The biology of lung cancer. *Curr Opin Oncol* 1992; **4**: 292–8.
18. Harada M, Dosaka-Akita H, Miyamoto H et al, Prognostic signficance of the expression of *ras* oncogene product in non-small cell lung cancer. *Cancer* 1992; **69**: 72–7.
19. Lee JS, Ro JY, Sahin AA et al, Expression of blood-group antigen A: a favourable prognostic factor in non-small cell lung cancer. *N Engl J Med* 1991; **324**: 1084–90.
20. Rusch V, Klimstra D, Venkatraman E et al, Aberrant p53 expression predicts clinical resistance to cisplatin-based chemotherapy in locally advanced non-small cell lung cancer. *Cancer Res* 1995; **55**: 5038–42.

21. Giatromanolaki A, Koukourakis M, O'Byrne K et al, Prognostic value of angiogenesis in operable non-small cell lung cancer. *J Pathol* 1996; **179**: 80–8.
22. Bakowski MT, Crouch JD, Chemotherapy of non-small cell lung cancer: a reappraisal and a look to the future. *Cancer Treat Rev* 1983; **10**: 159–72.
23. Joss RA, Cavalli F, Goldhirsch A et al, New agents in non-small cell lung cancer. *Cancer Treat Rev* 1984; **11**: 205–36.
24. Gralla RJ, Casper ES, Kelsen DP et al, Cisplatin and vindesine combination chemotherapy for advanced carcinoma of the lung: a randomized trial investigating two dosage schedules. *Ann Intern Med* 1981; **95**: 414–20.
25. Gandara D, Crowley J, Livingston R et al, Evaluation of cisplatin intensity in metastatic non-small cell lung cancer: a phase III study of the Southwest Oncology Group. *J Clin Oncol* 1993; **11**: 873–8.
26. Sculier JP, Klastersky J, Giner V et al, A phase II randomized trial comparing high-dose cisplatin with moderate-dose cisplatin and carboplatin in patients with advanced non-small cell lung cancer. *J Clin Oncol* 1994; **12**: 353–9.
27. Soresi E, Clerici M, Grilli R et al, A randomized clinical trial comparing radiation therapy versus radiation therapy plus *cis*-dichlorodiamine-platin (II) in the treatment of locally advanced non-small cell lung cancer. *Semin Oncol* 1988; **15**(Suppl 7): 20–5.
28. Schaake-Koning C, Bartelink H, Hara Adema B et al, Radiotherapy and cisdiamminedichloroplatinum (II) as a combined treatment modality for inoperable non-small cell lung cancer, a dose finding study. *Int J Radiat Oncol Biol Phys* 1986; **12**: 379–83.
29. Bunn PA, Review of therapeutic trials of carboplatin in lung cancer. *Semin Oncol* 1989; **16**(Suppl 5): 27–33.
30. Green M, Kreisman H, Soll D et al, Carboplatin in non-small cell lung cancer: an update on the Cancer and Leukemia Group B experience. *Semin Oncol* 1992; **19**(Suppl 2): 44–9.
31. Johnson DH, Overview of ifosfamide in small cell and non-small cell lung cancer. *Semin Oncol* 1990; **17**(Suppl 4): 24–30.
32. Eberhardt W, Niederle N, Ifosfamide in non-small cell lung cancer: a review. *Semin Oncol* 1992; **19**(Suppl 1): 40–8.
33. Depierre A, Lemarie E, Dabouis G et al, A phase II study of Navelbine (vinorelbine) in the treatment of non-small cell lung cancer. *Am J Clin Oncol* 1991; **14**: 115–19.
34. Spain RC, Neo-adjuvant mitomycin C, cisplatin and infusion vinblastine in locally and regionally advanced non-small cell lung cancer: problems and progress from the perspective of long-term follow-up. *Semin Oncol* 1988; **15**(Suppl 4): 6–15.
35. Slevin ML, Clark PI, Joel SP et al, A randomized trial to evaluate the effect of schedule on the activity of etoposide in small cell lung cancer. *J Clin Oncol* 1989; **7**: 1333–40.
36. Splinter TAW, Sahmoud T, Festen J et al, Two schedules of teniposide with or without cisplatin in advanced non-small-cell lung cancer: a randomized study of the European Organization for Research and Treatment of Cancer Lung Cancer Cooperative Group. *J Clin Oncol* 1996; **14**: 127–34.
37. Ettinger D, Overview of paclitaxel (Taxol) in advanced lung cancer. *Semin Oncol* 1993; **4**(Suppl 3): 46–9.
38. Cortes JE, Pazdur R, Docetaxel. *J Clin Oncol* 1995, 13: 2643–55.
39. Shepherd FA, Phase II trials of single-agent activity of gemcitabine in patients with advanced non-small cell lung cancer: an overview. *Anti-Cancer Drugs* 1995; **6**: 19–25.
40. Shepherd FA, Abratt RP, Anderson H et al, Gemcitabine in the treatment of elderly patients with non-small cell lung cancer. *Semin Oncol* 1997; **24**(2): S7-50–5.
41. Feld R, Wierzbicki R, Walde D et al, Phase I–II study of high dose epirubucin in advanced non-small cell lung cancer. *J Clin Oncol* 1992; **20**: 297–303.
42. Fukuoka M, Niitani H, Sizuki A et al, A phase II study of CPT-11, a new derivative of camp-

tothecin, for previously untreated non-small cell lung cancer. *J Clin Oncol* 1992; **10**: 16–20.
43. Asakawa M, Fujita A, Fukuoka M et al, Phase II study of CPT-11, a new camptothecin derivative in previously untreated non-small cell lung cancer. *Lung Cancer* 1991; 7: 125–9 (Abst 465)
44. Perez-Solar R, Fossella F, Glisson BS et al, Phase II study of topotecan in patients with advanced non-small cell lung cancer not treated previously with chemotherapy. *J Clin Oncol* 1996; **14**: 503–13.
45. Lynch T, Kalish L, Strauss G et al, Phase II study of topotecan in non-small cell lung cancer. *J Clin Oncol* 1994; **12**: 347–52.
46. Cahill A, White INH, Reductive metabolism of 3-amino-1,2,4-benzotriazine-1,4-dioxide (SR4233) and the induction of unscheduled DNA synthesis in rat and human derived cell lines. *Carcinogenesis* 1990; **11**: 1407–11.
47. Rodriguez G, Valdivvieso M, Von Hoff D et al, A phase I/II trial of the combination of tirapazamine and cisplatin in patients with non-small cell lung cancer. *Proc Am Soc Clin Oncol* 1996; **15**: 382 (Abst 1144).
48. Rapp E, Pater J, Willan A et al, Chemotherapy can prolong survival in patients with advanced non-small cell lung cancer. A report of the Canadian multicenter trial. *J Clin Oncol* 1988; **6**: 633–41.
49. Osoba D, Rusthoven JJ, Turnbull KA et al, Combination chemotherapy with bleomycin, etoposide and cisplatinum in metastatic non-small cell lung cancer. *J Clin Oncol* 1985; **3**: 1478–85.
50. Bunn PA, The expanding role of cisplatin in the treatment of non-small cell lung cancer. *Semin Oncol* 1989; **16**(Suppl 6): 10–21.
51. Gurney H, de Campos ES, Dodwell D et al, Ifosphamide and mitomycin in combination for the treatment of patients with progressive advanced non-small cell lung cancer. *Eur J Cancer* 1991; **27**: 565–8.
52. Drings P, European experience with ifosfamide in non-small cell lung cancer. *Semin Oncol* 1989; **16**: 22–30.
53. Cullen MH, Joshi R, Chetiyawardna A, Mitomycin, ifosfamide and cisplatin in non-small cell lung cancer: treatment good enough to compare. *Br J Cancer* 1988; **9**: 359–61.
54. Van Zandwijk N, ten Bokkel Huinink WW, Wanders J et al, Dose-finding studies with carboplatin, ifosfamide, etoposide and mesna in non-small cell lung cancer. *Semin Oncol* 1990; **17**: 16–21.
55. Shepherd FA, Evans WK, Goss PE et al, Ifosfamide, cisplatin and etoposide (ICE) in the treatment of advanced non-small cell lung cancer. *Semin Oncol* 1992; **19**(Suppl 1): 54–8.
56. Shepherd FA, Anglin G, Abratt RP et al, Influence of gemcitabine and cisplatin schedule on response and survival in advanced non-small cell lung cancer. *Proc Am Soc Clin Oncol* 1998; **17**: 472a (Abst 1816).
57. Bonomi P, Kim K, Chang A, Johnson D, Phase III trial comparing etoposide (E) cisplatin (C) versus taxol (T) with cisplatin–G-CSF (G) versus taxol–cisplatin in advanced non-small cell lung cancer. An Eastern Cooperative Oncology Group (ECOG) trial. *Proc Am Soc Clin Oncol* 1996; **15**: 382 (Abst 1145).
58. Giaccone G, Splinter T, Postmus P et al, Paclitaxel–cisplatin versus teniposide–cisplatin in advanced non-small cell lung cancer. *Proc Am Soc Clin Oncol* 1996; **15**: 373 (Abst 1109).
59. Wozniak AJ, Crowley JJ, Balcerzak GR et al, Randomized phase III trial of cisplatin (CDDP) vs. CDDP plus Navelbine in treatment of advanced non-small cell lung cancer (NSCLC): report of a Southwest Oncology Group study (SWOG-9308). *Proc Am Soc Clin Oncol* 1996; **15**: 374 (Abst 1110).
60. Depierre A, Chastang C, Quoix E et al, Vinorelbine versus vinorelbine plus cisplatin in advanced non-small cell lung cancer: a randomized trial. *Ann Oncol* 1994; **5**: 37–42.
61. Gil Deza E, Balbiani L, Coppola F et al, Phase II study of Navelbine (NVB) versus NVB plus cisplatin in non-small cell lung cancer stage III or IV. *Proc Am Soc Clin Oncol* 1996; **15**: 394 (Abst 1193).

62. Le Chevalier T, Brisgand D, Douillard JY et al, Randomized study of vinorelbine and cisplatin versus vinorelbine alone versus vindesine and cisplatin in advanced non-small cell lung cancer: results of a European multicenter trial including 612 patients. *J Clin Oncol* 1994; **12**: 360–7.
63. Holmes EC, Gail M, Lung Cancer Study Group, Surgical adjuvant therapy for stage II and stage III adenocarcinoma and large-cell undifferentiated carcinoma of the lung. *J Clin Oncol* 1986; **4**: 710–15.
64. Lad T, Rubinstein L, Fadeghi A, The benefit of adjuvant treatment for resected locally advanced non-small cell lung cancer. *J Clin Oncol* 1988; **6**: 9–17.
65. Feld R, Rubenstein L, Thomas P (Lung Cancer Study Group), Adjuvant chemotherapy with cyclophosphamide, doxorubicin, and cisplatin in patients with completely resected stage I non-small cell lung cancer. *J. Natl Cancer Inst* 1993; **85**: 299–306.
66. Niiranin AS, Niitamo-Korhonen S, Kouri M et al, Adjuvant chemotherapy after radical surgery for non-small cell lung cancer: a randomized study. *J Clin Oncol* 1992; **10**: 1927–32.
67. Dautzenberg B, Chastang C, Arriagada R et al, Adjuvant radiotherapy versus combined sequential chemotherapy followed by radiotherapy in the treatment of resected non-small cell lung carcinoma. *Cancer* 1995; **75**: 779–86.
68. Wada H, Hitomi S, Teramatsu T, Adjuvant chemotherapy after complete resection in non-small cell lung cancer. *J Clin Oncol* 1996; **14**: 1048–54.
69. Ohta M, Tsuchiya R, Shimoyama M et al, Adjuvant chemotherapy for completely resected stage III non-small-cell lung cancer. Results of a randomized prospective study. The Japan Clinical Oncology Group. *J Thorac Cardiovasc Surg* 1993; **106**: 307–8.
70. Ichinose Y, Hara N, Ohta M et al, Postoperative adjuvant chemotherapy in non-small cell lung cancer: prognostic value of DNA ploidy and postrecurrent survival. *J Surg Oncol* 1991; **46**: 15–20.
71. Non-Small Cell Lung Cancer Collaborative Group, Chemotherapy in non-small cell lung cancer: a meta-analysis using updated data on individual patients from 52 randomized clinical trials. *BMJ* 1995; **311**: 899–909.
72. Le Chevalier T, Brisgand D, Douillard JY et al, Randomized trial of vinorelbine and cisplatin versus vindesine and cisplatin versus vinorelbine alone in advanced non-small cell lung cancer. *J Clin Oncol* 1996; **14**: 687–8.
73. Morton RF, Jett JR, McGinnis WL et al, Thoracic radiation therapy alone compared with combined chemoradiotherapy for locally unresectable non-small cell lung cancer. *Ann Intern Med* 1991; **115**: 681–6.
74. Mattson K, Holsti LR, Holsti P et al, Inoperable non-small cell lung cancer: radiation with or without chemotherapy. *Eur J Clin Oncol* 1988; **24**: 477–82.
75. Dillman RO, Seagren SL, Propert KJ et al, A randomized trial of induction chemotherapy plus high-dose radiation vs. radiation alone in stage III non-small cell lung cancer. *N Engl J Med* 1990; **323**: 940–5.
76. Dillman RO, Herndon J, Seagren SL et al, Improved survival in stage III non-small cell lung cancer: seven-year follow-up of Cancer and Acute Leukemia Group B (CALGB) 8433 trial. *J Natl Cancer Inst* 1996; **88**: 1210–15.
77. Le Chevalier T, Arriagada R, Tarayre M et al, Significant effect of adjuvant chemotherapy on survival in locally advanced non-small cell lung cancer. *J Natl Cancer Inst* 1991; **83**: 417–23.
78. Sause W, Kolesar P, Taylor S et al, Five-year results: phase III trial of regionally advanced, unresectable non-small cell lung cancer, RTOG 8808, ECOG 4588, SWOG 8992. *Proc Am Soc Clin Oncol* 1998; **17**: 435a (Abst 1743).
79. Planting A, Helle P, Drings P et al, A randomized study of high-dose split course radiotherapy preceded by high-dose chemotherapy versus high-dose radiotherapy only in locally advanced non-small cell lung cancer. An EORTC Lung Cancer Cooperative Group trial. *Ann Oncol* 1996; **7**: 139–44.

80. Vokes EE, Leopold KA, Herndon JE et al, A CALGB randomized phase II study of gemcitabine or paclitaxel or vinorelbine with cisplatin as induction chemotherapy (Ind CT) and concomitant chemoradiotherapy (XRT) in stage IIIB non-small cell lung cancer (NSCLC): feasibility data. *Proc Am Soc Clin Oncol* 1997; **16**: 455a (Abst 1636).
81. Furuse K, Fukuoka Y, Takada Y et al for the West Japan Lung Cancer Group, A randomized phase III study of concurrent versus sequential thoracic radiotherapy (TRT) in combination with mitomycin (M), vindesine (V), cisplatin (P) in unresectable stage III non-small cell lung cancer (NSCLC). *Proc Am Soc Clin Oncol* 1997; **16**: 459a (Abst 1649).
82. Marino P, Preatone A, Cantone A, Randomized trials of radiotherapy alone versus combined chemotherapy and radiotherapy in stages IIIa and IIIb non-small cell lung cancer: a meta-analysis. *Cancer* l995; **76**: 593–601.
83. Pritchard R, Anthony S, Chemotherapy plus radiotherapy in the treatment of locally advanced, unresectable non-small cell lung cancer: a meta-analysis. *Ann Intern Med* 1996; **125**: 723–9.
84. Albain KS, Induction chemotherapy followed by definitive local control for stage III non-small cell lung cancer. a review with focus on recent trimodality trials. *Chest* 1993; **103**: 43s–50s.
85. Friedland DM, Comis RL, Perioperative therapy of non-small cell lung cncer: a review of adjuvant and neoadjuvant approaches. *Semin Oncol*, l995; **22**: 571–81.
86. Johnson DH, Piantidosi S, Chemotherapy for resectable stage III non-small cell lung cancer – can *that* dog hunt? *J Natl Cancer Inst* 1994; **86**: 650–1.
87. Shepherd FA, Induction chemotherapy for locally advanced non-small cell lung cancer. *Ann Thorac Surg* 1993; **55**: 1585–92.
88. Pass HI, Pogrebniak HW, Steinberg SM et al, Randomized trial of neoadjuvant therapy for lung cancer: interim analysis. *Ann Thorac Surg* 1992; **53**: 992–8.
89. Rosell R, Gomez-Codina J, Camp C et al, A randomized trial comparing preoperative chemotherapy plus surgery with surgery alone in patients with non-small cell lung cancer. *N Engl J Med* 1994; **330**: 153–8.
90. Roth JA, Atkinson EN, Fossella F et al, Long-term follow-up of patients enrolled in a randomized trial comparing perioperative chemotherapy and surgery with surgery alone in resectable stage IIIA non-small cell lung cancer. *Lung Cancer* 1998; **21**: 1–6.
91. Shepherd FA, Johnston MR, Payne D et al, Randomized study of chemotherapy and surgery versus radiotherapy for stage IIIA non-small-cell lung cancer: a National Cancer Institute of Canada Clinical Trials Group study. *Br J Cancer* 1998; **78**: 683–5.
92. Elias A, Herndorn J, Kumar P et al, for the Cancer and Acute Leukemia Group B, A phase III comparison of 'best local-regional therapy' with or without chemotherapy (CT) for stage IIIA T1–3N2 non-small cell lung cancer (NSCLC): preliminary results. *Proc Am Soc Clin Oncol* 1997; **16**: 448a (Abst 1611).
93. Depierre A, Milleron B, Lebeau B et al, An ongoing randomized study of neoadjuvant chemotherapy in resectable non-small cell lung cancer. *Semin Oncol* 1994; **21**(Suppl 14), 16–19.
94. Ellis PA, Smith IE, Hardy JR et al, Symptom relief with MVP (mitomycin C, vinblastine and cisplatin) chemotherapy in advanced non-small cell lung cancer. *Br J Cancer* 1995; **71**: 366–70.
95. Cormier Y, Bergeron D, La Forge J et al, Benefits of polychemotherapy in advanced non-small-cell bronchogenic carcinoma. *Cancer* 1982; **50**: 845–9.
96. Ganz PA, Figlin RA, Haskell CM, Supportive care versus supportive care and combination chemotherapy in metastatic non-small cell lung cancer. *Cancer* 1989; **63**: 1271–8.
97. Woods RL, Williams CJ, Levi J et al, A randomized trial of cisplatin and vindesine versus supportive care only in advanced non-small cell lung cancer. *Br J Cancer* 1990; **61**: 608–11.
98. Cellerino R, Tummarello D, Guidi F, A randomized trial of alternating chemotherapy versus best supportive care in advanced non-small cell lung cancer. *J Clin Oncol* 1991; **9**: 1453–61.

99. Kaasa S, Lund E, Thorud E et al, Symptomatic treatment versus combination chemotherapy for patients with extensive non-small cell lung cancer. *Cancer* 1991; **67**: 2443–7.
100. Quoix E, Dietemann A, Charbonneau J et al, La chimiothérapie comportant du cisplative est-elle utile dans le cancer bronchique non microcelluleve au stad IV? Resultats d'une étude randomisée. *Bull Cancer* 1991; **78**: 341–6.
101. Souquet P, Chauvin F, Boissel JP et al, Polychemotherapy in advanced non-small cell lung cancer: a meta-analysis. *Lancet* 1993; **342**: 19–21.
102. Jaakkimainen L, Goodwin PJ, Pater J et al, Counting the costs of chemotherapy in a National Cancer Institute of Canada randomized trial in non-small cell lung cancer. *J Clin Oncol* 1990; **8**: 1301–9.
103. Smith TJ, Hillner BE, Neighbors DM et al, Ecomonic evaluation of a randomized clinical trial comparing vinorelbine, vinorelbine plus cisplatin and vindesine plus cisplatin for non-small cell lung cancer. *J Clin Oncol* 1995; **13**: 2166–73.
104. Sandler A, Nemunaitis J, Denham C et al, Phase III study of cisplatin (C) with or without gemcitabine (G) in patients with advanced non-small cell lung cancer (NSCLC). *Proc Am Soc Clin Oncol* 1998; **17**: 454a (Abst 1747).
105. von Pawel J, von Roemeling R, Survival benefit from tirazone (tirapazamine) and cisplatin in advanced non-small cell lung cancer (NSCLC) patients: final results from the international phase III CATAPULT 1 trial. *Proc Am Soc Clin Oncol* 1998; **17**: 454a (Abst 1749).
106. Gatzemeier U, von Pawel J, Gottfried M et al, Phase III comparative study of high-dose cisplatin (HD-Cis) versus a combination of paclitaxel (TAX) and cisplatin (Cis) in patients with advanced non-small cell lung cancer (NSCLC). *Proc Am Soc Clin Oncol* 1998; **17**: 454a (Abst 1748).
107. Manegold C, Bergman B, Chemaissani A et al, Single agent gemcitabine versus cisplatin–etoposide: early results of a randomized phase II study in locally advanced or metastatic non-small cell lung cancer. *Ann Oncol* 1997; **8**: 525–9.
108. Perng RP, Chen Y, Ming-Liu J et al, Gemcitabine versus the combination of cisplatin and etoposide in patients with inoperable non-small cell lung cancer in a phase II randomized study. *J Clin Oncol* 1997; **15**: 2097–102.
109. Belani CP, Natale RB, Lee JS et al, Randomized phase 3 trial comparing cisplatin/etoposide versus carboplatin/paclitaxel in advanced and metastatic non-small cell lung cancer (NSCLC). *Proc Am Soc Clin Oncol* 1998; **17**: 455a (Abst 1751).
110. Cardenal F, Rosell, R, Anton A et al, Gemcitabine + cisplatin versus etoposide + cisplatin in advanced non-small cell lung cancer patients: preliminary randomized phase III results. *Proc Am Soc Clin Oncol* 1997; **16**: 458a (Abst 1648).
111. Crino L, Conte P, De Marinis F et al, A randomized trial of gemcitabine cisplatin (GP) versus mitomycin, ifosfamide and cisplatin (MIC) in advanced non-small cell lung cancer (NSCLC). A multi-centre phase III study. *Proc Am Soc Clin Oncol* 1998; **17**: 455a (Abst 1751).
112. Comella P, Panza N, Frasci G et al, Gemcitabine (GEM)–cisplatin (CDDP)–vinorelbine (VNR) combination in advanced non-small cell lung cancer (NSCLC). A phase II randomized study. *Proc Am Soc Clin Oncol* 1997; **16**: 449a (Abst 1616).
113. Frasci G, Panza N, Comella P et al, Cisplatin, gemcitabine and vinorelbine in locally advanced or metastatic non-small cell lung cancer: a phase I study. *Ann Oncol* 1997; **8**: 1045–8.

12 Treatment of Small Cell Lung Cancer

12.1 Treatment of SCLC: Surgery

Hisao Asamura, Robert J Ginsberg

Contents

INTRODUCTION

The role of surgery in the management of small cell lung cancer (SCLC) remains a controversial and as yet undecided issue despite re-examination of this role over the past 15 years. In 1969, the report by the British Medical Research Council demonstrated the failure of surgery alone to control this disease when compared to radiotherapy.[1,2] Although the results of this trial set the standards for non-surgical treatment for SCLC thereafter, this study must be criticized from the present view point for the following issues:

- SCLC located in the peripheral lung was excluded from the study, since only tumors diagnosed by rigid bronchoscopy prior to the treatment were enrolled.
- Complete resection of the tumor could be achieved in only 48% of the patients assigned to the 'surgery' arm.
- No intraoperative staging was done.
- Modern clinical staging techniques (CT scan and mediastinoscopy) were not used.

In the late 1960s and mid-1970s, surgery for early stage SCLC was championed by other reports, where survival was significant for tumors located in the periphery of the lung confined to the lung, with N0 status, and treated by lobectomy.[3,4] Reports in the late 1970s and early 1980s further demonstrated that surgical therapy alone could provide curative treatment in up to 25% of such patients.[5,6] A report by the Veterans Administration Surgical Oncology Group showed a 23% five-year survival rate for 132 patients resected, and concluded that resection was definitely indicated in patients with T1N0 lesions and probably indicated in those with T1N1 or T2N0 lesions.[6]

With the addition of postoperative chemotherapy, even better long-term survival in this very early stage of the disease has been reported. In stage I disease, up to 70% of patients will be cured. In more advanced disease (stages II and IIIa), when the tumor is totally excised at surgery and treated with postoperative chemotherapy, five-year survivals in the range of 20–30% can be expected.[7,8] However, like non-small cell lung cancer (NSCLC), the prognosis of patients with N2 disease is quite poor, and the chance of successful surgical intervention is least.[9,10]

The role of surgery in multimodality therapy to improve control of the primary site has been investigated by utilizing induction chemotherapy prior to surgical resection.[11–13] These programs have also included consolidation chemotherapy as well as mediastinal radiotherapy with or without prophylactic cranial irradiation.

The final role that has been suggested for surgery in the treatment of SCLC is that of 'salvage' treatment when primary chemoradiation fails to control the local disease or when recurrence occurs and only the primary site is affected.[14] In these instances, surgical treatment after reinduction chemotherapy has been utilized as a 'salvage' procedure.

Presently, chemoradiotherapy is the standard treatment for limited-stage SCLC.[15] However, preoperatively undiagnosed tumors, especially clinical T1 and T2N0 disease in peripheral locations, have continued to be resected by surgeons.

PRIMARY SURGERY

Complete resection of SCLC, often without prior knowledge of the cell type, will result in significant five-year survival. Several reports have suggested that early stage SCLC can be cured by surgical resection alone (Table 12.1.1). For instance, Shah et al[16] retrospectively analyzed the prognosis of 28 patients who received surgery alone for SCLC, and reported a five-year survival rate of 43.3%, and have stated that the prospects of cure by operation are similar to those with NSCLC. However, the most recent series reporting their data suggest that postoperative chemotherapy is a necessary part of treatment (Table 12.1.1). In most centers, following surgical resection, a minimum of four to six courses of adequate two- or three-drug regimen chemotherapy is advised. In a cooperative international lung cancer multimodality treatment trial, 112 patients with SCLC underwent initial surgical resection and were then randomized to receive one of two intensive postoperative chemotherapy regimens.[17] The projected 36-month survival rate for 43 patients with N0 disease was 65%; for 43 with N1 disease, it was 52%; and for 26 with N2 disease, it was 29%. If hilar and mediastinal lymph node disease is found at the time of surgery, postoperative mediastinal irradiation is also advised, although its role is not certain. The role of prophylactic cranial irradiation has also yet to be decided.

It is difficult to compare this multimodality surgical approach versus chemoradiation alone, since medical oncologists on the whole do not classify these 'very limited' tumors as a separate entity.[18] However, despite this, some retrospective analyses have been performed. Osterlind et al[19] in a retrospective analysis failed to demonstrate any beneficial effect for surgical resection. While they demonstrated a significantly better prognosis of 79 patients who met criteria for surgical resectability prior to treatment than that of 696 patients who did not, there was no significant difference in survival between 33 operated and 46 non-operated patients. Again in this study, however, only 33% of the operated patients underwent complete resection, which suggested that the criteria for resectability were not predictive enough and the unfavorable statement by Osterlind et al regarding the benefit of surgery was not conclusive. On the other hand, the Toronto Group,[13] in a retrospective analysis, has suggested a twofold improvement in survival when surgery is part of the treatment, by improving control of the primary site. It must be emphasized that the description of stage of patients in such a study by not only limited disease (LD)–extensive disease (ED) but also the tumor, node, metastasis (TNM) system is crucial to make the comparison possible between primary surgery and chemoradiation alone.

INDUCTION CHEMOTHERAPY PLUS ADJUVANT SURGERY

The role of surgery in more-proximal tumors with clinical N1 or minimal N2 disease (but still resectable by NSCLC criteria) is less apparent.

Table 12.1.1 Primary surgery for SCLC

Author	Number of patients	Median survival (months)	Five-year survival rate (%)
(a) Surgery + chemotherapy			
ISC–LCSG[23]	183		63[a] (TN0M0)
			37[b] (TN2M0)
Coolen[24]		15	27
			60 (stage I)
Davis[25]	37		50 (stage I)
			35 (stage II)
			21 (T3N2)
Muller[26]	45	18	36
			57 (stage I)
			28 (stage II)
			34 (stage IIIa)
Toronto Group[12]	79	21	40
Salzer[10]	25		25 (N2 disease)
Osterlind (1989)[27]	25		23[b]
Ohta[28]	52		31
SWOG[29]	15	25	44
[a]30-month survival. [b]3-year survival.			
(b) Surgery ± chemotherapy			
Lucchi[30]	127	18	22.6
			47.2 (stage I)
			14.8 (stage II)
			14.4 (stage III)
Miyazawa[31]	12		50 (latter period)
	25		8 (former period)
Merkle[32]	170		18
Maassen[33]	124		20
(c) Surgery alone			
Coolen[24]	15		13
			12 (stage I)
Shah[16]	28		43.3
			57.1 (stage I)
			55.5 (stage II)
Sorensen[34]	76		12
Shore[35]	40		27

Table 12.1.2 Induction chemotherapy followed by surgery for SCLC: the Toronto Group results

Stage	Number of patients	Median survival (years)	Estimated five-year survival rate (%)
Overall	38	1.8	38
N0	11	Not reached	45
N1	13	1.3	30
N2	14	1	40

Very few induction chemotherapy trials have been reported. The experiences of the Toronto Group[12] and the Innsbruck Group[10] suggest that, with this combined-modality treatment, utilizing surgery as an adjuvant, five-year survival rates in the rage of 40% can be obtained (Table 12.1.2). Those tumors with good responses to chemotherapy, having been downstaged by the time of surgery to an N0 level, have a five-year survival rate as high as a 60–70%. Persisting nodal disease yields a less satisfactory 20–30% five-year survival rate. An interesting side-light of such therapy is the fact that many of the resected tumors contain no remaining SCLC, but do contain persisting elements of NSCLC.

The North American Lung Cancer Study Group[20] reported the results of a randomized trial comparing the non-surgical with the adjuvant surgical approach in limited disease (Figure 12.1.1). Although most of the 146 patients randomized following induction chemotherapy were initially staged as 'limited' (versus 'very limited'), the results of this randomized trial showed no difference in survival of either arm. In 70 patients in the surgery group, complete resection was possible in 77%, and the pathologic complete response rate after induction chemotherapy was 19% compared with the clinical complete response rate of 40%. This study also failed a subset analysis that attempted to isolate the 'very limited' group, although very few patients were included in this subset.

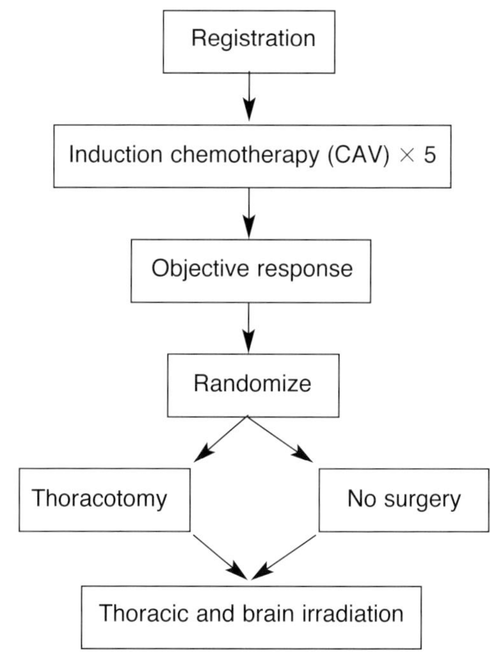

Figure 12.1.1
Study design of Lung Cancer Study Group Study 832.

It is fair to say that certain centers still believe in the value of surgery as an adjuvant treatment to control the primary site in 'very limited' SCLC where surgical resection would have been advised for patients had they had non-small cell disease. In our opinion, it still is appropriate to investigate adjuvant surgery in a prospective randomized trial confined to this 'very limited' small cell group.

Recently, Eberhardt et al[21] have reported an excellent local control and remarkable long-term survival in LD-SCLC patients undergoing aggressive trimodality treatment. Of 46 patients with LD-SCLC undergoing induction therapy (chemotherapy for stage I/II; chemoradiotherapy including hyperfractionated accelerated radiotherapy for stage IIIA/IIIB), 32 patients underwent surgical resection, with a complete resection rate of 72%. Eberhardt et al have reported that the median survival and the five-year survival rate of all 46 patients were 36 months and 46%, respectively. In particular, for 32 completely resected patients, 68 months and 63% were reported, as well as a 100% local control rate. This kind of aggressive multimodality approach using intensive local therapy such as surgery and hyperfractionated accelerated radiotherapy might be promising in the treatment of potentially resectable LD-SCLC, and may be one of the future directions for trials for these patients. However, morbidity and mortality must be carefully audited when using this aggressive approach.

SALVAGE SURGERY

The Toronto Group has promulgated the concept of 'salvage' surgery for SCLC persisting in the primary site after induction treatment or recurring only in the primary site following a complete response.[14] Patients with mixed SCLC/NSCLC at diagnosis and persistent NSCLC after induction chemotherapy are also prime candidate for this type of surgery. In such instances, mediastinoscopy is utilized to eliminate patients with unresectable disease. In the Toronto study, 28 patients with limited SCLC who did not have a complete remission with standard treatment, or who had only local recurrence after treatment and appeared to be completely resectable, underwent surgery. Pathologic examination showed only SCLC in 18 patients, mixed SCLC and NSCLC in 4 and only NSCLC in 6. A median survival of 74 weeks and a five-year survival rate of 23% were reported. This report by the Toronto Group suggests the existence of occasional SCLC patients who will benefit from salvage surgery after relapse or failure to respond to chemotherapy and radiotherapy.

Although this 'salvage' type of operation has only allowed a handful of long-term survivors, it is rare that reinduction chemotherapy and radiotherapy in locally recurrent or persistent disease even result in long-term disease-free survival.

DISCUSSION

The role of surgery in the treatment of SCLC has yet to be clearly defined. As stated earlier, surgery for SCLC may be employed in three different situations:

- primary surgery followed by chemo(radio)-therapy in N0 disease;
- adjuvant surgery following induction chemo(radio)therapy in N2 disease;
- salvage surgery for local persistence or recurrence.

There is no doubt that surgeons will continue to operate on peripheral nodules when the diagnosis is uncertain or in question. Also, until the results of non-surgical treatment for these peripheral tumors are known, surgery still offers the best hope of permanent cure. Following surgical excision, postoperative chemotherapy appears to be advantageous. The exact role of 'adjuvant surgery' for central 'very limited' disease clinically staged as I, II or IIIa has yet to be fully defined. Certainly, the report of the North American Lung Cancer Study Group suggests no difference in survival benefit in those patients with limited (versus 'very limited') disease treated with the addition of surgery. Finally, there will be patients who have failed at the primary site and still have disease of a limited nature. In these rare individuals, 'salvage' surgery may be indicated.

The International Association for the Study of Lung Cancer (IASLC) has published a consensus report regarding SCLC,[22] in which the following important points were stated:

- The contribution of surgery, postoperative chemotherapy or postoperative radiotherapy to survival has not been well defined.
- There may be a role for surgery in the small proportion of patients with very localized tumors, especially if they are in the peripheral lung.

Future clinical trials should be aimed at clarifying the role of surgery in each individual setting of treatment as primary surgery, adjuvant surgery and salvage surgery.

REFERENCES

1. Miller AB, Fox W, Tall R, Five-year follow-up of the Medical Research Council's comparative trial of surgery and radiotherapy for the primary treatment of small-celled or oat-celled carcinoma of the bronchus. *Lancet* 1969; **ii**: 501–5.
2. Fox W, Scadding JG, Medical Research Council comparative trial of surgery and radiotherapy for primary treatment of small-celled or oat-celled carcinoma of the bronchus: ten year follow-up. *Lancet* 1973; **ii**: 63–5.
3. Lennox SC, Flavell G, Pollock DJ, Results of resection for oat-cell carcinoma of the lung. *Lancet* 1968; **ii**: 925–7.
4. Higgins GA, Shields TW, Keehn RJ, The solitary pulmonary nodule. Ten year follow-up of Veterans Administration Armed Forces Cooperative Study. *Arch Surg* 1975; **110**: 570–5.
5. Mountain CF, Clinical biology of small cell lung cancer: relationship to surgical therapy. *Semin Oncol* 1978; **5**: 272–9.
6. Shields TW, Higgins GA, Matthews NJ, Kiihn RJ, Surgical resection in the management of small-cell carcinoma of the lung. *J Thorac Cardiovasc Surg* 1982; **84**: 481–8.
7. Karrer K, Shields TW, Denck H et al, The importance of surgical and multimodality treatment for small cell bronchial carcinoma. *J Thorac Cardiovasc Surg* 1989; **97**: 168–76.
8. Shepherd FA, Ginsberg RJ, Evans WK et al, Reduction in local recurrence and improved survival in surgically treated patients with small cell lung cancer. *J Thorac Cardiovasc Surg* 1983; **89**: 498–506.
9. Meyer JA, Gullo JJ, Ikins PM et al, Adverse prognostic effect of N2 disease in treatment of small cell carcinoma of the lung. *J Thorac Cardiovasc Surg* 1984; **88**: 495–501.
10. Salzer GM, Muller LC, Huber H et al, Operation for N2 small cell lung carcinoma. *Ann Thorac Surg* 1990; **49**: 759–62.
11. Shepherd FA, Ginsberg RJ, Patterson GA et al, A prospective study of adjuvant surgical resection after chemotherapy for limited small cell lung cancer: a University of Toronto Lung Oncology Group study. *J Thorac Cardiovasc Surg* 1989; **97**: 177–86.
12. Shepherd FA, Ginsberg RJ, Feld R et al, Surgical treatment for limited small-cell lung cancer. The University of Toronto Lung Oncology Group experience. *J Thorac Cardiovasc Surg* 1991; **101**: 385–93.
13. Prager RL, Foster JM, Hainworth JD et al, The feasibility of adjuvant surgery in limited-stage small cell carcinoma: a prospective evaluation. *Ann Thorac Surg* 1984; **38**: 622–6.
14. Shepherd FA, Ginsberg R, Patterson GA et al, Is

there ever a role for salvage operations in limited small-cell lung cancer? *J Thorac Cardiovasc Surg* 1991; **101**: 196–200.
15. Livingston RB, Current chemotherapy of small cell lung cancer. *Chest* 1986; **89**: 2585–625.
16. Shah SS, Thompson J, Goldstraw P, Results of operation without adjuvant therapy in the treatment of small cell lung cancer. *Ann Thorac Surg* 1992; **54**: 498–501.
17. Karrer K, Shields TW, Denck H, The importance of surgical and multimodality treatment for small cell bronchial carcinoma. *J Thorac Cardiovasc Surg* 1989; **97**: 168–76.
18. Shepherd FA, Ginsberg R, Evans WK et al, 'Very limited' small cell lung cancer (SCLC): results of non-surgical treatment. *Proc Am Soc Clin Oncol* 1984; **2**: 223 (Abst C-870).
19. Osterlind K, Hansen M, Hansen HH et al, Treatment policy of surgery in small cell carcinoma of the lung: retrospective analysis of a series of 874 consecutive patients. *Thorax* 1985; **40**: 272–7.
20. Lad T, Piantadosi S, Thomas P et al, A prospective randomized trial to determine the benefit of surgical resection of residual disease following response of small cell lung cancer to combination chemotherapy. *Chest* 1994; **106**: 320s–3s.
21. Eberhardt W, Stamatis G, Stuschke H et al, Aggressive trimodality treatment including chemoradiation induction and surgery (S) in LD-small-cell lung cancer (LD-SCLC) (stages I–IIIB). Long-term results. *Proc Am Soc Clin Oncol* 1998; **17**: 450a
22. Ihde D, Souhami B, Comis R et al, Consensus report: small cell lung cancer. *Lung Cancer* 1997; **17**: 19s-21s.
23. Karrer K, Ulsperger E, Surgery for cure followed by chemotherapy in small cell carcinoma of the lung. *Acta Oncol* 1995; **34**: 899–906.
24. Coolen L, van den Eeckhout A, Deneffe G et al, Surgical treatment of small cell lung cancer. *Eur J Cardio-thorac Surg* 1995; **9**: 59–64.
25. Davis S, Crino L, Tonato M et al, A prospective analysis of chemotherapy following surgical resection of clinical stage I–II small-cell lung cancer. *Am J Clin Oncol* 1993; **16**: 93–5.
26. Muller LC, Salzer G, Huber H et al, Multimodal therapy of small cell lung cancer in TNM stages I through IIIa. *Ann Thorac Surg* 1992; **54**: 493–7.
27. Osterlind K, Hansen M, Hansen HH et al, Influence of surgical resection prior to chemotherapy on the long-term results in small cell lung cancer. A study of 150 operable patients. *Eur J Cancer Clin Oncol* 1986; **22**: 589–93.
28. Ohta M, Hara N, Ichinose Y, The role of surgical resection in the management of small cell carcinoma of the lung. *Jpn J Clin Oncol* 1986; **16**: 289–96.
29. Friess GG, McCracken JD, Troxell ML et al, Effect of initial resection of small-cell carcinoma of the lung: a review of Southwest Oncology Group Study 7628. *J Clin Oncol* 1985; **3**: 964–8.
30. Lucchi M, Mussi A, Chella A et al, Surgery in the management of small cell lung cancer. *Eur J Cardio-thorac Surg* 1997; **12**: 689–93.
31. Miyazawa N, Tsuchiya R, Naruke T et al, A clinicopathological study of surgical treatment of small cell carcinoma of the lung. *Jpn J Clin Oncol* 1986; **16**: 297–307.
32. Merkle NM, Mickisch GH, Kayser K et al, Surgical resection and adjuvant chemotherapy for small cell carcinoma. *Thorac Cardiovasc Surg* 1986; **34**: 39–42.
33. Maassen W, Greschuchna D, Small cell carcinoma of the lung – to operate or not? Surgical experience and results. *Thorac Cardiovasc Surg* 1986; **34**: 71–6.
34. Sorensen HR, Lund C, Alstrup P, Survival in small cell lung carcinoma after surgery. *Thorax* 1986; **41**: 478–82.
35. Shore DF, Paneth M, Survival after resection of small cell carcinoma of the bronchus. *Thorax* 1980; **35**: 819–22

12.2 Treatment of SCLC: Radiotherapy

Anna Gregor, William T Sause

Contents Introduction • Where are we now? • Current recommendations • Radiotherapy for symptom control • Future directions

INTRODUCTION

Radiotherapy has provided the single most significant incremental survival improvement for patients with small cell lung cancer (SCLC) in the last decade. The chemosensitivity and often disseminated nature of SCLC make systemic chemotherapy the logical first-line treatment choice, and for a long time it directed efforts in clinical research. Currently available and previously tested chemotherapy strategies, such as maintenance and the use of hybrid non-cross-resistant regimens, have not led to major improvements in long-term survival (see Chapter 12.3), and over 90% of SCLC patients continue to relapse and ultimately die with chemoresistant and widespread tumors. SCLC is known to be highly radiosensitive, and radiotherapy has been widely used in the treatment of this disease entity for a decade. Furthermore, important prognostic factors predicting long-term survival have been identified, and allow patient categorization at the time of diagnosis and first-line induction therapy.

In the 'good-prognosis' group of patients with limited disease (LTD), good performance status, normal biochemistry, no significant weight loss and major response to induction chemotherapy, intrathoracic relapse at the primary site of the tumor and brain metastases are two common sites of failure. Thoracic irradiation (TI) and prophylactic cranial irradiation (PCI) have been known for more than a decade to halve the incidence of relapse at these sites.[1–3] The lack of demonstrable survival benefit in individual clinical trials, as well as legitimate concerns about the increased short-term toxicity of TI and significant long-term side-effects associated with the use of PCI, have tempered enthusiasm for their routine use.

Two events changed the scenario. The first was a series of overviews[1–6] and a meta-analysis[7] that demonstrated that a 30% reduction in intrathoracic failure rate led to a 7% improvement in two-year survival. The second was a series of PCI trials[8–11] and a meta-analysis[12] that confirmed the ability of moderate doses of PCI to significantly reduce brain metastases with no demonstrable increase in central nervous system (CNS) toxicity as well as the small, but consistently observed, survival benefits associated with PCI. Both TI and PCI are therefore recommended as a standard treatment policy for the subgroup of SCLC patients with realistic prospects of long-term survival.

WHERE ARE WE NOW?

Thoracic irradiation

Many practical issues, such as radiation dose, volume, fractionation and optimal integration with chemotherapy, remain unresolved. Trying to 'fine-tune' combined-modality treatment for

SCLC is a formidable challenge. The individual benefits attributable to the different parts of this puzzle are likely to be numerically small, and manipulation of one aspect may produce a cascade of events with conflicting effects on overall outcome. These methodological problems have resulted in real difficulty in designing appropriate and randomized trials addressing these questions.

No large randomized trials have looked at *radiation dose* as the only variable. Retrospective analyses of studies of thoracic radiation used after cyclophosphamide- and doxorubicin-containing chemotherapy regimens suggest that radiation doses as high as 50–60 Gy are necessary for durable local control.[2,5] Using concurrent TI and cisplatin/etoposide (PE) chemotherapy, lower doses such as 45 Gy in 25 fractions appear to be adequate.[13] Whether this will achieve durable local control with prolonged survival is unknown.

A further practical question concerns the *target volume* for thoracic irradiation. The tradition of irradiating large volumes covering all 'prechemotherapy tumor involvement' with generous margins or prophylactic irradiation of distant lymphatic drainage sites may not be necessary, and more modest radiation treatment volumes will lead to lower rates of serious pulmonary toxicity.[5,13–17]

Several phase II studies of radiation given in multiple daily fractions (MDF),[17,18] either concurrently with cisplatin and etoposide or in an interdigitated sequence, have been followed in a large intergroup randomized trial.[19] In this study, 417 patients were treated with concurrent TI starting with the first cycle of PE chemotherapy and randomized between a standard schedule (1.8 Gy in 25 daily fractions over five weeks) or hyperfractionated schedule (45 Gy in 1.5 Gy fractions twice daily over three weeks). With mature follow-up (median eight years) the two-year survival rate is 43.8% overall, 40.8% for the daily and 46.6% for the twice-daily fractionation arm ($p=0.067$), with an estimated hazard ratio of 1.23 (95% confidence interval 0.99–1.54). The hyperfractionated arm had higher rates of esophagitis, but overall only 2.7% treatment-associated mortality was reported. This suggests that a regimen of four courses of PE chemotherapy and concurrent irradiation is safe in a multicenter intergroup setting. The five-year survival rates were 16% and 26% respectively, which is highly encouraging, and provides a benchmark that needs to be replicated in non-trial clinical treatment setting.

The issue of *radiotherapy timing* is also not resolved. An early three-arm randomized Cancer and Acute Leukemia Group B (CALGB) trial[20] suggested that best survival/toxicity ratio can be obtained by delaying radiation until the fourth cycle of chemotherapy. This was due to high rates of treatment-related fatalities in schedules using concurrent radiation and cyclophosphamide, methotrexate, lomustine and doxorubicin. More recently, a Canadian trial produced significant survival advantage for early (cycle 2) concurrent radiotherapy with a schedule of alternating cycloposphamide, doxorubicin (Adriamycin) and vincristine (CAV) and PE.[21] An ongoing Japanese study[22] also suggests improvement with early scheduling of TI, while such an effect has not been observed in other studies (Table 12.2.1)

Attempts to introduce radiotherapy early into the overall treatment scheme increase toxicity and limit the choice of chemotherapy to these agents without sensitizing properties for critical normal tissues. Strategies aimed at reducing the risks of toxicity have included evaluation of alternating schedules. Series of non-randomized studies by French collaborative groups[23,24] have reported encouraging results, and the concept has been tested in a randomized trial by the European Organization for Research and Treatment of Cancer (EORTC) Lung Cancer Group.[25] In this

Table 12.2.1 Trials testing the timing of thoracic irradiation

Trial	Number of patients	Start of radiotherapy (day)	Two-year survival rate (%)	Significance
CALGB	125	1	24	0.08
	145	64	30	
NCIC	155	22	40	0.008
	153	106	33	
Aarhus	97	1	20	ns[a]
	98	126	18	
Ljubljana	52	1	71	0.052
	51	36	53	
Takada	115	2	36 months[b]	
	116	84	21 months[b]	

[a]ns, not significant.
[b]Median survival.

trial, the survival of the 286 randomized patients was similar in both arms, and acute toxicities were more frequent and severe using the alternating approach, which was also more demanding for patients and health care resources. Thus alternating schedules cannot be recommended for use in routine clinical practice.

Brain metastases

Brain metastases are common sites of failure in SCLC. At diagnosis, 20% of patients have evidence of spread into the brain, which rises to 50% at two years and to more than 80% at post mortem.[26] The concept of PCI, taken from settings such as acute lymphoblastic leukemia, demonstrated 20 years ago that moderate radiation doses can significantly reduce the rate of brain metastases.[11,20,27,28] In these small historical trials, no evidence of survival benefit was seen, and the short overall survival underestimated the size of the observed risk. In addition, emerging reports of CNS morbidity[29] tempered the enthusiasm for PCI. Nevertheless, the problem of CNS disease and its control has continued to involve clinical practice. The modest effectiveness of radiotherapy or chemotherapy for patients with established brain metastases as well as their functional consequences[3,29–33] and negative impact on quality of life has lead to re-evaluation of PCI in a series of second-generation trials. These were designed to address issues of effectiveness as well as morbidity.

The choice of radiation dose in these trials was empirical. The relative radioresponsiveness of SCLC and the presumption that subclinical, small-volume disease will be sterilized by modest radiation doses informed the first generation of PCI trials. Concerns about toxicity led to further reductions in total dose and individual fraction sizes. The optimal dose of PCI remains unknown. The only trial designed to address this issue showed a radiation dose–response relationship, and demonstrated the lack of effectiveness of 24 Gy in 2 Gy fractions.[11] The biological effectiveness of total radiation dose can possibly be augmented by increasing the individual radiation fraction size,[3,8,10] but this strategy may lead to increased risk of late CNS toxicity.

The optimal timing of PCI administration is also unknown, and will be governed by the choice of the chemotherapy regimen as well as by patient characteristics. No randomized comparisons have been performed. Most of the available studies used postchemotherapy PCI administration, which allows selection of patients with good response to chemotherapy and reasonably good predicted survival.

Most of the low-to-moderate PCI dose schedules reduce and delay, but do not abolish, the risk of CNS metastases. Their effectiveness and how it is perceived will be influenced by the length of observation, i.e. length of patient survival, which is in turn critically dependent on patient selection and the effectiveness of systemic therapy. A review of available studies suggests that halving the actuarial risk at any time point should be the minimum effect achievable – for example from 50% to 25% at two years.

Toxicity of PCI is a major concern – particularly late CNS morbidity, which has a profound impact on functional outcome and quality of life. Most of the available evidence comes from non-randomized retrospective surveys or recall assessments and is limited to small numbers of highly selected long-term survivors. Most of these patients were treated with neurotoxic chemotherapy regimens as well as radiation. More recent studies have failed to confirm the high rates and severity of impairment.[8,11] Interestingly a large proportion (40%) of patients with SCLC have neuropsychometric deficits before PCI.[32,33]

CURRENT RECOMMENDATIONS

Radiotherapy plays an important role in the treatment of SCLC patients. Its optimal utilization requires close collaboration between all the specialists involved in the care of these patients, and thoracic radiation oncologists should be an intrinsic part of the multidisciplinary team. Only in this way can safe and speedy progress be made.

'Good-prognosis' patients with SCLC should be managed by specialists using a formal multimodality protocol of treatment, and preferably in the context of a clinical trial. The clinical practice in many centers is to use concurrent chemotherapy with PE chemotherapy and 45 Gy of irradiation delivered in daily fractions of 1.8–2 Gy and starting with or shortly after the second course of chemotherapy. Concurrent chemoradiotherapy with drugs other than cisplatin and etoposide may necessitate dose modifications and reductions on the grounds of toxicity.

Outside clinical trials, an alternative approach to combined-modality treatment would be for TI at a dose of 50–55 Gy in 2–2.5 Gy fractions to be delivered to responding patients no later than four to five months from the start of therapy. As chemotherapy programs utilize increasingly short and intensive schemes, this should be achievable at the end of chemotherapy. Outside clinical trials, we would recommend once-daily fractionation and avoidance of concurrent chemotherapy on the grounds of safety. These considerations apply to PCI as well as to TI, but the doses are lower (24 Gy in eight fractions, 25 Gy or 30 Gy in ten fractions). TI and PCI can be delivered concurrently.

Having selected the patients who are likely to go on to TI and possibly PCI, it is important to obtain a prechemotherapy radiological series that will inform subsequent radiotherapy planning. As a minimum, this should be a chest X-ray taken supine to mimic the anatomical positions during radiotherapy treatments, but preferably a computed tomography (CT) scan of the thorax and upper abdomen. These must be available, together with a contemporary and comparable series of radiological investigation, to the radiation oncologist at the time of treatment planning.

The decision on what radiotherapy treatment volume to use will depend on:

- the extent of original tumor involvement;
- the degree of response to and the choice of chemotherapy;
- the patient's lung function and performance status;
- the dose, fractionation and timing of the radiotherapy course.

In practice, most radiation oncologists would irradiate areas of prechemotherapy involvement with a margin consistent with safety. This is a minimum of 1 cm on the transverse and 2 cm in the sagittal plane of involvement. Prophylactic irradiation of nodal sites remote from the initial sites of involvement, such as routine irradiation of supraclavicular fossae in patients with upper lobe tumors, is probably not necessary, and adds considerably to toxicity.

Because SCLC often presents with a bulky central tumor and extensive mediastinal involvement, these treatment volumes are large. Irradiation of large intrathoracic tumor volume to a high and homogeneous dose represents a technical challenge. The main trade-offs are between the radiation dose delivered to surrounding normal lung and the radiation tolerance of the spinal cord.

A safe approach requires composite and sophisticated planning techniques, similar to those used in the treatment of NSCLC, often using phased or 'shrinking' field techniques (Figures 12.2.1 and 12.2.2, and see Appendix to Chapter 11.2 on pages 210–12).

The choice of volume for PCI is simple. The entire cranial cavity and contents need to be irradiated, usually using opposing lateral portals. The areas needing particular attention are the meningeal reflections of the cribriform fossa and middle fossa.

TI and PCI administered using conventional doses and fractionation after chemotherapy lead to trivial acute side-effects. Tiredness, esophagitis and lymphopenia are the most common. They are self-limiting, and do not as a rule need anything more than simple symptomatic measures. Administration of concurrent chemotherapy and hyperfractionated accelerated TI regimens are much more toxic, with esophagitis and hematological toxicity often being dose-limiting. These may be slow to recover from, and may compromise further treatment tolerance.

The most significant side-effects are:

- late pulmonary toxicity;
- late CNS toxicity of PCI and spinal cord damage;
- cardiac failure due to irradiation of large areas of the heart and to anthracyclines.

RADIOTHERAPY FOR SYMPTOM CONTROL

The radioresponsiveness of SCLC makes radiotherapy a useful agent for treatment of metastatic recurrent disease in patients resistant to or unsuitable for chemotherapy. The approach will

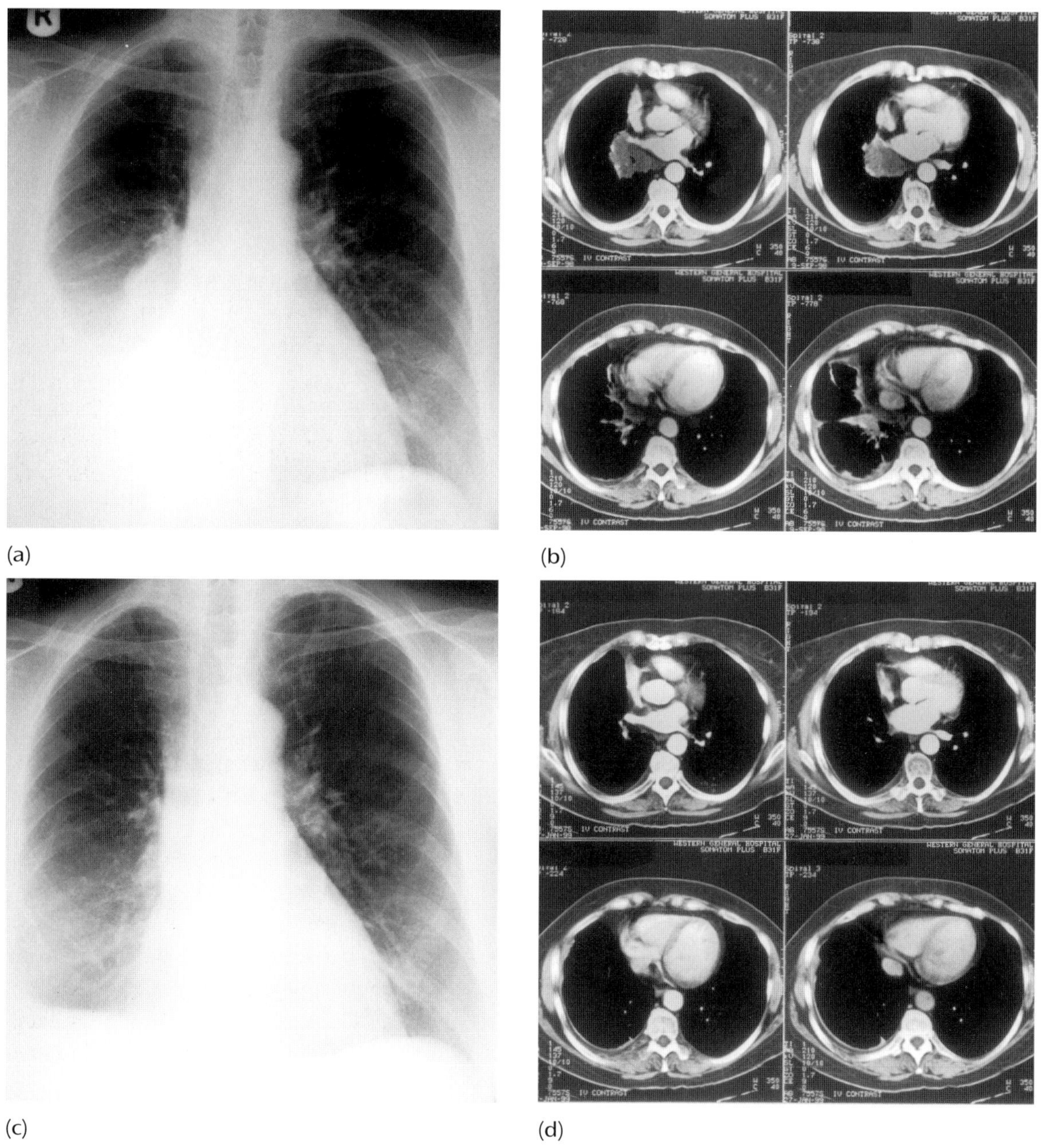

Figure 12.2.1
(a) Prechemotherapy chest X-ray; (b) prechemotherapy CT scan; (c) postchemotherapy chest X-ray; (d) postchemotherapy CT scan.

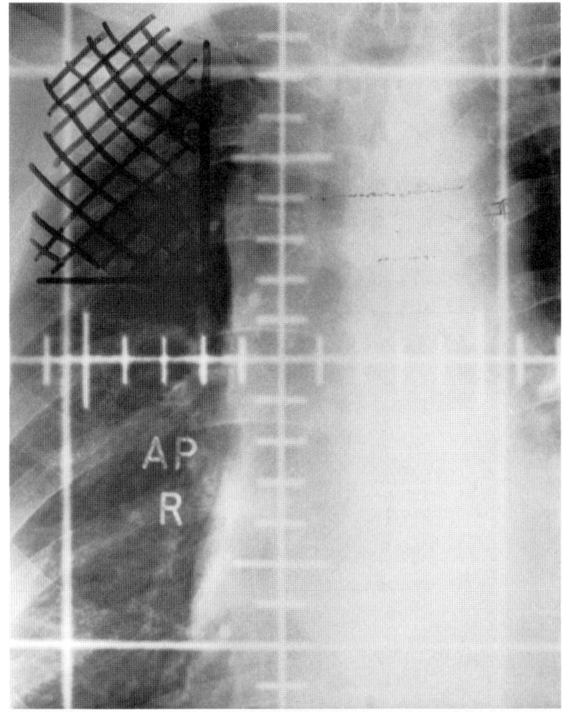

(a)

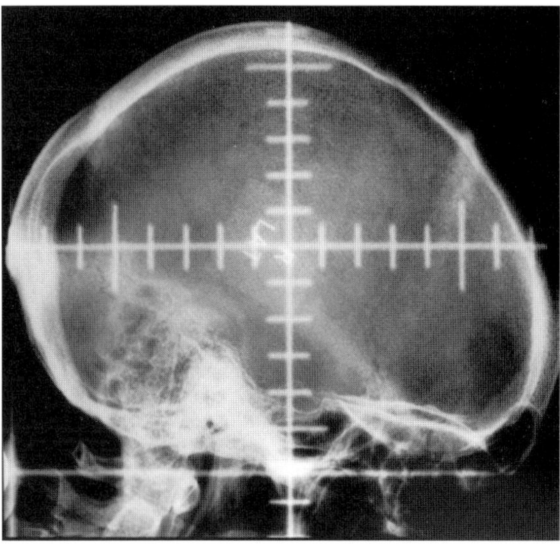

(b)

Figure 12.2.2
(a) TI portal simulator film; (b) PCI portal simulator film.

best be individualized and similar to that used in non-small cell lung cancer. In general, short and undemanding courses of irradiation including single-fraction treatments can be used, aimed at symptom control through tumor shrinkage and associated with little or no additional toxicity. Commonly used regimens include 20 Gy in five fractions or single treatments of 8–10 Gy.

FUTURE DIRECTIONS

Clinical trials are necessary to evaluate optimal *TI schedules*. The current vogue for accelerated hyperfractionated regimens, with their additional levels of acute toxicity, needs to be critically evaluated. The optimization of *scheduling of TI and chemotherapy* is another area where further work is needed. The current evidence suggests that earlier is better – but how early is unknown, and concurrent radiochemotherapy from days 1 to 21 determines the choice of chemotherapy regimen and limits patient eligibility.

Prospective randomized trials of large versus small *treatment volumes* of TI would help to inform planning decision as well as facilitate the introduction of newer radiation techniques, such as conformal radiotherapy planning and beam-intensity modulation.

The use of radiosensitizing agents, particularly if they have tumor specificity, would be welcome in helping to reduce pulmonary toxicity.

In PCI, the question of dose and schedule needs second- and third-generation clinical trials, which are being planned. Continual toxicity surveillance of long-term survivors is needed to monitor late effects.

Formal evaluation of the palliative role of radiotherapy in relapsing patients would help to define the role and value of second- and third-line chemotherapy. Having confirmed the value of irradiation in the management of patients with SCLC, the challenge is to optimize its use.

REFERENCES:

1. Cay P, Hodson I, Murray N et al, Patterns of failure following loco-regional radiotherapy in the treatment of limited stage small cell lung cancer. *Int J Radiat Oncol Biol Phys* 1993; **28**: 355–62.
2. Liengswangwong JA, Bonner EG, Shaw RL et al, Limited stage small cell lung cancer: patterns of intrathoracic recurrence and the implications of thoracic radiotherapy. *J Clin Oncol* 1994; **12**: 496–502.
3. Gregor A, Cranial irradiation in small cell lung cancer. *Br J Cancer* 1991; **63**: 13–14.
4. Warde P, Payne D, Does thoracic irradiation improve survival and local control in limited-stage small cell carcinoma of the lung? *J Clin Oncol* 1992; **6**: 890–5.
5. Turrisi AT, Thoracic radiotherapy variables: influence on local control in small cell lung cancer limited disease. *Int J Radiat Oncol Biol Phys* 1990; **19**: 1473–9.
6. Payne DG, The role of thoracic irradiation therapy in small cell carcinoma of the lung: a consensus report. *Lung Cancer* 1989; **5**: 135–8.
7. Pignon JP, Arriagada R, Ihde D et al, A meta-analysis of thoracic radiotherapy for small cell lung cancer. *N Engl J Med* 1992; **327**: 1618–24.
8. Arriagada R, Le Chevalier T, Borie F et al, Prophylactic cranial irradiation for patients with small cell lung cancer in complete remission. *J Natl Cancer Inst* 1995; **87**: 183–90.
9. Bunn PA, Kelly K, Prophylactic cranial irradiation for patients with small cell lung cancer. *J Natl Cancer Inst* 1995; **87**: 161–2.
10. Brewster AE, Hopwood P, Stout R et al, Single fraction prophylactic cranial irradiation for small cell carcinoma of the lung. *Radiother Oncol* 1995; **34**: 132–6.
11. Gregor A, Cull A, Stephens RJ et al, Prophylactic cranial irradiation is indicated following complete response to induction therapy in small cell lung cancer: results of a multicentre randomized trial. *Eur J Cancer* 1997; **33**: 1752–8.
12. Arriagada R, Auperin A, Pignon J-P et al, Prophylactic cranial irradiation overview in patients with small cell lung cancer in complete remission. *Proc Am Soc Clin Oncol* 1998; **17**: 4571 (abst).
13. Johnston BE, Salen C, Nesbitt J et al, Limited stage small cell lung cancer treated with concurrent hyperfractionated chest radiotherapy etoposide/cisplatin. *Lung Cancer* 1993; **9**: 215–65.
14. Hoskin PJ, Partin D, Yarnold JR et al, Intercalated radiochemotherapy in small cell lung cancer toxicity and implications for future regimens. *Radiother Oncol* 1991; **20**: 177–80.
15. Arriagada R, Kramar A, Le Chevalier T et al, Competing events determining relapse-free survival in limited small-cell lung carcinoma. The French Cancer Centres' Lung Group. *J Clin Oncol* 1992; **10**: 447–51.
16. Brooks BJ Jr, Seifter EJ, Walsh TE et al, Pulmonary toxicity with combined modality therapy for limited stage small-cell lung cancer. *J Clin Oncol* 1986; **4**: 200–9.
17. Kies MS, Mira JC, Livingston RB, Multimodal therapy for limited small cell lung cancer. A randomized study of induction combination chemotherapy with or without thoracic irradiation in complete responders; and with widefield vs reduced volume radiation in partial responders. *J Clin Oncol* 1987; **5**: 592–600.
18. Frytak S, Shaw E, Eagan R et al, Accelerated, hyperfractionated split course thoracic radiotherapy and infusion cisplatin based chemotherapy for small cell lung cancer. *Lung Cancer* 1991; 7(Suppl): 157.
19. Turrisi III AT, Kyungmann K, Blum R et al, Twice-daily compared with once-daily thoracic radiotherapy in limited small-cell lung cancer treated concurrently with cisplatin and etoposide. *N Engl J Med* 1999; **340**: 265–71.

20. Perry MC, Eaton WL, Proport KJ et al, Chemotherapy with or without radiation therapy in small cell carcinoma. *N Engl J Med* 1987; **316**: 912–18.
21. Murray N, Coy P, Pater J et al, Importance of timing for thoracic irradiation in the combined modality treatment of limited stage small cell lung cancer. *J Clin Oncol* 1991; **11**: 336–44.
22. Takada M, Fukuoka M, Furuse K et al, Phase III study of concurrent versus sequential thoracic radiotherapy in combination with cisplatin and etoposide for limited stage small cell lung cancer. *Proc Am Soc Clin Oncol* 1996; **15**: 372.
23. Arriagada R, Le Chevalier T, Baldeyrou P et al, Alternating radiotherapy and chemotherapy schedules in small cell lung cancer limited disease. *Int J Radiat Oncol Biol Phys* 1985; **11**: 1461–7.
24. Arriagada R, Le Chevalier T, Ruffie P et al, Alternating radiotherapy and chemotherapy in 173 consecutive patients with limited small cell lung carcinoma. GROP and the French Cancer Centre's Lung Group. *Int J Radiat Oncol Biol Phys* 1990; **19**: 1135–8.
25. Gregor A, Drings P, Burghouts J et al, Randomized trial of alternating versus sequential radiotherapy/chemotherapy in limited disease patients with small cell lung cancer: an EORTC study. *J Clin Oncol* 1997; **15**: 2840–9.
26. Nugents JL, Bunn PA, Matthews MJ et al, CNS metastases in small-cell bronchogenic carcinoma. Increasing frequency and changing pattern with lengthening survival. *Cancer* 1979; **44**: 1885–93.
27. Hansen HH, Should initial treatment of small cell carcinoma include systemic chemotherapy and brain irradiation? *Cancer Chemother Rep* 1973; **4**: 239–41.
28. Kristjansen PEG, Kristensen CA, The role of prophylactic cranial irradiation in the management of small cell lung cancer. *Cancer Treat Rev* 1993; **19**: 3–16.
29. Lucas CF, Robinson B, Hoskin PJ et al, Morbidity of cranial relapse in SCLC and the impact of radiation therapy. *Cancer Treat Rep* 1986; **70**: 565–70.
30. Felletti R, Souhami RL, Piro SG, Social consequences of brain or liver relapse in small cell carcinoma of the bronchus. *Radiat Oncol* 1985; **4**: 335–9.
31. Komaki R, Prophylactic cranial irradiation for small cell carcinoma of the lung. *Cancer Treat Symp* 1985; **2**: 35–9.
32. Cull A, Gregor A, Hopwood P et al, Neurological and cognitive impairment in long-term survivors of small cell lung cancer. *Eur J Cancer* 1994; **30**: 1067–74.
33. Komaki R, Neurological sequelae in long-term survivors of small cell lung cancer. *Int J Radiat Oncol Biol Phys* 1996; **34**: 1181–3.

12.3 Treatment of SCLC: Chemotherapy

Desmond N Carney, Frances A Shepherd

Contents

INTRODUCTION

Small cell lung cancer (SCLC) accounts for approximately 20–25% of all new cases of lung cancer. The majority of cases are due to cigarette smoking.

At diagnosis, almost 60% of patients will have extensive disease (radiologically or clinically identifiable metastatic disease), while the remainder will have limited-stage disease. Among all cell types of lung cancer, SCLC is the most sensitive to both radiation therapy and many different chemotherapeutic agents. Before the use of combination chemotherapy with or without radiation therapy, few patients survived beyond 12 weeks. Currently, with appropriate combination chemotherapy, there has been a fivefold increase in median survival, and a long-term disease-free survival is achieved in 5–10% of patients.[1,2]

Over the past decade, there has been an explosion in our knowledge of the biology of SCLC[3,4] (see Chapter 3). This new information has helped us to consider alternative or different strategies for treating this disease, namely monoclonal antibodies, gene therapy, etc. However, such approaches, while holding hope for the future, are not yet ready to be introduced as standard treatments for this disease.

In the overview in this chapter, the current standard therapeutic options with chemotherapy in the management of SCLC will be discussed. While such approaches utilizing combination chemotherapy with or without radiation therapy have greatly improved the overall survival of patients with this disease, few patients currently are cured. There remains an urgent need to develop therapeutic approaches for treating patients with SCLC and for preventing this disease.

STAGING

The staging of patients with SCLC is based on the recognition that this is a systemic disease from the outset. While it is recognized that patients can be subdivided into distinct prognostic groups based on biochemical evaluation, including lactate dehydrogenase (LDH) and alkaline phosphatase, the continued use of an anatomic staging classification is of value both in terms of prognosis and more importantly in the design of therapeutic strategies (e.g. the role of chest radiation for limited-stage disease).[5–10] Although the traditional tumor, node and metastases (TNM) staging system has generally not been useful in SCLC, with modifications a revised TNM system has recently been introduced in this disease and may be used. The classic Veterans' Administration Lung Cancer Study Group (VALSG) staging system of limited and extensive stage remains the most universally utilized staging system for SCLC.[11]

Limited-stage disease includes patients with disease restricted to one hemithorax, with regional lymph node metastases including hilar, ipsilateral or contralateral mediastinal lymph node and/or supraclavicular lymph node involvement. Patients with cytologically positive or negative ipsilateral pleural effusions are also included in limited-stage disease. Extensive disease includes all patients with disease beyond the confines of limited disease. In general, at the time of presentation, approximately 40% of patients will have limited disease and the remaining patients extensive disease.

As therapeutic considerations will depend upon the stage of disease at diagnosis, most patients undergo detailed staging procedures following the histologic confirmation of SCLC (Table 12.3.1). The minimum staging procedures should include a detailed history and physical examination, chest radiograph, a computed tomography (CT) scan of thorax and upper abdomen (to include liver and adrenal glands), a radionuclide bone scan, and a unilateral bone aspirate and biopsy. Other more detailed procedures, including brain CT scan or magnetic resonance imaging (MRI), lumbar puncture with cerebrospinal fluid (CSF) analysis, etc., should depend upon the clinical situation, and are not standard tests outside the realms of a clinical trial. While more detailed testing, including in vitro culture techniques, monoclonal antibody staining or MRI examination, may increase the detection of tumor cells in the bone marrow, the impact of these tests on outcome remains to be determined, and as yet they are not universally carried out on newly diagnosed patients.[12,13]

A number of serum biochemical markers have been evaluated in patients with SCLC, such as neuron-specific enolase and chromogranin A.[14] While levels in general correlate with tumor burden – and indeed sequential analysis of these levels may reflect responsiveness to chemotherapy – their overall lack of sensitivity and specificity limits their usefulness in the staging of patients with SCLC.

PROGNOSTIC FACTORS (Table 12.3.2)

Several key prognostic factors have been identified in SCLC, the most important of which include the

Table 12.3.1 Staging procedures for newly diagnosed patients with SCLC

Complete history and physical examination
Complete full blood count
Serum biochemistry (including LDH)
Chest radiograph
CT scan of thorax and upper abdomen
Radionuclide bone scan
Bone marrow aspirate and biopsy
Pathology/cytology review
Brain CT scan/MRI[a]

[a]If clinically indicated.

Table 12.3.2 Prognostic factors in SCLC

Stage of disease
Performance status
Age
Serum biochemistry (LDH)
Histologic subtype[a]
Bone marrow metastases
Liver metastases
CNS metastases

[a]Mixed tumors (e.g. small cell/large cell) appear to have a poorer prognosis.

stage of the disease at presentation and the performance status of the patient.[1,9] Both of these factors accurately predict outcome in terms of responsiveness to therapy, and medium- and long-term survival. Other important prognostic factors include age, sites of metastatic disease (including central nervous system (CNS) and liver metastases), initial LDH levels and sex. Several studies also suggest that elderly patients have a poorer prognosis. However, this may be a reflection of compromised chemotherapy administration (i.e. dose reduction or delayed schedules, etc.), rather than a lower chemosensitivity in this age group. Studies have also suggested that young female patients have a better prognosis and survival than their male counterparts. The biological reasons for this remains to be determined. Finally, it should be noted that SCLC is frequently associated with paraneoplastic syndromes (e.g. SIADH, ectopic ADH, etc.). The presence of these at diagnosis is a poor prognostic factor.

TREATMENT OF SCLC

The mainstay of treatment of SCLC is the use of combination systemic chemotherapy with the goal of achieving the highest response rate and long-term disease-free survival ('cure') with the lowest possible and acceptable morbidity. It must be recognized that in the prechemotherapy days, when treatment for SCLC was usually palliative radiation, the medial survival for patients with limited disease was just 12 weeks, while for those with extensive disease it was approximately 6 weeks, with few patients ever achieving long-term (then over two years) survival. With current therapeutic approaches, an overall initial response rate of 80–90% will be achieved, with 30–60% of patients achieving a complete (radiological and clinical) remission.[1] The median survival for all patients is approximately 11 months, with 5–10% of patients achieving long-term survival. As might be expected, higher complete remission rates and median (18–24 months) and long-term (20–25% over two years) survival will be observed in patients with limited disease and good performance status.

Table 12.3.3 Chemotherapy agents active in SCLC
Cyclophosphamide
Ifosfamide
Vincristine
Vindesine
Etoposide
Teniposide
Cisplatin
Carboplatin
Doxorubicin
Methotrexate

SCLC is highly chemosensitive at diagnosis. As indicated in Table 12.3.3, a large number of chemotherapy agents are active in this disease, achieving response rates as high as 50–60%, even when used as single agents. More recently, a small number of newer agents with different modes of action have been added to this list.[15]

The majority of suitable patients with SCLC are treated with combinations of two to four drugs. The most commonly used regimens are indicated in Table 12.3.4. While earlier studies have suggested that four-drug combinations or schedules of alternating regimens might be superior, an analysis of more recent results suggests that etoposide in a two-drug combination with either cisplatin or carboplatin is as effective as any other multidrug combination in producing clinical and radiological responses.[15–18] Carboplatin can be substituted for

Table 12.3.4 Commonly used chemotherapy regimens in SCLC

EP	Etoposide	100 mg/m^2	days 1–3	i.v.
	Cisplatin	75 mg/m^2	day 1	i.v.
CAV	Cyclophosphamide	1 g/m^2	day 1	i.v.
	Doxorubicin (Adriamycin)	50 mg/m^2	day 1	i.v.
	Vincristine	1.4 mg/m^2	day 1	i.v.
CDE	Cyclophosphamide	1 g/m^2	day 1	i.v.
	Doxorubicin	45 mg/m^2	day 1	i.v.
	Etoposide	100 mg/m^2	days 1, 3, 5	i.v.
EC	Etoposide	100 mg/m^2	days 1–3	i.v.
	Carboplatin	300 mg/m^2	day 1	i.v.

cisplatin without any loss of activity, but allows for greater ease of administration with a more favorable toxicity profile.

With combination chemotherapy a response rate of 80–90% will be observed in both limited-disease and extensive-disease patients. Complete remission will be observed in 40–60% of patients with limited disease and 20–30% of patients with extensive disease. The median survival for limited-disease patients is now almost 18 months, while that for extensive-disease patients remains between 7 and 9 months. It should be noted that, while the combination of etoposide with either cisplatin or carboplatin can be recommended for newly diagnosed patients, there is some recent evidence suggesting that the improved survival with this combination is also associated with increased toxicity, including toxic deaths, when compared with older regimens.

Survival beyond five years may be achieved in up to 10–20% of patients with limited disease and 0–5% of patients with extensive disease. Results from large national and cooperative studies are less encouraging when compared with dedicated single-institution studies, suggesting some degree of selection bias for inclusion of patients into the studies that may be reflected in the somewhat better treatment results at those institutions.

In general, chemotherapy is administered every three to four weeks for approximately six months. There are no convincing data suggesting that maintenance chemotherapy has any role to play in the management of SCLC.

IMPROVING RESPONSES TO CHEMOTHERAPY

While improvements in the response to chemotherapy were observed in the late 1970s and early 1980s, over the past decade, with a few minor exceptions, no significant improvements in outcome or long-term survival have been noted.[19] Indeed, since patients now entering clinical trials undergo more rigorous staging procedures than in the past, the improvements that have been made might be a result of the stage migration effect, and – particularly in patients with limited disease – might simply be a reflection of more detailed staging.[20] In addition, the inclusion of a greater number of female patients in trials may also give a more favorable outcome to treatment assessments when comparing current results with historical data.

In a similar fashion to other solid tumors, many approaches have been attempted to improve outcome for patients with SCLC receiving chemotherapy. These include:

- the use of alternating non-cross-resistant chemotherapy;
- the use of high-dose chemotherapy with or without growth factor support, bone marrow transplantation or peripheral blood stem cell transplantation;
- new scheduling of drug administration.

Alternating chemotherapy regimens[21–28]

(Table 12.3.5)

The emergence of drug-resistant clones of SCLC, which develop either at the time of diagnosis or during chemotherapy, account for treatment failures in most patients. It has been postulated that the use of alternating non-cross-resistant regimens would reduce the emergence of drug-resistant clones. However, a review of 13 randomized phase III trials of alternating versus sequential combination chemotherapy provides no convincing data suggesting a benefit from alternating chemotherapy regimens in particular in patients with extensive-stage disease.

Table 12.3.5 Alternating chemotherapy in SCLC[23]

Combination[a]	EP	CAV	EP/CAV
No. of patients	148	146	143
Stage	ED	ED	ED
Median survival (months)	8.6	8.3	8.1

[a]See Table 12.3.4.

Dose intensification[29–32]

Several approaches for increasing the dose intensity of chemotherapy have been evaluated in SCLC. These include:

- the use of modestly higher doses (two- to fourfold) of chemotherapy without growth factor support;
- the administration of chemotherapy at shorter (i.e. weekly) intervals, with or without growth factor support;
- the use of high-dose chemotherapy schedules with autologous bone marrow transplantation (ABMT) or peripheral blood stem cell transplantation (PBSCT) and growth factor support.

When chemotherapy is administered in standard doses (as indicated in Table 12.3.4) and on schedule, there is little evidence to suggest that for most patients the use of higher doses leads to any meaningful improvement in overall survival. While increasing dose intensity may be associated with a higher initial response rate, this does not appear to translate into improved overall survival, and conversely is associated with increasing toxicity and cost. The small number of studies of increasing dose intensity that appear to yield positive results have in most cases entered patients into the studies with an excellent performance status (0/1), with the majority of patients having small-volume limited-stage disease. Thus the applicability of these studies to large national populations remains to be determined.

In a similar fashion, studies of high-dose chemotherapy with ABMT or PBSCT rescue have been carried out on very small numbers of patients, all with excellent performance status and minimum-stage disease.[33] The impact of these studies on overall survival is marginal when compared with results of standard chemotherapy.

Further studies are required to evaluate the potential value of high-dose chemotherapy and dose intensification as part of induction or consolidation treatment in SCLC. Moreover, given that many patients (almost 50%) with SCLC are more than 65 years of age at diagnosis and frequently have co-morbid tobacco-induced medical problems, SCLC patients, with few exceptions, are not optimum candidates for dose-intensity studies including high-dose chemotherapy and stem cell transplantation.

Weekly chemotherapy

Based on data obtained from the use of weekly chemotherapy in aggressive lymphomas, and in other tumors, several investigators have evaluated the weekly use of active regimens in SCLC. The CODE regimen (cyclophosphamide, vincristine (Oncovin), doxorubicin and etoposide) reported by Murray et al[34] in 48 extensive-stage SCLC patients was associated with an overall response rate of 94%, including a 40% complete remission rate and a median survival of 61 weeks. Grade 4 myelosuppression was significant, and was noted in almost 50% of patients. While these results appear to be better than historical data, a subsequent randomized trial of CODE versus CAV alternating with cisplatin and etoposide failed to demonstrate the survival advantage for the more toxic CODE regimen.[35] In most circumstances, the use of such a toxic regimen for patients with SCLC has fallen out of favor.

Maintenance/duration of chemotherapy[36–43]

While early studies of chemotherapy in patients with SCLC advocated a prolonged use of chemotherapy (i.e. 12–18 months), the increased toxicity associated with its use and the appearance of second cancers led to questions regarding the need for such prolonged treatment in this disease. In newly diagnosed patients, maximum responses are most frequently observed within the first two to three cycles of treatment. It is rare to see improved responses beyond that time. Among responding patients, the continuation of chemotherapy beyond six to eight courses of treatment (i.e. four to six months) does not appear to confirm any advantage in survival to the patient, but rather adds to the toxicity and morbidity. Among several randomized studies, two UK studies showed a modest improvement in survival for maintenance chemotherapy after four to six months, while a large EORTC study revealed no benefit. The consensus among investigators is that maintenance chemotherapy beyond four to six months of initial chemotherapy is of no added benefit to the patient. Studies utilizing biological response modifiers or anticoagulants (including interferons) as maintenance in SCLC after standard induction chemotherapy have yielded conflicting results, and would not be considered standard care in the management of patients with this disease.[39–43]

Chemotherapy in relapsed patients

With few exceptions, the majority of the 80–90% of patients who respond to initial combined chemotherapy and radiation therapy will relapse and develop progressive disease. In general, while relapses may initially appear to be localized or confined to one organ, rapid dissemination is the rule. For localized thoracic metastases and patients who have not yet received radiation, thoracic irradiation is a treatment of choice. The use of systemic chemotherapy in patients in relapse and who are not part of a clinical trial may be dictated by (i) the response to initial systemic chemotherapy and (ii) the chemotherapy-free interval from initial chemotherapy cessation to subsequent relapse. Those patients who have had either a complete or partial remission with induction chemotherapy and have had a greater than six-month chemotherapy-free interval will have response rates of 25–75% with further chemotherapy (either the same or different regimens).[44,45] However, in general, response durations are usually much shorter: about two to four months. The choice of chemotherapy will depend upon the initial drugs used, the response achieved and the current performance status of the patient, and will include EP, CAV, chronic low-dose etoposide and newer agents such as topotecan. In a recent randomized trial of CAV versus topotecan in relapsed SCLC patients, the response to topotecan was similar to that to CAV, with no difference in survival noted between the two regimens.[46] It should be noted that patients who have had an initial excellent response to chemotherapy and who are more than six months off chemotherapy in general have a higher response rate and are more chemosensitive than patients who either progress while on standard induction chemotherapy or relapse within a couple of months of completing it.

Chemotherapy of elderly patients or patients with poor performance status

Among all patients who present with SCLC, only those with limited disease and good performance (ECOG 0–1) and who are 65 years old or less at diagnosis are in general suitable candidates for treatment with a curative intent. In such patients, the use of combined-modality therapy with chemotherapy and radiation has recently been reported to be associated with a two-year disease-free survival rate of 25–40% and a significant long-term survival. However, in a review of more than 400 unselected patients with SCLC referred to a university hospital medical oncology department, less than 25% of newly diagnosed patients fell into that 'suitable' category.[47] The remainder were either elderly patients (with limited or extensive disease), limited-disease patients with poor performance status (ECOG 2/4) or extensive-stage patients. With the most optimistic approach, the majority of oncologists would accept that, by current standards, such patients (who represent 75% of all newly diagnosed SCLC patients) are incurable with current treatment standards and that the treatment goal is to achieve optimum palliation of the disease with improved quality of life and improved overall survival. While many of these patients will be candidates for standard treatment approaches (i.e. chemotherapy including etoposide/carboplatin with or without radiation), some (approximately 20–25% of the total) are either too elderly or too unfit for such combined-modality treatment approaches to be considered. For such patients, chemotherapy strategies have been designed to use chemotherapy in a palliative approach. Reports of single-agent oral etoposide given over five days in such patients indicated a response rate of 50–80% and a median survival of seven to nine months with acceptable toxicity.[48] However, two recently reported randomized trials comparing single-agent etoposide with combination chemotherapy given intravenously have both demonstrated superiority for the combination-chemotherapy arm in terms of response rate, median survival and quality of life.[49,50] Based on these data, unless medically contraindicated, combination chemotherapy remains the treatment of choice even for the elderly or unfit patient with SCLC.

Chemotherapy in unique clinical situations

CNS metastases[51–54]

For SCLC patients who have CNS metastases at initial presentation, the standard approach includes concomitant cranial irradiation and chemotherapy. Recent evidence suggests that, for previously untreated patients, chemotherapy alone would be associated with an intracranial response rate of up to 75%, including complete resolution of the disease. Indeed, for such patients where the sole site of metastatic disease is cranial, their median survival will approximate that of patients with limited disease. For patients relapsing from prior chemotherapy, responses of CNS metastases to chemotherapy are much lower than for newly diagnosed patients. For these patients, radiation treatment is the recommended treatment. Leptomeningeal metastases are also common in SCLC patients – particularly in patients with progressive disease. Systemic chemotherapy is uniformly poor, and treatment with intrathecal methotrexate, with or without local radiation to symptomatic regions, is the treatment of choice.

For patients who develop spinal cord compression (up to 3%), a standard treatment approach utilizing high-dose steroids plus irradiation is recommended. Surgical intervention is rarely required, owing to the sensitivity of this tumor to radiation.

SECOND LUNG CANCERS IN PATIENTS AFTER TREATMENT FOR AN INITIAL LUNG CANCER[55]

Patients who have been successfully treated for either SCLC or non-small cell lung cancer remain at risk for developing second smoking-related lung or other cancers. In a recent review of SCLC patients surviving more than two years from initial diagnosis, the risk of developing a second lung cancer was 2–14% per patient per year, and that risk increased two- to sevenfold at 10 years from initial diagnosis. The majority of second cancers are squamous cell, and fewer than 20% can be resected. Of note, survivors who continued to smoke cigarettes had a greater risk of developing a second cancer. Overall, fewer than 20% of these patients survived five years. The recognition that the risk of second cancers remains a problem for those few SCLC patients initially cured of their disease means that such patients may be candidates for more intensive surveillance from completion of treatment, and may also be candidates for chemoprevention studies.

NEW DRUGS IN SCLC[56–66]

The relatively modest improvement in overall survival for patients with SCLC stresses the important need for the evaluation of new agents in the treatment of this disease (Table 12.3.6). Several phase I/II studies have identified agents with activity in SCLC. These include the taxanes, the topoisomerase inhibitors, the antimetabolites and vinorelbine. In studies of previously untreated patients using these compounds as single agents, response rates ranging from 5% to 39% have been observed, with lower rates being observed in previously treated patients. The single-agent activities of some of these compounds compare favorably with those of some of the established active

Table 12.3.6 New active drugs in SCLC

Agent	No. of patients	Response rate (%)
Topotecan	48	39
Paclitaxel	79	34–41
Docetaxel	14	8
Gemcitabine	29	27
Vinorelbine	22	5

agents in SCLC. The evaluation of these agents in combination with established agents needs urgent assessment in phase II/III clinical trials.

SUMMARY AND FUTURE DIRECTIONS

1. Four to six months of initial chemotherapy is effective treatment for both limited- and extensive-stage SCLC. Maintenance chemotherapy beyond this time does not improve survival.
2. In patients with limited disease, combined-modality therapy would appear to be the treatment of choice, leading to improved response rates, local control and overall survival. The optimum use of radiation, including its integration with chemotherapy, fractionation and total dose, still remains to be determined. Studies do suggest that the early use of combined-modality therapy appears to be associated with an improved outcome. (See Chapter 12.2.)
3. The use of etoposide with cisplatin or carboplatin as initial chemotherapy appears to allow the integration of radiation therapy (in combined-modality therapy) with acceptable toxicity compared with doxorubicin-containing regimens.
4. There are no data supporting the use of dose-intensive therapy requiring cytokine support, bone marrow support or peripheral blood stem cell support outside clinical trials.
5. The use of prophylactic cranial irradiation (PCI) should be reserved for patients (both limited-disease and extensive-disease) who achieve a complete remission with induction treatment. Delaying PCI until completion of chemotherapy may also decrease long-term neurological sequelae. (See Chapter 12.2.)
6. Late recurrences (i.e. later than six months after completion of initial chemotherapy) may be chemosensitive, and such patients should be considered for further chemotherapy.
7. The development of second cancers in SCLC patients two years after initial diagnosis continues to be a problem. As a significant proportion of very late relapses may be non-small cell lung cancer, further biopsies of such patients for histologic evaluation is indicated before the institution of further specific therapy.
8. The evaluation of newer cytotoxic agents and their integration with currently proven active regimens offer some hope for the future treatment of SCLC.
9. The elimination of cigarettes from our society provides the best hope for reducing the number of new cases of SCLC and deaths from this disease in the future.

REFERENCES

1. Hansen HH, Management of small cell cancer of the lung. *Lancet* 1992; **339**: 846–9.
2. Kristensen CA, Jensen PB, Poulson HS et al, Small cell lung cancer: biological and therapeutic aspects. *Crit Rev Oncol Hematol* 1996; **22**: 27–60.
3. Salgia R, Skarin AT, Molecular abnormalities in lung cancer. *J Clin Oncol* 1998; **16**: 1207–17.
4. Carney DN, Biology of small cell lung cancer. *Lancet* 1992; **339**: 843–9.
5. Cerny T, Blair V, Anderson H et al, Pretreatment prognostic factors and system in 407 small cell lung cancer patients. *Int J Cancer* 1987; **39**: 146–9.
6. Cohen MH, Makuch R, Johnston-Early A et al, Laboratory parameters as an alternative to performance status in prognostic stratification of patients with small cell lung cancer. *Cancer Treat Rep* 1981; **65**: 187–95.
7. Sagman U, Maki E, Evans WK et al, Small-cell carcinoma of the lung – derivation of a prognos-

tic staging system. *J Clin Oncol* 1991; **9**: 1639–49.

8. Souhami RL, Bradbury I, Geddes DM et al, Prognostic significance of laboratory parameters measured at diagnosis in small cell carcinoma of the lung. *Cancer Res* 1985; **45**: 2878–82.
9. Wolf M, Holle R, Hans K et al, Analysis of prognostic factors in 766 patients with small cell lung cancer (SCLC): the role of sex as a predictor for survival. *Br J Cancer* 1991; **63**: 986–92.
10. Lassen U, Osterlind K, Hansen M et al, Long-term survival in small cell lung cancer: posttreatment characteristics in patients surviving 5 to 18+ years – an analysis of 1714 consecutive patients. *J Clin Oncol* 1995; **13**: 1215–20.
11. Mountain CF, Staging of lung cancer. The new international system. *Lung Cancer* 1987; **3**: 4–11.
12. Beiske K, Myklebust AT, Aamdal S et al, Detection of bone marrow metastases in small cell lung cancer patients. Comparison of immunologic and morphologic methods. *Am J Clin Pathol* 1992; **141**: 531–8.
13. Jelinek JS, Redmond J, Perry JJ et al, Small cell lung cancer: staging with MR imaging. *Radiology* 1990; **177**: 837–42.
14. Jorgensen LGM, Osterlind K, Cooper EH, Serum neuron specific enolase (NSE) is determinant of response in small cell lung cancer (SCLC). *Br J Cancer* 1992; **66**: 594–8.
15. Edelman MJ, Gandara DR, Small cell lung cancer: current status of new chemotherapeutic agents. *Crit Rev Oncol Hematol* 1998; **27**: 211–28.
16. Evans WK, Shepherd FA, Feld R et al, VP.1b and cisplatin as first line therapy for small cell lung cancer. *J Clin Oncol* 1985; **3**: 1471–7.
17. Lassen U, Kristjansen PEG, Osterlind K et al, Superiority of cisplatin or carboplatin in combination with teniposide and vincristine in the induction chemotherapy of small cell lung cancer. A randomized trial with 5 years follow up. *Ann Oncol* 1996; **7**: 365–71.
18. Kosmidis PA, Samantas E, Fountzilas G et al, Cisplatin/etoposide versus carboplatin/etoposide chemotherapy and irradiation in small cell lung cancer. A randomized phase III study. *Semin Oncol* 1994; **21**: 23–30.
19. Souhami RL, Law K, Longevity in small cell lung cancer. *Br J Cancer* 1990; **61**: 584–9.
20. Dearing MP, Steinberg SM, Phelps R et al, Outcome of patients with small cell lung cancer: effect of changes in staging procedures and imaging technology on prognostic factors over 14 years. *J Clin Oncol* 1990; **8**: 1042–9.
21. Osterlind K, Sorenson S, Hansen HH et al, Continuous versus alternating combination chemotherapy for advanced small cell carcinoma of the lung. *Cancer Res* 1983; **43**: 6085–9.
22. Pedersen AG, Osterlind K, Vindelov LL, Alternating or continuous chemotherapy of small cell lung cancer. A three armed randomized trial. *Proc Am Soc Clin Oncol* 1987; **6**: 187.
23. Roth BJ, Johnson DH, Einhorn LH et al, Randomized study of cyclophosphamide, doxorubicin, and vincristine versus etoposide and cisplatin versus alternation of these two regimens in extensive small cell lung cancer: a phase II trial of the Southeastern Cancer Study Group. *J Clin Oncol* 1992; **10**: 282–91.
24. Evans WK, Feld R, Murray N et al, Superiority of alternating non-cross-resistant chemotherapy in extensive small cell lung cancer. A multicenter, randomized clinical trial by the National Cancer Institute of Canada. *Ann Intern Med* 1987; **107**: 451–8.
25. Ettinger DS, Finkelstein DM, Abeloff MD et al, A randomized comparison of standard chemotherapy versus alternating chemotherapy and maintenance versus no maintenance therapy for extensive stage small cell lung cancer: a phase III study of the Eastern Cooperative Oncology Group. *J Clin Oncol* 1990; **8**: 230–40.
26. Goodman GE, Crowley JJ, Blasko JC et al, Treatment of limited small cell lung cancer with etoposide and cisplatin alternating with vincristine, doxorubicin and cyclophosphamide versus concurrent etoposide, vincristine, doxorubicin and cyclophosphamide and chest radiotherapy: a Southwest Oncology Group Study. *J Clin Oncol* 1990; **8**: 39–47.
27. Wolf M, Prithch M, Drings P et al, Cyclic alternating versus response oriented chemotherapy in small

cell lung cancer: a German multicenter randomized trial of 321 patients. *J Clin Oncol* 1991; **9**: 614–24.

28. Fukuoka M, Furuse K, Saijo N et al, Randomized trial of cyclophosphamide, doxorubicin, and vincristine versus cisplatin and etoposide versus alternation of these regimens in small cell lung cancer. *J Natl Cancer Inst* 1991; **83**: 855–61.
29. Klasa RJ, Murray N, Coldman AJ, Dose intensity meta analysis of chemotherapy regimens in small cell carcinoma of the lung. *J Clin Oncol* 1991; **9**: 499–508.
30. Pujol J-L, Douillard JY, Riviere A et al, Dose intensity of a four drug chemotherapy regimen with or without recombinant human granulocyte colony stimulating factor in small cell lung cancer. *J Clin Oncol* 1997; **15**: 2082–9.
31. FuruseK, Fukuda M, Nishiwaki Y et al, Phase III study of intensive weekly chemotherapy with recombinant human granulocyte colony stimulating factor versus standard chemotherapy in extensive disease small cell lung cancer. *J Clin Oncol* 1998; **16**: 2126–32.
32. Steward WP, von Pwel J, Gatzemeier U et al, Effects on granulocyte macrophage colony stimulating factor and dose intensification of V-ICE chemotherapy in small cell lung cancer: a prospective randomized study of 300 patients. *J Clin Oncol* 1998; **16**: 642–50.
33. Elias A, Ayash C, Frei E et al, Intensive combined modality therapy for small cell lung cancer. *J Natl Cancer Inst* 1993; **85**: 559–66.
34. Murray N, Shah A, Osoba D, Intensive weekly chemotherapy for the treatment of extensive stage small cell lung cancer. *J Clin Oncol* 1991; **9**: 1632–8.
35. Murray N, Livingston RB, Shepard FA et al, A randomized study of CODE plus thoracic irradiation versus alternating CAV/EP for extensive stage small cell lung cancer (ESCLC). *Proc Am Soc Clin Oncol* 1997; **16**: 456.
36. Spiro SG, Souhami RL, Geddes DM et al, Duration of chemotherapy in small cell lung cancer: a Cancer Research Campaign trial. *Br J Cancer* 1989; **59**: 578–83.
37. Giaccone G, Dalexio O, McVie JG et al, Maintenance chemotherapy in small cell lung cancer: long term results of a randomized trial. *J Clin Oncol* 1993; **11**: 1230–40.
38. Sculier J-P, Paesmans M, Bureau G et al, Randomized trial comparing induction chemotherapy versus chemotherapy followed by maintenance chemotherapy in small cell lung cancer. *J Clin Oncol* 1997; **14**: 2237–44.
39. Mattson K, Niiranen A, Ruotsalainen T et al, Interferon maintenance therapy for small cell lung cancer: improvement in long-term survival. *J Interferon Cytokine Res* 1997; **17**: 103–5.
40. Jett JR, Maksymiuk AW, Su JQ et al, Phase III trial of recombinant interferon gamma in complete responders with small cell lung cancer. *J Clin Oncol* 1994; **12**: 2321–6.
41. Zarogoulidis K, Ziogas E, Papagiannis A et al, Interferon alpha-2a and combined chemotherapy as first line treatment in SCLC patients: a randomized trial. *Lung Cancer* 1996; **15**: 197–205.
42. Zacharski LR, Henderson WG, Rickles FR, Effect of warfarin on survival in small cell lung cancer of the lung. *JAMA* 1998; **245**: 831–5.
43. Chahinian AP, Prospert KJ, Ware JH et al, A randomized trial of anticoagulation with warfarin and of alternating chemotherapy in extensive small cell lung cancer. *J Clin Oncol* 1989; **7**: 993–1002.
44. Chute JP, Kelley MJ, Verzon D et al, Retreatment of patients surviving cancer free 2 or more years after initial treatment of small cell lung cancer. *Chest* 1996; **110**: 165–70.
45. Anderson M, Kristjansen PEG, Hansen HH, Second line chemotherapy in small cell lung cancer. *Cancer Treat Rev* 1990; **17**: 427–36.
46. Schiller J, Von Pawel J, Shepard FA et al, Topotecan versus cyclophosphamide, doxorubicin and vincristine for the treatment of patients with recurrent small cell lung cancer: a phase III study. *Proc Am Soc Clin Oncol* 1998; **17**: 456.
47. Carney DN, Carboplatin/etoposide combination chemotherapy in the treatment of poor prognosis patients with small cell lung cancer. *Lung Cancer* 1995; **12**(S3): 77–83.
48. Carney DN, Byrne A, Etoposide in the treatment of elderly/poor-prognosis patients with small cell

lung cancer. *Cancer Chemother Pharmacol* 1994; **34**: s96–100.

49. Souhami RL, Spiro SG, Rudd RM et al, Five day oral etoposide treatment for advance small cell lung cancer: randomized comparison with intravenous chemotherapy. *J Natl Cancer Inst* 1997; **89**: 577–80.
50. Girling DJ, Thatcher N, Clark PI et al, Comparison of oral etoposide and standard multidrug intravenous chemotherapy for small cell lung cancer: a stopped multicentre randomised trial. *Lancet* 1996; **348**: 563–6.
51. Kristjansen PEG, Sorensen PS, Hansen MS et al, Prospective evaluation of the effect on initial brain metastates from small cell lung cancer of platinum/etoposide based induction chemotherapy followed by an alternating multidrug regimen. *Ann Oncol* 1993; **4**: 579–83.
52. Kristensen CA, Kristjansen PEG, Hansen HH, Systemic chemotherapy of brain metastases from small cell lung cancer: a review. *J Clin Oncol* 1992; **10**: 1498–502.
53. Postmus PE, Sleijfer DTH, Haaxma-Reiche H, Chemotherapy for central nervous system metastates from small cell lung cancer. A review. *Lung Cancer* 1989; **5**: 254–63.
54. Pedersen AG, Bach F, Melgaard B, Frequency, diagnosis and prognosis of spinal cord compression in small cell bronchogenic carcinoma. A review of 817 consecutive patients. *Cancer* 1985; **55**: 1818–1822.
55. Johnston BE, Second lung cancers in patients after treatment for initial lung cancer. *J Natl Cancer Inst* 1998; **90**: 1335–45.
56. Ettinger DS, Finkelstein DM, Abeloff MD, Justification for evaluating new anticancer drugs in selected untreated patients with extensive stage small cell lung cancer: an Eastern Cooperative Oncology Group randomized study. *J Natl Cancer Inst* 1992; **84**: 1077–84.
57. Ardizzoni A, Hansen HH, Dombernowsky P et al, Topotecan, a new active drug in the second line treatment of small cell lung cancer: a phase II trial in patients with refractory and sensitive disease. *J Clin Oncol* 1997; **15**: 2090–6.
58. Perez-Soler R, Glisson BS, Lee JS et al, Treatment of patients with small cell lung cancer refractory to etoposide and cisplatin with the topoisomerase I poison topotecan. *J Clin Oncol* 1996; **14**: 2785–90.
59. Schiller J, Kim K, Hutson P et al, Phase II study of topotecan in patients with extensive stage small cell lung carcinoma of the lung: an Eastern Cooperative Oncology Group trial. *J Clin Oncol* 1996; **14**: 2345–52.
60. Masuda N, Fukuoka M, Kusunoki Y et al, CPT-11: a new derivative of camptothecin for treatment of refractory or relapsed small cell lung cancer. *J Clin Oncol* 1992; **10**: 1225–9.
61. Negoro S, Fukuoka M, Niitani H et al, Phase II study of CPT-II, a new camptothecin derivative in small cell lung cancer. *Proc Am Soc Clin Oncol* 1991; **10**: 241.
62. Ettinger DS, Finkelstein DM, Sarma R et al, Phase II study of paclitaxel in patients with extensive disease small cell lung cancer: an Eastern Cooperative Oncology Group study. *J Clin Oncol* 1995; **13**: 1431–5.
63. Hainsworth JD, Gray JR, Stoup SL et al, Paclitaxel, carboplatin, and extended schedule etoposide in the treatment of small cell lung cancer: comparison of sequential phase II trials using different dose-intensities. *J Clin Oncol* 1997; **15**: 3463–70.
64. Latreille J, Cormier Y, Martina H et al, Phase II study of docetaxel in patients with previously untreated extensive small cell lung cancer. *Invest New Drugs* 1996; **13**: 342–5.
65. Cormier Y, Eisenhaues EA, Muldal A et al, Gemcitabine is an active new agent in previously untreated extensive small cell lung cancer. A study of the National Cancer Institute of Canada clinical trial. *Ann Oncol* 1994; **5**: 283–5.
66. Higano CS, Crowley JJ, Veith RV et al, A phase II trial of intravenous vinorelbine in previously untreated patients with extensive small cell lung cancer, a SWOG study. *Invest New Drugs* 1997; **15**: 153–6.

13 Malignant mesothelioma

Bernadette Scott, Sutapa Mukherjee, Richard Lake, Blair McLaren, Bruce Robinson

Contents Introduction • Epidemiology • Pathogenesis • Pathobiology • Immunobiology • Clinical presentation and course • Diagnosis • Management • Future directions

INTRODUCTION

Malignant mesothelioma (MM) is an aggressive malignant tumour of serosal surfaces. It most commonly affects the pleura, but also involves peritoneal and occasionally other serosal surfaces. It was considered a rare disease before about 1960, but has increased dramatically in incidence since that time, almost certainly owing to the widespread use of asbestos fibres in the post-war industrial boom.

A lot has been written about MM, and our aim in this chapter is not to repeat what has already been well described but rather to summarize the main features of the disease and provide an update of recent developments. The latter should be of substantial interest to the reader, since there have been a number of recent publications in mesothelioma research that not only have begun to unravel the mysteries of the disease but have also provided the prospect of new approaches to therapy for this otherwise treatment-resistant problem. Advances have been in the area of pathogenesis and mechanisms, particularly the identification of the growth factors involved in the disease, the potential role of non-asbestos agents such as the SV40 virus, and the identification of tumour suppressor gene lesions in this disease. Advances have also been made in the immunobiology and immunotherapy of the disease, in the development of new chemotherapy trials, and in the areas of epidemiology and medicolegality. There have also been recent developments in the area of disease prevention, particularly with the use of retinoic acid.

In this chapter, we shall begin by reviewing the epidemiology and biology of MM, particularly with regard to its pathogenesis and immunobiology. We shall then summarize the clinical aspects of the disease, and finish the chapter with a discussion of possible future directions based upon these recent advances.

EPIDEMIOLOGY

In 1960 Wagner et al[1] reported an association between asbestos and both pleural and peritoneal MM in a case series of the North Western Cape Province of South Africa, where blue asbestos (crocidolite) was mined. Since then, many reports supporting the relationship between occupational or environmental exposure to asbestos and the subsequent development of MM have been published from all parts of the world.[2,3] The relationship is clearly one of cause and effect. This has been shown in case series and cohort studies.

Wagner's initial study identified the difference in risk from direct occupational exposure and brief or indirect exposure to asbestos. The risk of development of MM is directly related to the duration and intensity of exposure to asbestos. Therefore if asbestos exposure occurred at a young age then the lifetime risk of development of MM is higher than in someone whose exposure occurred at a later age. Asbestos workers had direct occupational exposure to asbestos, and their families received brief or indirect exposure via clothes and hair brought home from the workplace.[4] Other employees working in the same area as asbestos workers were also subject to greater risk.

Epidemiological studies have shown that 50–80% of individuals with MM have an identifiable exposure to asbestos.[5] Therefore in 20–50% of cases there is no obvious exposure to asbestos, and examination of the lung mineral fibre content shows that in many of these subjects there is a lower lung fibre burden than seen in subjects with asbestosis.[6] This supports the evidence that MM may occur after brief and indirect exposure to asbestos. As a group, however, patients with MM have markedly increased lung fibre burdens when compared with a reference population.

Asbestos fibre dimensions and type play an important role in the development of MM, with longer and thinner asbestos fibres causing more damage than shorter and wider fibres because they can deposit within and penetrate the lungs (see below). The critical fibre dimensions appear to be less than 0.25 mm in diameter and greater than 5 mm in length to produce MM, and, while the risk of developing MM from exposure to chrysotile fibres is lower than that from amphibole fibres, large amounts of chrysotile can cause MM, possibly because of contaminating tremolite fibres.[7] A potential role for SV40 is also described.

PATHOGENESIS

Mesothelial tissues

Mesothelial tissues include all those that line the cavities that were derived from the embryonic mesodermal coelomic cavity. The tissue develops as a continuous epithelial layer, which covers the pleura, the pericardium and the peritoneal cavity. In the pleura, it exists as a single layer of mesothelial cells, resting on a basement membrane. The cells are variable in shape, from flat to cuboidal to columnar. Their rate of division is generally slow, but it is increased in response to inflammatory damage. Mesothelial cells are actively phagocytic in culture, and they can take up asbestos fibres.[8] This may be important in their susceptibility to transformation, since they are not normally exposed to chronic insults.

Etiological agents

Asbestos

Asbestos is a collective name for a group of fibrous minerals composed of hydrated magnesium silicate. They divide into serpentines, which are short and curved, such as chrysotile, and amphiboles, which are long and needle-like, such as crocidolite. Not all of the different forms have had widespread commercial use – in fact, 90% of industrial asbestos is chrysotile. The mining and use of asbestos were maximal in 1973, and are now in decline because it has become clear that exposure to asbestos can cause a number of pulmonary conditions. These include pleural plaques, diffuse pleural thickening, rounded atelectasis and asbestos-related pleural effusions. As mentioned above, there is an association between asbestos and MM, and it now seems reasonably clear that the duration and dose of exposure to asbestos correlate with the risk of developing MM.[9]

The physical characteristics of the asbestos fibres are important in the development of MM.

It is generally thought that the amphiboles, particularly crocidolite, are more carcinogenic.[5] Some cases of MM occur following exposure to chrysotile, although this apparent association may be due to contamination of this form with amphiboles. However, in experimental situations, the two groups of asbestos fibres are equally mutagenic to mesothelial cells. In these studies, the chrysotile was introduced intrapleurally, and it may be that the shape of these fibres makes it less likely that they would penetrate the intact lung after inhalation. Consistent with this hypothesis, the most carcinogenic fibres in animal studies have been shown to have a diameter of less than 1.5 μm and a length of greater than 8 μm, i.e. a high length-to-width ratio.[10] The disease progresses through the formation of granulomatous lesions that have a surface layer of mesothelium, with subsequent neoplastic transformation.

Mesothelial cells have been shown to be 10 times more sensitive than bronchial epithelial cells to the direct cytotoxic effects of asbestos fibres,[11] but, after intraperitoneal injection of asbestos, the initial response is from macrophages, with resultant inflammation and cytokine production.[12] The fibres cause iron-catalysed generation of reactive oxygen metabolites, which have a direct toxic effect, causing DNA point mutations and strand and chromosomal breaks.[13] These events usually lead to cellular apoptosis, but particular mutations, combined with the direct mitotic damage of cells by asbestos fibres[14] and the increased proliferation induced by inflammation, may increase the risk that these cells survive despite their genetic changes. The end result is malignant transformation.

SV40

The double-stranded DNA virus SV40 has been suggested as a possible etiological agent in the development of mesothelioma. In 1994, Carbone and co-workers found SV40-like sequences in 60% of frozen mesothelioma specimens by polymerase chain reaction (PCR). The majority of these patients also had a history of asbestos exposure, raising the possibility of SV40 acting as a co-carcinogen. SV40 is a papovavirus whose normal host is the monkey. As a small virus, it is dependent on its host for the enzymes of replication except for the large T antigen (TAG). When the virus infects a cell, the TAG is transcribed from the viral genome. TAG binds to the specific SV40 origin of replication, pulling apart the DNA strand, allowing viral DNA synthesis. In this way, the virus is able to bypass the normal cellular controls on replication, and will even do so in quiescent cells. This process is facilitated by TAG binding to both p53 and the retinoblastoma protein (pRb), with inactivation of these cell cycle checkpoints.

It is presumed that SV40 was introduced into humans as a result of the Salk polio vaccines used in the 1950s. It has been estimated that up to 30% of vaccines used were contaminated by SV40 as a result of culturing the poliovirus in rhesus monkey kidney cells. SV40 had long been known to be tumorigenic in rodents, but in 1992 Bergsagel et al[15] found evidence of TAG sequences in childhood tumours. This discovery was followed by evidence obtained by Carbone's group,[16] suggesting an oncogenic role of SV40 in causing mesothelioma in hamsters. They found that 100% of hamsters that were injected with intrapleural SV40 developed mesothelioma, and this led to the sequencing of SV40 in human mesothelioma by this group.[17]

Since then, a number of other studies have confirmed Carbone's findings, with the proportion of cases ranging from 44% to 86% of mesotheliomas tested. One dissenting group has been that of Strickler,[18] who examined mesothelioma tissue from 50 patients with two separate primer sets and did not detect any SV40 sequences. This group also undertook a retrospective cohort study comparing those people who were likely to have received contaminated polio virus against those who did not, and found no increase in the incidence of a number of cancers, including mesothelioma.[19] As Strickler's group concede, the cohort studied has not yet reached the age of peak incidence for mesothelioma.

In two separate studies, Carbone's group have gone on to study possible mechanisms by which SV40 may contribute to the pathogenesis of mesothelioma. They have found that the SV40 sequences present in mesothelioma tissue samples retain the ability to inactivate both p53[20] and pRb.[21] The potential to overcome these checkpoints in cellular proliferation could be crucial in enabling a tumour to survive and progress. While such speculation is inviting, reservations remain about the place of SV40 in cancer. Clearly it is not essential in the development of mesothelioma, since many cases do not express TAG sequences. Are such tumours different in their behaviour – and what of those that do not express TAG? There may be as-yet undiscovered cofactors that are more important for tumorigenesis. If we are to accept the polio vaccine contamination hypothesis then why is TAG expressed in tumours of children who were too young to be immunized in this setting? Artefactual presence would call into question all of the above research, but there must otherwise be previously undescribed vertical transmission of the virus or some other means of human infection. Further investigations are therefore required to determine more clearly how SV40 fits into the pathogenesis of mesothelioma.

Other agents

One-quarter of people who develop MM have had no known exposure to asbestos. While some of these cases may arise from occult exposure, a number of other possible agents have been proposed to cause the disease. These include thoracic radiotherapy, intrapleural thorium dioxide, and other silicates, including erionite and zeolite. The numbers of cases attributed to radiation exposure are very small. A genetic predisposition has also been suggested by occasional reports of clusters of disease within a family, but again numbers are small and co-exposure is difficult to exclude. Although asbestos exposure and smoking have been shown to be synergistic in terms of the likelihood of development of bronchogenic carcinoma, there is no known association between smoking and MM.[22]

Molecular lesions

The pathogenesis of most tumours is currently believed to follow that of the classic model described for the development of colon cancer by Volgelstein et al.[23] In this model, a single cell develops a genetic mutation that enables it to proliferate despite absent or even negative growth-stimulatory signals from normal tissue. Such mutations can occur in response to a carcinogen such as asbestos in MM, as discussed above. The multistep accumulation of further mutations to cells in this clone leads to the development of the hallmarks of a frank malignancy, namely autocrine growth, invasion and the ability to metastasize. This whole process may occur over a period of many years. Alterations enabling this malignant pattern of growth to occur may include oncogene activation or mutation, loss of tumour suppressor genes, and autocrine or paracrine secretion of growth factors. Determining which changes a cell undergoes to develop this malignant phenotype has the potential to provide insights into new methods of treatment for a tumour. In MM, considerable progress has been made over the last ten years in elucidating candidate factors, but no clear single pathogenic pathway has yet been found.

Chromosomal abnormalities

Asbestos is known to induce chromosomal mutations directly. This may occur by the production of reactive metabolites as mentioned above, by interference with the mitotic spindle at division, or by direct chromosomal adherence resulting in fragmentation. The majority of cases of MM subjected to cytogenetic study have shown karyotypic changes,[24] and a wide range of complex and heterogeneous chromosomal abnormalities have been described. Chromosomal gains have been found to be as frequent as losses, and some of these are relatively common, such as loss of 4, 22, 9p and 3p, and gain of 7, 5 and 20.[25] Significant correlation between certain losses (1 and 4) and a high content of asbestos fibres in lung tissue has been shown. The mean chromosomal number has also been shown to correlate with survival in patients with MM. Those patients with a normal chromosome number and no clonal abnormalities had the longest average survival.[26]

Of the many abnormalities described, there are some alterations that are of particular interest in terms of pathogenesis. Monosomy 22 is the most common numerical cytogenetic change, and has been correlated with mutations in the neurofibromatosis type 2 (*NF2*) gene.[27] The loss of at least one locus in 1p (nearly all in 1p22) was found in 74% of examined specimens,[28] and 42–62.5% of cases of MM have been found to have loss of heterozygosity of one or more loci on chromosome 3p.[29] These changes are of interest in that there is a gene for cellular senescence on chromosome 1 and a tumour suppressor gene located on chromosome 3.[13] Polysomy of chromosome 7 is common, and the number of copies of the short arm of this chromosome has been found to be an adverse prognostic feature.[24] The loci for the epidermal growth factor receptor (EGFR) and the platelet-derived growth factor A chain (PDGF-A) are both present on this chromosome (see below). In one study, 83% of cell lines had deletions of 9p,[30] which is the location of the gene for $p16^{ink4}$ (see below). Sixty-one per cent of MM specimens were also found to have allelic losses in 6q in four discrete locations, most of which had losses in more than one of these regions.[31] As was postulated by Bell et al,[31] the consistent losses seen in certain areas may imply that these regions are the sites of tumour suppressor genes, the loss of which is central to the development of the tumour.

Oncogenes

Specific oncogenes have been found to be central to the progression of many malignancies, but as yet this has not been particularly well studied in MM. Of interest, however, are the findings that the v-*src* gene has been shown to cause MM in chickens[32] and that the EJ-*ras* gene causes tumorigenic transformation of mesothelial cells when transfected.[33] There is no evidence that these oncogenes play a role in human MM. The most promising candidates have been c-*fos* and c-*jun*, which have been implicated in animal models. The levels of both c-*fos* and c-*jun* mRNA have been shown to be upregulated when rat pleural mesothelial cells are exposed to asbestos.[34] This pathway has been further investigated by showing that these changes are prevented by the use of *N*-acetylcysteine[35] and by calphostin C, a protein kinase C inhibitor.[36] Such findings could implicate these proto-oncogenes in the pathogenesis of MM, but the levels of c-Fos protein were found to be similar in MM and non-neoplastic mesothelial tissue.[37] Wild-type K-Ras was found in all 20 MM cell lines examined by Metcalf et al.[38] c-Myc immunocytochemical expression is common,[39] but c-*myc* was not found to be amplified in murine MM cell lines.[40]

Tumour suppressor genes

In order for a tumour to continue to proliferate in the face of genomic damage, it is necessary that it avoid the normal cellular processes for the detection of such damage. Tumour suppressor genes enable the cell either to arrest the cell cycle with the possibility of repair or to undertake programmed cell death (apoptosis). Mutation or loss of a tumour suppressor gene enables an altered cell to continue through the cell cycle unchecked, and allows further proliferation. The most well-described of the tumour suppressors is *p53*, which is known to be mutated in a majority of human cancers.[41] Alterations in *p53* have been found in 75% of murine MM cell lines,[42] but wild-type p53 was normally expressed in most human MM cell lines[38] and demonstrated by immunohistochemistry in primary tumours.[43]

The retinoblastoma protein pRb prevents progression of a damaged cell into S phase when it is hypophosphorylated. Its level of expression in human MM cell lines has been shown to be normal.[44] Mouse double-minute 2 (MDM2), a protein that can inhibit the function of both p53 and pRb, is not overexpressed in human MM,[45] although a proportion has been shown to have positive staining for MDM2.[46] The possibility of expressed pRb being abnormal in this tumour has been raised by the finding that a monoclonal antibody specific for the epitopes between exons 21 and 27 showed no immunoreactivity by immunohistochemistry, whereas a polyclonal antiserum showed staining in all MMs examined.[47]

In keeping with the frequent loss of chromosome 9, the product of the *CDKN2* gene, $p16^{INK4}$, was found to be abnormally expressed in 12 of 12 primary mesotheliomas and 15 of 15 MM cell lines.[48] $p16^{INK4}$ normally inhibits phosphorylation of pRb, and thus its loss would allow uncontrolled progress through this stage of the cell cycle. Deletions of the portion of chromosome 9 containing *CDKN2A*, but not *CDKN2B*, were also found in MM cell lines,[49] whereas *p16* has previously been found to be deleted in 85% of MM cell lines but only 22% of primary tumours.[50] Seventy-two percent of primary MMs have also been found to have co-deletions of *p15* and *p16*.[51]

The third tumour suppressor of particular interest in MM is the *NF2* gene. This was found to be mutated in 41% of MM cell lines examined by Sekido et al[52] and 53% of cell lines examined by Bianchi et al.[53] This latter group also found that three-quarters of these mutations were confirmed to be present in the primary tumour. This finding for MM in humans does not correlate with the disease in rats, where mutations were not found.[54]

The Wilms' tumour gene (*WT1*) is expressed in normal mesothelium during embryogenesis. It is potentially interesting in view of the fact that one of the actions of the WT1 protein is to control the transcription of genes such as those for PDGF-A,[55] insulin-like growth factor (IGF)-II,[56] transforming growth factor β (TGF-β)[57] and the IGF-I receptor (IGF-IR).[58] All of these have been described as potential autocrine growth factors in MM, and the deletion of *WT1* could allow excessive production. Expression of *WT1* mRNA has been found in most human MM cell lines examined and in most primary tumours.[59,60] The level of expression has been found to be variable, but there was no inverse correlation found between expression of WT1 and IGF-II or PDGF-A.[61] A further study using mutational screening found no significant changes to *WT1*, and also found no correlation between WT1 immunostaining and EGFR or IGF-IR levels.[62]

PATHOBIOLOGY

The diagnosis of MM is usually made on the basis of histological analysis, from which the tumour can be classified as follows:

1. *Epithelial:* the tumour mass consists of papillary, tubular, acinar-like or solid tissue in which cuboidal tumour cells form a pave-

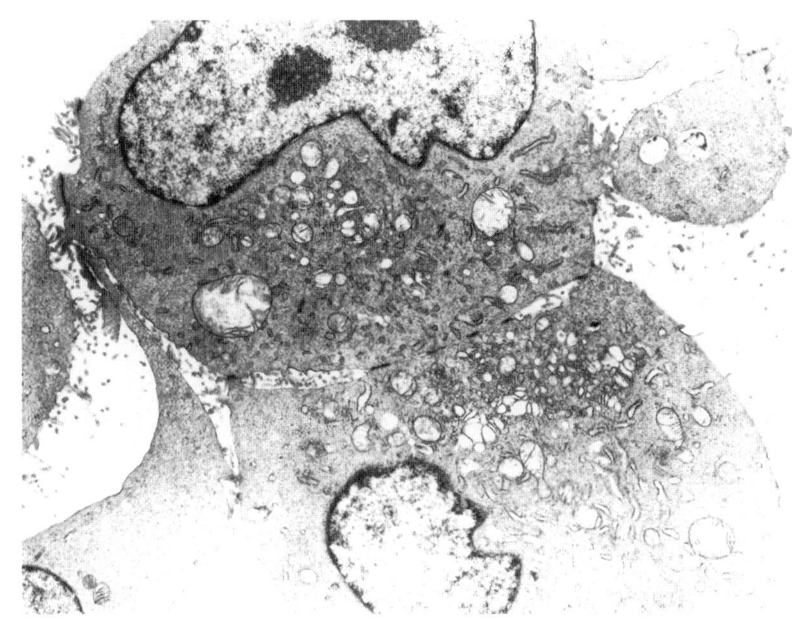

Figure 13.1
Electron micrograph of malignant mesothelioma cells maintained in cell culture, demonstrating typical ultrastructural features, including long microvilli, glycogen granules, swollen mitochondria, desmosomes and prominent nucleoli

ment-like appearance. The amount of stroma within the tumour is variable.

2. *Sarcomatous:* the tumour mass consists of spindle-shaped cells forming organized bundles, though whirls, 'herring bone' or irregular patterns of tumour cells also occur.
3. *Desmoplastic:* the tumour mass consists of a sizable connective tissue component with variable cellularity and pleomorphism. Epithelium-like structures are not present in this form.
4. *Biphasic:* the tumour mass consists of a mix of the epithelial and sarcomatous forms. This is the most common type.

Differential diagnosis of MM from reactive mesothelium or adenocarcinoma is an important aspect of analysis of biopsy samples. Cytological diagnosis is based first on the malignant nature of the samples by generally applicable criteria (nuclear polymorphism, irregularity of nuclear membrane, chromatin distribution), followed by confirmation of the mesothelial characteristics. These characteristics include a characteristic cytoplasmic appearance, a brushlike border and multinucleation. Further confirmation can be obtained by ultrastructural analysis, showing long microvilli and numerous intermediate filaments[63] (Figure 13.1). Additional immunohistological analysis, such as the use of the ME monoclonal antibodies that differentiate mesothelial-derived cells from adenocarcinoma,[64] and the use of special stains are also useful tools in the accurate diagnosis of this malignancy. Typically, mesothelioma are positive for epithelial membrane antigen (EMA) and WT1, but negative for carcinoembryonic antigen (CEA).

IMMUNOBIOLOGY

The human disease

In contrast to many other tumours, there is little evidence in MM that specific immune responses are initiated against the tumour during the course of the disease. Some descriptions of leukocytic infiltrations have been reported in the literature, but these examples are rather non-systematic and use very broad characterizations. What is evident is that the extent of infiltration depends on the individual tumour.[65,66] One unusual form of MM is termed lymphohistiocytoid mesothelioma – so called because there is evidence of lymphocytes infiltrating the tumour mass.[67] Although suggestive of specific immune recognition of the tumour, there is no direct evidence that supports this hypothesis, and these cells may simply reflect a non-specific inflammatory response. In fact, early attempts to isolate MM-reactive killer cells from patients proved unsuccessful.[68] Overall, the lack of tumour-infiltrating lymphocytes (TILs), as with many other tumours, has been attributed either to a lack of tumour antigen expression or to other factors, such as the secretion of immunosuppressive cytokines, that diminish the overall immunogenicity of the tumour.

However, more recent work has suggested that an immune response is generated in a significant proportion (28%) of MM patients.[69] In these studies, patient sera reacted with a panel of human MM cell lines as determined by Western blot analysis. When sequential sera were analysed, it was found that the titre increased with the progression of the disease. Importantly, the MM-reactive antibodies within the sera were of the IgG class, indicative of immunoglobulin class switching and hence the involvement of the cellular arm of the immune response, which is obligatory for this process. These are important data, which will lead to identification of a number of potential tumour-associated antigens (TAAs), the characterization of which will be invaluable in the context of potential vaccination strategies or immunotherapeutic treatments.

In addition, clinical studies have suggested that, even if an immune response is not a normal event in the disease process, this malignancy may be susceptible to immunotherapy. In a small trial using intralesional therapy with granulocyte–macrophage colony-stimulating factor (GM-CSF), while there was no direct evidence of a tumour-specific immune response, the one patient who showed a partial response also had an intense lymphocytic infiltration in biopsy samples.[70] Apart from using this direct administration of a cytokine, efforts have been made to utilize gene therapy techniques in treatment. In particular, the use of genes encoding cytokines have been the most prevalent, in the hope that they will boost or enhance any ongoing anti-tumour response. Although gene therapy has provided some encouraging results in animal models, the difficulty with this technique in solid tumours, such as MM, is the inability to transduce all tumour cells with the gene of interest. Therefore some emphasis has been placed on trials in which cytokine genes are transferred via viral vectors such as vaccinia.

The growth of tumours is often considered to be immunosuppressive, and MMs have been shown to secrete a number of cytokines or factors that are known to modulate immune responses, including PDGF, TGF-β and interleukin-6 (IL-6). As is quite often the case with such products, they are responsible for coordinating or mediating a number of processes, and PDGF and TGF-β have also been shown to be growth factors for MMs. The role of these molecules in influencing the immune response to MM has not been investigated deeply, and what we know has been elucidated in animal models (see below).

Another potential mechanism whereby MMs might evade immune recognition is by the down-regulation of HLA class I molecules, such as has been reported for melanoma. However, a survey of a panel of human and murine lines has shown that these tumours all express class I molecules, and therefore they can still be targets for the immune response.

Animal models

A number of different models of MM have been established in animals, predominantly in an effort to understand the pathogenesis of the disease and to test potential therapeutic agents. Such models include the xenografting of human tumour tissue or cell lines into immune-deficient rodents, as well as the establishment of rodent MM lines using the known inducing agents, asbestos and SV40. With such little information available as to the extent and type of immune response induced by MM in patients, it is not surprising that the bulk of our knowledge concerning the immunobiology of MM is derived from animal models, in particular a murine asbestos-induced model. These MM cells exhibit the diagnostic characteristics of the human tumour. Upon subcutaneous inoculation into mice, solid tumours form and grow rapidly. There is little evidence of lymphocytic infiltration, although those cells that are present appear at the periphery of the tumour mass and are of both the $CD4^+$ and $CD8^+$ phenotype. The most prominent infiltrating leukocyte is the macrophage, making up to 50% of the tumour mass. These macrophages are predominantly class II negative, and are therefore of an unactivated phenotype and unlikely to contribute to the initiation of an effective antitumour response. In fact, in the absence of exogenous factors, T-cell-mediated antitumour responses cannot be detected in mice inoculated with these tumours, which is indicative of an inherent lack of immunogenicity.

These same murine MM lines have been transfected with a number of immunologically relevant molecules, including the co-stimulatory molecule B7.1 and the cytokines IL-2 and IL-12. Such experiments indicate that, while the tumour itself does not generally induce an effective antitumour response, it is susceptible to eradication by the immune system. Transduction of B7.1 can lead to the induction of cytolytic T cells, which can recognize and destroy both the transfectant and the parental cell line.

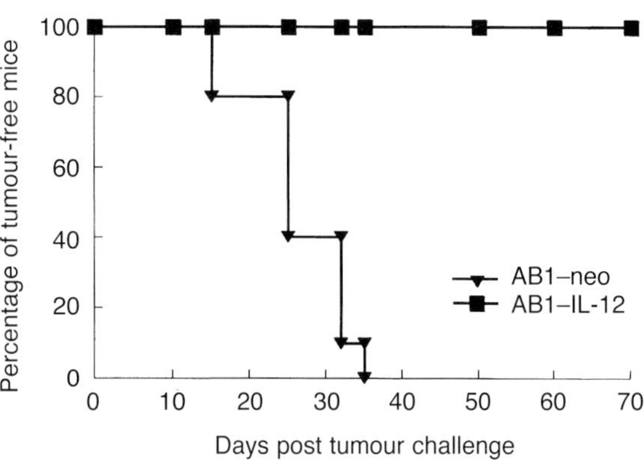

Figure 13.2
Mesothelioma cell line AB1 transfected with the IL-12 gene fails to grow in immune-competent mice. BALB/c mice were inoculated with AB1 tumour cells that were transfected with either the neomycin-resistance gene only (AB1–neo; n = 10) or with the gene encoding IL-12 (ABI–IL-12; n = 10), and tumour growth was then monitored.

MMs transfected with the productive IL-12 gene do not grow in syngeneic recipients (Figure 13.2). This is an immune-mediated phenomenon, since the tumorigenicity of the transfected line is unaffected in immune-deficient mice. Both $CD4^+$ and $CD8^+$ cells are required, and can be seen to heavily infiltrate the site of tumour inoculation prior to complete tumour eradication. The potency of IL-12, a cytokine associated with the differentiation of T-cell-mediated cytolytic responses, is also evident when administered systemically to established tumours. In this case, IL-12 can cause stagnation of tumour growth and even disappearance of the tumour. However, these effects – profound for such an aggressive tumour – require the continual presence of the cytokine, and cessation of treatment leads to progression of tumour growth (Figure 13.3).

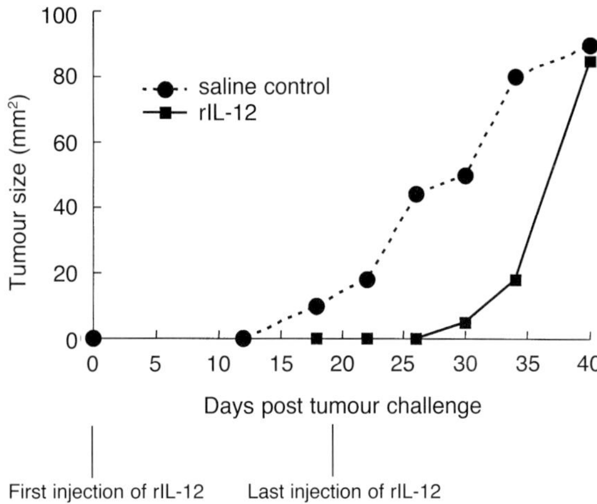

Figure 13.3
Systemic administration of IL-12 prevents and delays tumour emergence. BALB/c mice were injected with a syngeneic mesothelioma tumour AB1. Starting on day 0, ten mice were injected daily intraperitoneally with 0.5 μg of recombinant (r) IL-12 or saline, five times per week for three weeks. The graph shows the tumour growth rate of these two experimental groups.

Applications to therapy

As mentioned above, immunomodulatory molecules such as TGF-β are produced by mesothelioma cells as obligate growth factors. One could therefore hypothesize that interventions that target such factors may be very effective from two aspects: first, by interfering with the growth cycle of the tumour cells, and, second, by allowing an immune response to be generated. In experiments in which TGF-β production was reduced by inhibiting translation of these proteins using antisense DNA technology, tumour growth could be inhibited but not eradicated.[71] Inhibition of tumour growth was concomitant with treatment – the effects were lost on cessation of treatment. No evidence of an improved antitumour response was noted in these experiments. This result may have several explanations, including that the amount of TGF-β required for tumour cell growth is significantly greater than that required for immunosuppression. Such approaches are worthy of further investigation – possibly in combination with other treatments. See the section below on 'Future directions'.

CLINICAL PRESENTATION AND COURSE

MM usually develops in males with a history of occupational exposure to asbestos. The latency period between asbestos exposure and the development of MM is at least 20 years.[1,72] Therefore patients are usually over 50 years of age.[73] However, non-occupational exposure does occur, and in some of these cases the exposure occurred in childhood. Patients with pleural mesothelioma usually present with symptoms of chest pain or discomfort, dyspnoea and cough. In fact, the presence of chest wall pain in any at-risk patient is a strong clue to the possible presence of mesothelioma. Early in the course of the disease, dyspnoea is the commonest symptom, and is due to the presence of an effusion. The majority of patients with pleural mesothelioma will have a malignant pleural effusion, which is usually bloodstained, often loculated and of large volume. As the tumour progresses, chest discomfort or tightness may occur. The dyspnoea may improve because of fusion of the pleural surfaces and resolution of the effusion. Unremitting chest pain may occur as the tumour locally invades the intercostal nerves. Eventually, the lung becomes encased by tumour, leading to worsening of dyspnoea and chest tightness. The tumour commonly spreads by direct extension to involve the chest wall, the mediastinum, other pleura or the diaphragmatic surface, the pericardium and the liver. Invasion of the pericardium leads to a pericardial effusion, which worsens the dyspnoea.

Spread to local lymph nodes occurs in 40% of cases, but haematogenous spread is not usually of much clinical significance. Weight loss occurs in the late stages of the disease.

Examination findings in the early stages of the disease usually reflect the presence of a pleural effusion, with dullness to percussion and reduced breath sounds. As the tumour progresses and encases the entire hemithorax, chest expansion becomes noticeably restricted, and dullness to percussion and reduced breath sounds are found over the hemithorax. Breathing sounds can be 'harsh' rather than reduced, and sometimes are frankly 'bronchial' in nature. Protrusion of tumour through the intercostal spaces tends to occur at sites of previous thoracocentesis, chest tube insertion or thoracotomy incision. Supraclavicular lymphadenopathy and ascites may be present if the tumour has spread to these areas. Paraneoplastic syndromes are rare, but can include hypercalcaemia, autoimmune haemolytic anaemia and inappropriate secretion of antidiuretic hormone (SIADH).[74] Thrombocytosis with a platelet count of greater than 400 000/μl occurs in approximately 30% of cases,[73] but does not seem to lead to increased thrombotic events. Those with peritoneal disease experience abdominal pain and distension, weight loss, anorexia and bloating. Peritoneal mesothelioma rarely invades superiorly through the diaphragm.

DIAGNOSIS

Radiology

The most common chest X-ray abnormality in early stage disease is the presence of a large pleural effusion. Pleural thickening or small focal pleural masses may be seen on computed tomography (CT) of the chest, and CT is useful in differentiating pleural fluid from pleural thickening,[75] although ultrasound is often required. CT scanning also provides information on the state of the pulmonary parenchyma, the mediastinum and invasion of the chest wall.[76,77] As the disease progresses there is diffuse involvement of the pleura and larger pleurally based masses may become obvious. The pleural effusion often becomes loculated. Eventually, the lung becomes encased in a thick pleural rind of tumour that compresses the underlying lung. Magnetic resonance imaging (MRI) is useful for delineation of chest wall invasion.

Histopathology

Accurate diagnosis of MM can be time-consuming, and may require more than one diagnostic procedure because of the difficulty in obtaining malignant tissue for histopathological assessment. Pleural biopsies, obtained via closed or open (thoracoscopy/thoracotomy) procedures, improve the diagnostic yield. Pleural biopsy samples should be assessed by immunohistochemistry and electron microscopy, since these are the important studies to assist in making a definitive diagnosis.[78,79] The major problems associated with closed pleural biopsies are:

- lack of useful pleural tissue;
- difficulty in interpretation of small biopsy samples;[80]
- the need to distinguish malignant mesothelioma from reactive mesothelial inflammation and metastatic pleural tumours.

Cytology

Most patients with MM present with a pleural effusion, and therefore thoracocentesis is often the first diagnostic procedure. Large amounts of pleural fluid should be obtained and sent for cytological examination; this will be diagnostic in 30–50% of cases.[74] The fluid should be examined using light microscopy and immunochemical stains for cytokeratins and vimentin and immunohistochemical stains (especially CEA and EMA) to differentiate adenocarcinoma from mesothelioma (see above). The combination of cytological assessment of pleural fluid and histopathology on closed pleural biopsy specimens can increase diagnostic accuracy for pleural malignancy, including MM.[81]

MANAGEMENT

MM is a uniformly fatal disease that is not usually curable with surgery, chemotherapy or radiotherapy. The potential treatment options are the same as for other malignancies, namely surgery, radiotherapy, chemotherapy, immunotherapy, gene therapy, supportive care, or combination therapy utilizing some or all of the above treatments. However, there are major differences from other cancers, because in mesothelioma it is often difficult to objectively quantify the location and extent of disease, and the patients are older and often have underlying illness that makes them unfit for aggressive, rigorous treatment plans. The rarity of the condition means that few large prospective clinical trials have been published, and clinicians must rely on retrospective clinical trials with small numbers of patients. Also, different centres seem to favour different treatment regimens, which are often difficult to compare. In any case, it is clear that MM is a treatment-resistant disease, and therefore there is no standard treatment regimen.

Surgery

Four types of operation have been performed as treatment for mesothelioma: pleuropneumonectomy, pleurectomy/decortication, limited pleurectomy, and thoracoscopy with talc pleurodesis. Pleuropneumonectomy involves an en bloc resection of the pleura, lung, ipsilateral hemidiaphragm and pericardium. Butchart[82] reported that this procedure carried an operative mortality rate of 30%, but since then there have been a few studies reporting a reduction in operative mortality rate to 6–9%.[83–86] This was most likely due to improved patient selection, experience and better postoperative care. Median survival in these studies ranged from 8 to 16 months. Pleurectomy/decortication involves attempting to remove all obvious pleural disease without removing the underlying lung. The operative mortality rate is 1.8%;[87] however, long-term survival is not significantly increased in most patients. Limited pleurectomy is a palliative procedure designed to resect part of the parietal pleura to control a pleural effusion. Thoracoscopy with talc pleurodesis is an effective palliative procedure for control of effusion.

Overall, in most cases, surgical procedures alone will not lead to any significant improvement in survival. However, Sugarbaker[88] showed that combination therapy (resection of tumour, chemotherapy followed by radiotherapy) in selected patients can lead to some improvement in survival. In this study, operative morbidity rate was measured at 17%, mortality rate was 6%, and overall survival was 16 months. Generally, surgery is not recommended except for diagnostic or palliative reasons (such as control of effusions).

Radiotherapy

Mesothelioma is a radioresistant tumour,[89] and radiotherapy has usually been given in combination with surgery. It is therefore difficult to evaluate the success of radiation as a single treatment. Radiation doses are usually limited to 4500 cGy or less to prevent damage to vital structures, such as the lungs, heart, oesophagus and spinal cord. Localized foci for radiation delivery have been tried (e.g. colloids), but with little success.

Chemotherapy

Numerous chemotherapy trials (>120) have been undertaken in mesothelioma. Unfortunately, very few chemotherapeutic agents have consistently shown a response rate greater than 20%.[90] Active agents include cyclophosphamide, doxorubicin, detorubicin, edatrexate, epirubicin, ifosfamide, cisplatin, carboplatin, mitomycin, methotrexate, 5-azacytidine and 5-fluorouracil. In the past, combination chemotherapy regimens have shown no clear advantage over single-agent treatment.[91] However, a recent phase II study using cisplatin and gemcitabine for MM reports a response rate of 47.6% based on treatment of 21 patients with significant symptomatic improvement.[92]

Immunotherapy and gene therapy

These are relatively new treatment options, and their role alone or in combination with surgery or radio- or chemotherapy has not yet been adequately evaluated. It is known that systemic interferon-α (IFN-α),[93,94] IL-2[95] and GM-CSF[70] have some activity in selected cases of MMs but none has achieved a response rate sufficient to warrant their recommendation in all patients. Combining IFN-α with chemotherapy has also produced no added benefit.[96]

FUTURE DIRECTIONS

In this section, we shall highlight directions in which mesothelioma research is heading, focusing on aspects that could prove to be clinically useful.

Diagnosis

An interesting recent development has been the use of serological screening of recombinant cDNA expression libraries ('SEREX') to identify mesothelioma antigens. A number have been characterized, and at this preliminary stage it appears that the majority of patients presenting with MM express one or more at diagnosis.[69] This is very exciting, because it may represent a useful diagnostic tool and one that can be fairly simply applied (all it requires is the patient's serum). Equally importantly, the fact that these antibody reactivities can be detected at presentation implies that they will be detectable prior to presentation. At present, it is not known whether this represents a few months or a few years, but it is possible that the use of this technology will generate a screening test for mesothelioma. It is unlikely that this would be entirely specific, but it might be useful for patients at high risk – if the tests are positive, the patient would undergo more detailed investigations, perhaps even including pleuroscopy.

The molecular pathogenic events underlining asbestos-induced cancer are being progressively analysed. None of the changes so far described are specific for MM, but it is possible that patterns will emerge that will make the application of molecular techniques useful in terms of establishing a diagnosis of MM, in particular enabling pathologists to distinguish MM from reactive mesothelium and from other malignancies (e.g. adenocarcinoma).

Therapy

Future therapies in mesothelioma will have two aims. The first is to alleviate symptoms. Patients with MM often experience profound weight loss, fevers, hypoalbuminaemia and pain. Recent studies have identified cytokines that are likely to contribute to this, particularly IL-6. In animal studies, blockade of IL-6 has had a profound effect on animals' clinical status, although the actual antitumour effect was modest, and possibly related to the improvement in the host's well-being. If a simple method of inhibiting IL-6 activity in vivo can be established, it is likely that this could be given to patients with mesothelioma to alleviate their systemic symptoms. Such therapy might involve receptor blockade or IL-6-signalling blockade (e.g. via the SOCS molecules).[97]

The second area in which new developments in therapy might occur is in the generation of antitumour effects.

Development of new single agents

MM is largely resistant to chemotherapy,[98] although some recent effective combinations have been discovered (e.g. cisplatin and gemcitabine).[92] A number of investigators have begun to analyse the mechanisms whereby MM is resistant to chemotherapy. In general, it appears that it is de novo resistant to chemotherapy, in contrast to other tumours such as small cell lung cancer that are largely sensitive to chemotherapy initially but develop resistance following treatment. It does not appear that the multidrug resistance gene is the major mechanism for resistance to chemotherapy in MM. Once the mechanisms of resistance have been identified, new therapeutic strategies are likely to combine blockade of these with chemotherapeutic agents. In addition, as new agents are developed, they will continue to be tried in MM. The recent success of the cisplatin–gemcitabine combination suggests that some of these approaches will be effective in this disease – at least at reducing tumour bulk.

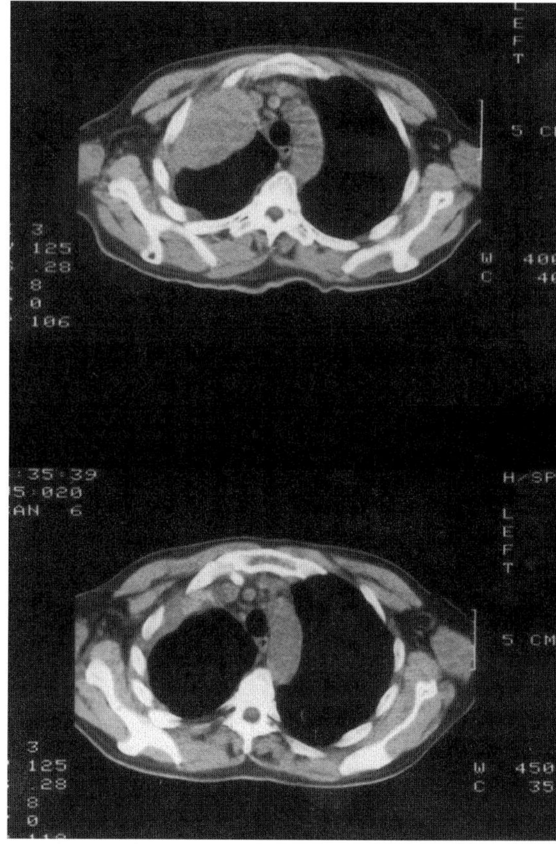

Figure 13.4
Thoracic CT scan before and after interferon therapy. CT scans showing an extensive right-sided pleural mesothelioma (upper scan), which showed marked shrinkage following three months' therapy with subcutaneous recombinant IFN-α (lower scan).

Immunotherapy in its various forms has begun to be tried in MM, and it is likely that in the future the limited but clear success of this approach will be augmented, probably in combination with other therapies. While established agents such as recombinant IFN-α have had limited but surprising effects[93] (Figure 13.4), combining this approach with chemotherapy has not proved more efficacious.[96] This may be partly because of the toxicity of chemotherapeutic approaches. It is therefore likely that future immunotherapeutic approaches to MM will involve other strategies, particularly the local administration of immunomodulatory agents into the tumour and/or into distal local sites. The continuous infusion of GM-CSF into MM produced some tumour shrinkage and mononuclear cell infiltrates, but proved technically demanding.[70] Future developments aimed at improving delivery of these agents to the tumour that are less technically demanding are likely to occur. There are three possibilities: improved continuous-infusion technology, depot release preparations and gene therapy.

The last is the most advanced. Initial studies using immunological gene therapy in MM have involved the administration of virus–cytokine constructs. In one pilot study, this approach was shown to be feasible, to produce a T-cell infiltrate in the tumour and to be free of side-effects in the patient and in contacts.[99] These are very early days for the immunological gene therapy of MM, and there is no doubt that in the future we shall see further developments in this area. Other gene therapy strategies that have been utilized have included herpes simplex TK 'suicide gene' therapy, which has produced some responses and which may be working by a combination of tumour shrinkage and necrosis generating antitumour immune effects. Other gene therapy approaches that have been utilized preclinically include the use of antisense oligonucleotides to block mesothelioma growth factors such as PDGF and TGF-β. This approach has proved most efficacious in vivo, and has caused a profound reduction in tumour growth in animal models.[71] It is likely that future treatment of MM will involve such gene therapy approaches, provided that the concentration of antisense oligonucleotides can be increased within tumours to a level sufficient to cause the required biological effects.

Combination therapies

It seems likely that the most effective treatment of MM will require combination therapy. Combinations include some of those described above, for example molecular approaches to increase the sensitivity of tumour cells to chemotherapeutic agents combined with systemic administration of such agents, or a combination of suicide gene therapy with immunotherapy. In addition, it is possible that chemotherapy can be strategically combined with immunotherapy in a way that augments the efficacy of each; for example, it is possible that cycles of drug therapy may alter the antigenic profile of tumour cells so that they provide new targets for immunotherapy.

The future development of effective therapies in MM is likely to rely on two fundamental principles. First, it will be essential to understand the basic biology and immunology of the disease before optimal therapies can be developed. MM is a disease that has remained mysterious for many years, yet over the past five years or so the underlying pathogenic mechanisms and immunobiology have begun to be elucidated. Secondly, it is likely that combined therapy will be necessary, and that each component will need to have independently proven efficacy, i.e. it will be important to build on treatments that already have a track record of clear success at reducing tumour bulk.

Tumour biology and epidemiology

Detecting the basic molecular and protein abnormalities in mesothelioma cells has required the use of rather laborious laboratory techniques. Molecular techniques aimed at generating high-throughput screening have recently been developed, partly as a result of the Human Genome Project. When these technologies are applied to MM, it is likely that the spectra of molecular and protein differences between benign and malignant cells, and between malignant cells with different types of clinical behaviour, will be identified. Such technologies include improve analysis of mRNA expression difference between cells, for example using representational difference analysis (RDA) and serial analysis of gene expression (SAGE).[100] In addition, DNA chip technology is being developed, and, although it cannot analyse differences in all cellular mRNAs expressed, it is useful for rapid analysis of differences in limited gene numbers.[101]

In terms of epidemiology, it would be interesting to see whether in the future other agents besides asbestos are either sole etiological agents in MM or act as cofactors with asbestos. The recent identification of the SV40 virus as a potential factor in the development of MM is of interest,[20] and it will also be interesting to see if other infectious agents that have known oncogenic effects are identified. A number of viruses are at least partially trophic to the pleural mesothelium (e.g. causing the clinical syndrome of viral pleurisy), and a potential role for such viruses in the generation of MM may be identified in the future. Similarly, there are a large number of cases of MM in whom the level of asbestos exposure is no higher than that of the background population. It has been assumed that these cases represent the unfortunate small proportion of patients who develop a tumour with low levels of carcinogen (similar to the small proportion of sun-exposed individuals who develop UV-induced skin cancers). Nevertheless, it remains possible that other agents may be identified as etiological agents in MM. For example, many patients with MM are farmers, and, while it has always been assumed that this is because they have been exposed to asbestos in their farming activities, it would be interesting to determine whether or not inhalation of potentially carcinogenic pesticides may contribute to the development of the disease.

Finally, the future may see the development of preventive measures in mesothelioma. There are some populations that are at extremely high risk of developing mesothelioma, for example, those exposed to crocidolite as children. A number of studies have been undertaken in an attempt to reduce their risk, such as the use of prophylactic vitamin A. This has shown some efficacy, but many of these individuals still develop MM.[102] The above-mentioned identification of mesothelioma antigens raises the possibility that a tumour vaccine may be developed for MM. Such at-risk groups would welcome such a vaccine. However, there are two major hurdles to overcome. First, these vaccines are difficult to test because they need to be given to large numbers of patients and followed for a long period of time before any valid efficacy can be determined: for example something like 5000–10 000 patients, followed over a period of five years or so. Secondly, as most tumour antigens are self-antigens, the risk of autoimmune disease in vaccinated patients would be substantial. This may cause pleurisy, peritonitis or pericarditis. It is thus possible that the development of a mesothelioma vaccine may be limited by the almost inevitable occurrence of such side-effects in a significant proportion of those vaccinated. If these side-effects are minimal then the benefit may outweigh the risk, but the logistics of determining this are substantial. Most tumour vaccines are used in an adjuvant setting, i.e. they are used in patients once the disease is already diagnosed.

In many ways, the future directions in mesothelioma research and treatment will parallel those for other tumours, and yet, in other ways, in view of the rather unusual clinical and biological behaviour of MM, they will be unique to that disease. Certainly MM is a very aggressive disease that has been largely resistant to all therapeutic attempts tried. In view of the increasing incidence of this disease and the poor success rate with current therapies, it is hoped that in the future the application of modern molecular and biological techniques to the problem, in association with the commitment of managing clinicians to utilize novel therapeutic approaches, combined with the courage of the afflicted population, will lead to the development of improved methods of diagnosis, therapy and prevention of MM.

ACKNOWLEDGEMENTS

The authors thank the following individuals for technical or administrative assistance: Dr Irene

Caminischi, Dr Terry Robertson, Mrs Christine Bundell, Mrs Janeeka Watters and Mrs Trudy Turner.

REFERENCES

1. Wagner JC, Sleggs CA, Marchand P, Diffuse pleural mesothelioma and asbestos exposure in the North Western Cape Province. *Br J Ind Med J* 1960; **17**: 260–71.
2. Mossman BT, Bignon J, Corn M et al, Asbestos: scientific developments and implications for public policy. *Science* 1990; **247**: 294–301.
3. Becklake MR, Asbestos-related diseases of the lung and other organs: their epidemiology and implications for clinical practice. *Am Rev Respir Dis* 1976; **114**: 187–227.
4. Antman KH, Natural history and epidemiology of malignant mesothelioma. *Chest* 1993; **103**: 373S–6S.
5. McDonald JC, McDonald AD, The epidemiology of mesothelioma in historical context. *Eur Respir J* 1996; **9**: 1932–42.
6. Roggli VL, Mineral fibre content of lung tissue in patients with malignant mesothelioma. In: *Malignant Mesothelioma* (Henderson D, Shilken K, Langlois S, Whitaker D, eds). New York: Hemisphere: New York, 1992: 210–22.
7. Churg A, Chrysotile, tremolite, and malignant mesothelioma in man. *Chest* 1988; **93**: 621–8.
8. Jaurand MC, Kaplan H, Thiollet J et al, Phagocytosis of chrysotile fibers by pleural mesothelial cells in culture. *Am J Pathol* 1979; **94**: 529–38.
9. Hansen J, Deklerk NH, Musk AW, Hobbs MST, Environmental exposure to crocidolite and mesothelioma – exposure–response relationships. *Am J Respir Crit Care Med* 1998; **157**: 69–75.
10. Rom WN, Travis WD, Brody AR, Cellular and molecular basis of the asbestos-related disease. *Am Rev Respir Dis* 1991; **143**: 408–22.
11. Lechner JF, Tokiwa T, LaVeck M et al, Asbestos-associated chromosomal changes in human mesothelial cells. *Proc Nat Acad Sci USA* 1985; **82**: 3884–8.
12. Branchaud RM, Garant LJ, Kane AB, Pathogenesis of mesothelial reactions to asbestos fibers. Monocyte recruitment and macrophage activation. *Pathobiology* 1993; **61**: 154–63.
13. Walker C, Everitt J, Barrett JC, Possible cellular and moleculr mechanisms for asbestos carcinogenicity. *Am J Ind Med* 1992; **21**: 253–73.
14. Yegles M, Saint-Etienne L, Renier A et al, Induction of metaphase and anaphase/telophase abnormalities by asbestos fibers in rat pleural mesothelial cells in vitro. *Am J Respir Cell Mol Biol* 1993; **9**: 186–91.
15. Bergsagel DJ, Finegold MJ, Butel JS et al, DNA sequences similar to those of simian virus 40 in ependymomas and choroid plexus tumors of childhood. *N Engl J Med* 1992; **326**: 988–93.
16. Cicala C, Pompetti F, Carbone M, SV40 induces mesotheliomas in hamsters. *Am J Pathol* 1993; **142**: 1524–33.
17. Carbone M, Pass HI, Rizzo P et al, Simian virus 40-like DNA sequences in human pleural mesothelioma. *Oncogene* 1994; **9**: 1781–90.
18. Strickler HD, Goedert JJ, Fleming M et al, Simian virus 40 and pleural mesothelioma in humans. *Cancer Epidemiol Biomarkers Prev* 1996; **5**: 473–5.
19. Strickler HD, Rosenberg PS, Devesa SS et al, Contamination of poliovirus vaccines with simian virus 40 (1955–1963) and subsequent cancer rates. *JAMA* 1998; **279**: 292–5.
20. Carbone M, Rizzo P, Grimley PM et al, Simian virus-40 large-T antigen binds p53 in human mesotheliomas. *Nature Med* 1997; **3**: 908–12.
21. Deluca A, Baldi A, Esposito V et al, The retinoblastoma gene family Prb/P105, P107, Prb2/P130 and simian virus-40 large T-antigen in human mesotheliomas. *Nature Med* 1997; **3**: 913–16.
22. Muscat JE, Wynder El, Cigarette smoking, asbestos exposure, and malignant mesothelioma. *Cancer Res* 1991; **51**: 2263–7.
23. Vogelstein B, Fearon ER, Hamilton SR et al, Genetic alterations during colorectal-tumor development. *N Engl J Med* 1988; **319**: 525–32.
24. Knuutila S, Tiainen M, Tammilehto L et al, Cytogenetics of human malignant mesotheliomas. *Eur Respir Rev* 1993; **3**: 25–8.

25. Hagemeijer A, Versnel MA, Van Drunen E et al, Cytogenetic analysis of malignant mesothelioma. *Cancer Genet Cytogenet* 1990; **47**: 1–28.
26. Tiainen M, Rautonen J, Pyrhonen S et al, Chromosome number correlates with survival in patients with malignant pleural mesothelioma. *Cancer Genet Cytogenet* 1992; **62**: 21–4.
27. Huncharek M, Genetic factors in the aetiology of malignant mesothelioma. *Eur J Cancer* 1995; **31A**: 1741–7.
28. Lee WC, Balsara B, Liu Z et al, Loss of heterozygosity analysis defines a critical region in chromosome 1p22 commonly delected in human malignant mesothelioma. *Cancer Res* 1996; **56**: 4297–301.
29. Zeiger MA, Gnarra JR, Zbar B et al, Loss of heterozygosity on the short arm of chromosome 3 in mesothelioma cell lines and solid tumors. *Genes Chromosomes Cancer* 1994; **11**: 15–20.
30. Cheng JQ, Jhanwar SC, Lu YY, Testa JR, Homozygous deletions within 9p21–p22 identify a small critical region of chromosomal loss in human malignant mesotheliomas. *Cancer Res* 1993; **53**: 4761–3.
31. Bell DW, Jhanwar SC, Testa JR, Multiple regions of allelic loss from chormosome arm 6q in malignant mesothelioma. *Cancer Res* 1997; **57**: 4057–62.
32. England JM, Panella MJ, Ewert DL, Halpern MS, Induction of a diffuse mesothelioma in chickens by intraperitoneal inoculation of v-src DNA. *Virology* 1991; **182**: 423–9.
33. Reddel RR, Malan-Shibley L, Gerwin BI et al, Tumorigenicity of human mesothelial cell line transfected with EJ-ras oncogene. *J Natl Cancer Inst* 1989; **81**: 945–8.
34. Heintz NH, Janssen YM, Mossman BT, Persistent induction of c-fos and c-jun expression by asbestos. *Proc Natl Acad Sci USA* 1993; **90**: 3299–303.
35. Janssen YMW, Heintz NH, Mossman BT, Induction of c-fos and c-jun proto-oncogene expression by asbestos is ameliorated by N-acetyl-L-cysteine in mesothelial cells. *Cancer Res* 1995; **55**: 2085–9.
36. Fung H, Quinlan TR, Janssen YMW et al, Inhibition of protein kinase C prevents asbestos-induced c-fos and c-jun protooncogene expression in mesothelial cells. *Cancer Res* 1997; **57**: 3101–5.
37. Ramael M, Vandenbossche J, Buysse C et al, Immunoreactivity for c-Fos and c-Myc protein with the monoclonal antibodies 14eio and 6e10 in malignant mesothelioma and nonneoplastic mesothelium of the pleura. *Histol Histopathol* 1995; **10**: 639–43.
38. Metcalf RA, Welsh JA, Bennett WP et al, p53 and Kirsten-ras mutations in human mesothelioma cell lines. *Cancer Res* 1992; **52**: 2610–15.
39. Suzuki Y, Weston A, Ashley R, Immunocytochemical analysis of oncoproteins and growth factors in human malignant mesothelioma. *Oncol Rep* 1995; **2**: 897–902.
40. Moyer VD, Cistulli CA, Vaslet CA, Kane AB, Oxygen radicals and asbestos carcinogenesis. *Environ Health Perspect* 1994; **102**: 131–6.
41. Hollstein M, Sidransky D, Vogelstein B, Harris CC, p53 mutations in human cancers. *Science* 1991; **253**: 49–53.
42. Cora EM, Kane AB, Alterations in a tumour suppressor gene, p53 in mouse mesotheliomas induced by crocidolite asbestos. *Eur Respir Rev* 1993; **3**: 148–50.
43. Mor O, Yaron P, Huszar M et al, Absence of p53 mutations in malignant mesotheliomas. *Am J Respir Cell Mol Biol* 1997; **16**: 9–13.
44. Van de Meeren A, Seddon MB, Kispert J et al, Lack of expression of retinoblastoma gene is not frequently involved in the genesis of human mesothelioma. *Eur Respir Rev* 1993; **3**: 177–9.
45. Ungar S, Vandemeeren A, Tammilehto L et al, High levels of Mdm2 are not correlated with the presence of wild-type p53 in human malignant mesothelioma cell lines. *Br J Cancer* 1996; **74**: 1534–40.
46. Segers K, Backhovens H, Singh SK et al, Immunoreactivity for p53 and Mdm2 and the detection of p53 mutations in human malignant mesothelioma. *Virchows Arch Int J Pathol* 1995; **427**: 431–6.

47. Ramael M, Segers K, Vanmarck E, Differential immunohistochemical staining for retinoblastoma protein with the antibodies C15 and 1f8 in malignant mesothelioma. *Pathol Res Pract* 1994; **190**: 138–41.
48. Kratzke RA, Otterson GA, Lincoln CE et al, Immunohistochemical analysis of the p16(Ink4) cyclin-dependent kinase inhibitor in malignant mesothelioma. *J Natl Cancer Inst* 1995; **87**: 1870–5.
49. Prins JB, Williamson KA, Kamp MML et al, The gene for the cyclin-dependent-kinase-4 inhibitor, Cdkn2a, is preferentially deleted in malignant mesothelioma. *Int J Cancer* 1998; **75**: 649–53.
50. Cheng JQ, Jhanwar SC, Klein WM et al, p16 alterations and deletion mapping of 9p21–p22 in malignant mesothelioma. *Cancer Res* 1994; **54**: 5547–51.
51. Xiao S, Li DZ, Vijg J et al, Codeletion of p15 and p16 in primary malignant mesothelioma. *Oncogene* 1995; **11**: 511–15.
52. Sekido Y, Pass HI, Bader S et al, Neurofibromatosis type 2 (NF2) gene is somatically mutated in mesothelioma but not in lung cancer. *Cancer Res* 1995; **55**: 1227–31.
53. Bianchi AB, Mitsunaga SI, Cheng J et al, High frequency of inactivating mutations in the neurofibromatosis type 2 gene (NF2) in primary malignant mesotheliomas. *Proc Nat Acad Sci USA* 1995; **92**: 10854–8.
54. Kleymenova EV, Bianchi AA, Kley N et al, Characterization of the rat neurofibromatosis 2 gene and its involvement in asbestos-induced mesothelioma. *Mol Carcinogen* 1997; **18**: 54–60.
55. Wang ZY, Madden SL, Deuel TF, Rauscher FJ, The Wilms' tumor gene product, WT1, represses transcription of the platelet-derived growth factor A-chain gene. *J Biol Chem* 1992; **267**: 21999–2002.
56. Drummond IA, Madden SL, Rohwer-Nutter P et al, Repression of the insulin-like growth factor II gene by the Wilms' tumor suppressor WT1. *Science* 1994; **57**: 11–25.
57. Dey BR, Sukhatme VP, Roberts AB et al, Repression of the transforming growth factor-beta 1 gene by the Wilms' suppressor WT1 gene product. *Mol Endocrinol* 1994; **8**: 595–602.
58. Werner H, Re GG, Drummond IA et al, Increased expression of the insulin-like growth factor I receptor gene, IGFIR, in Wilms' tumor is correlated with modulation of IGFIR promoter activity by the WT1 Wilms' tumor gene product. *Proc Natl Acad Sci USA* 1993; **90**: 5828–32.
59. Walker C, Rutten F, Yuan XQ et al, Wilms' tumor suppressor gene expression in rat and human mesothelioma. *Cancer Res* 1994; **54**: 3101–6.
60. Amin KM, Litzky LA, Smythe WR et al, Wilms' tumor 1 susceptibility (Wt1) gene products are selectively expressed in malignant mesothelioma. *Am J Pathol* 1995; **146**: 344–56.
61. Langerak AW, Williamson KA, Miyagawa K et al, Expression of the Wilms' tumor gene Wt1 in human malignant mesothelioma cell lines and relationship to platelet-derived growth factor a and insulin-like growth factor 2 expression. *Genes Chromosomes Cancer* 1995; **12**: 87–96.
62. Kumarsingh S, Segers K, Rodeck U et al, Wt1 mutation in malignant mesothelioma and Wt1 immunoreactivity in relation to p53 and growth factor receptor expression, cell-type transition, and prognosis. *J Pathol* 1997; **181**: 67–74.
63. Whitaker D, Manning LS, Robinson BWS, Shilken KB, The pathobiology of the mesothelium. In: *Malignant Mesothelioma* (Henderson D, Shilken K, Langlois S, Whitaker D, eds). New York: Hemisphere: New York, 1992: 25–68.
64. Stahel RA, O'Hara CJ, Waibel R, Martin A, Monoclonal antibodies against mesothelial membrane antigen discriminate between malignant mesothelioma and lung adenocarcinoma. *Int J Cancer* 1988; **41**: 218–23.
65. Corson JM, Pathology of malignant mesothelioma. In: *Asbestos-Related Malignancy* (Antman K, Aisner J, eds). Orlando: Grune and Stratton, 1987: 176–200.
66. Henderson DW, Shilken KB, Whitaker D, The pathology of malignant mesothelioma, including immunohistochemistry and ultrastructure. In: *Malignant Mesothelioma* (Henderson D, Shilken K, Langlois S, Whitaker D, eds). Hemisphere: New York, 1992: 69–139.

67. Henderson DW, Shilken KB, Whitaker D, Unusual histological types and anatomic sites of mesothelioma. In: *Malignant Mesothelioma* (Henderson D, Shilken K, Langlois S, Whitaker D, eds). Hemisphere: New York, 1992: 140–66.
68. Embleton MJ, Wagner JC, Wagner MM et al, Assessment of cell-mediated immunity to malignant mesothelioma by microcytotoxicity tests. *Int J Cancer* 1976; **17**: 597–601.
69. Robinson C, Robinson BW, Lake RA, Sera from patients with malignant mesothelioma can contain autoantibodies. *Lung Cancer* 1998; **20**: 175–84.
70. Davidson JA, Musk AW, Wood BR et al, Intralesional cytokine therapy in cancer: a pilot study of GM-CSF infusion in mesothelioma. *Hum Gen Ther* 1998; **9**: 2121–33.
71. Marzo AL, Fitzpatrick DR, Robinson BWS, Scott B, Antisense oligonucleotides specific for transforming growth factor beta-2 inhibit the growth of malignant mesothelioma both in vitro and vivo. *Cancer Res* 1997; **57**: 3200–7.
72. Selikoff IJ, Churg J, Hammond EC, Relation between exposure to asbestos and mesothelioma. *N Engl J Med* 1965; **272**: 560–5.
73. Ruffie P, Feld R, Minkin S et al, Diffuse malignant mesothelioma of the pleura in Ontario and Quebec: a retrospective study of 332 patients. *J Clin Oncol* 1989; **7**: 1157–68.
74. Rusch V, Clinical features and current treatment of diffuse malignant pleural mesothelioma. *Lung Cancer* 1995; **12**(Suppl 2): S127–46.
75. Law MR, Gregor A, Husband JE, Kerr H, Computed tomography in the assessment of malignant mesothelioma of the pleura. *Clin Radiol* 1982; **33**: 67–70.
76. Mirvis S, Dutcher JP, Haney PJ et al, CT of malignant pleural mesothelioma. *Am J Roentgenol* 1983; **140**: 655–70.
77. Rusch VW, Godwin JD, Shuman WP, The role of computed tomography scanning in the initial assessment and the follow up of malignant pleural mesothelioma. *J Thorac Cardiovasc Surg* 1988; **96**: 171–7.
78. Battifora H, Kopinski MI, Distinction of mesothelioma from adenocarcinoma. *Cancer* 1985; **55**: 1679–85.
79. Wirth PR, Legier J, Wright GL Jr, Immunohistochemical evaluation of seven monoclonal antibodies for differentiation of pleural mesothelioma from lung adenocarcinoma. *Cancer* 1991; **67**: 655–62.
80. Whitaker D, Shilkin KB, Diagnosis of pleural malignant mesothelioma in life – a practical approach. *J Pathol* 1984; **143**: 147–75.
81. Salyer WR, Eggleston JC, Erozan YS, Efficacy of pleural needle biopsy and pleural fluid cytopathology in the diagnosis of malignant neoplasm involving the pleura. *Chest* 1975; **67**: 536–9.
82. Butchart EG, Ashcroft T, Barnsley WC, Holden MP, Pleuropneumonectomy in the management of diffuse malignant mesothelioma of the pleura. Experience with 29 patients. *Thorax* 1976; **31**: 15–24.
83. Sugarbaker DJ, Heher EC, Lee TH et al, Extrapleural pneumonectomy, chemotherapy, and radiotherapy in the treatment of diffuse malignant pleural mesothelioma. *J Thorac Cardiovasc Surg* 1991; **102**: 10–15.
84. DeLaria GA Jr, Faber LP, Kittle CF, Surgical management of malignant mesothelioma. *Ann Thorac Surg* 1978; **26**: 375–82.
85. DeValle MJ, Faber LP, Kittle CF, Jensik RJ, Extrapleural pneumonectomy for diffuse, malignant mesothelioma. *Ann Thorac Surg* 1986; **42**: 612–18.
86. Pass H, Kranda K, Temeck BK et al, Surgically debulked malignant pleural mesothelioma: results and prognostic factors. *Ann Surg Oncol* 1997; **4**: 215–22.
87. Rusch VW, Piantadosi S, Holmes EC, The role of extrapleural pneumonectomy in malignant pleural mesothelioma. *J Thorac Cardiovasc Surg* 1991; **102**: 1–9.
88. Sugarbaker DJ, Strauss GM, Lynch TJ et al, Node status has prognostic significance in the multimodality therapy of diffuse, malignant mesothelioma. *J Clin Oncol* 1993; **11**: 1172–8.
89. Robinson BWS, Davidson JA, Garlepp MJ, The immunology and immunopathology of malignant

mesthelioma. In: *Immunopathology of Lung Disease* (Kradin RL, Robinson BWS, eds). Butterworth-Heinemann: Stoneham, MA, 1996: 491–513.

90. Ong ST, Vogelzang NJ, Chemotherapy in malignant pleural mesothelioma. A review. *J Clin Oncol* 1996; **14**: 1007–17.
91. Ryan CW, Herndon J, Vogelzang NJ, A review of chemotherapy trials for malignant mesothelioma. *Chest* 1998; **113**(1 Suppl): 66S–73S.
92. Byrne MJ, Davidson JA, Musk AW et al, Cisplatin and gemcitabine treatment for malignant mesothelioma: a phase II study. *J Clin Oncol* 1999; **17**: 25–30.
93. Christman TI, Manning LS, Garlepp MJ et al, Effect of interferon-alpha 2a on malignant mesothelioma. *J Interferon Res* 1993; **13**: 9–12.
94. Morene de la Santa P, Butchart EG, Therapeutic options in malignant mesothelioma. *Curr Opin Oncol* 1995; **7**: 134–7.
95. Astoul P, Picat-Joossen D, Viallat JR, Boutin C, Intrapleural administration of interleukin-2 for the treatment of patients with malignant pleural mesothelioma: a phase II study. *Cancer* 1998; **83**: 2099–104.
96. Upham JW, Musk AW, van Hazel G et al, Interferon alpha and doxorubicin in malignant mesothelioma: a phase II study. *Aust NZ J Med* 1993; **23**: 683–7.
97. Nicholson SE, Hilton DJ, The SOCS proteins: a new family of negative regulators of signal transduction. *J Leukoc Biol* 1998; **63**: 665–8.
98. Bowman RV, Manning LS, Davis MR, Robinson BW, Chemosensitivity and cytokine sensitivity of malignant mesothelioma. *Cancer Chemother Pharmacol* 1991; **28**: 420–6.
99. Robinson BW, Mukherjee SA, Davidson A et al, Cytokine gene therapy or infusion as treatment for solid human cancer. *J Immunother* 1998; **21**: 211–17.
100. Velculescu VE, Zhang L, Vogelstein B, Kinzler KW, Serial analysis of gene expression. *Science* 1995; **270**: 484–7.
101. Wallace RW, DNA on a chip: serving up the genome for diagnostics and research. *Mol Med Today* 1997; **3**: 384–9.
102. de Klerk NH, Musk AW, Ambrosini GL et al, Vitamin A and cancer prevention II: comparison of the effects of retinol and beta-carotene. *Int J Cancer* 1998; **75**: 362–7.

14 Therapeutic bronchoscopic palliation of lung tumours

Anton JM van Boxem, Thomas G Sutedja, Pieter E Postmus

Contents Introduction • Indications • Techniques to remove endobronchial tumours • Bronchoscopic treatment of extrabronchial tumours • General remarks, economic aspects and recommendations

INTRODUCTION

The therapeutic possibilities with curative intent for non-small cell lung cancer (NSCLC) have not changed significantly during the last decade; surgical resection is still the treatment for choice in stage I and II tumours.[1] Unfortunately, many patients will develop local recurrence or a second primary. For small cell lung cancer (SCLC), symptoms secondary to distant metastases are more prominent, but local recurrence occurs in 20–30% of all cases in spite of the use of local treatment modalities, such as chest irradiation and, in rare cases, surgery.

For the large majority of lung cancer patients, palliative treatment is the only possibility, which is often needed to treat pulmonary symptoms affecting quality of life. For patients with symptoms due to the irresectable primary tumour, external radiotherapy is considered standard to achieve tumour reduction and improvement of symptoms.[2] However, despite the use of various radiation schedules, there is a high degree of local tumour persistence, with variable results regarding atelectasis and relief of airway obstruction.[3] As tumour persistence or progression may affect quality of life, the currently available bronchoscopic techniques are often used to palliate airway obstruction.[4]

INDICATIONS

Tumours obstructing the larger airways can be treated by endobronchial therapy. The clinical tumour (TNM) classification, and the patient's general, cardiac and pulmonary condition, are important factors for the treatment strategy.

Important factors for the decision to try to improve the symptoms due to tumour obstruction are as follows:

- Only tumours obstructing the larger airways are accessible to bronchoscopic instruments.
- The integrity of the tracheobronchial wall has to be respected to prevent airway collapse.
- Current endoscopic techniques do not enable us to assess tumour dimensions accurately. An 'iceberg tumour' is a common phenomenon for every bronchoscopist, and therefore additional investigations such as computed tomography (CT) are often needed.
- Extraluminal tumour bulk resulting in airway obstruction is only treatable by the insertion of a stent.

For the majority of patients, relief of dyspnoea, haemoptysis, severe cough or obstructive pneumonia is the major treatment goal. Improvement of gas exchange is the aim of airway reopening, but regions with low gas exchange (e.g. after radiation or due to significant peribronchial disease) may improve little if treated. Any bronchoscopic treatment may only enhance the dead-space ventilation if local perfusion is hampered by tumour growth. A disproportionate loss of regional perfusion together with CT findings of extensive peribronchial disease are good indicators for gross extraluminal involvement.[5]

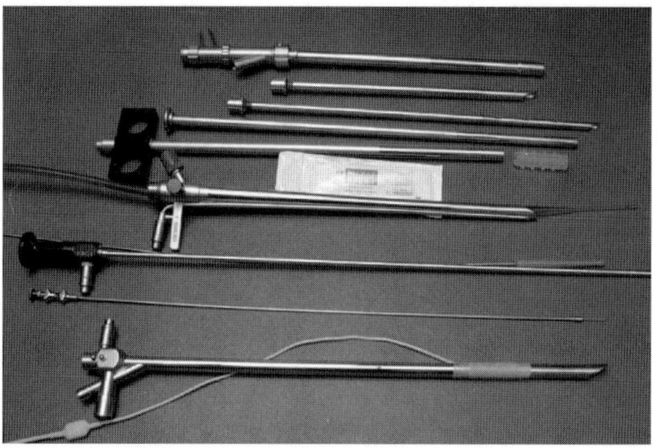

Figure 14.1
Instruments for bronchoscopic therapy with a rigid bronchoscope.

TECHNIQUES TO REMOVE ENDOBRONCHIAL TUMOURS

Mechanical tumour removal

Removal of foreign bodies is an old bronchoscopic technique, which may be used for tumour tissue extraction, but the risk of bleeding after tumour manipulation may be considerable.[6,7] A biopsy forceps and the rigid bronchoscope can be used to remove and core-out less-vascularized and necrotic tumour (Figure 14.1). Immediate symptomatic relief has been reported using this technique.[7] Bleeding is easily managed using various methods such as balloon occlusion catheters, adrenaline (epinephrine)-soaked pledgets, and irrigation with adrenaline solution.[6] Symptomatic and radiographic improvement has been achieved in up to 90% of cases. Complications such as pneumonia, bleeding, pneumothorax and arrhythmias have also occurred. Mechanical tumour removal can result in an immediate symptomatic relief in the hands of an experienced bronchoscopist who can successfully deal with possible complications. Nowadays, this technique is frequently used in combination with other techniques such as the Nd–YAG laser or electrocautery.[8–10]

Nd–YAG laser resection

The neodymium–yttrium aluminium garnet (Nd–YAG) laser is the best known tool for bronchoscopic intervention. Argon and carbon dioxide lasers are less popular in tracheobronchial malignancies, because the argon laser is strongly absorbed by haemoglobin and penetrates less deeply in tissue, while the carbon dioxide laser has a shallow tissue effect and requires a rigid optical system to transmit the laser beam.[11] The Nd–YAG laser beam enables easier manipulation using a flexible quartz fibre. Wide experience with the Nd–YAG laser for relief of central airway malignancies has been published.[9,12,13] The Nd–YAG laser is an excellent tool for tissue coagulation and evaporation.[9] Uncontrolled application of high power can lead to disastrous effects, such as perforation of the bronchial wall and too-extensive necrosis, because the depth effect of the Nd–YAG laser is not always immediately apparent. Therefore it is necessary to know the extent of the endobronchial mass to define the treatment area. Bronchography has been used prior to treatment to assess the length of the bronchial obstruction.[14,15] CT scanning might also be useful for defining the extent of the endobronchial and peribronchial tumour mass. Whether the choice of general anaesthesia is an important factor in

Table 14.1 Summary of three large series of Nd–YAG laser treatment

Ref	Numbers	Method	Response	Complications	Survival rate (%)
9	839 pts 1503 Rx	GA 76.9% RB 100%	Previous series 96.3%	35 Rx (2.3%) *M* = 5 (0.4%)	NS
12	1000 pts 1396 Rx	GA 77.9% RB 92%	92.4%	27 Rx (1.9%) *M* = 5 (0.5%)	50 (6 months) 26 (12 months)
13	1310 pts 2284 Rx	GA RB High jet	NS	42 Rx (1.8%) *M* = 16 (1.2%)	25 (12 months)

Abbreviations: pts, patients; Rx, treatment sessions; GA, general anaesthesia; RB, rigid bronchoscope; FB, flexible bronchoscope; *M*, mortality; NS, not specified.

Nd–YAG laser treatment remains controversial.[16–18] The use of muscle relaxants, duration of anaesthesia and the age of the patient are predictive variables for post-treatment complications.[17] Any bronchoscopic technique has a significant effect on the deterioration of blood gases, regardless of the type of anaesthesia. Many investigators obviously prefer general anaesthesia, using the rigid bronchoscope to have an optimal treatment setting,[9,12,13] and it is clear that significantly more treatment sessions are necessary if the Nd–YAG laser treatment is performed under local anaesthesia.[16] Table 14.1 summarizes the details given in the large series previously reported.[9,12,13] However, as well as being safe and effective, a palliative treatment should avoid prolonged hospital stay, and should provide an ambulant approach whenever feasible.[18] Awareness of possible post-treatment complications is also important in the treatment strategy. The immediate and long-term results of Nd–YAG laser treatment are good. The mortality rate can be as low as 2.7%.[13] A high success rate of 92.4% has been reported, with remission duration more than six months, and a one-year survival rate of 25%.[12]

Electrocautery

Despite its use in every operating room during surgery, endobronchial electrocautery or diathermy has received little attention. Heat is generated by a high-frequency electrical current passing through tissue with a high resistance, and can be applied to coagulate, vaporize or cut tumour tissue, using a probe or a snare.[19,20] Hooper and Jackson[19] discussed the significant potential of this technique to remove tumour tissue and mentioned this as a practical and less costly alternative to the laser.[9] Complete endobronchial tumour removal using a snare and a fiberoptic bronchoscope can be achieved under general anaesthesia, in which a single treatment is sufficient to achieve long-standing results.[21] Electrocautery has also been used to remove tumour bulk, while the mural and extramural tumour compartments were subsequently irradiated by interstitial implantations of ^{198}Au grains.[8] Recent data indicate that electrocautery is equally

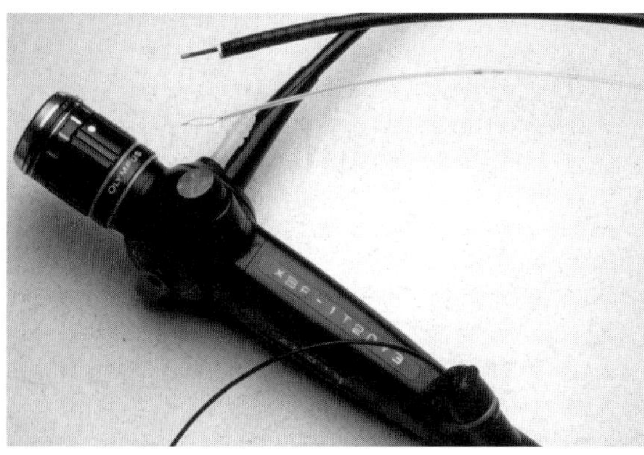

Figure 14.2
Flexible bronchoscope with electrocautery probe and snare.

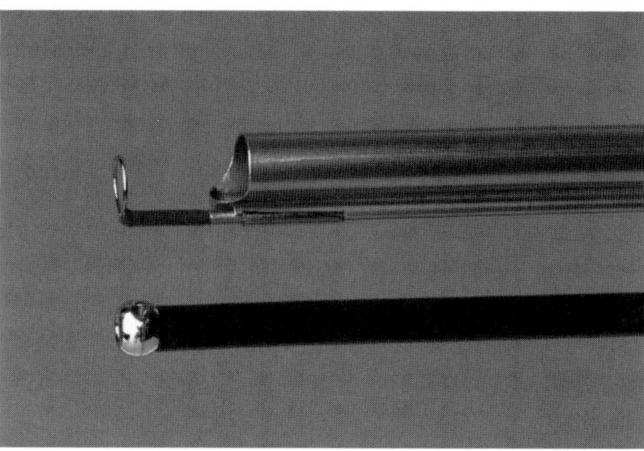

Figure 14.3
Electrocautery snare and probe for a rigid bronchoscope.

effective and less costly than the Nd–YAG laser for tumour debulking.[22]

General anaesthesia with a rigid system[8] or local anaesthesia with a fibre-optic system can be performed for palliation (Figures 14.2 and 14.3).[23] Electrocautery is standard equipment in every surgical ward, and this facility is cheap. Tissue effect during coagulation and vaporization is clearly visible for the endoscopist, and corresponds to superficial necrosis of 2–3 mm depth.

Cryotherapy

Repetitive rapid freezing and slow thawing are maximally lethal for tumour tissue, achieving durable result.[24–26] The impedance metric method is used to give better control of the process of cooling and thawing.[24] Haemoptysis can be treated successfully. Data show that good results are achieved with regard to the treatment of post-obstruction infections, dyspnoea, haemoptysis and atelectasis, with success rates of 40–93%.[25] A fibre-optic bronchoscopy is performed afterwards to remove tumour slough. Cryotherapy requires special applicators, although equipment is less costly than lasers. It is also safe for the cartilage; however, repeated treatments, debris removal post-treatment and secondary necrosis are relative disadvantages in cases with imminent respiratory failure.

Endobronchial brachytherapy

Endobronchial brachytherapy (EBT) is the application of tiny radioactive seeds for irradiation intraluminally by the afterloading technique, using remote control and an automatic stepper-device motor.[27–29] This makes this technique of local irradiation less hazardous for health-care personnel. The Nd–YAG laser and a special applicator are sometimes used to facilitate positioning of the catheter.[28,30] High-dose-rate (HDR) brachytherapy using ^{192}Ir has gained wider acceptance, because the treatment duration is short, and up to 5–20 Gy can be given in less than 20 minutes at a 1 cm distance from the source. In low-dose-rate (LDR) brachytherapy, 30 Gy is delivered in a period of 20–40 hours.[31]

Many phase II reports have shown the efficacy of EBT for the palliation of patients with inoperable NSCLC, and also in patients with recurrences after previous therapy. HDR and LDR have been applied with different doses and fractions.[28,32–34] Different parameters have been used to evaluate response,[35] but the results are strikingly similar. Palliation has proved significant in achieving symptomatic relief (Table 14.2).

It is logical that results were correlated to tumour volume, with better results being obtained in patients with mainly intraluminal small-volume tumours.[31,36] It is interesting that a single treatment of HDR seemed to be equally palliative also in comparison with a hypofractionated external radiation scheme.[32,38,41]

Although, theoretically, LDR causes less damage to normal tissue than HDR,[31] both fistula and haemorrhage occurred in 11% of the cases after treatment,[34] while several reports indicated a lower rate of complications.[33,38] The incidence of more serious complications such as haemorrhage and fistula is also variable.[30,42,43] Radiation bronchitis and stenosis were also reported to occur in up to 13% of patients.[43] It is difficult to say whether this complication rate is acceptable in terms of palliation. Late normal tissue damage and prior therapies such as Nd–YAG laser, external radiotherapy and local disease progression may all increase the risk of pulmonary haemorrhage.[30,42]

Brachytherapy has been shown to improve survival, compared with patients who received Nd–YAG laser treatment alone.[34] A similar survival rate was reported for three groups of patients after HDR, with or without additional external radiotherapy, whether the HDR was given with curative or palliative intent.[35] The cause of death appeared to be similar in all groups, with 40% due to intrathoracic cancer and 40% as a result of metastatic disease, in which case death was due to progressive disease outside the treated area. It was therefore concluded that future dose escalation of HDR will not significantly improve the results.

Overall, HDR brachytherapy is a simple and reliable treatment method that can be performed in an outpatient setting under local anaesthesia, whereas LDR treatment needs a short hospital admission. There has been borderline significant improvement in local control with HDR in addition to external radiotherapy alone; better local control can be achieved in particular in patients with squamous cell cancer.[39] HDR alone seems to be inferior to external radiotherapy alone.[40]

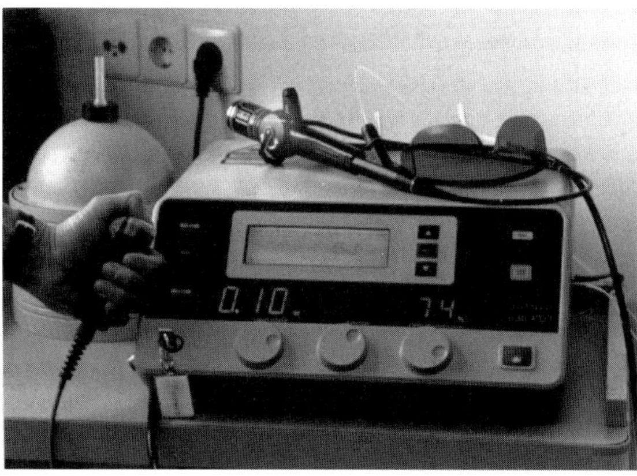

Figure 14.4
Photodynamic therapy equipment.

Photodynamic therapy

Photodynamic therapy (PDT) is the activation of photosensitizer molecules in tumour tissue by laser light (Figure 14.4).[44,45] In vivo, PDT causes vascular shut-off, with subsequent hypoxia and secondary tumour necrosis, while damaged normal tissue regenerates after PDT.[46] Tracheal cartilage after PDT is undamaged and the mechanical strength of the trachea remains normal.[47] All these factors contribute positively to the tissue-sparing potential of PDT in causing more selective tumour damage. PDT can be performed using a fibre-optic bronchoscope under local anaesthesia. Early clinical experience has shown significant tumour necrosis up to 15 mm deep. The degree of intra- and extraluminal tumour mass and tumour location may limit the efficacy of PDT, since optimal or homogeneous illumination is difficult to

Table 14.2 Endobronchial brachytherapy

Ref	No. of patients	Method[a]	Results		Follow-up
32	50	1 × HDR	Haemoptysis	24/28 (86%)	Earliest recurrence at 4 months
		15–20 Gy	Dyspnoea	21/33 (64%)	
			Cough	9/18 (50%)	
		4 patients	Collapse	11/24 (46%)	
		plus ER	X-rays	16/41 (39%)	
			BR	15/17 (88%)	
36	20	1 × HDR	Haemoptysis	6/6 (100%)	16 pts > 3 months
		15 Gy	Dyspnoea	19/19 (100%)	11 pts > 6 months
			Cough	7/19 (37%)	3 pts > 1 year
			Collapse	9/13 (70%)	Median tumour volume 10 cm^3 (range 6–12
			Tumour mass reduction	2/6 (33%)	months)
33	87	LDR 105 Rx 30 Gy (0.5–1 cm)	BR	42/71 (59%)	Better >25 Gy/2 cm Two haemorrhages Four fistulas
28	56	3 × HDR	Dyspnoea	44/56 (79%)	Four haemorrhages
		7.5 Gy	Atelectasis	22/25 (88%)	Two fistulas
37	64	3 × HDR 15 Gy/3 mm 60 Gy/3 mm	66% complete up to 800 days		22.8% haemorrhage 5.3% fistula
38	32	LDR 38 Rx	(including SD):		Three haemorrhages
		25 Gy	Symptoms	30/34 (88%)	One fistula
			X-rays	22/24 (92%)	
			BR	10/12 (83%)	
29	20	1 × HDR	Palliation	17/20 (94%)	18 haemoptysis
		10 Gy	Cough	14/15 (93%)	Five tumour-related
			Haemoptysis	9/9 (100%)	
			Dyspnoea	6/6 (100%)	
34	65	LDR 30 Gy	Haemoptysis	19/24 (80%)	11% haemorrhage
		at 0.5–1 cm	Cough	50%	11% fistula abscesses and necrosis
			Dyspnoea	50%	
			BR	24/40 (60%)	

Table 14.2 Continued

Ref	No. of patients	Method[a]	Results		Follow-up
35	141	3 × HDR 10 Gy	Various parameters	70–86%	3% complications 4% radiation stenosis
30	31	2–3 × HDR 10 Gy	Dyspnoea BR	18/22 (82%) 22/31 (71%)	Eight haemorrhages Three fistulas
39	99	HDR 1 × 15 ER 30 Gy/8 fractions	ER better symptom control and modest survival gain		ER more oesophagitis
40	98	HDR 2 × 4.8 Gy ER 60 Gy	Additional HDR improves local control and median survival		+ HDR 18.9% fatal haemoptysis versus 14.2% ER alone

Abbreviations: ER, external radiotherapy; HDR/LDR, high/low-dose rate; Rx, number of treatment sessions; BR, bronchoscopic response; SD, stable disease.
[a]Dose at 1 cm radius if unstated.

achieve.[48,49] Cautious interpretation of apparent complete responses by bronchoscopy is advocated, since microscopic study may reveal residual tumour. A cure cannot be expected in patients with tumour infiltration of the cartilage and bronchial muscular layer.[50–52] Secondary necrosis due to tumour hypoxia and fibrin plug formation make it necessary to perform a 'clean-up' bronchoscopy to prevent respiratory failure.[53,54] Especially in patients with poor pulmonary condition, the complication rate may be high, if a 'clean-up' bronchoscopy is not routinely performed.[55] One randomized study in a limited number of patients reported the benefit of PDT additional to external radiotherapy, with regard to the quality of life and physiological scores. PDT plus external radiotherapy provided a better and more durable local control compared with external radiotherapy alone.[56] Skin photosensitivity occurred in 20–40% of patients, but did not lead to irreversible skin damage.[57] Fatal bleeding after PDT has been reported.[44,53,54,58] As the PDT effect is known to be mainly vascular, caution is necessary in treating tumours close to the large vessels.

PDT laser equipment is relatively expensive and complicated. The need for a 'clean-up' bronchoscopy and the skin photosensitivity issue limit its potential for palliative treatment (Table 14.3).

BRONCHOSCOPIC TREATMENT OF EXTRABRONCHIAL TUMOURS

The above-mentioned techniques cannot be used for the relief of extraluminal airway compression by

Table 14.3 Photodynamic therapy (PDT) of locally advanced tumours

Ref	No. of patients	Method	Response	Complications	Survival
53	81	CD 200 J/cm^2	BR 80/81	Ten sunburn Five haemorrhages	KPS-related, median 7 months
51	13	CO 200 mW; 10–40 min 5 + surgery	BR 100% PR microscopy 5/14, advanced stage no CR	Eleven sunburn	NS
56	11	Randomized ER alone vs PDT + ER 30 Gy	+PDT significantly better and longer remission	None	124–309 days
58	26	CD 200 J/cm^2	PR 11/15 stage III CR 10/11 stage I	Four skin redness	Median 4 months Median 7 months
55	17	CD 200–300 J/cm^2	6 partial necrosis, 7 tumour reduction	Eight intensive care, various complications	Mean 40 days

Abbreviations: CD, cylindrical diffuser fibre; CO, cut-off fibre; BR, bronchoscopic response; CR/PR, complete/partial response; ER, external irradiation; KPS, Karnofsky performance scale; NS, not specified.

a tumour. In particular cases, brachytherapy may have a limited effect on the tumour mass within the radiation field of the catheter.[27,31] Placing a stent is the only choice for major airway obstruction by an extraluminal tumour. Hood and Montgomery silicone stents have had long-term use for the management of tracheobronchial obstruction and anastomosis disruption.[59,60] After tumour debulking, the stents are inserted either through a tracheostoma or through the larynx. Various stents are available – all for the purpose of restoring the dimension and rigidity of the tracheobronchial tree in resisting inward tumour pressure.[10,59–63] Stents can be made from metal, silicone, semicircular metal rings or meshwork imbedded in silicone; they can be 'semi' fixed diameter or expandable. The method of placement depends on the type of stent. Direct visual placement or placement under fluoroscopic guidance is possible if some types of stents are used. Metal stents become gradually imbedded in bronchial

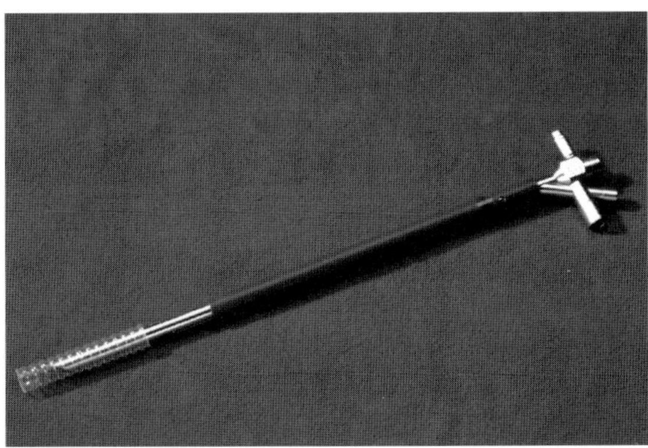

Figure 14.5
Rigid bronchoscope with a stent applicator.

mucosa after placement, and are therefore more difficult to remove (Orlowski, Gianturco, Palmaz and Wall stents). The success rate obviously depends on the proper indication and placement by an experienced bronchoscopist.[10]

Many patients present with imminent respiratory failure due to a life-threatening airway obstruction. Therefore general anaesthesia is needed, allowing the use of Nd–YAG laser or airway dilatation prior to stenting, when necessary. Meticulous assessment of the stenosis can be carried out before placing the stent. Endobronchial sonography as well as bronchography have been used to assess airway stenosis prior to bronchoscopic intervention.[14,15,64] Some expandable stents (Wall, Palmaz) shorten after dilatation during placement, and this should be anticipated.

The excellent work of Dumon has led to increased interest in the use of stent insertion for malignant airway obstruction (Figure 14.5).[10] The median follow-up period of his patients was 3.5 months. Fixed-diameter stents will not easily compress during a cough manoeuvre, and remain relatively 'wide'. The lower shear force causes mucostasis; this has led to the recent development of the 'dynamic' airway stent by Freitag et al.[61]

The benefit of stenting is excellent, but it requires experience and skill to be successful. Tumour growth above and beneath the stent can obviously cause subsequent problems that need to be solved separately. Stenting has also been used for benign cases, such as for stenosis after lung transplantation, to close a broncho-oesophageal fistula or for bronchomalacia. The development of a foldable stent with memory, to ease the method of insertion, is under way (Nitinol stent, Novastent).

GENERAL REMARKS, ECONOMIC ASPECTS AND RECOMMENDATIONS

Current bronchoscopic techniques provide the bronchoscopist with alternatives for local palliation. Each technique has its own merits and limitations. Treatment choice is based upon the following: clinical presentation, the experience and skill of the bronchoscopist, the availability of additional bronchoscopic instruments, anaesthetic care, intensive care for the post-treatment period and technical support in each hospital. Economic aspects may further influence the choice (Table 14.4).

It is understandable that every bronchoscopist is inclined to use the technique considered most suitable and available at that particular moment, since skill and experience are important matters. It is also obvious that a bronchoscopist will have a preference for a familiar technique that is easily available in the clinic, although theoretically the technique itself may not seem ideal.

When the indications have been properly assessed, any treatment can be equally successful in dealing with an emergency situation, whether the treatment chosen is the Nd–YAG laser, mechanical tumour removal, electrocautery or a combination of these. Techniques

Table 14.4 Treatment costs of bronchoscopic interventions in the Netherlands

	Price of equipment (US$)	Cost refund (US$)[a]
One-visit consultancy		56
Second-visit consultancy		23
One day hospital stay		190
Bronchoscopy		309
Anaesthesia		318
Nd–YAG laser	215 200	880
PDT laser	282 200	1077
Cryotherapy	30 000	309
Electrocautery	20 000	309
Stent placement: 1 set	10 000	1123
1 stent	250	
Brachytherapy (HDR)	250 000	539
Brachytherapy (LDR)	250 000	729

[a]Based on old tariffs of the 'COTG' (Government Health Insurance Tariff).

that cannot provide immediate symptomatic improvement because of late/secondary effects, such as brachytherapy, photodynamic therapy and cryotherapy, are less suitable for patients with imminent respiratory failure. But, as long as the bronchoscopist does realize the limitations and danger of each approach and is confident about the benefit of treatment, any treatment may be equally successful. In patients with a high chance of haemorrhage and respiratory failure, the use of general anaesthesia and the Nd–YAG laser is most sensible. Stent insertion provides an immediate solution in patients with airway compression due to extraluminal tumour mass. The advantages and disadvantages of the bronchoscopic techniques are summarized in Table 14.5.

Treatments that cause late effects with or without secondary necrosis and fibrinous exudate, such as cryotherapy, photodynamic therapy and brachytherapy, are less suitable for immediate palliation and for emergency situations. For non-emergency situations, brachytherapy is a good choice. A guideline for doctors dealing with patients having malignant airway obstruction is shown in Figure 14.6. After solving the emergency situation, additional treatment (e.g. stenting, brachytherapy and external radiotherapy) may be considered in order to consolidate airway patency or for the improvement of local control. This is certainly the case if it is considered worthwhile to prolongate palliation.

The frequent occurrence of emergency situations in patients with poor prognosis makes it impractical to perform a randomized study to look for the best palliative technique. The population at risk is not homogeneous, and the follow-up period is relatively short. Many patients will die because of disease progression outside the treatment area. So, the question about the best

Table 14.5 Advantages and disadvantages of various bronchoscopic intervention techniques

Technique	Advantages	Disadvantages
Mechanical removal	Standard equipment, immediate results	Requires skill, bleeding management, only short-term control
Cryotherapy	Lethal effect of several millimetres depth, safe for the cartilage	Special equipment, repeated treatments, necrotic removal
Electrocautery	Standard equipment, simple treatment, immediate results	Superficial necrosis
Nd–YAG laser	Coagulation and vaporization, deep necrosis, immediate results	Usually general anaesthesia, risk of perforation, requires expertise, late complications
HDR/LDR brachytherapy	Simple treatment, short duration (HDR), reliable device, use of fibre-optic scope	Nd–YAG pre-canalization, normal tissue damage, late results
Photodynamic therapy	Simple treatment, deep necrosis, multiple lesions	Complex dosimetry, complex equipment, clean-up bronchoscopy, skin photosensitivity
Stenting	The only alternative for extraluminal tumour obstruction	General anaesthesia, requires expertise, migration, granuloma and mucus plugging, extraluminal disease progression

palliative technique will remain more or less academic. The use of a simple technique that can be performed in an outpatient setting, causing the least morbidity, is preferable but not always feasible.

Photodynamic therapy is a 'tissue-sparing' treatment. This concept is appealing for the treatment of early stage lung cancer(s). Ample data have shown its curative potential in patients with occult or early stage squamous cell cancer(s). Current developments of fluorescence techniques (and ultrasonography) may provide the bronchoscopist with an excellent tool for early tumour detection and accurate tumour assessment. Data are accumulating, however, showing that the technique per se is not the determinant of cure in treating patients with early stage lung cancer.[65] The size of the tumour and the presence

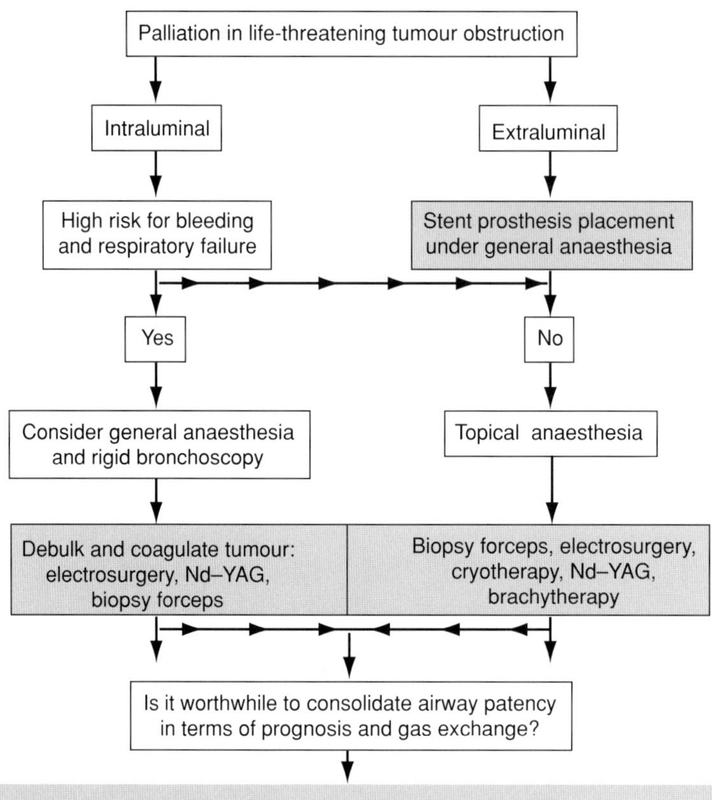

Figure 14.6
Guidelines for palliative treatment of airway obstruction.

of nodal disease are limits for the curative potential of any kind of bronchoscopic treatment. The problem has shifted towards finding more early stage lung cancers and accurately assessing the true stage of small intraluminal tumours. The cost-effectiveness of any bronchoscopic therapy also depends on the availability of the necessary equipment in each hospital and whether or not this equipment is used in a multidisciplinary setting (see Table 14.4).

REFERENCES

1. Bains MS, Surgical treatment of lung cancer. *Chest* 1991; **100**: 826–37.
2. Bleehen NM, Girling DJ, Machin D, Stephens RJ, A Medical Research Council (MRC) randomized trial of palliative radiotherapy with two fractions or a single fraction in patients with inoperable non-small cell lung cancer (NSCLC) and poor performance status. *Br J Cancer* 1992; **65**: 934–41

3. Chetty KG, Moran EM, Sasoon CS et al, Effect of radiation therapy on bronchial obstruction due to bronchogenic carcinoma. *Chest* 1989; **95**: 582–4.
4. Cortese DA, Edell ES, Role of phototherapy, laser therapy, brachytherapy and prosthetic stents in the management of lung cancer. *Mayo Clin Proc* 1993; **14**: 149–59.
5. Lam S, Muller NL, Miller RR et al, Laser treatment of obstructive endobronchial tumours: factors which determine response. *Lasers Surg Med* 1987; **7**: 29–35.
6. Mathisen DJ, Grillo HC, Endoscopic relief of malignant airway obstruction. *Ann Thorac Surg* 1989; **48**: 469–75.
7. Mehta AC, Livingstone DR, Biopsy excision through a fibreoptic bronchoscope in the palliative management of airway obstruction. *Chest* 1987; **91**: 774–5.
8. Petrou M, Kaplan D, Goldstraw P, Bronchoscopic diathermy resection and stent insertion: a cost effective treatment for tracheobronchial obstruction. *Thorax* 1993; **48**: 1156–9.
9. Dumon JF, Shapsay S, Bourceraou J et al, Principles for safety in application of neodymium–YAG laser in bronchology. *Chest* 1984; **86**: 163–8.
10. Dumon JF, A dedicated tracheobronchial stent. *Chest* 1990; **97**: 328–32.
11. Sliney DH, Laser–tissue interactions. *Clin Chest Med* 1985; **2**: 203–8.
12. Cavaliere S, Foccoli P, Farina PL. Nd:YAG laser bronchoscopy. A five-year experience with 1396 applications in 1000 patients. *Chest* 1988; **94**: 15–21.
13. Personne C, Colchen A, Leroy M, Indications and technique for endoscopic laser resections on bronchology. *J Thorac Cardiovasc Surg* 1986; **91**: 710–15
14. George PJ, Pearson MC, Edwards D et al, Bronchography in the assessment of patients with lung collapse for endoscopic laser therapy. *Thorax* 1990; **45**: 503–8.
15. Joyner LR, Maran AG, Sarama R, Yakaboski A. Neodymium–YAG laser treatment of intrabronchial lesions. A new mapping technique via the flexible fiberoptic bronchoscope. *Chest* 1985; **87**: 419–27.
16. George PJ, Barret CPO, Nixon C et al, Laser treatment for tracheobronchial tumours: local or general anaesthesia? *Thorax* 1987; **42**: 656–60.
17. Hanowell LH, Martin WR, Savelle JE, Foppiano LE, Complications of general anesthesia for Nd:YAG laser resection of endobronchial tumours. *Chest* 1991; **99**: 72–6.
18. Sutedja G, Koppenol W, Stam J, Nd–YAG laser under local anaesthesia in obstructive endobronchial tumours. *Respiration* 1991; **58**: 238–40.
19. Hooper RG, Jackson FN, Endobrochial electrocautery. *Chest* 1985; **87**: 712–14.
20. Jackson R, Basic principles of electrosurgery: a review. *Can J Surg* 1970; **13**: 354–61.
21. Gerasin VA, Shafirovsky BB, Endobronchial electrosurgery. *Chest* 1988; **93**: 270–4.
22. Sutedja G, van Boxem T, Schramel F et al, Endobronchial electrocautery is an excellent alternative for Nd–YAG laser to treat airway tumours. *J Bronchol* 1997; **4**: 101–5.
23. Sutedja G, van Kralingen K, Schramel F, Postmus PE, Fibreoptic bronchoscopic electrosurgery under local anaesthesia for rapid palliation in patients with central airway malignancies: a preliminary report. *Thorax* 1994; **49**: 1243–6.
24. Homasson JP, Renault P, Angebault M et al, Bronchoscopic cryotherapy for airway strictures caused by tumours. *Chest* 1986; **90**: 159–64.
25. Marasso A, Gallo E, Massaglia GM et al, Cryosurgery in bronchoscopic treatment of tracheobronchial stenosis. *Chest* 1993; **103**: 472–4.
26. Walsh DA, Maiwand MO, Nath AR et al, Bronchoscopic cryotherapy for advanced bronchial carcinoma. *Thorax* 1990; **45**: 509–13.
27. Krell WS, Overview of endobronchial brachytherapy. In: *Brachytherapy HDR and LDR. Proceedings Brachytherapy Meeting. Remote Afterloading: State of the Art* (Martinez AA, ed). Nucletron: Columbia, 1990: 3–9.
28. Macha HN, Koch K, Stadler M et al, New technique for treating occlusive and stenosing

tumours of the trachea and main bronchi: endobronchial irradiation by high dose iridium-192 combined with laser canalization. *Thorax* 1987; **42**: 511–15.

29. Seagren SL, Harrell JH, Horn RA, High dose rate intraluminal irradiation in recurrent endobronchial carcinoma. *Chest* 1985; **88**: 810–14.
30. Sutedja G, Baris G, Schaake-Koning C, van Zandwijk N, High dose rate brachytherapy in patients with local recurrences after radiotherapy of non-small cell lung cancer. *Int J Radiat Oncol Biol Phys* 1992; **24**: 551–3.
31. Fowler JF, The radiobiology of brachytherapy. In: *Brachytherapy HDR and LDR. Proceedings Brachytherapy Meeting. Remote Afterloading: State of the Art* (Martinez AA, ed). Nucletron: Columbia, 1990: 121–37.
32. Burt PA, O'Driscoll R, Maeve Notley H et al, Intraluminal irradiation for the palliation of lung cancer with high dose rate micro-Selectron. *Thorax* 1990; **45**: 765–8.
33. Lo TC, Beamis JF Jr, Weinstein RS et al, Intraluminal low-dose rate brachytherapy for malignant endobronchial obstruction. *Radiother Oncol* 1992; **23**: 16–20.
34. Shaw EG, Bonner JA, Foote RL et al, Role of radiation therapy in the management of lung cancer. *Mayo Clin Proc* 1993; **68**: 597.
35. Speiser B, Spratling L, High dose rate remote afterloading brachytherapy in the control of endobronchial carcinoma. In: *Brachytherapy HDR and LDR. Proceedings Brachytherapy Meeting. Remote Afterloading: State of the Art* (Martinez AA, ed). Nucletron: Columbia, 1990: 10–23.
36. Goldman JM, Bulman AS, Rathmel AJ et al, Physiological effect of endobronchial radiotherapy in patients with major airway occlusion by carcinoma. *Thorax* 1993; **48**: 110–14.
37. Macha HN, Wahlers B, Endobronchiale Brachytherapie: Die Endoluminale Kleinraumbestrahlung von Bronchialtumoren mit dem Afterloading HDR-verfahren. *Pneumologie* 1991; **45**: 95–9.
38. Paradelo JC, Waxman MJ, Throne BJ et al, Endobronchial irradiation with Ir-192 in the treatment of malignant endobronchial obstruction. *Chest* 1992; **102**: 1072–4.
39. Huber R, Fischer R, Hautmann H et al, Does additional brachytherapy improve the effect of external irradiation? A prospective randomised study in central lung tumours. *Int J Radiat Oncol Biol Phys* 1997; **38**: 533–40.
40. Hopwood P, Swindell R, But P, Clinically relevant quality of life outcomes in the first UK randomised trial of endobronchial brachytherapy versus external beam radiotherapy in patients with inoperable non-small cell cancer. *Lung Cancer* 1997; **18s**: 131.
41. Stout R, Single dose brachytherapy for endobronchial cancer. In: *Program and Abstracts 7th International Brachytherapy Working Conference*. Nucletron: Baltimore/Washington, 1992: 105–8.
42. Khanavkar B, Stern P, Alberti W, Nakhosteen JA, Complications associated with brachytherapy alone or with laser in lung cancer. *Chest* 1991; **99**: 1062–5.
43. Speiser BL, Spratling L, Radiation bronchitis and stenosis secondary to high dose rate endobronchial irradiation. *Int J Radiat Oncol Biol Phys* 1993; **25**: 580–97.
44. Dougherty TJ, Photodynamic therapy – new approaches. *Semin Surg Oncol* 1989; **5**: 6–16.
45. Gomer CJ, Rucker N, Ferrario A, Wong S, Review. Properties and applications of photodynamic therapy. *Radiat Res* 1989; **120**: 1–18.
46. Star WM, Marijnissen HPA, van den Berg-Blok E et al, Destruction of rat mammary tumor and normal tissue microcirculation by hematoporphyrin derivative photoradiation observed in vivo in sandwich observation chambers. *Cancer Res* 1986; **46**: 2532–40.
47. Smith SGT, Bedwell J, MacRobert AJ et al, Experimental studies to assess the potential of photodynamic therapy for the treatment of bronchial carcinomas. *Thorax* 1993; **48**: 474–80.
48. Furuse K, Fukuoka M, Kato H et al, A prospective phase II study on photodynamic therapy with Photofrin II for centrally located early-stage lung cancer. *J Clin Oncol* 1993; **11**: 1852–7.
49. Sutedja G, Lam S, LeRiche JC, Postmus PE,

Response and pattern of failure after photodynamic therapy for intraluminal stage I lung cancer. *J Bronchol* 1994; **1**: 295–8.
50. Okunaka T, Kato H, Konaka C et al, Photodynamic therapy for multiple primary bronchogenic carcinoma. *Cancer* 1991; **68**: 253–8.
51. Hayata Y, Kato H, Konaka C et al, Hematoporphyrin derivative and laser photoradiation in the treatment of lung cancer. *Chest* 1982; **81**: 269–77.
52. Hayata Y, Kato H, Konaka C et al, Photoradiation therapy with hematoporphyrin derivative in early and stage I lung cancer. *Chest* 1984; **86**: 169–77.
53. Balchum OJ, Doiron DR, Huth GC, Photoradiation therapy of endobronchial lung cancer. Large obstructing tumours, non-obstructing tumours and early stage bronchial cancer lesions. *Clin Chest Med* 1985; **6**: 255–75.
54. McCaughan JS, Hawley PC, Walker J, Management of endobronchial tumours: a comparative study. *Semin Surg Oncol* 1989; **5**: 38–47.
55. Vincent RG, Dougherty TJ, Rao U et al, Photoradiation therapy in advanced carcinoma of the trachea and bronchus. *Chest* 1984; **85**: 29–33.
56. Lam S, Kostashuk EC, Coy P, A randomized comparative study of the safety and efficacy of photodynamic therapy using Photofrin II combined with palliative radiotherapy versus palliative radiotherapy alone in patients with inoperable obstructive bronchogenic carcinoma. *Photochem Photobiol* 1987; **46**: 893–7.
57. Dougherty TJ, Cooper MT, Mang TS, Cutaneous phototoxic occurrences in patients receiving Photofrin. *Lasers Surg Med* 1990; **10**: 485–8.
58. Sutedja G, Baas P, Stewart F, van Zandwijk N, A pilot study of photodynamic therapy in patients with inoperable non-small cell lung cancer. *Eur J Cancer* 1992; **28A**: 1370–3.
59. Cooper DJ, Pearson GA, Todd TR et al, Use of silicone stents in the management of airway problem. *Ann Thorac Surg* 1989; **47**: 371–8.
60. Montgomery WW, T-tube tracheal stent. *Arch Otolaryngol* 1965; **82**: 320–1.
61. Freitag L, Eicker R, Linz B, Greschuchna D, Development of a dynamic airway stent. In: *Proceedings of the 7th World Congress of Bronchology*. Mayo Clinic: Rochester, 1992: 80.
62. Orlowski TM, Palliative intubation of the tracheobronchial tree. *J Thorac Cardiovasc Surg* 1987; **94**: 343–8.
63. Simonds AK, Irving JD, Clarke SW, Dick R, Use of expandable metal stents in the treatment of bronchial obstruction. *Thorax* 1989; **44**: 680–1.
64. Hürter T, Hanrath P, Endobronchial sonography: feasibility and preliminary results. *Thorax* 1992; **47**: 565–7.
65. van Boxem AJM, Postmus PE, Venmans BWJ, Sutedja G, Curative endobronchial therapy in early stage non-small cell lung cancer. A review. *J Bronchol* 1999; **6**: 198–206.

Complications of lung cancer

Maurizio Tonato, Vincenzo Minotti

Contents Introduction • Infections • Major haemoptysis • Chest pain • Pleural effusion • Superior vena cava syndrome • Cardiac tamponade • Extrathoracic complications • Paraneoplastic syndromes

INTRODUCTION

Complications in lung cancer patients depend on the location of the tumour, its locoregional spread and the presence of metastatic growth. Moreover, lung cancer, especially small cell lung cancer (SCLC), is associated with paraneoplastic syndromes more frequently than any other type of cancer is.

Clinicians must keep in mind the most frequent complications of lung cancer, since a timely diagnosis and adequate treatment are essential in order to ameliorate symptoms.

Although a multitude of signs and symptoms may be manifested by patients with lung cancer, the focus of this chapter will be on the more frequent and severe complications due to intrathoracic growth of tumour and to remote effects that are not related to direct invasion or metastasis (Table 15.1).

Table 15.1. Most frequent and severe complications of lung cancer

- Infections
- Major haemoptysis
- Chest pain
- Pleural effusion
- Superior vena cava syndrome
- Cardiac tamponade
- Paraneoplastic syndromes

INFECTIONS

Pulmonary infections frequently complicate the course of patients with lung cancer, and are often the direct cause of death. The local and systemic effects of the tumour, as well as the immunosuppression induced by anticancer treatment, predispose the patient to develop pulmonary infections. To determine the factors involved, Nagata and colleagues[1] reviewed the case records and autopsy data of 304 patients who died of lung cancer. They showed that the local and systemic effects of the lung cancer itself were probably more important than either antineoplastic agents or corticosteroids in predisposing the patient to bacterial infections. Perlin and colleagues[2] reviewed retrospectively a cohort of 121 lung cancer patients in an attempt to identify the frequency of infection and to determine its impact on the survival of those patients. In 85 patients (70%), infections were documented; the most common organisms were streptococci, *Staphylococcus aureus*, *Klebsiella pneumoniae*, *Enterobacter aerogenes* and *Pseudomonas aeruginosa*. The median survival of all infected patients was 4.2 months, which was significantly shorter than that of uninfected patients, who had a median survival of 12.9 months. In the only prospective study done to date, involving 96 consecutive lung cancer patients at diagnosis, Putinati and colleagues[3] reported an incidence of secondary respiratory infections in 33 patients (34%). Major pathogens responsible for infection were *Haemophilus* spp., *S. aureus* and *P. aeruginosa*.

Pulmonary infections depend on the particular pattern of growth of the lung cancer. Centrally located tumours produce airway obstruction, which may cause an obstructive pneumonitis, while large tumour masses occasionally cavitate and present as malignant abscesses. Such patients suffer from typical symptoms of pneumonia, including fever, chills, and a productive cough with streaky haemoptysis. Non-small cell lung cancer (NSCLC), particularly squamous cell carcinoma, may present with a shaggy cavitary density indistinguishable from a conventional anaerobic lung abscess on chest radiograph. Extensive central necrosis is responsible for the cavitary appearance. Several clinical clues may suggest the presence of cancer, including persistent haemoptysis, relative absence of fever and leukocytosis, and radiographic location in a region of the lung with minimal surrounding pneumonitis. A rare and severe complication of lung cancer is the formation of a tracheo- or broncho-oesophageal fistula, which can manifest by paroxysmal violent cough after meals and recurrent aspiration pneumonia.

Bronchoscopy is useful to establish a microbiological diagnosis[4] and to search for an underlying lung cancer in patients with atypical resolution of pneumonia by chest radiography. In 115 cases with a clinical profile of chronic bacterial pneumonia, bronchoscopy disclosed newly diagnosed NSCLC in 14% of cases.[5] Identification of a definitive etiological agent is of great importance for rational antimicrobial treatment of pulmonary infections. Endobronchial obstruction with distal uncontrolled pneumonia or a lung abscess can be treated by endoscopic removal of tumour or, in the case of an abscess, percutaneous or bronchoscopic drainage of the abscess. It is rare that a palliative, incomplete surgical resection is required for patients presenting with these complications.

MAJOR HAEMOPTYSIS

Haemoptysis occurs in more than 50% of patients with lung cancer. However, massive haemoptysis is a rare event, with most patients experiencing blood-streaked sputum. Santiago and colleagues[6] reviewed the records of 264 patients who underwent bronchoscopy for unexplained haemoptysis in order to determine the various causes of haemoptysis. Bronchogenic carcinoma was the most common cause, accounting for 29% of the cases. The diagnosis of bronchogenic carcinoma was established endoscopically in 65 (82%) of 78 patients. Four patients with carcinoma had normal chest radiographs. These four patients had centrally located lesions that were diagnosed endoscopically. Massive haemoptysis is arbitrarily defined as expectoration of at least 600 ml of blood in a 24-hour period or intrabronchial bleeding at such a rate as to present a threat to life.[7] Death from haemoptysis is usually attributed to asphyxia rather than exsanguination. In a series of 58 lung cancer patients with massive haemoptysis reported by Panos et al,[8] 36% of patients died from the haemoptysis. This horrific complication is associated more frequently with central squamous cell carcinoma. These tumours tend to be large and angioinvasive, and to undergo spontaneous necrosis and cavitation. Haemoptysis results from necrosis and destruction of lung parenchymal support for vessels, as well as from neovascularization of the tumour.

The primary goals of therapy are to maintain the airway to optimize oxygenation and to stabilize the haemodynamic status. Clinically stable patients should be positioned with the bleeding side in a dependent position, to reduce aspiration of blood into the contralateral lung. Supplemental oxygen, sedatives, bed rest, mild cough suppression and avoidance of excessive thoracic manipulation are helpful. Traditionally, a rigid rather than a flexible bronchoscope is generally preferred with massive bleeding, when the need to remove large clots is anticipated. Because of its larger diameter, a rigid bronchoscope is particularly effective in suctioning, oxygen administration and airway control. Usually the airway can be protected from blood aspiration by inflating a Fogarty balloon catheter proximal to the bleeding site. The balloon can be left in place while the patient is stabilized and considered for resectional therapy.

Another approach to protect functional airways involves placing a special endotracheal tube with inflatable distal cuff into the non-bleeding right or left mainstem bronchus. The use of a double-lumen tube permits adequate suctioning of blood. However, placement of the tube requires experienced personnel.

Urgent surgical intervention should be considered when bleeding is associated with persistent haemodynamic and respiratory compromise. Patients with uncontrolled haemorrhage taken to surgery have an overall lower mortality than those treated with conservative non-surgical therapy.

In patients who are not candidates for surgery because of their overall prognosis, extensive neoplasm, co-morbid conditions, prior pulmonary resection or inadequate pulmonary reserve (predicted postoperative FEV_1 less than 0.8–1 l), several non-operative techniques have been reported to control massive haemoptysis. Prolonged tamponade with a Fogarty balloon catheter, ice–saline lavage, and arteriography with therapeutic embolization of bronchial arteries have been reported to be successful in controlling bleeding. However, no prospective comparative trials have been conducted on the efficacy of these various techniques, and it is well known that conservative non-surgical management of massive haemoptysis carries a mortality rate of 50–100%.

Radiation therapy (endobronchial or external-beam) and laser therapy may be useful in controlling bleeding lung tumours. Palliative management should also be aimed at reducing awareness and fear. A combination of a parenterally administered strong opioid and a benzodiazepine is usually required.

CHEST PAIN

Chest pain is reported at presentation in one-quarter to one-half of patients with lung cancer,[9] and usually arises via direct invasion or metastatic involvement of pain-sensitive intrathoracic structures (mediastinum, pleura or chest wall). Marino and colleagues[10] reported early thoracic pain in 40% of 164 patients with lung cancer without extrathoracic or distant metastasis. Pain was present on the side of the neoplasm in 80% of the patients.[10] Peripheral tumour invading the costal parietal pleura and chest wall gives rise to sharp, intermittent, pleuritic pain. This type of pain may also be caused by obstructive pneumonitis or associated pulmonary embolus. Other patients suffer from a poorly localized, vague, persistent discomfort, sometimes associated with central tumours with mediastinal extension and possible involvement of perivascular and peribronchial nerves. It is important to distinguish the chest pain that accompanies direct contiguous chest wall extension from rib metastases.

A characteristic pain syndrome is caused by local extension of an apical lung tumour at the superior thoracic inlet. Such a tumour is called a superior pulmonary sulcus tumour, and the associated pain is known as *Pancoast's syndrome* (Figure 15.1). The most common initial symptom

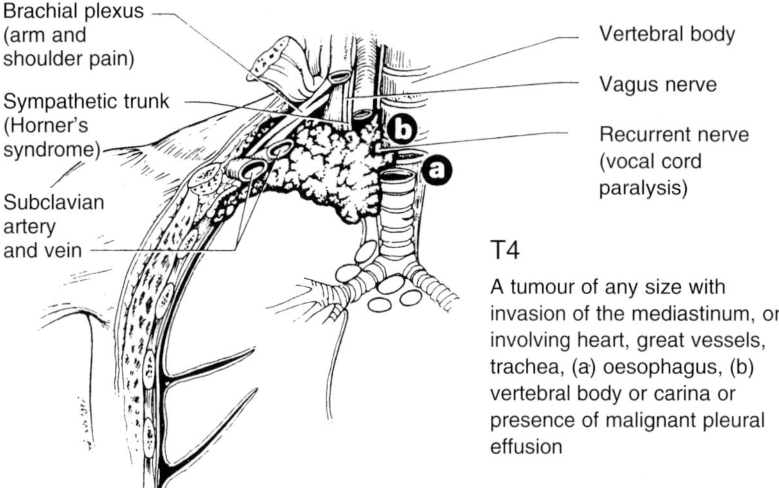

Figure 15.1 Schematic of International Staging System definitions for superior sulcus tumours, including Pancoast's syndrome. (Reproduced with permission from Mountain CF, A new international staging system for lung cancer. Chest 1986; **89**: 225S.)

is shoulder pain, produced by neoplastic involvement of the brachial plexus, parietal pleura, endothoracic fascia, vertebral bodies, and first, second and third ribs.[11] The pain is often severe and unrelenting; while initially confined to the shoulder and scapula, it later radiates down the arm, following an ulnar distribution, reflecting involvement of the C8 and T1 nerve roots. Pulmonary symptoms and signs are conspicuously absent, while arm weakness signifies advanced branchial plexus invasion. With further extension through the intervertebral foramina in 5% of patients initially, but in as many as 25% later in the course of the disease, compression of the spinal cord and paraplegia may result.[12] The majority of cases of Pancoast's syndrome are caused by NSCLC, most commonly squamous, followed by adenocarcinoma and large cell carcinoma. SCLC is only rarely associated with this syndrome.

Although in the past a histological diagnosis was not considered necessary before therapy, the wide variety of diseases that can result in Pancoast's syndrome (other primary thoracic neoplasms, metastatic and haematological neoplasms, infectious processes, neurogenic thoracic outlet syndrome) now mandates a conclusive diagnosis before definitive treatment is started. The chest radiograph may show an obvious apical mass, but frequently only a subtle increase in density is visible at the apex, and is often missed. Magnetic resonance imaging (MRI) has become the diagnostic modality of choice, because of its superiority to CT in delineating tumour extension to vascular and neural structures, vertebrae and the spinal canal.

Therapeutic modalities for superior sulcus tumours involve combinations of preoperative, intraoperative and postoperative radiotherapy, and either surgery or radiotherapy alone. Surgical resection after preoperative radiotherapy has been the most common treatment of superior sulcus tumours. However, there is no conclusive scientific evidence to recommend the standard use of preoperative radiotherapy for such tumours. Proponents of these treatment modalities based their recommendations on retrospective data. Standard resection is usually performed by en bloc resection of the tumour, generally by lobectomy, including chest wall, and may also be accompanied by resection of the involved paravertebral sympathetic chain, stellate ganglion, lower trunks of the brachial plexus, and, in some cases, the subclavian artery and portions of the thoracic vertebrae. Contraindications to surgical treatment include extensive involvement of the brachial plexus and paraspinal region, especially the intervertebral foramina, bodies and laminae of the vertebrae. Radiotherapy at doses of at least 60 Gy (dose range 20–70 Gy) can be used alone as a primary treatment, especially for inoperable superior sulcus tumours, palliating pain in up to 90% of patients.[13] The role of intraoperative and postoperative radiotherapy is unclear at present, and they should be used mainly in patients who are found to have unresectable tumours after a surgical attempt.[14] Despite recent interest in the use of neoadjuvant chemotherapy for locally advanced NSCLC, its efficacy in the treatment of superior sulcus tumours has not been studied prospectively. Clinical factors associated with improved survival include good performance status, a weight loss of less than 5% of total body weight, and achievement of local control and pain relief after treatment.[15]

PLEURAL EFFUSION

Approximately 25% of patients with lung carcinoma develop a malignant effusion during the course of their disease. Impaired drainage from the pleural space is the predominant mechanism for the accumulation of fluid associated with malignancy. Tumour cells either seed the mesothelial surface or invade the subserous layer. When the mesothelial surface is involved, tumour cells are abundant in pleural fluid; with subserous involvement, only a few malignant cells are exfoliated into the pleural space. Peripheral tumours, most commonly adenocarcinomas, may directly seed the pleural space.

Patients usually present symptoms that compromise their quality of life, including progressive dyspnoea, cough and/or chest pain.[16] Symptoms appear to be closely related to the rate of pleural fluid accumulation rather than the total volume. Accompanying fever usually represents atelectasis and infection. About one-quarter of patients with malignant pleural effusions are asymptomatic. The fluid itself may be serous, serosanguineous or grossly bloody, and typically it is ipsilateral to the main tumour and of moderate to large volume. The finding of malignant cells in the fluid confirms stage IIIB disease and a relatively poor prognosis. However, not all pleural effusions associated with lung cancer are due to pleural metastasis. Occasionally, fluid formation is only indirectly related to the tumour. Patients are at increased risk for pleural effusions from postobstructive pneumonia, atelectasis, pulmonary emboli, and drug or radiation reactions. In one series, 4 of 73 NSCLC patients with pleural effusion had surgically resectable tumours and survived for intervals ranging from 3 to 14 years.[17]

The diagnosis should be made on physical examination and confirmed by chest radiograph. The latter may be the only clue to the presence of pleural effusion. Approximately 300 ml of fluid is required for detection of a pleural effusion on a standard posteroanterior chest film. The lateral decubitus chest film is extremely useful in cases of subpulmonic effusion, detecting significantly smaller quantities of pleural fluid. Loculated effusions can be localized with ultrasonography or CT scan. The most definitive and simplest method of identifying a malignant pleural effusion is by cytological examination. A sample of 250–1000 ml of fresh pleural fluid should be sent to the cytology laboratory for examination. The diagnostic efficacy increases on repeat aspirations, from approximately 50% positivity on initial thoracentesis to 65% on the second sample and to 70% on the third.[18]

The management of malignant pleural effusions depends on the treatment potential of the primary malignancy. Systemic treatment may control pleural effusion due to SCLC, although therapeutic thoracentesis may still be required to improve symptoms. Patients with SCLC who present ipsilateral effusions as their only manifestation of metastatic spread beyond the primary tumour and regional lymph nodes have an overall response rate, complete response rate and survival equivalent to patients staged as having limited disease.[19]

If effective systemic treatment is not available, treatment is often palliative, usually consisting of sequential thoracentesis or tube thoracostomy with or without sclerotherapy. Therapeutic thoracentesis may improve patient comfort and relieve dyspnoea. The subjective response to drainage and the rate of fluid reaccumulation should be monitored. Repeated thoracenteses are reasonable if they achieve symptomatic relief, if fluid reaccumulation is slow, and if the patients expected remaining lifespan is very short. Used alone it is not an effective means for preventing recurrence. The mean time to fluid reaccumulation in one series was as short as 4 days, with a 98% recurrence rate at 39 days.[20]

The most cost-effective method of controlling a malignant pleural effusion is chest tube drainage and intrapleural instillation of a chemical agent. A number of antineoplastic and non-antineoplastic chemical agents have been used for pleurodesis, with variable success. The ideal sclerosing agent has not yet been identified, but at present talc seems to be the most effective. The traditional method of treatment, namely tube thoracostomy with large-bore chest tubes connected to continuous wall suction, requires hospitalization, is expensive, limits patient mobility, and can cause significant discomfort. More recent trials have explored new techniques, including small-bore catheters and thoracoscopic insufflation of talc. Pleural drainage and sclerosis with small-bore catheters have been shown to be successful.[21] Preliminary results suggest that sclerotherapy with small-bore chest tubes for management of malignant pleural effusion is feasible on an outpatient basis.[22] Such treatment offers important potential benefits to patients, including a better quality of life and a reduction in overall health-care costs.

As talc appears to be the most efficacious and cost-effective sclerosant, controversies centre on the route of delivery. There are many studies demonstrating the effectiveness of talc insufflation at thoracoscopy using general or local anaesthesia. Several authors have demonstrated that thoracoscopic talc poudrage does not require general anaesthesia,[23] and most of them felt that this treatment modality should be reserved only for patients with a prospect for survival of longer than one month.[24]

Successful pleurodesis includes distribution of the sclerosing agent on all pleural surfaces and the ability of the lung to re-expand against the chest wall. Pleurodesis will fail if the lung is unable to re-expand following fluid removal, as is the case with bronchial obstruction or 'trapped lung' due to encapsulated visceral pleura.

Thoracoscopy itself adds an advantage to pleurodesis in that trapped lung can be identified and the appropriateness of pleurodesis ascertained. Moreover, multiloculated effusions can be evacuated and adhesions lysed. Although talc for pleurodesis is most often used as an atomized powder via thoracoscopy, it has been successfully employed as a slurry that can be instilled into a chest tube. A prospective, randomized trial of operative talc poudrage versus bedside talc slurry sclerosis is under way within the cooperative cancer groups throughout North America.[25]

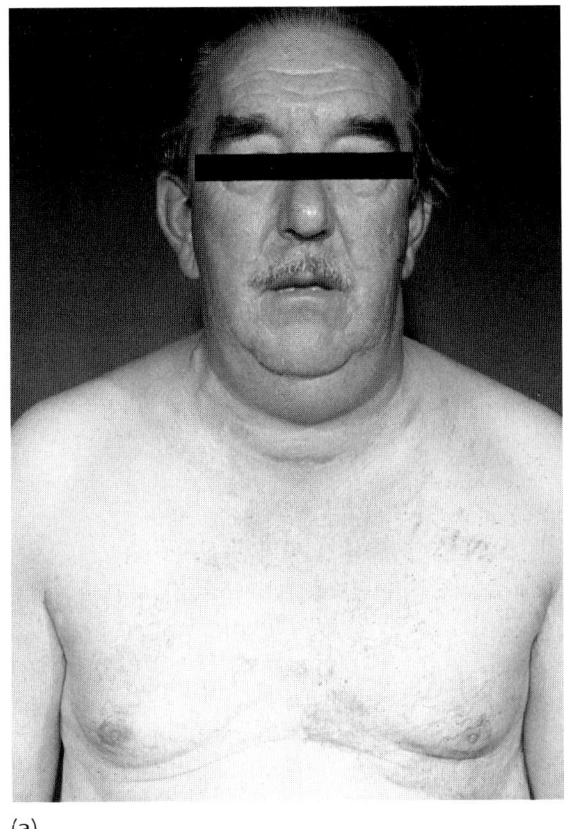

(a)

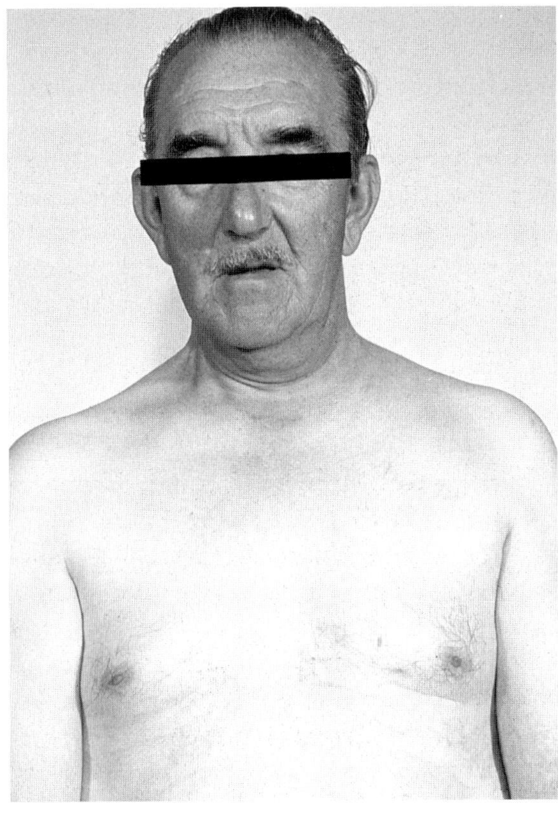

(b)

(c)

Figure 15.2
Superior vena cava syndrome: Clinical picture, before (a) and after (b) treatment; (c) X-ray of the chest, before (left) and after (right) treatment.

SUPERIOR VENA CAVA SYNDROME

The principal vascular syndrome associated with extension of lung cancer into the mediastinum is superior vena cava syndrome (SVCS), most commonly from invasion of the vein and extrinsic compression by a large primary tumour or its mediastinal lymph node metastases, but also from intraluminal thrombosis (Figure 15.2). Patients characteristically complain of headache, swelling of the face, neck and upper extremities, or a host of thoracic symptoms, such as dyspnoea, cough, chest pain and dysphagia. Physical examination may show facial oedema, neck vein distension, and striking collateral engorgement over the anterior chest wall and upper abdomen. The degree of collateral formation reflects the time over which superior vena cava obstruction has developed and the relative anatomical site of the blockade, since obstruction above the azygos vein is better tolerated. Signs of airway obstruction (e.g. stridor) or intracranial pressure (stupor or convulsion) should prompt rapid evaluation and treatment. When typical signs are present, complete SVC obstruction is easily diagnosed. The CT scan is likely to show tumour masses, and can also reveal the presence of thrombi and collateral vessels.

Lung cancer accounts for 65–90% of patients with SCVS, with approximately 85% of primary lung tumours occurring on the right, primarily in the right upper lobe or right mainstem bronchus. Among 2000 patients presenting lung cancer, 4% had SVCS.[26] By cell type, SCLC predominates as the cause of SVCS, followed by squamous cell carcinoma. In addition to lung cancer, lymphoma and other malignancies, benign causes of obstruction of the SVC include fibrosing mediastinitis, thrombosis, inflammatory adenopathy, postirradiation fibrosis and aneurysms.

Contrary to prior clinical wisdom, it has been convincingly demonstrated that the SVCS does not constitute a true medical emergency requiring urgent treatment without a tissue diagnosis.[27] The immediate causes of death directly related to SVC obstruction are airway obstruction and intracerebral haemorrhage. In the absence of significant airway obstruction and signs of severely elevated intracranial pressure, definite diagnosis can be obtained before therapy. An accurate diagnosis is also especially important in view of the diverse etiological considerations mentioned above. Bronchoscopy and, depending on the clinical circumstances, node biopsy, mediastinoscopy or even thoracotomy can be employed safely and effectively to diagnose lung cancer in this setting.

Most patients with SVCS secondary to lung cancer have resolution of symptoms after initiation of radiation or chemotherapy.[28] Before instituting radiotherapy in SVCS, general medical manoeuvres, including oxygen support, bed rest with elevation of the head of the bed, and corticosteroids, may be used as temporizing measures.

Chemotherapy is particularly useful when SVC obstruction is secondary to SCLC, although radiotherapy has been used in selected series. There is no difference in outcome or in time to resolution between the two,[29] but chemotherapy offers the advantage of simultaneous management of systemic disease and avoidance of large-field irradiation to the heart and lung. Resolution of the syndrome is prompt (7–10 days), and is achieved in 43–100% of cases.[30] If the chemotherapy drugs include vesicants, these should not be injected into the dilated, high-pressure, upper-extremity veins. The right upper extremity should be avoided for any drug administration, since the rate of blood flow is markedly decreased, and thrombosis, phlebitis and erratic drug distribution are likely.

Radiation is generally indicated in the management of the patient with SVCS secondary to NSCLC. Initial treatment with two to four fractions of 300–400 cGy, followed by conventional fractionation to a total dose of 3000–5000 cGy, has been advocated on the basis of limited evidence suggesting a prompter response with this schedule. A recent study evaluated the efficacy of treating patients with SVCS with a short course of hypofractionated irradiation.[31] The study compared a regimen of 8 Gy fractions once a week (to a total dose of 24 Gy) within two weeks, versus a programme of delivering only two fractions of 8 Gy (to a total dose of 16 Gy) within a week. In both regimens, a good palliative result was established; however, the results of the 24 Gy regimen were superior. Using the 24 Gy regimen, partial responses were obtained in 96% of patients, and 56% achieved complete response. The 16 Gy regimen yielded a complete response in only 28% of patients. Median overall survival was longer with the higher-dose regimen (nine months), compared with the low-dose regimen (three months).

Anticoagulation with heparin may be of benefit in SVCS resulting from intraluminal thrombosis of the SVC. Operative therapy is rarely indicated. Some authors believe that surgery with bypass grafting has a role in treating highly selected patients such as those with acute SVC occlusion and severe symptoms, or those with complete occlusion of the SVC, severe refractory symptoms and thrombosis of venous collaterals. The alternative surgery involves insertion of an SVC stent, a method that has been used experimentally in a few institutions throughout the world. The decision for surgery must be made with regard to the severity of the underlying disease, the patient's overall health, the risk of surgical intervention, the patient's life expectancy and the anatomy of the receptive vein.[32]

CARDIAC TAMPONADE

Neoplastic cardiac tamponade is one of the true emergencies of clinical oncology. It may appear abruptly and cause death in a patient who otherwise has good short-term life expectancy. Carcinoma of the lung is associated with the highest frequency of malignant pericardiac effusion, accounting for 37% of reported cases.[33] Haskell and French[34] reported on 23 patients in whom cardiac tamponade was the initial presentation in malignancy: 7 of these patients had lung cancer. Pericardial involvement arises either from direct extension of the tumour or because of retrograde spread through mediastinal and epicardial lymphatics. Cardiac tamponade may also be caused by postirradiation pericarditis with fibrosis or by encasement of the heart by tumour. The amount of fluid necessary to cause tamponade may be small (less than 200 ml) when the effusion accumulates rapidly or when the pericardium is uncompliant owing to fibrosis. When the pericardial effusion is chronic, over 1 l may accumulate before causing tamponade.

The symptoms of cardiac tamponade are non-specific. The most frequent complaints are apprehension, chest pain and dyspnoea. Occasionally, cough, hoarseness, hiccups, nausea and abdominal pain are prominent complaints. Elevated jugular venous pressure, tachycardia and narrow arterial pulse pressure are almost always seen. Pulsus paradoxus, an abnormally large drop in arterial systolic pressure during inspiration (>10 mmHg), is a hallmark of cardiac tamponade. The chest radiograph may show a large globular ('water bottle') heart, but cardiac silhouette may appear normal when the effusion has accumulated rapidly or is less than 250 ml. Sinus tachycardia and low voltage (QRS complex <5 mV) are usually present on a 12-lead electrocardiogram. QRS complex electrical alternans, pathognomonic of cardiac tamponade, is infrequently seen. A pericardial effusion may be quickly and accurately diagnosed by echocardiogram. Two-dimensional echocardiography is more sensitive than M-mode, because it displays virtually the entire circumference of the heart. Certain two-dimensional echocardiographic findings help to determine the functional significance of a pericardial effusion. Diastolic right atrial and right ventricular collapse occur early during the development of cardiac tamponade. However, physical examination and non-invasive tests may not elucidate the functional significance of pericardial effusion, particularly in patients with associated cardiopulmonary disease. In such cases, right heart catheterization or diagnostic pericardiocentesis is indicated.

Definitive treatment of cardiac tamponade requires decompression of the heart either surgically or by pericardiocentesis. Supportive therapy, including intravenous fluids, pressor agents and oxygen, is of limited benefit. Acute pericardial tamponade with haemodynamic instability is life-threatening, and must be alleviated by prompt fluid removal – most rapidly by pericardiocentesis. If the patient develops cyanosis, dyspnoea, shock or impaired consciousness, a pulsus paradoxus greater than 50% of pulse pressure, or a decrease of more than 20 mmHg in pulse pressure, emergency pericardiocentesis must be performed. If the patient is haemodynamically stable, a more definitive procedure should be performed. Zwischenberger and Bradford[35] recommend echocardiography or CT-guided percutaneous tube pericardiotomy to accomplish both diagnosis and therapy at the initial intervention. Once the pericardium has been drained, these authors use doxycyclin or bleomycin for sclerotherapy. If sclerotherapy does not control the effusion, they proceed with subxiphoid pericardiotomy for evacuation of the effusion. A subxiphoid pericardial window can be performed under local anaesthesia, and is reported to control the effusion in almost all patients. The high control rate and low incidence of complications with subxiphoid pericardiotomy have also led other investigators to conclude that this procedure can be used instead of pericardiocentesis for initial treatment of cardiac tamponade.[36]

EXTRATHORACIC COMPLICATIONS

Lung cancer frequently metastasizes to distant organs. More than 60% of patients with SCLC and approximately 30–40% of those with NSCLC have stage IV metastatic disease. The usual sites of distant metastatic disease include the adrenals, brain, liver, lung and bone, although virtually any organ can be affected. Metastases may present at the same time as the primary tumour or may occur much later, and they may be single or multiple, clinically silent or requiring urgent diagnosis and treatment. Manifestations resulting from distant metastases depend on the specific organ involved, and are similar to those for other kinds of cancer.

Brain metastases

The most frequent metastatic neurological complications of lung cancer are metastases to the brain. Clinically diagnosed brain metastases are present at initial presentation in 4–19% of SCLC patients,[37] and the incidence rises to 50% in patients not receiving prophylactic cranial irradiation.[38] Patients with NSCLC, especially those with adenocarcinoma, often develop brain metastases during the course of their disease.[39]

Brain metastases may be detected before the primary tumour is found or at the same time (synchronous presentation), but more commonly (80%) the diagnosis of the lung cancer antedates the development of the brain metastases (metachronous presentation). Focal neurological abnormalities and global deficit of higher mental function are the commonest findings, with headaches being the most frequent symptom at presentation. Headaches occur in approximately 50% of patients with brain metastases – more commonly in those with multiple metastases and with metastases in the posterior fossa. They may be associated with other symptoms characteristic of increased intracranial pressure, such as vomiting, visual blurring and confusion. Focal weakness is the presenting symptom in 20–40% of patients. Deficits of higher mental function (memory problems and mood or personality changes) are reported by one-third of patients, whereas cognitive dysfunction as detected by standard tests of mental status may be present in as many as 75%. Seizures occur in approximately 10% of patients as the first sign of metastases. CT and MRI are the primary radiographic means of evaluating patients suspected of having brain metastases. MRI is more sensitive in detecting multiple lesions, and allows improved visualization of the brainstem.

The prognosis for patients with brain metastases is very poor, and depends on their functional and neurological status, evidence of systemic tumour involvement and whether the brain metastasis is truly solitary. Steroids alone can temporarily improve symptoms in around 60% of patients, but without treatment half of the patients die in about two months. This average survival is derived from a heterogeneous group of patients with very different ages, primary sites and levels of functioning. Advances in surgery and in radio- and chemotherapy have led us to pursue other strategies to improve control in the brain, with the hope of impacting upon survival.

Surgical resection plus postoperative whole brain radiation therapy (WBRT) is currently the treatment of choice for patients with surgically accessible single brain metastases. The data supporting surgery for single brain metastases come from many retrospective studies[40] and two randomized prospective trials,[41,42] the results of which show that surgical resection is of benefit in selected patients. In the first randomized trial, by Patchell et al,[41] 48 patients with known systemic cancer were treated either with biopsy of the suspected brain metastases plus WBRT or with complete surgical resection of the metastases plus WBRT. A statistically significant increase in survival time was found in the surgical group (40 weeks versus 15 weeks). In addition, patients receiving surgery also had a significant decrease in recurrence at this surgical site and an improved quality of life. A second randomized study[42] evaluated 63 patients randomized either to complete surgical resection plus WBRT or to WBRT alone. Survival was significantly longer in the surgical group (10 months versus 6 months), and a non-significant trend towards longer duration of functional independence was seen in the surgically treated patients.

On the basis of these data, surgery and radiotherapy are usually recommended for good-performance-status patients with a solitary cerebral metastasis. However, over 50% of isolated brain lesions are not amenable to surgery. Stereotactic radiosurgery (SRS) is an alternative method able to deliver a highly focused single dose of radiation to a well-defined small intracranial target, thus minimizing exposure to the normal surrounding brain. To date, no randomized trial comparing radiosurgery with any of the conventional methods of therapy has been reported, although many uncontrolled series have been published.[43,44] The median survival ranged from 6 to 11 months, and one year control rates of 75–88% were reported in three studies. In the majority of these studies, SRS was performed for recurrent metastases after previous radiation. One trial[45] reviewed the outcome for 122 patients who met the same selection criteria used by Patchell et al[41] and who received WBRT followed by a radiosurgery boost. The overall median survival (56 weeks) and the duration of functionally independent survival (44 weeks) were similar to those in the surgical arm of the randomized trial of Patchell et al. Whether SRS will be superior to surgery will have to be determined by randomized trials.

The majority of patients with brain metastases present with multiple lesions, and are not candidates for aggressive local therapy. The mainstay of treatment is palliative WBRT.[46] Many studies have compared different radiation schedules and doses. Final results from the Royal College of Radiologists' trial[47] suggest that a hypofractionated course of WBRT could palliate symptoms with minimal toxicity. Patients with NSCLC who are elderly or have a poor performance status could benefit from a short course of treatment. Recent studies indicate that chemotherapeutic agents may cross the blood–brain barrier in patients with brain metastases.[48] The observed response rate to chemotherapeutic agents was similar in the brain (16–35%) as in other organs.[49,50] Two studies on concomitant radiotherapy and chemotherapy for brain metastases in NSCLC reported higher objective rates (58–76%).[51,52] Moreover, both studies demonstrated a neurological improvement in more than 50% of patients. Whether there is a definitive role for chemotherapy or combined chemoradiotherapy in the treatment of brain metastases in patients with NSCLC will have to be determined by prospective studies taking account of survival and quality of life as their main endpoints. Patients with SCLC and brain metastases at presentation should be treated with primary chemotherapy. Whether consolidating cranial radiotherapy should be given after a few courses of initial chemotherapy is unclear. In patients who are unfit for chemotherapy or who have brain relapses during or immediately after chemotherapy, some palliative effect can be obtained with a short course of WBRT. As with NSCLC, combined chemoradiotherapy should be considered only in the context of a clinical trial.

Spinal cord compression

After brain metastases, spinal cord compression (SCC) is the most frequent neurological complication of lung cancer. Five per cent of patients with lung cancer develop spinal cord compression, more frequently at an interval after the diagnosis, usually six months.[53] In a retrospective study on metastatic SCC secondary to lung cancer, Bach et al[54] observed some variations between the different types of lung cancer. In SCLC, 75% of the cases of SCC were diagnosed during the first month after the primary malignant diagnosis was established, which contrasts with 12 months for adenocarcinoma and 21 months for squamous subtypes. Lung cancer has a predeliction to metastasize to the vertebral column. The most common mode of SCC is that due to expansion or collapse of the vertebral body (85%) or neural arch. Paraspinal lung cancer may also directly invade the extradural space through the intervertebral foramen, producing SCC without body involvement.

Malignant spinal cord compression is a medical emergency, and the key to successful management is early diagnosis and prompt treatment. All too often, the diagnosis is made too late for useful treatment. Those patients who present paraparesis, sensory symptoms and sphincteric dysfunction usually pose no difficulty in diagnosis. Patients with more subtle presentations must be identified, and an appreciation of the earliest clinical manifestation is therefore essential.

Isolated back pain is the initial symptom in 70–95% of patients, and it always antedates diagnosis of SCC by several days to many months. Pain can be local or radicular. Symptoms other than pain suggest compromise of neural structures. Weakness is present in approximately 80% of patients, and may be most evident when it affects proximal muscles of the lower extremity, creating difficulty when climbing stairs or rising from chairs. Non-painful sensory symptoms include paraesthesias, which in SCC usually begin in the feet and gradually ascend, ultimately stopping at a specific level that the patient may indicate. Loss of proprioception, producing ataxia, and sphincteric dysfunction are often late manifestations. Careful neurological examination usually identifies the neurological level and establishes the diagnosis.

The evaluation of the patient with SCC must be speedy and decisive. Although 80% of patients show abnormalities on plain spinal radiography, normal spine films do not exclude epidural metastases. MRI is being recognized as the diagnostic method of choice in SCC. Patients diagnosed with epidural cord compression should be treated urgently. Loss of ambulation or sphincter function before treatment is associated with a poor response to treatment and an adverse prognosis. About 80% of patients with little or no ambulatory dysfunction retain the ability to walk. Patients who are paraparetic recover ambulation in 20–60% of cases. Paraplegia improves in response to treatment in no more than 16% of cases.[55,56]

When the diagnosis of epidural compression has been made, dexamethasone should be administered. There is good evidence that the administration of high-dose steroids (dexamethasone 96 mg intravenous bolus, then 24 mg orally four times a day for three days, then taper over ten days) improves the postradiation ambulatory rate compared with those who do not receive any steroids.[57] However, the utility of moderate-dose steroids (dexamethasone 10 mg intravenous bolus, then 4 mg intravenously, with a taper over two weeks) remains unclear. There is fair evidence that dexamethasone does not need to be given to asymptomatic ambulatory patients with radiographic cord compression who are receiving radiotherapy.[58] The decision to proceed with surgery or radiotherapy is based on the individual patient's specific circumstances. Although based on inconclusive evidence, some general treatment recommendations can be suggested.[59] Patients who present spinal instability or bony compression of their spinal cord, with no histological diagnosis, with redevelopment of epidural compression in a previously radiated site, and with neurological deterioration during radiotherapy, should be considered for surgical resection. Ambulatory patients postsurgically may benefit from postoperative radiotherapy. Other patients can be treated effectively with radiotherapy alone, specifically those with life expectancy of three months or less, more than one level of simultaneous SCC, paraplegia of greater than 12–24 hours duration, and co-morbid conditions that preclude surgery.

PARANEOPLASTIC SYNDROMES

Complications of lung cancer that are not related to direct invasion, obstruction or metastatic effects of the tumour are generally termed paraneoplastic. Paraneoplastic syndromes comprise a group of disorders mediated by the production of circulating factors by, or in response to, lung cancer. These syndromes are numerous and occur in 10–20% of lung cancer patients, and include endocrine, neurological, cardiovascular, skeletal and cutaneous manifestations (Table 15.2).

In this review, we focus only on the most common syndromes.

Paraneoplastic endocrine syndromes

Syndrome of inappropriate antidiuretic hormone (SIADH)

SIADH results from inadequate secretion of antidiuretic hormone (ADH, vasopressin), which is almost exclusively associated with small cell histology. SCLC is estimated to account for 75% of tumour-associated SIADH. The main features of SIADH are water intoxication and hyponatraemia. Diagnostic criteria include:

- hypo-osmotic hyponatraemia;
- inappropriately concentrated urine (urine osmolarity $>$100 mosmol/kg);
- euvolaemia;
- normal renal, adrenal and thyroid function.

The clinical features are related to osmotic water shift that leads to increased intracellular fluid (ICF) volume, specifically brain cell swelling. More often, hyponatraemia develops

Table 15.2. Paraneoplastic syndromes of lung cancer

Syndrome	Clinical frequency (%)	Isotypes
Endocrine		
Inappropriate ADH	5–10	SCLC
Ectopic ACTH	3–7	SCLC
Humoral hypercalcaemia	10	Most frequently with squamous cell types
Neurological		
Lambert–Eaton	6	SCLC
Peripheral neuropathy	Rare	
Encephalopathy	Rare	
Myelopathy	Rare	
Cutaneous and musculoskeletal		
Clubbing/hypertrophic pulmonary osteoarthropathy	10	More with adenocarcinoma
Dermatomyositis	Rare	
Acanthosis nigricans	Rare	
Vascular and haematological		
Hypercoagulable state	10–15	More with adenocarcinoma
Thrombophlebitis	Uncommon	
Non-bacterial thrombotic endocarditis	Uncommon	

insidiously, and adaptive mechanisms tend to minimize the increase in the ICF volume and its symptoms. Most patients experience minimal symptoms, and are discovered on routine laboratory evaluation when they have hyponatraemia. Symptoms most frequently associated with hyponatraemia include anorexia, nausea, vomiting, headache and mildly altered mental status. In severe or rapid-onset hyponatraemia, patients may experience symptoms related to cerebral oedema, resulting in confusion, irritability, seizures, coma and ultimately respiratory arrest.

In evaluating a patient with hyponatraemia, the physician must carefully exclude other causes and non-malignant conditions associated with SIADH. The first step in the diagnostic process is to assess volume status. As SIADH is one of the so-called euvolaemic hyponatraemic states, the physician must recognize all diseases associated with volume overload, such as congestive heart failure, nephrotic syndrome and severe liver disease. On the other hand, it is also important to exclude causes of hypovolaemic hyponatraemia that develops as a consequence of electrolyte-free water retention. Once the patient has been determined to be euvolaemic, other causes of hyponatraemia associated with a normal extracellular fluid volume must be ruled out, including glucocorticoid deficiency, hypothyroidism and renal disease. Finally, other causes of SIADH must be excluded before the disorder is accepted as a paraneoplastic syndrome. Well-known nonmalignant conditions associated with SIADH include pulmonary infections, central nervous system disorders (e.g. head trauma, space-occupying lesions and cerebrovascular accidents) and drugs (most commonly chlorpropamide, carbamazepine, tricyclic antidepressants, thiazide diuretics, morphine, cyclophosphamide and vincristine). List and colleagues[60] reviewed 350 cases of SCLC and noted that 40 (11%) met a strict definition of SIADH similar to that outlined above, and 33 of them had the syndrome at initial presentation.

Chemotherapy of the associated SCLC is generally associated with improvement in the syndrome. SIADH has not been shown to be a negative prognostic factor in terms of response to chemotherapy. In 80% of patients, the serum sodium returns to normal within three weeks of the start of chemotherapy, and this may predate other indices of response. Supportive measures such as fluid restriction and pharmacological therapy can be undertaken to treat SIADH. For patients with sodium levels below 130 mmol/l, placement on free-water restriction (500 ml/day) is generally recommended, in addition to treatment of the primary malignancy. In the event that this measure does not bring the serum sodium level above 130 mmol/l, the tetracycline antibiotic demeclocycline (150–300 mg, 6–8 hourly) can be used, which induces nephrogenic diabetes insipidus such that the distal tubule becomes refractory to the effect of arginine vasopressin. In patients with more severe or life-threatening symptoms related to hyponatraemia (serum sodium less than 115 mmol/l), treatment consists of intravenous fluids with 0.9% saline (rarely, hypertonic saline) and diuresis with a loop diuretic such as intravenous frusemide (furosemide).

The rate of correction of hyponatraemia depends on the absence or presence of neurological dysfunction. This is in turn related to the rapidity of onset and magnitude of the fall of the serum sodium. The rate of correction of the sodium is best limited to 1–2 mmol/l/h or a maximum of 20 mmol/l/day until a level of 120–130 mmol/l is reached. More rapid correction has been associated with the development of central pontine myelinolysis, which is characterized by flacid paralysis, dysarthria and dysphagia.

Ectopic adrenocorticotrophic hormone syndrome

Cushing's syndrome is due to the chronic effects of an excess of glucocorticoid hormone, most often iatrogenic resulting from therapy with glucocorticoid drugs. Adrenocorticotrophic hormone (ACTH)-secreting pituitary microadenomas (Cushing's disease) account for some 80% of cases of endogenous Cushing's syndrome. About 15–20% of cases of Cushing's syndrome are due to ectopic ACTH or corticotrophin-releasing hormone (CRH) production. SCLC and bronchial carcinoid tumours account for most of these cases.[61] The classic signs and symptoms include truncal obesity, cutaneous striae, moon face, buffalo hump, proximal myopathy and weakness, osteoporosis, diabetes mellitus, hypertension and personality changes. However, lung cancer patients with Cushing's syndrome often do not have the classic clinical finding. The commonest physical findings are oedema (83%) and proximal myopathy (61%).[62] Myopathy with weakness and muscle wasting is much more common in ectopic ACTH production. Moreover, hyperpigmentation is found in ectopic ACTH production, but not in Cushing's disease. Most patients will have a hypokalaemic alkalosis, and about half will be hyperglycaemic. This difference in presentation may be due to the rapid growth of the malignancy, relatively high levels of ACTH, and the fact that patients may not live long enough to develop the more classic features of the syndrome.

Cushing's syndrome occurs in approximately 5% of cases of SCLC, although raised concentrations of immunoreactive corticotrophin can be detected in as many as 50%. In a review of more than 500 patients with SCLC, 23 cases (4.5%) of Cushing's syndrome were identified.[62] Thirteen patients had the syndrome at initial diagnosis, and ten developed it at the time of relapse of their disease after therapy. All of these patients had a shorter survival compared with patients without the syndrome. This may be due in part to the observed complications (infections and gastrointestinal ulceration) related to prolonged exposure to high levels of corticosteroids secondary to ectopic ACTH production. The diagnosis of Cushing's syndrome is best established by 24-hour urine-free cortisol measurements or low-dose dexamethasone suppression testing (0.5 mg every six hours for eight doses).[63]

The most effective treatment of this syndrome is treatment of the tumour, but inhibition of adrenal steroid synthesis is said to be beneficial. Drugs that are able to inhibit cortisol production include mitotane, aminoglutethimide, metyrapone and ketoconazole. Because of its rapid onset of action and favourable toxicity profile, ketoconazole (300–400 mg twice as day) has become the therapy of choice for ectopic ACTH.[64]

Humoral hypercalcaemia

Hypercalcaemia is probably the most common metabolic complication of cancer and, since determination of the serum calcium level became routine, the recognition of patients with hypercalcaemia associated with cancer has increased. Hypercalcaemia may be related to direct bone destruction or to secretion of a parathyroid hormone (PTH)-related protein or other bone-resorbing substances (cytokines) secreted by the tumour. A PTH-related protein that shares an N-terminal sequence with PTH but has a unique C-terminal portion has been shown to be responsible for most cases of hypercalcaemia of malignancy. Elevated levels of PTH-related protein by radioimmunoassay were found in 30 of 42 patients (71%) with hypercalcaemia of malignancy, but only in 3 of 23 patients with cancer (13%) but with normal calcium levels.[65] In a study of 200 consecutive patients with untreated bronchogenic carcinoma, the overall frequency of hypercalcaemia was 12.5%.[66] Of these 25 patients, 14 did not have evidence of bony metastases. Humoral hypercalcaemia was most commonly observed in those with squamous cell histology, and was uncommonly observed with adenocarcinoma and SCLC.

The symptoms associated with hypercalcaemia generally correlate with the magnitude and rapidity of the rise in serum calcium. Mild hypercalaemia is generally asymptomatic. More severe hypercalcaemia is frequently associated with neurological, gastrointestinal and renal symptoms. The neurological manifestations range from mild drowsiness, progressing to weakness, depression, lethargy, stupor and coma. Gastrointestinal symptoms may include constipation, nausea, vomiting, anorexia and peptic ulcer disease. Hypercalcaemia-induced nephrogenic diabetes insipidus often results in polyuria, leading to extracellular fluid (ECF) volume depletion and a reduction in the glomerular filtration rate (GFR), which may lead to a further increase in calcium concentration. Cardiovascular effects include shortened QT interval, broadened T wave, heart block, ventricular arrhythmia and asystole. Individual patients may manifest any combination of these signs and symptoms to varying degrees.

Hypercalcaemia may be completely reversible with effective treatment of the underlying cancer; it is important to recognize that hypercalcaemia per se does not rule out the possibility of curative therapy, including surgery, if indicated. The prognosis for patients with hypercalcaemia and no further treatment of the underlying malignancy is extremely poor, with median survivals of 30–45 days.[67] The symptoms and the magnitude of the hypercalcaemia are key considerations in determining the need for aggressive therapy. If the serum calcium concentration is greater than 14 mg/dl, immediate treatment is indicated, even if symptoms are absent. In the case of mild calcium elevation (<12 mg/dl) in patients with widely metastatic and incurable malignancy, it may be most appropriate to give supportive care only, without specific therapy for the hypercalcaemia. Otherwise, most patients with serum calcium values of 12–14 mg/dl should be treated. The approaches to the management of hypercalcaemia can be divided into four specific areas:

- treating the underlying tumour;
- correcting dehydration;
- enhancing renal excretion of calcium;
- inhibiting accelerated bone resorption.

The intravenous administration of isotonic saline is an important component, and is the first step in the management of severe hypercalcaemia with associated symptoms. A widely used regimen is to administer 3 l of isotonic saline daily, recognizing that the rate of fluid administration may need to be varied if symptoms and signs of fluid overload appear. The next step is to add a loop diuretic, such as frusemide, that will increase calcium excretion.

This initial treatment usually has little effect on calcium levels, effecting a median decrease of only 1.0 mg/dl. Specific therapy to inhibit accelerated bone resorption is often necessary. Bisphosphonates are potent inhibitors of bone resorption that have dramatically changed the therapeutic approach to hypercalcaemia. These compounds have poor gastrointestinal absorption, and are best used intravenously. Etidronate is usually given as a two- to four-hour infusion for three to five days. Pamidronate has been tested most often, and is the most useful of the commercially available compounds. On the basis of a review of the literature and a few published dose–response trials, Body and associates[68] recommend a total dose of 60–90 mg (or 1.0–1.5 mg/kg), either as a single infusion or in divided doses over two or three days. With such doses, 90% of the patients become normocalcaemic, and the response to pamidronate is not significantly influenced by the tumour type or the presence of metastatic bone involvement. With this therapeutic scheme, normalization of serum calcium is obtained after three days (range 1–11 days), and normocalcaemia is maintained for a variable length of time (median of one to two weeks). Bisphosphonates are well tolerated; the only clinically detectable side-effect is transient fever in about 20% of the cases.

Other inhibitors of osteoclast activity include calcitonin, plicamycin and gallium nitrate. Calcitonin inhibits bone resorption, increases renal calcium excretion and has a rapid onset of action. The hypercalcaemia effect begins within hours, with a nadir in serum calcium within 12–24 hours, but the effect on calcium concentrations is modest and transient, and calcitonin alone has no place in the treatment of severe hypercalcaemia. However, in very severe cases, it is an excellent addition to the later-acting bisphosphonates or plicamycin.

Plicamycin (mithramycin) inhibits osteoclastic RNA synthesis. It lowers the serum calcium more quickly than bisphosphonates do, but significant side-effects (raised transaminases, nephrotoxicity with proteinuria, thrombocytopenia, nausea, and local inflammation or cellulitis at sites of extravasation) decrease enthusiasm for this agent unless the calcium concentration needs to be lowered very rapidly.

Gallium nitrate also inhibits bone resorption. As with bisphosphonates, it takes several days before a nadir in serum calcium is reached, and this lasts about a week. Side-effects are frequent and severe, and include nephrotoxicity, hypophosphataemia and anaemia. The need to treat patients for five days with a continuous infusion and its toxicity limit the use of this compound in the treatment of hypercalcaemia.

Paraneoplastic neurological syndromes

Paraneoplastic neurological syndromes have long been recognized, and these disorders are now thought to result from the cross-reaction of antitumour antibodies with antigen also present in neural tissue.[69] One such antigen is the nuclear-associated HuD protein, which has been cloned by use of high-titre antibodies from the serum of patients with paraneoplastic syndromes.[70] In health, the antigen is expressed only in neural tissue, but is expressed by all SCLCs, perhaps reflecting the apparent neuroendocrine origin of this tumour. Why high titres of anti-HuD antibodies develop in some patients with SCLC is unknown. What is known is that these antibodies are strongly associated with paraneoplastic sensory neuropathy/encephalitis. The pathogenesis of neural injury here is also uncertain, since the presence of antibodies may simply be an index of a cell-mediated immune response.

Neurological paraneoplastic syndromes include sensory, sensorimotor and autonomic neuropathies and encephalomyelitis. Neurological symptoms of encephalomyelitis include dementia (limbic encephalitis), cerebellar degeneration, brain-stem encephalitis and myelitis. Sensory neuropathy and encephalomyelitis often occur together, and are associated primarily with SCLC.

Symptoms may precede the diagnosis of lung cancer by many months, or they may be the first sign of tumour recurrence. Direct metastatic effects as well as metabolic or infectious processes must be excluded as contributors to the neurological findings. The severity of neurological symptoms is not related to tumour bulk; in fact, a primary malignant lesion may be undetected before death, despite disabling symptoms. In a patient with the appropriate neurological findings, positive anti-Hu antibody and significant smoking history, a diligent diagnostic evaluation should be undertaken. The most helpful diagnostic test is probably CT of the chest, with careful attention to mediastinal or hilar nodes.

Lambert–Eaton myasthenic syndrome

The neurological syndrome most commonly recognized is the Lambert–Eaton myasthenic syndrome, reported to occur in up to 6% of cases of SCLC. Clinically, this syndrome is characterized by muscle weakness, hyporeflexia and autonomic dysfunction due to impaired release of acetylcholine from the cholinergic nerve terminals. Symptoms are most pronounced in the pelvic girdle and thigh muscles, making it difficult for patients to climb stairs or get out of a bathtub. Other symptoms, such as dysarthria, dysphagia, diplopia and ptosis, may occur. It is distinguished from myasthenia gravis by the absence or minor involvement of bulbar or extraocular muscles. Standard electromyography characteristically demonstrates a reduced amplitude of the compound muscle action potential, which increases immediately after 10–15 seconds of maximal voluntary contraction or during high-frequency nerve stimulation, while there is a steady decrease in classic myasthenia. The manifestations of the disease may occur as long as two to four years before the diagnosis of SCLC.

The syndrome is thought to result from autoantibody-mediated impairment of presynaptic neuronal calcium channel activity, which impairs the nerve stimulus-induced release of acetylcholine.[71] Treatment-induced remission of the SCLC may cause attenuation or remission of the syndrome in some patients. The use of acetylcholinesterase inhibitors is of limited benefit. 3,4-Diaminopyridine enhances the release of acetylcholine, and has been shown to be effective in treating both the motor and the autonomic deficits of the syndrome.[72] Immunosuppressive treatment may provide benefit, but its effects are usually delayed and incomplete. Many patients become severely debilitated from their motor dysfunction, regardless of the status of their lung cancer.

Peripheral neuropathy

Patients with cancer who suffer from a peripheral neuropathy usually do so from causes other than paraneoplastic syndromes (e.g. neoplastic invasion, chemotherapeutic agents, and nutritional and metabolic disorders). Therefore a careful evaluation for other causes of peripheral neuropathy should be made before the disorder is accepted as a paraneoplastic syndrome.

One exception is the *subacute sensory neuropathy* occurring in patients who have the anti-Hu antibody, where the presence of the antibody establishes the diagnosis as a paraneoplastic syndrome and the cancer as highly likely to be SCLC. In about 20% of all patients with a subacutely developing pure sensory neuropathy, cancer is the underlying cause. Subacute sensory neuropathy is usually a rapidly developing severe disorder in which patients lose all modalities of sensation, usually in all four extremities. The disorder is clinically distinguishable from cisplatin sensory neuropathy, because cisplatin neuropathy causes loss of proprioception and spares pain and temperature sensation. Although the disorder may begin in the face or trunk, it commonly begins distally in the extremities and extends proximally. The sensory loss is so severe that patients may be unable to walk, use their hands or coordinate movements. The neurological symptoms may precede the diagnosis of SCLC by several months.[73] Electrodiagnostic tests show absent sensory potentials. Motor nerve conduction and F waves may be entirely normal. The neuropathological findings include drop-out of neurons in the dorsal root ganglia, inflammatory infiltrates mainly composed of T cells, and anti-Hu antibody on the surface and in the nuclei of the remaining sensory neurons.

Other neurological syndromes

Among the other SCLC-associated neurological syndromes are *limbic encephalopathy, necrotizing myelopathy* and *intestinal dysmotility syndrome*.

Anti-Hu antibody has been noted in patients with SCLC presenting these rare neurological paraneoplastic syndromes.[74] Limbic encephalopathy is characterized by memory loss and behavioural changes, including dementia, which often antedate the diagnosis of cancer. Necrotizing myelopathy is an unusual neurological paraneoplastic syndrome, and is characterized by a relatively acute, rapidly ascending paraplegia that culminates in rapid deterioration and death.

Intestinal pseudo-obstruction of the bowel is the most well-defined isolated autonomic symptom. Patients may suffer weight loss, refractory constipation and abdominal distension. Neurological studies show loss of neurons in myenteric plexus with inflammatory infiltrates. Serum antibodies to myenteric and submucosal neural plexus of the jejunum and stomach have been found in patients with SCLC.[75]

Paraneoplastic cutaneous and musculoskeletal syndromes

Digital clubbing and hypertrophic pulmonary osteoarthropathy are the other major paraneo-

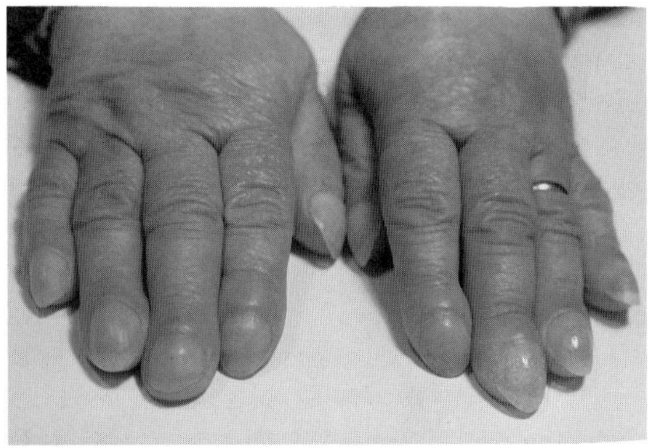

Figure 15.3
Digital clubbing.

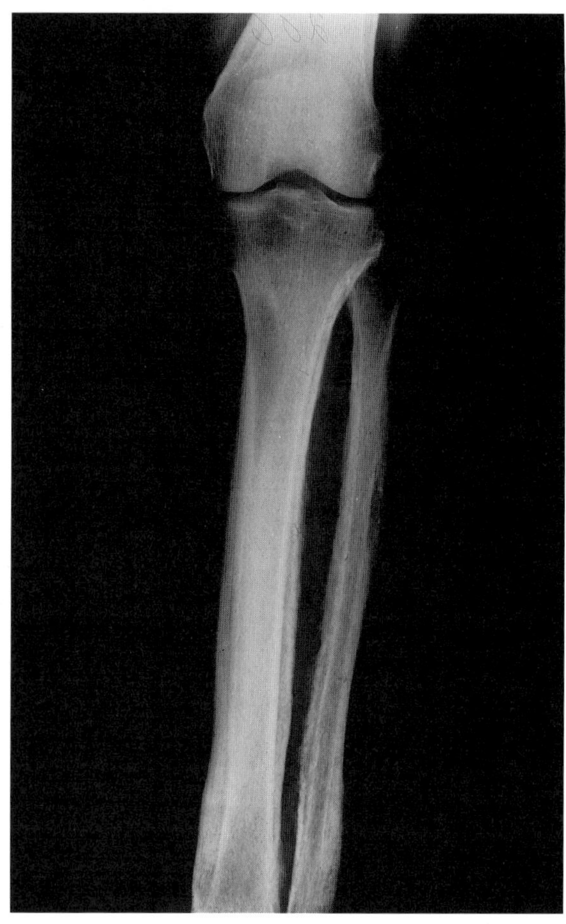

Figure 15.4
Hypertrophic pulmonary osteoarthropathy.

plastic syndromes that are associated with lung cancer, almost exclusively with NSCLC.[76]

Digital clubbing is characterized by subungual soft tissue thickening, most commonly involving the fingernails, which are often bulbous in appearance (Figure 15.3). Clubbing of the digits is one of the most commonly discussed findings on pulmonary medicine clinical rounds. Etiological factors include hereditary and both non-pulmonary and pulmonary diseases, including bronchogenic carcinoma.

Hypertrophic pulmonary osteoarthropathy (HPO) is less common than digital clubbing, and is usually associated with intrathoracic malignancy, especially lung cancer, and often resembles rheumatoid arthritis (Figure 15.4). It is characterized by painful symmetric polyarthritis that generally involves the ankles, wrists and knees. HPO is due to proliferative periostitis of the long bones, often with little or no evidence of clubbing. The onset of HPO is often acute, may precede the diagnosis of cancer by months, and usually, but not invariably, is associated with inoperability. The cause of HPO is not known, but may be due to a humoral agent. Patients with HPO frequently have consulted a rheumatologist or orthopaedic specialist before the ultimate diagnosis of lung cancer is suspected and a chest radiograph is obtained. In patients who smoke and present arthralgia, HPO must be included in the differential diagnosis. Radionuclide bone scans typically show increased uptake at the distal ends of the affected long bones, and this may be confirmed by evidence of new bone formation on plain-film radiographs. The spine is spared. The syndrome may resolve with response of the cancer; however, no effective form of treatment is recognized, including aspirin and non-steroidal anti-inflammatory agents.

Other cutaneous paraneoplastic syndromes include dermatomyositis, acanthosis nigricans, and hyperkeratosis of the palm and soles. These conditions are rarely seen in patients with lung cancer.

Dermatomyositis is a rare but very disabling complication of lung cancer. The patient presents weakness and a characteristic rash. Sometimes the disease presents as a cardiac or pulmonary disease. Weakness usually moves gradually and progressively. Although they do not occur in all patients, muscle tenderness and aches may be very striking. The inflammation characteristically causes elevations of serum levels of aldolase and creatinine kinase, and liver function tests. Although most patients respond initially to corticosteroids, cytotoxic drugs are sometimes added when steroid toxicity or refractoriness develops.

Paraneoplastic vascular and haematological syndromes

The association between cancer and venous thromboembolism is well known. Over 100 years ago, Trousseau reported cases of episodic migratory *thrombophlebitis* in patients with cancer. The pathogenic mechanisms for the association include hypercoagulability due to activation of clotting by tumour cells, vessel wall injury and stasis. Occasionally, the thromboembolic event occurs before the diagnosis of cancer, and it has been suggested that deep venous thrombosis may be a predictor of the subsequent diagnosis of cancer. Two studies have noted a significant association between primary venous thrombosis and the subsequent development of cancer.[77,78] This link seems particularly strong in patients with recurrent deep venous thrombosis. Lung cancer and other malignancies, especially those of the gastrointestinal tract (e.g. the pancreas), are commonly associated with Trousseau's syndrome. Pulmonary embolism has been observed at autopsy in 20% of patients with lung cancer, and may precede the diagnosis of cancer;[79] 25% of adult patients with acute pulmonary embolism may develop cancer within five years.[80] There appears to be a general activation of the clotting system in patients with lung cancer, the clinical consequence much more often being thrombosis rather than bleeding.

Disseminated intravascular coagulation (DIC) is another state of haemostatic disarray, characterized by the inappropriate coexistence of enhanced fibrin production and fibrinolysis. DIC has been reported as a complication of many neoplastic disorders, but is most likely to occur in carcinoma of the lung, prostate, breast and gastrointestinal tract, in melanoma, and in leukaemia. In its grossest form, DIC is readily recognized by prolongation of the thrombin time, prothrombin time and partial thromboplastin time, by a decrease in the concentration of plasma fibrinogen and other clotting factors, by thrombocytopenia, and by the presence in serum of antigens reacting with antiserum to fibrinogen or its derivatives. However, apparent DIC, with consumption of platelets and clotting factors and bleeding, is rare and is most commonly associated with acute promyelocytic leukaemia and adenocarcinoma.

Non-bacterial thrombotic endocarditis (NBTE), also known as marantic endocarditis, probably relates to this hypercoagulable state, and is generally defined as vegetations on the heart valves or wall that contain fibrin and platelets, but without evidence of infection. It is particularly associated with bronchoalveolar carcinoma and adenocarcinoma of the lung. At autopsy, the incidence of NBTE in each of these cell types is approximately 7%. The mitral valve is commonly involved, and clinically significant emboli to the central nervous system, kidneys and coronary arteries have been described in what previously was thought to be a syndrome of only pathological interest at autopsy.[81] Although some patients may have heart murmurs, most do not. Echocardiography picks up vegetations larger than 2 mm. In a review of cerebrovascular complications in patients with cancer, Graus and colleagues[82] observed cerebral embolic infarction in 42 of 86 patients with pathologically documented NBTE and careful autopsy examination of the brain. NSCLC was the most common malignancy in this group. Cerebral infarction was symptomatic in 32 (76%) of these patients ante mortem, and was associated with clinical evidence of other systemic emboli in 19 patients. The definitive diagnostic test is cerebral angiography, which shows multiple arterial occlusions.

Tumour embolization to the lungs and brain is another cause of emboli in cancer patients, in addition to venous thrombosis and NBTE. Tumour emboli are an unusual clinical event, although autopsy series have reported tumour emboli in up to 23% of solid tumours.[83] Lung cancer and breast cancer were the most common malignancies in these patients, but in only one patient was the tumour embolism correctly diagnosed ante mortem.

The management of thromboembolic complications in patients with lung cancer is difficult. Typically, such patients are resistant to anticoagulation, especially with warfarin. Long-term administration of subcutaneous heparin or use of oral antiplatelet drugs may be more effective approaches, but no controlled trials have been performed as yet.

REFERENCES

1. Nagata N, Nikaido Y, Kido M et al, Terminal pulmonary infections in patients with lung cancer. *Chest* 1993; **103**: 1739–42.
2. Perlin E, Bang KM, Shah A et al, The impact of pulmonary infections on the survival of lung cancer patients. *Cancer* 1990; **66**: 593–6.
3. Putinati S, Trevisani L, Gualandi M et al, Pulmonary infections in lung cancer patients at diagnosis. *Lung Cancer* 1994; **11**: 243–9.
4. Thorpe JE, Baugham R-P, Frame PT et al, Bronchoalveolar lavage for diagnosis acute bacterial pneumonia. *J Infect Dis* 1987; **155**: 855–61.
5. Kirdand SH, Winterbauer RH, Dreis DF et al, A clinical profile of chronic bacterial pneumonia – a report of 115 cases. *Chest* 1994; **106**: 15–22.
6. Santiago S, Tobias J, Williams AJ, A reappraisal of the causes of hemoptysis. *Arch Intern Med* 1991; **151**: 2449–51.
7. Spain RC, Whittlesey D, Respiratory emergencies in patients with cancer. *Semin Oncol* 1989; **16**: 471–89.
8. Panos RJ, Barr LF, Walsh TJ, Silverman HJ, Factors associated with fatal hemoptysis in cancer patients. *Chest* 1988; **94**: 1008–13.
9. Chute CG, Greenberg ER, Baron J et al, Presenting conditions of 1539 population-based lung cancer patients by cell type and stage in New Hampshire and Vermont. *Cancer* 1985; **56**: 2107–11.
10. Marino C, Zoppi M, Morelli F et al, Pain in early cancer of the lungs. *Pain* 1986; **27**: 57–62.
11. Arcasoy SM, Jett JR, Current concepts: superior pulmonary sulcus tumors and Pancoast's syndrome. *N Engl J Med* 1997; **337**: 1370–6.
12. Kauner RM, Martini N, Foley KM, Incidence of pain and other clinical manifestations of superior pulmonary sulcus (Pancoast) tumors. In: *Advances in Pain Research Research and Therapy*, Vol 4 (Bonica JJ, Ventafridda V, Pagni CA, eds). Raven Press: New York, 1982: 27–39.
13. Komaki R, Roh J, Cox JD et al, Superior sulcus tumors: results of irradiation of 36 patients. *Cancer* 1981; **48**: 1563–8.
14. Fuller DB, Chambers JS, Superior sulcus tumors: combined modality. *Ann Thorac Surg* 1994; **57**: 1113–19.
15. Anderson TM, Moy PM, Holmes EC, Factors affecting survival in superior sulcus tumors. *J Clin Oncol* 1986; **4**: 1598–603.

16. Tattersall M, Pleural effusions. *Curr Opin Oncol* 1992; **42**: 642–6.
17. Decker DA, Dines DE, Payne WS et al, The significance of a cytologically negative pleural effusion in bronchogenic carcinoma. *Chest* 1978; **74**: 640–2.
18. Salyer WR, Eggleston JC, Erozan YS, Efficacy of pleural needle biopsy and pleural fluid cytopathology in the diagnosis of malignant neoplasm invading the pleura. *Chest* 1975; **67**: 536–9.
19. Livingston RB, McCracken JD, Trauth CJ et al, Isolated pleural effusion in small cell lung carcinoma: favorable prognosis. A review of the Southwest Oncology Group experience. *Chest* 1982; **81**: 208–11.
20. Anderson CB, Philpott GW, Ferguson TB, The treatment of malignant pleural effusions. *Cancer* 1974; **33**: 916–22.
21. Parker LA, Charnock GC, Delany DJ, Small bore catheter drainage and sclerotherapy for malignant pleural effusions. *Cancer* 1989; **64**: 1218–21.
22. Patz EF, Malignant pleural effusions. Recent advances and ambulatory sclerotherapy. *Chest* 1998; **113**: 74S–7S.
23. Aelony Y, King R, Bautin C, Thorascopic talc poudrage for chronic recurrent pleural effusion. *Ann Intern Med* 1991; **115**: 778–82.
24. Hausheer FH, Yarbo JW, Diagnosis and treatment of malignant pleural effusion. *Semin Oncol* 1985; **12**: 54–75.
25. De Camp M, Mentzer SJ, Swanson SJ et al, Malignant effusive disease of the pleura and pericardium. *Chest* 1997; **112**: 291S–5S.
26. Neito AF, Doty DB, Superior vena cava obstruction: clinical syndrome, etiology, and treatment. *Curr Probl Cancer* 1986; **20**: 443–84.
27. Ahmann FR, A reassessment of the clinical implications of the superior vena cava syndrome. *J Clin Oncol* 1984; **2**: 961–9.
28. Sculier JP, Evans WK, Feld R et al, Superior vena cava obstruction syndrome in small cell lung cancer. *Cancer* 1986; **57**: 847–51.
29. Yahalom J, Superior vena cava syndrome. In: *Cancer: Principles and Practice of Oncology*, 5th edn (DeVita VT, Hellman S, Rosenberg SA, eds). Lippincott-Raven: Philadelphia, 1997: 2469–76.
30. Maddox AM, Valdivesio M, Lukeman J et al, Superior vena cava obstruction in small-cell bronchogenic carcinoma. *Cancer* 1983; **52**: 2165–72.
31. Rodriguez CI, Njo KH, Karim ABMF, Hypofractionated radiation therapy in the treatment of superior vena cava syndrome. *Lung Cancer* 1993; **10**: 221–8.
32. Nesbitt JC, Surgical management of superior vena cava syndrome. In: *Lung Cancer: Principles and Practice* (Pass HI, Mitchell JB, Johnson DH, Turrisi AT, eds). Lippincott-Raven: Philadelphia, 1996: 671–81.
33. Press OW, Livingston R, Management of malignant pericardial effusion and tamponade. *JAMA* 1988; **255**: 1088–93.
34. Haskell RJ, French WJ, Cardiac tamponade as the initial presentation of malignancy. *Chest* 1985; **88**: 70–3.
35. Zwischenberger JB, Bradford DW, Management of malignant pericardial effusion. In: *Lung Cancer: Principles and Practice* (Pass HI, Mitchell JB, Johnson DH, Turrisi AT, eds). Lippincott-Raven: Philadelphia, 1996: 655–62.
36. Alcan KE, Zabetakis PM, Marino ND et al, Management of acute cardiac tamponade by subxiphoid pericardiotomy. *JAMA* 1982; **247**: 1143–8.
37. Nugent JL, Bunn PA, Mathews MJ et al, CNS metastases in small cell bronchogenic carcinoma. *Cancer* 1979; **44**: 1885–93.
38. Hirsch FR, Paulson OB, Hansen HH et al, Intracranial metastases in small cell carcinoma of the lung and correlation of clinical and autopsy findings. *Cancer* 1982; **90**: 2433–7.
39. Sorensen JB, Hansen HH, Hansen M et al, Brain metastases in adenocarcinoma of the lung: frequency, risk groups, and prognosis. *J Clin Oncol* 1988; **6**: 1474–80.
40. Burt M, Wronski M, Arbit E et al, Resection of brain metastases from non-small cell lung carcinoma. *J Thorac Cardiovasc Surg* 1992; **103**: 399–411.
41. Patchell RA, Tibbs PA, Walsh JA et al, A randomized trial of surgery in the treatment of single metastases to the brain. *N Engl J Med* 1990; **322**: 494–500.

42. Noordijk EM, Vecht CJ, Haaxma-Reiche H et al, The choice of treatment of single brain metastases should be based on extracranial tumor activity and age. *Int J Radiat Oncol Biol Phys* 1994; **29**: 711–17.
43. Flickinger JC, Kondziolka D, Lunsford LD et al, A multi-institutional experience with stereotactic radiosurgery for solitary brain metastases. *Int J Radiat Oncol Biol Phys* 1994; **28**: 797–802.
44. Engenhart R, Kimming BN, Hover K-H et al, Long-term follow-up for brain metastases treated by percutaneous stereotactic single high-dose irradiation. *Cancer* 1993; **71**: 1353–61.
45. Auchter RM, Lamond JP, Alexander E III et al, A multiinstitutional outcome and prognostic factor analysis of radiosurgery for resectable single brain metastases. *Int J Radiat Oncol Biol Phys* 1996; **35**: 27–35.
46. Ellis R, Gregor A, The treatment of brain metastases from lung cancer. *Lung Cancer* 1998; **20**: 81–4.
47. Priestman TJ, Dunn J, Brada M et al, Final results of the Royal College of Radiologists trial comparing two different radiotherapy schedules in the treatment of cerebral metastases. *Clin Oncol* 1996; **8**: 308–15.
48. Kelly K, Bunn PA, Is it time to reevaluate our approach to the treatment of brain metastases in patients with non-small cell lung cancer? *Lung Cancer* 1998; **20**: 85–91.
49. Minotti V, Crino' L, Meacci ML et al, Chemotherapy with cisplatin and teniposide for cerebral metastases in non-small cell lung cancer. *Lung Cancer* 1998; **20**: 93–8.
50. Cotto C, Cerille J, Souquet PJ et al, A phase II trial of fotemustine and cisplatin in central nervous system metastases from non-small cell lung cancer. *Eur J Cancer* 1996; **32**: 69–71.
51. Reboul F, Vincent P, Brewer Y et al, Chemotherapy for brain metastases of lung origin. Results of a phase II study. *Proc Am Soc Clin Oncol* 1996; **15**: 373–5 (Abst 1106).
52. Furuse K, Kamimori T, Kawahara M, A pilot study of concurrent whole-brain radiotherapy and chemotherapy combined with cisplatin, vindesine and mitomycin in non-small cell lung cancer with brain metastasis. *Br J Cancer* 1997; **75**: 614–18.
53. Bach F, Larsen BH, Rohode K et al, Metastatic spinal cord compression. Occurrence, symptoms, clinical presentations and prognosis in 398 patients with spinal cord compression. *Acta Neurochir* 1990; **107**: 37–43.
54. Bach F, Agerlin N, Sorensen JB, Metastatic spinal cord compression secondary to lung cancer. *J Clin Oncol* 1992; **10**: 1781–7.
55. Maranzano E, Latini P, Effectiveness or radiation therapy without surgery in metastatic spinal cord compression: final results from a prospective trial. *Int J Radiat Oncol Biol Phys* 1995; **32**: 959–67.
56. Young RF, Post EM, King GA, Treatment of spinal epidural metastases. Randomized prospective comparison of laminectomy and radiotherapy. *J Neurosurg* 1980; **53**: 741–8.
57. Sorensen S, Helweg-Larsen S, Mouridsen H et al, Effect of high-dose dexamethasone in carcinomatous metastatic spinal cord compression treated with radiotherapy: A randomized trial. *Eur J Cancer* 1994; **1**: 22–7.
58. Maranzano E, Latini P, Beneventi S et al, Radiotherapy without steroids in selected metastatic spinal cord compression patients. A phase II trial. *Am J Clin Oncol* 1996; **19**: 179–83.
59. Loblaw A, Laperriere NJ, Emergency treatment of malignant extradural spinal cord compression: an evidence-based guideline. *J Clin Oncol* 1998; **16**: 1613–24.
60. List AF, Hainsworth JD, Davis BW et al, The syndrome of inappropriate secretion of antidiuretic hormone (SIADH) in small cell lung cancer. *J Clin Oncol* 1986; **4**: 1191–8.
61. Orth DN, Medical progress: Cushing's syndrome. *N Engl J Med* 1995; **332**: 791–803.
62. Sheperd F, Laskey J, Evans W et al, Cushing's syndrome associated with ectopic corticotrophin production and small cell lung cancer. *J Clin Oncol* 1992; **10**: 21–7.
63. Kaye TB, Crapo L, The Cushing's syndrome: an update on diagnostic tests. *Ann Intern Med* 1990; **112**: 434–44.

64. Hoffman D, Brigham B, The use of ketoconazole in ectopic adrenocorticotrophic hormone syndrome. *Cancer* 1991; **67**: 1447–9.
65. Bydayt AA, Nissenson RA, Klein RF et al, Increased serum levels of parathyroid hormone-like protein malignancy-associated hypercalcemia. *Ann Intern Med* 1989; **111**: 807–12.
66. Bender RA, Hansen H, Hypercalcemia in bronchogenic carcinoma. *Ann Intern Med* 1974; **80**: 205–12.
67. Ralston SH, Gallacher SJ, Patel U et al, Cancer-associated hypercalcemia: morbidity and mortality. *Ann Intern Med* 1990; **112**: 499–504.
68. Body JJ, Medical treatment of tumor-induced hypercalcemia and tumor-induced osteolysis: challenges for future research. *Support Care Cancer* 1993; **1**: 26–33.
69. Kornguth S, Neuronal proteins and paraneoplastic syndromes. *N Engl J Med* 1989; **321**: 1607–8.
70. Szabo A, Dalman J, Manley G et al, HuD: a paraneoplastic encephalomyelitis antigen, contains RNA-binding domains and is homologous to Elav and sex-lethal. *Cell* 1991; **67**: 325–33.
71. Lambert EH, Lennon VA, Selected IgG rapidly induces Lambert–Eaton myasthenic syndrome in mice: complement independence and EMG abnormalities. *Muscle Nerve* 1988; **11**: 1133–6.
72. McEvoy KM, Windebank AJ, Daube JR et al, 3,4 Diaminopyridine in the treatment of Lambert–Eaton myasthenic syndrome. *N Engl J Med* 1989; **321**: 1567–71.
73. Graus F, Elkan KB, Cordon-Cardo C et al, Sensory neuropathy and small cell lung cancer. *Am J Med* 1986; **80**: 45–7.
74. Patel AM, Davile DG, Peters SG, Paraneoplastic syndrome associated with lung cancer. *Mayo Clin Proc* 1993; **68**: 278–81.
75. Lennon VA, Sas DF, Busk MF et al, Enteric neuronal autoantibodies in pseudo-obstruction with small cell lung carcinoma. *Gastroenterology* 1991; **100**: 137–40.
76. Hansen-Flaschen J, Nordberg J, Clubbing and hypertrophic osteoarthropathy. *Clin Chest Med* 1987; **8**: 287–94.
77. Nordstrom M, Lindblad B, Anderson H et al, Deep venous thrombosis and occult malignancy: an epidemiological study. *BMJ* 1994; **308**: 891–4.
78. Prandoni P, Lensin AWA, Buller HR et al, Deep-vein thrombosis and the incidence of subsequent symptomatic cancer. *N Engl J Med* 1992; **327**: 1128–33.
79. Coon WW, Risk factors in pulmonary embolism. *Surg Gynecol Obstet* 1976; **143**: 385–8.
80. Gore JM, Appelbaum JS, Greene HL et al, Occult cancer in patients with acute pulmonary embolism. *Ann Intern Med* 1982; **96**: 556–61.
81. Mac Donald RA, Robbins SL, The significance of nonbacterial thrombotic endocarditis: an autopsy and clinical study of 78 cases. *Ann Intern Med* 1957; **46**: 255–9.
82. Graus F, Rogers LR, Posner JB, Cardiovascular complications in patients with cancer. *Medicine* 1985; **64**: 16–35.
83. Goldhaber SZ, Dricker E, Buring JE et al, Clinical suspicion of autopsy-proven thrombotic and tumor pulmonary embolism in cancer patients. *Am J Heart* 1987; **114**: 1432–5.

16 Quality of life and supportive care

Jean-Paul Sculier, Isabelle Mancini, Marianne Paesmans, Jean Klastersky

Contents

INTRODUCTION

During the last decade, there has been great interest in the well-being of patients, especially among oncologists. Quality-of-life (QoL) assessment is a way to obtain objective data in order to 'measure' a patient's condition and to evaluate the global impact of therapies administered to improve his or her situation. Unfortunately, there are considerable methodological difficulties in designing adequate universal instruments for comprehensive measurement of QoL. Most of the investigations performed so far in this field have in fact assessed the symptoms in a semiquantitative way.

Specific anticancer treatment is in many situations the obvious way to control the disease and thus to improve the patient's condition but it can be associated with side-effects and complications; it may act with some delay or may not always be applicable or effective. The purpose of supportive care is to manage the problems for which anticancer therapy is often not effective or sufficient. The field covered by supportive care is very large, ranging from critical care to terminal care, and includes management of complications, symptomatic treatment, psychosocial support and palliative care.

In this chapter, we shall first review QoL assessment of lung cancer patients, with an analysis of the published data, indications and principles of critical care in oncology, management of the most common symptoms related to bronchial neoplasms (dyspnoea and pain) and treatment of the usual complications of anticancer treatment (emesis and febrile neutropenia).

QUALITY-OF-LIFE ASSESSMENT

Since the mid-1980s, increasing attention has been paid to QoL evaluation in oncology and for lung cancer patients in particular. Progress in improving survival (the traditional endpoint for phase III clinical trials) for small cell lung cancer (SCLC) as well as for unresectable non-small cell lung cancer (NSCLC) has been disappointing, justifying the need to pay more attention to the identification of less toxic treatments, achieving optimal palliation of symptoms and improving the overall QoL of patients. QoL assessments are especially appealing for patients with advanced NSCLC: although the survival benefit obtained with cisplatin-based chemotherapy versus supportive care alone has been established by several meta-analyses, its magnitude is not very large, and some clinicians are still reluctant to propose chemotherapy to their patients, arguing that the benefits do not counterbalance the side-effects of the treatment. Since QoL was not assessed in most of the trials incorporated in these meta-analyses, the controversy remains open. It is important to know whether chemotherapy is detrimental or beneficial to the QoL of these patients. However, incorporating QoL assessment in clinical research presents several strong theoretical and practical problems, which explain why, up to now, only a few randomized trials have addressed QoL issues.

The first of the problems consists in defining 'quality of life'. While there is a clear consensus on the multidimensional aspects of the concept, there is no universal agreement on the dimensions to be included. In medical research, most often, there is a restriction of the concept to the dimensions directly related to the disease, its symptoms and its treatment, and we shall deal here with a health-related QoL, with frequent inclusion of the following dimensions: physical function, occupational function, psychological or emotional function, and social function.

Once a definition has been adopted, a second difficulty lies in determining how to measure QoL, taking into account that the assessment has to be made by the patient (owing to its subjective nature, physicians, nurses or other people involved in patient care are poor raters of QoL), and it has to be reproducible (an unchanged measure has to be obtained when the patient's condition is stable) and sensible (able to capture any change in the patient's condition). Much research has been successfully devoted to the development of general as well as disease-specific instruments, and various validated questionnaires to measure QoL have become available. Among those that have been tested for lung cancer patients, the following have been found in a recent review to be the most popular:[1]

- the European Organization for Research and Treatment of Cancer (EORTC) Quality of Life Questionnaire, including a core (QLQ C30) and a lung cancer module assessing disease-specific symptoms and toxicities (QLQ LC13);
- the Rotterdam Symptom Check List (RSCL);
- the Functional Living Index–Cancer (FLIC);
- the Hospital Anxiety and Depression Scale (HADS);
- the Daily Diary Card (DDC).

There were three lung-cancer-dedicated measures:[2]

- the already-mentioned EORTC QLQ LC13;
- the Lung Cancer Symptom Scale (LCSS);
- the Functional Assessment of Cancer Therapy–Lung (FACT-L).

The properties of these instruments have been compared with those of the first measure, to be introduced (in 1949), the Karnofsky performance index, which takes physical function into account and is recognized to provide too limited an assessment of QoL. However, it is strongly correlated with global QoL, with a clear worsening in performance status when the lung-cancer-related symptoms increase in number and/or in intensity and a possible decrease of the index in the case of psychiatric disorders.

Finally but not least importantly, the analysis of QoL data is difficult for several reasons. Indeed, QoL assessment generates a huge amount of data owing to its multifactorial definition and to the need to study it longitudinally: a baseline measurement is required, since each patient is his or her own control, and this must be followed by repeated measures at times depending on the disease and the treatment. Therefore classical statistical techniques lead to multiple testing and to high probabilities of getting false-positive comparisons. Possible solutions are to adjust significance probabilities as proposed by Bonferroni and/or to reduce the data by calculating summary parameters and global test statistics (O'Brien's approach). This results in loss of information and to effects going in opposite directions being undetected, and requires analysis of variance models for repeated measures, adjustment of the data with chronological series allowing autocorrelated stochastic processes, and/or analysis of survival times adjusted for QoL. The application of these models is complicated by an important, not completely solved problem, namely the missing data, which cannot be assumed to be missing at random (deteriorating patients being, for instance, less compliant than other patients) – an assumption underlying most of the statistical models. This difficulty is particularly crucial in advanced NSCLC patients, a non-negligible proportion of whom die during anticancer treatment. Patient compliance can be improved by carefully monitoring the study and by having specialized research personnel taking care of the QoL data collection. However, censoring of information will persist and, although some methods for analysing longitudinal data with an informative drop-out process have already been proposed, the most important progress in QoL research methodology will probably come from further developments in this area.

Therefore, as already mentioned and despite its recognized value as a tool to assess new treatment approaches, QoL is not a frequently studied outcome in published randomized clinical trials. It is often assessed in only a subgroup of patients, and is almost never used as a primary endpoint. It has been used more often as a way to characterize lung cancer at presentation or as a prognostic factor for tumour response to therapy or for survival.

In SCLC, fatigue and malaise have been shown as QoL indicators,[3] and QoL has been considered as an endpoint for testing conventional chemotherapy against less-intensive palliative chemotherapy or against intensive chemotherapy. In the first type of trials, if no survival disadvantage was demonstrated using the palliative option, QoL was shown to be improved with conventional therapy together with a better tumour response and improvement in palliation of the symptoms. In the latter group of trials, however, it was suggested that pursuing the treatment results in worsening of QoL.

In patients with NSCLC treated by surgery, no real QoL assessment has been made. In inoperable disease, aggressive radiotherapy was shown to result in a slightly improved survival, but was similar with regard to side-effects and in achieving relief of symptoms, with QoL being assessed using RSCLC and HADS.[4] In a large randomized trial comparing a 2-fraction palliative thoracic radiotherapy against a 13-fraction schedule in more than 500 patients,[5] the same group, using HADS, RSCLC and daily diary cards, concluded that there was better survival in the hyperfractionated regimen, together with less psychological distress, but with more dysphagia and slower palliation of symptoms. Testing adjuvant chemotherapy combined with thoracic irradiation versus radiotherapy alone, a meta-analysis has shown survival improvement with the use of cisplatin-based chemotherapy regimens, but no conclusion about QoL can be drawn from the studies incorporated in the aggregation. However, in an English trial testing the addition of an MIC (mitomycin C, ifosfamide and cisplatin) chemotherapy to radiotherapy in more than 400 patients, survival was improved together with QoL with better palliation of symptoms in the chemotherapy arm.[6] The impact of chemotherapy on QoL was assessed by the Cancer and Leukemia Group B, comparing chemotherapy with cisplatin and vinblastine and with hydrazine sulfate versus placebo in 291 patients with advanced NSCLC. The QoL component of the trial was reported[7] in a paper illustrating the methodological difficulties encountered with that particular endpoint. The instruments were the EORTC questionnaire and the Duke–UNC social support scale. With no survival difference between the two arms, QoL was improved at two months in the hydrazine group (a better EORTC total score, but also improvements in physical functioning, fatigue and lung-cancer-specific subscales), but the difference did not persist in the later assessments (months 4 and 6). In metastatic disease, it is now established that cisplatin-based chemotherapy improves survival slightly compared with the best supportive care. One of the trials included in the meta-analyses[8] incorporated QoL as an endpoint in the trial design, using the FLIC questionnaire. However, difficulties in collecting the QoL data were encountered, with high missing rates even at the baseline assessment (13%), preventing the authors from estimating a treatment effect on QoL. They confirmed the positive correlation between Karnofsky performance index and FLIC scores. More recent studies tested QoL in chemotherapy-treated patients with a MIC regimen,[6] with single-agent gemcitabine[9] or with carboplatin combined with etoposide.[10] The results all tend in the same direction, leading to the conclusion that global QoL scores are increased by chemotherapy together with improved symptomatic palliation, providing valuable information for the evaluation of the role of chemotherapy for metastatic NSCLC.

CRITICAL CARE OF THE LUNG CANCER PATIENT

Intensive care is becoming more and more important in the management of cancer patients and major cancer hospitals have developed intensive care units (ICUs) not only for surgical patients but also for medical patients. However, there is limited information in the medical literature about intensive care in oncology, especially concerning the description of the types of patients admitted to such units. An international inquiry performed in anticancer centres[11] has shown that 70% of cancer hospitals have at least one ICU especially devoted to patients with neoplastic diseases. Whether general, surgical or medical, these units do not depart from the recommended guidelines for intensive care, in so far as the number of beds, the nursing staff and the main critical care techniques performed are concerned.

Admission of patients to an ICU is usually based on the following three principles.[12] First, the patients have to be 'salvageable': patients whose chances of being cured or having their disease put into remission are minimal should not be admitted or should not stay in an ICU. Secondly, the patient's 'autonomy' must be respected: a patient who refuses intensive supportive therapy because he or she understands the potential poor prognosis of the underlying cancer should not be admitted to the ICU. Finally, since medical resources are limited, even in highly developed countries, 'distributive justice' should be taken into account: patients with the best chances of benefiting from intensive therapy should be admitted as a priority.

The assumption that patients with active malignant disease should not be admitted to an ICU often predominates in general hospitals, and causes problems in the management of critically ill cancer patients. This negative opinion is not supported by scientific data. It results from the bias of many physicians, who refuse critical care to cancer patients although they are willing to provide it to patients with serious non-neoplastic diseases such as advanced heart failure or liver cirrhosis who have no better short- and long-term prognoses.[13]

There are four main reasons to admit a cancer patient to the ICU:

1. This allows postoperative recovery with facilities as for any high-risk postoperative patient (availability of continuous haemodynamic monitoring, early identification of

cardiovascular and respiratory disturbances, facilities for respiratory support, and constant skilled nursing care).

2. The critical complications of the cancer and its treatment are very numerous, and can be very specific to oncology. Their management must always take into consideration the presence of a severe chronic underlying disease.
3. It is possible to administer treatment with strict monitoring and control. This is important in a number of situations, for example when there is an increased risk related to the patient's condition, when intensive chemotherapy requiring patient monitoring must be given, when it might be necessary to treat unknown toxicity arising in a phase I trial (when optimal conditions of surveillance are required for safety), or when treatment is given that is known to result frequently in severe acute toxicity.
4. Disease (such as myocardial infarction or severe asthma), possibly unrelated to the neoplastic disease or its treatment, might be present and require treatment.

Data specific to the critical care of lung cancer patients are very limited, and are usually devoted to airways and respiratory complications. A small series concerning artificial ventilation[14] in non-surgical patients has indicated poor prognosis for the lung cancer patients when it is applied because of respiratory failure due to the neoplastic disease itself in situations where no effective anticancer therapy is available. Respiratory distress can also be due to obstruction of the major airways by tumours involving the tracheobronchial tree. Since conventional treatments such as radiation therapy and/or chemotherapy will often be too slow to reopen the airway, endoscopic laser therapy should be used without delay, and might allow a very rapid relief of dyspnoea.[15] Another life-threatening emergency is massive haemoptysis, the etiology that must be identified rapidly in order to provide appropriate treatment such as surgery, endobronchial laser therapy or bronchial artery embolization. More information about the critical care of cancer patients can be obtained in specific reviews.[16]

MANAGEMENT OF SYMPTOMS

The signs and symptoms manifested by patients with lung cancer depend on the localization of the tumour, its locoregional spread and the effects of metastatic growth. Dyspnoea, pain and cough are common symptoms of lung cancer patients, with frequencies of 59%, 48% and 71% respectively.[17]

Pain

Direct tumour involvement is the most common cause of pain. In approximately two-thirds of patients, it explains the pain from metastatic cancer.[18] Bone destruction (direct or metastatic) is the cause in about 50% of cases. Pain in the remaining 50% is due to nerve compression or infiltration of soft tissue. Depending on the localization of the primary tumour, adjacent structures such as the chest wall and mediastinum may be involved by direct spread, resulting in radicular chest wall pain. In apical tumours, the classic Pancoast's syndrome (lower brachial plexopathy, Horner's syndrome and shoulder pain) occurs because of local invasion of the lower brachial plexus (T1 and C8 nerve roots), chest wall and stellate ganglion. Pleural invasion may cause pleural effusion and pleuritic pain. Non-specific and vague chest pains, generally referred to the ipsilateral hemithorax, are frequent in patients with lung cancer. This type of pain is visceral and is unrelated to invasion of local structures. Persistent post-therapy pain from long-term effects of surgery, radiotherapy and chemotherapy accounts for an additional 20% of patients who report pain with metastatic cancer. A small residual group experiences pain from non-cancer-related causes. A clear understanding of the characteristics of the pain and its pathophysiological basis for proper management is paramount.

Communication about pain is greatly aided by using a scale allowing the patient to report it. A simple rating scale ranges from 0 to 10, with 0 being 'no pain' and 10 being 'pain as bad as you can imagine'.This pain severity scale may be very helpful in titrating analgesics and in monitoring pain increase with progressive disease. Description by the patient of the area of pain on a drawing of a human figure may aid diagnosis. Careful questioning concerning the characteristics of the pain is essential. In addition to severity, these characteristics include the temporal pattern of the pain (constant or episodic) and its quality. Episodic or incident pain is much more difficult to control than continuous pain.[19] The physical examination of the patient includes the examination of the painful areas as well as neurological and orthopaedic assessments. Since bone metastases are common in lung cancer, bone scans and radiographs may be helpful. Computed tomographic (CT) scanning is useful in the evaluation of the spine, the base of the skull, and the retroperitoneal, paravertebral and pelvic areas. Identification of a treatable neoplastic lesion as the responsible factor for pain will call for radiotherapy (for example in cases of Pancoast's syndrome, chest wall involvement or bone metastases), chemotherapy or, in rare instances, surgical debulking.

There is a growing consensus concerning the types of analgesic drugs to use, their routes of administration and their optimal schedule.[18] The first step is the choice of the type of analgesic drug (non-opioid, opioid or a combination). The second step is the choice of adjuvant drugs, which can increase the analgesic effectiveness and can produce other palliative effects to counter the disruptive consequences of pain. Non-steroidal antiinflammatory drugs (NSAIDs) represent the majority of non-opioid analgesics. Their effect on the inflammatory process is a key to their analgesic property. The NSAIDs seem to exert their analgesic, antipyretic and antiinflammatory actions by blocking the synthesis of prostaglandins. Because of their different mechanisms of action and toxicity profiles, the NSAIDs and opioids are often administered together. NSAIDs have a number of serious side-effects, such as gastritis and gastrointestinal haemorrhage, bleeding due to platelet inhibition, and renal failure.

Opioid analgesics should be prescribed as soon as there is evidence that pain is not well controlled with non-opioid analgesics. Except in a minority of patients whose pain is clearly episodic, analgesics should be given around the clock, with the time interval based on the duration of effectiveness of the drug and on the patient's report of the duration of effectiveness. The so-called weak opioids, including codeine and oxycodone, usually formulated in combination with paracetamol (acetaminophen) or aspirin, can provide active patients with good pain relief for long periods. Oral morphine, either in immediate- or sustained-release preparation, is the analgesic of choice for moderate-to-severe cancer pain. A typical starting dose of immediate-release oral morphine is 10–30 mg every 4 hours in patients not previously taking opioids. The starting dose may not be sufficient, and relatively rapid upward titration may be needed, especially if pain is severe. When an effective dose of short-acting morphine has been established, the required dose for a long-acting preparation can be calculated. An additional supply of short-acting morphine, given when necessary, will help the patient to manage breakthrough pain. Consistent need for this additional morphine will dictate an upward adjustment of the dose of sustained-release drug. Appoximately 70% of patients will benefit from the use of an alternative route of opioid administration, which may be intravenous or subcutaneous, rectal or transdermal. As adjuvant drugs, tricyclic antidepressants have been found to be useful in a variety of neuropathic pain syndromes, especially when pain has a prominent dysaesthetic or burning character. Carbamazepine, phenytoin, valproate and clonazepam, alone or in combination with the tricyclic antidepressants, have been used successfully to treat neuropathic pain. Controlled studies suggest that the administration of corticosteroids to selected patients with advanced cancer results in decreased pain and improved appetite and activity. Unfortunately, the duration of their effects is short. The mechanism by which corticosteroids appear to produce beneficial symptom effects in patients with terminal cancer is unclear, but may involve their euphoriant effect or the inhibition of prostaglandin metabolism.

Dyspnoea

Dyspnoea or breathlessness is defined as an uncomfortable awareness of breathing. This symptom is actually complex, including physiological, psychological and social components, and is perceived as one of the most devastating symptoms by the patient and family. Its major physical evidence is tachypnoea.

The etiology of dyspnoea may be related to the primary or metastatic disease, or to cancer treatment, or it may be unrelated to the underlying disease (Table 16.1).[20] In lung cancer patients, the most common cause of dyspnoea is the cancer itself. The cause can be easily determined in most patients by an adequate history and physical examination. Chest radiography, digital oximetry and simple blood tests will rule out a significant number of causes of dyspnoea. Pulmonary function tests can be particularly

Table 16.1 Causes of dyspnoea in cancer patients

Direct effects of the tumour
- Primary and/or metastatic tumour
- Pleural/pericardial effusion
- Superior vena cava syndrome
- Carcinomatous lymphangitis
- Atelectasis
- Phrenic nerve palsy
- Tracheal obstruction or tracheo-oesophageal fistula
- Carcinomatous infiltration of the chest wall

Effects of therapy
- Postradiation fibrosis
- Postpneumectomy
- Bleomycin-induced fibrosis
- Doxorubicin (Adriamycin)- and cyclophosphamide-induced cardiomyopathy

Not directly due to the tumour or therapy
- Anaemia
- Cachexia
- Ascites
- Metabolic acidosis
- Muscle weakness/myasthenia/Eaton–Lambert syndrome
- Rib fracture
- Fever
- Chest wall deformity
- Chronic obstructive pulmonary disease
- Asthma
- Pulmonary embolism
- Heart failure
- Neuromuscular disease
- Obesity
- Pneumonia
- Pneumothorax
- Thyrotoxicosis
- Psychosocial distress

useful in the assessment of obstructive and restrictive pulmonary disorders.

In palliative care, it may be less important to discover the etiology than to make an appropriate assessment. The literature gives some useful tools, including the Linear Analogue Scale Assessment (LASA), the Borg Category Scale (which is only a 'verbal analogue' of the LASA scale), the Modified Medical Research Council Dyspnoea Scale (MMRCDS) or the Oxygen-Cost Diagram. The LASA is a horizontal or vertical line anchored with terms that characterize two extremes of a possible subjective status, such as 'no breathlessness' and 'worst possible breathlessness'. Individuals are asked to mark the portion of the line that best reflects the intensity of dyspnoea at a given time. The Borg Category Scale is a vertical scale labelled from 0 to 10, with corresponding verbal expression of progressively increasing sensation intensity, such as 'nothing at all' to 'maximal'. The MMRCDS is a four-point questionnaire that asks patients to assess their dyspnoea according to the limitations they are experiencing secondary to shortness of breath, from 'Not troubled with breathlessness except with strenuous exercise' to 'Too breathless to leave the house or breathless when dressing or undressing'. The Oxygen-Cost Diagram is a vertical visual analogue scale measuring 100 mm ('no breathlessness' to 'the greatest breathlessness'), with descriptive phrases of everyday activities (from sleeping to brisk walking uphill) that may cause shortness of breath.

With a thorough assessment of dyspnoea, including the patient's general assessment of his or her activities of daily living secondary to dyspnoea, and lastly the presence of concurrent other symptoms, an appropriate management regimen for this symptom can be approached. Management of dyspnoea in the cancer patient is often complex and difficult.[21] The first aim should be to correct the cause when possible and if appropriate. Examples are tapping pleural fluid, treating infections with antibiotics, treating the tumour with chemotherapy and radiotherapy, giving steroids to decrease inflammation and oedema, and correcting anaemia with blood transfusions. Environmental issues are essential in the management of dyspnoea. A calm atmosphere with a quiet setting often helps patients to prevent or reduce the anxiety that is associated with dyspnoea. A cool fan, or cool air blowing directly on the patient, can decrease the perception of dyspnoea. Paramedical interventions, including relaxation and breathing techniques, can often break the vicious cycle of shortness of breath and anxiety.

The use of oxygen is beneficial in providing subjective improvement of the symptoms of dyspnoea.[22] Opioids are very useful in its management by decreasing the perception of breathlessness. If an opioid is already prescribed for pain, the dose needs to be titrated to relieve dyspnoea. If the patient is opioid-naive, the advised starting morphine dose is 10 mg orally or 5 mg subcutaneously every 4 hours around the clock, and 5 mg orally or 2.5 mg subcutaneously every hour as required. More recently, nebulized opioids have been used. It is unclear whether or how nebulized opioids work, but it seems that they act peripherally, on receptors in lung tissue. Bronchodilators are useful when an obstructive component is present. Steroids used for the treatment of oedema and inflammation surrounding obstructive lesions can be very beneficial to open up airways, and can temporarily remove the cause of dyspnoea. Steroids are also important for the treatment of lymphangitic disease in patients with metastatic cancer. Hyoscine (scopolamine) or atropine given, for example, by subcutaneous injections, can be beneficial in drying up upper airway secretions. Lastly, benzodiazepines may be useful for intractable dyspnoea or when an anxious component is obvious.

Cough

Cough is a common symptom in lung cancer patients.[23] An incidence of 70–90% has been reported. A primary lung tumour or lung metastases may stimulate the cough reflex by impinging on irritant receptors. Radiation- or chemotherapy-induced fibrosis must also be considered when evaluating the cause of cough in these patients.

The other common causes of chronic cough include respiratory infections, postnasal drip, asthma, gastro-oesophageal reflux and chronic bronchitis. The control of cough is important, since it can lead to other problems, such as sleep disturbance, shortness of breath and pain. The usual treatment of cough aims at identifying the underlying cause and then choosing the appropriate therapy. The specific pharmacological approach for untractable cough includes the use of opioids such as morphine or hydromorphone acting centrally via opioid receptors, the use of nebulized cromoglycate disodium (two puffs every 4 hours) or a nebulized anaesthetic working essentially on small unmyelinated C-fibres by reducing sodium conductance in the plasma membrane of neurons (for example nebulized lignocaine (lidocaine) 40 mg every 4 hours). There are also reports on the use of lignocaine as an intravenous cough suppressant, with doses ranging from 0.3 to1.5 mg/kg. This route appears to be more effective but not as convenient as nebulization in the treatment of cough in patients with advanced cancer.

MANAGEMENT OF TREATMENT COMPLICATIONS

Infections

Infections in patients with lung cancer are extremely common, although no precise data are available. It has been demonstrated that infections under these circumstances are associated with a shortening of survival. This underlines the need for diagnosis, prevention and treatment of these complications.[24]

First, infection can be seen as part of the natural history of lung cancer. The tumour is often responsible for obstruction, aspiration, lung abcesses and nosocomial pneumonias. Once again, there is very little specific information about the incidence and consequences of these infections. Also, very little is known about the pathogens involved. Nevertheless, it is clear that common respiratory pathogens are often to blame, especially pneumococci. In our own studies, we have found lung cancer and chronic lymphocytic leukaemia to be the two most common underlying diseases associated with pneumococcal bacteraemia.

On the other hand, infection can be the consequence of the chemotherapy received by lung cancer patients. Most of these chemotherapeutic treatments cause neutropenia, and it has long been known that granulocytopenia increases the rate of bacterial infection.

Twenty years ago, most of the infections complicating neutropenia were caused by Gram-negative pathogens; today, there is a predominance of Gram-positive microorganisms as a cause of fever and infection in cancer patients. Most of these Gram-positive pathogens are coagulase-negative staphylococci, but streptococci and, in lung cancer patients, pneumococci are also very important.

Most of the chemotherapy regimens used in lung cancer patients cause short-lived neutropenia, which is complicated by infection in less than 10% of cases. Therefore there is little need for the use of growth factors or prophylactic antibiotics in patients treated with chemotherapy for lung cancer. However, there have been and will be attempts to intensify chemotherapy in lung cancer patients; under these circumstances, neutropenia becomes more common and more severe. In these patients, the frequency and types of infection associated with neutropenia are similar to those that complicate neutropenia in patients who receive more aggressive treatment, such as those with leukaemias or lymphomas.

The overall approach to the infection of patients with solid tumours under these circumstances is not different from that which has been well described in patients with haematological malignancies.

As already mentioned, chemoprophylaxis of infection in lung cancer patients is rarely necessary; nevertheless, there have been several studies showing that, in patients with SCLC treated with relatively aggressive chemotherapy, prophylactic treatment with co-trimoxazole could reduce the frequency of infection.

In any case, given the importance of pneumococci as pathogens in patients with lung cancer, prophylaxis or treatment of infection should provide adequate coverage for these pathogens. Vaccination against pneumocci might be another preventive measure for infections in lung cancer patients; unfortunately, as in other categories of cancer patients, antipneumococcal vaccinations have not been successful in lung cancer patients, presumably owing to the poor capacity of the patients to raise an adequate antibody response.

Nausea and vomiting

It was the development of cisplatin-based therapy for lung cancer patients that stimulated the search for adequate measures to control chemotherapy-induced nausea and vomiting.[25] The initial regimens that were able to control severe emesis caused by high-dose cisplatin chemotherapy consisted of high doses (2–4 mg/kg) of metoclopramide (a D2 dopamine receptor/5-HT_3 serotonin receptor antagonist) together with dexamethasone and lorazepam. That regimen, although complicated by a significant number of side-effects, such as extrapyramidal motor disturbances, proved to be highly effective in controlling nausea and vomiting in a majority in patients treated with a highly emetogenic therapy. Although their mechanism is still not fully understood, corticosteroids (dexamethasone or prednisone) definitely increase the anti-emetogenic effect of metoclopramide. The usefulness of the addition of lorazepam, acting perhaps through its anxiolytic and amnesia-causing effects, has also been clearly demonstrated. As well as the side-effects already mentioned, the major inconvenience of this triple-drug regimen was the neccessity of intravenous administration.

The introduction of the 'setrons' made antiemetic therapy in patients treated with cisplatin much easier. These drugs, which act as 5-HT_3 serotonin receptor antagonists, like high-dose metoclopramide, can control nausea and vomiting in most patients treated with highly emetogenic drugs. Once again, the addition of corticosteroids increases the effectiveness of all the setrons. The precise modality for their use is still not entirely clear. It seems that a single dose of these agents administered daily is sufficient; recently, it has been shown that 32 mg of ondansetron or 3 mg of granisetron, as a single administration, is highly effective in preventing nausea and vomiting in patients treated with highly emetogenic regimens. The exact dosage for these agents is not entirely known either; it is possible that a lower dosage can be as effective as that mentioned above.

Whether the anti-emetic combination should be repeated during the day following the administration of emetogenic therapy is also unclear. Most experts would recommend that it be repeated for two or three days, and, in the case of highly emetogenic therapy, that metoclopramide and corticosteroids be given orally for an extra few days, to prevent late emesis.

Another important consideration is the provision of effective anti-emetic treatment after the first course of chemotherapy, in order to avoid anticipatory nausea and vomiting, as a conditioned reflex, in the future. If anticipatory nausea and vomiting occur, psychotherapy and/or alprazolam might be effective.

REFERENCES

1. Montazeri A, Gillis CR, McEwen J, Quality of life in patients with lung cancer. A review of literature from 1970 to 1995. *Chest* 1998; **113**: 467–81.
2. Moinpour C, Measuring quality of life: an emerging science. *Semin Oncol* 1994; **21**: 48–63.
3. Hürny C, Bernhard J, Joss R et al, Fatigue and malaise as quality of life indicator in small cell lung cancer patients. *Support Care Cancer* 1993; **1**: 316–20.
4. Hopwood P, Stephens RJ, Quality of life assessment in a multicentre randomised clinical trial of two policies of radiotherapy in non small cell lung cancer. *Lung Cancer* 1994; **11**: S82–6.
5. Macbeth F, Bolger J, Hopwood P et al, Randomized trial of palliative two-fraction versus more intensive 13-fraction radiotherapy for patients with inoperable non small cell lung cancer and good performance status. *Clin Oncol* 1996; **8**: 167–75.
6. Billingham L, Cullen M, Woods J et al, Mitomycin, ifosfamide and cisplatin (MIC) in non-small cell lung cancer: results of a randomised trial evaluating palliation and quality of life. *Lung Cancer* 1997; **18**: S9.
7. Herdon J, Fleishman S, Kosty M, Green M, A longitudinal study of quality of life in advanced non small cell lung cancer: Cancer and Leukemia Group B (CALGB) 8931. *Controlled Clin Trials* 1997; **18**: 286–300.
8. Ganz P, Haskell M, Figlin R et al, For the UCLA Solid Tumour Study Group, Estimating the quality of life in a clinical trial of patients with metastatic lung cancer using the Karnofsky performance status and the functional living index–cancer. *Cancer* 1988; **61**: 849–56.
9. Anderson H, Cottier B, Nicolson M et al, On behalf of the Gemcitabine Study Group. *Lung Cancer* 1997; **18**: S9.
10. Helsing M, Bergman B, Chemotherapy with carboplatin and etoposide improves quality of life and survival in patients with advanced non small cell lung cancer. *Lung Cancer* 1997; **18**: S8.
11. Sculier JP, Markiewicz E, Intensive care in anticancer centers: an international inquiry. *Support Care Cancer* 1995; **3**: 130–4.
12. Chevrolet JCL, Jolliet Ph, An ethical look at intensive care for patients with malignancies. *Eur J Cancer* 1991; **27**: 210–12.
13. Wachter RM, Luce JM, Hearst N, Lo B, Decisions about resuscitation: inequities among patients with different diseases but similar prognoses. *Ann Intern Med* 1989; **111**: 525–32.
14. Ewer MS, Ali MK, Atta MS et al, Outcome of lung cancer patients requiring mechanical ventilation for pulmonary failure. *JAMA* 1986; **256**: 3364–6.
15. Dedhia HV, Le Roy N, Jain PR et al, Endoscopic laser therapy for respiratory distress due to obstructive airway tumours. *Crit Care Med* 1985; **13**: 464–7.
16. Sculier JP, Intensive care. In: *Handbook of Supportive Care in Cancer* (Klastersky J, Schimpff SC, Senn HJ, eds). Marcel Dekker: New York, 1995: 511–39.
17. Hollen PJ, Gralla RJ, Kris MG et al, Quality of life assessment in individuals with lung cancer: testing the Lung Cancer Symptom Scale. *Eur J Cancer* 1993; **29**: S51–8.
18. Cleeland CS, Bruera E, Pain and symptom management. In: *Manual of Clinical Oncology*, 6th edn (Love RR, ed). Springer-Verlag: New York, 1994: 556–69.
19. Mercadante S, Armata M, Salvaggio L, Pain characteristics of advanced cancer patients referred to a palliative care service. *Pain* 1994; **59**: 141–5.
20. Ripamonti C, Bruera E, Dyspnea: pathophysiology and assessment. *J Sympt Management* 1997; **13**: 220–32.
21. Farncombe M, Dyspnea: assessment and treatment. *Support Care Cancer* 1997; **5**: 94–9.
22. Bruera E, de Stoutz N, Velasco-Leiva A et al,

Effects of oxygen on dyspnoea in hypoxaemic terminal-cancer patients. *Lancet* 1993; **342**: 13–14.

23. Louie K, Bertolino M, Faisinger R, Management of intractable cough. *J Palliative Care* 1992; **8**: 46–8.
24. Klastersky J, Les complications infectieuses du cancer bronchique. *Rev Mal Respir* 1998; **15**: 451–9.
25. Tonato M, Roila F, Principles of supportive care: antiemetics. In: *Textbook of Medical Oncology* (Cavalli F, Hansen HH, Kaye SB). Martin Dunitz: London, 1997: 363–72.

17 Cost-effectiveness of lung cancer treatment

William K Evans, B Phyllis Will, Jean-Marie Berthelot

Contents Introduction • Types of economic evaluation • Methodological issues • Other considerations • Estimating costs of lung cancer care in Canada

INTRODUCTION

Lung cancer is the second most common cancer in men and women in North America and the leading cause of cancer death among both sexes in the industralized world. In North America, it was estimated that it was responsible for the deaths of over 200 000 individuals in 1997.[1,2] Lung cancer occurs mainly between the ages of 50 and 80 years, and there has been a marked increase in its incidence in women.[3] Worldwide, the problem of lung cancer is escalating as the peoples of the developing world succumb to the advertising of the tobacco industry. The resulting worldwide epidemic of lung cancer is a major public health concern, not only because of the enormous loss of life and the great morbidity caused by lung cancer, but also because of the large economic burden it places on health care systems and society in general.

It is estimated that expenditures on cancer care in the USA make up approximately 5% of the total direct health care expenditure in that country.[4] Studies by Brown and co-workers have estimated that the annual direct cancer care expenditure for diagnosis and treatment totalled US$27.4 billion in 1990.[5] Of these direct expenditures for cancer care, over 80% are attributable to just four cancers: breast US$6.6 billion, colorectal US$6.4 billion, lung US$5.1 billion and prostate US$4.7 billion. In the Canadian health care system, Statistics Canada estimated that approximately C$320 million (using 1988 Canadian dollars) was expended on the direct medical care costs of managing lung cancer patients diagnosed in 1988.[6,7] From these numbers, it can be easily appreciated that the cost of lung cancer will be high in those industrialized countries where there is a high incidence of lung cancer, widespread clinical expertise and adequate resources for aggressive clinical interventions. Extrapolated into the health care systems of developing countries, such large economic burdens could easily overwhelm the financial ability of a country to pay, or could result in failure to treat patients with this disease. Even in the so-called wealthy nations, fiscal constraint is increasingly causing physicians and health care administrators to critically examine the value of health care interventions and the efficiency of health care delivery systems.

This concern about the value for money expended is particularly relevant to the problem of lung cancer, where, despite some recent advances, the prognosis for the disease remains extremely grim.[3] New treatments for lung cancer are having a modest impact on the survival and quality of life of patients with inoperable lung cancer, particularly for those with locally advanced disease. However, the reputation of the disease as one with a very poor prognosis, coupled with the expense associated with the new treatment approaches, has created a barrier to the adoption of these new therapies. Economic evaluations of the old and new treatment interventions for lung cancer can shed light on their relative cost-effectiveness compared with other health care interventions. An understanding of the cost components of care can also help to inform health care providers on how to deliver treatments in the most efficient fashion. This chapter will describe some of the economic analyses that have been conducted on lung cancer management throughout the world, particularly in Canada. Although it is not possible to extrapolate health economic evaluations directly from one health care system to another easily, there are relevant lessons to be learned from a review of these studies.

Physicians have typically had little interest or training in health economics, and therefore may be relatively unaware of the types of health economic analyses that can be done and their application to the setting of lung cancer. Therefore, prior to presenting data from studies evaluating the economic burden of lung cancer, the cost components of lung cancer management and the cost-effectiveness of treatment, it is worthwhile first to provide some information on costing methodology and the types of economic evaluations that are commonly undertaken.

TYPES OF ECONOMIC EVALUATION

Economic evaluations provide a framework to systematically compare the cost and outcomes of alternative health care interventions.[8] In any economic evaluation, the alternatives must be clearly identified. In studies of lung cancer, it may be appropriate to explore the costs and outcome benefits of a 'do-nothing' or best supportive care (BSC) alternative compared with an intervention, such as chemotherapy for metastatic non-small cell lung cancer. For locally advanced disease, the comparison might be between standard radiotherapy and combined-modality therapy.

The perspective of the analysis will affect the range of costs and benefits included in the study and, ultimately, the conclusions of the evaluation. Ideally, economic evaluations should consider the cost and benefits to all sectors of society affected by the intervention. However, economic evaluations are often carried out from a specific perspective, such as that of the provider or the purchaser of the health care service. Even if the perspective is that of the health care system, this may ignore important costs to social service agencies or to family members, who may lose wages staying at home to provide care. Whatever the perspective, it should be explicitly stated, so that the reader of the study fully understands what is being described.

There are four principal types of economic evaluations (Table 17.1). Each involves a comparison of both the costs and consequences of alternative interventions. The main difference between each of these types of analysis is the method used to measure the consequence of the intervention.

Cost-minimization analysis

This type of economic evaluation assumes that the outcomes and effectiveness of the treatments are equal. The only significant difference between the options is the amount of resource used to obtain the outcome. Therefore the direct cost associated with each intervention is compared, and the least costly strategy is identified as the preferred choice. In such analyses, there is no need to assess the consequences of the treatment. Relatively few cost-minimization studies have been reported in the cancer literature.

Cost-effectiveness analysis

In such analyses, a comparison is made of outcomes that are different, as well as their cost.

Table 17.1 Types of economic analyses

Cost-minimization analysis	Compares strategies with equal outcomes to determine which is least expensive
Cost-effectiveness analysis	Compares ratios of the incremental cost over the incremental effectiveness of alternative strategies
Cost–utility analysis	Compares ratios of the incremental cost over the incremental utility. The utility is a measure of the value attributed to a health state – usually measured in quality-adjusted life-years (QALYs)
Cost–benefit analysis	Assigns monetary value to the health benefits of an intervention. If the cost–benefit ratio is less than 1, the intervention is attractive

The effectiveness of the alternatives is measured in natural units such as life-years gained, cases successfully treated or complications averted. These outcomes are then related to the direct costs of the interventions and expressed as ratios of cost per unit of effectiveness, such as cost per life year gained. This is the most common evaluation in the literature, and it is useful in providing a rough comparator between the value of different treatments assuming that similar cost elements are included in the studies being compared. A weakness of cost-effectiveness analyses is that they look only at survival as an outcome, and not at toxicity, inconvenience or quality of life. The major value of a cost-effectiveness analysis is that it may help to make choices between similar treatments for a specific disease, but not between dissimilar treatments and conditions.

Cost–utility analysis

A cost–utility analysis is very similar to a cost-effectiveness analysis, but it also includes information about morbidity. The life years gained are adjusted by the quality of the life gained and expressed as quality-adjusted life years (QALYs). This allows comparison of the relative efficiency of health care interventions for different conditions.

Quality of life can be approximated by a utility, which is a measure of preference for a given health state rated on a scale from 0 (worst imaginable health state, or death) to 1 (perfect health). The utility can be derived from a variety of techniques, such as the standard gamble and time trade-off techniques. The quality of the life gained can sometimes be weighted by using ratings on visual analog scales, as well as from instruments, such as the Health Utilities Index and the European Quality of Life (EuroQoL) scale.[8] Most quality-of-life instruments have not undergone the testing required to accurately convert their scores into utilities.

Cost–benefit analysis

A cost–benefit analysis takes a cost–utility evaluation one step further. It attempts to determine whether the benefits of an intervention outweigh its costs. The value in monetary terms of the QALY in the denominator of the cost–utility analysis is measured, and the intervention is considered cost-beneficial if the benefits are measurably greater than the costs in monetary terms. The problem is that placing a monetary value on the often intangible outcomes of health care is extremely difficult. As a result, true cost–benefit analyses are rare, and none has addressed the issue of lung cancer treatment.

METHODOLOGICAL ISSUES

As the primary purpose of a cost-effectiveness analysis is to introduce considerations of resource consumption into medical decision-making, an economic evaluation begins by identifying all the consequences of adopting one intervention over another.[8] This involves the identification of all of the resources used (medical care services, the costs of informal caregiving and other non-direct medical care costs) and the effects of the treatment intervention on the health state. There must be an explicit examination of all the resources consumed which consist of both direct and indirect health care costs. The term 'direct' refers to changes in resource use that are directly attributable to the medical intervention or treatment regimen. In health economics, the term 'indirect' refers to gains or losses in productivity related to the illness. Because indirect costs in accounting terminology refer to overhead or fixed costs of production, some health economists recommend the use of the term 'productivity costs' to define the indirect costs associated with the morbidity or mortality of an illness.[8]

Direct costs

Direct costs include the value of all goods and services and other resources that are used to provide the treatment or intervention or to deal with the consequences of the treatment, such as side-effects or complications. The most obvious direct costs are the costs of the tests, drugs, medical supplies, health care personnel time and the use of medical facilities. However, there are also direct non-health-care costs that should not be overlooked. These costs include such things as out-of-pocket expenses for transportation to health care facilities, parking, child care, and the time volunteered by family members and other volunteers in support of the patient. Such costs are often omitted from economic evaluations, in part because of the difficulty in documenting the amount of resource consumed and then in assigning a monetary value to it. If these costs are judged to be relatively small, or the alternatives being evaluated have similar direct non-health-care costs, they may reasonably be omitted from the analysis.

Indirect or 'productivity' costs

These are the costs that result from the inability to work or to engage in normal leisure activities due to morbidity resulting from the disease or its treatment, or that result from the loss of economic productivity because of death. The costs associated with the morbidity of a disease can be measured in monetary terms, or the impact of treatment-related morbidity on quality of life can be included in the calculation of the QALY. Changes in life expectancy resulting from a treatment intervention are included in the denominator of the cost-effectiveness ratio and are expressed in the natural unit of time.

Identifying the resources consumed

Ideally, an economic evaluation should collect resource utilization data in three steps. The first step is to identify the various types of resources consumed, the second step is to measure or quantify the resource utilization, and the third step is to place a value on the resources used. In undertaking a cost-effectiveness analysis involving a treatment intervention, it is necessary to understand the epidemiology of the disease and how affected individuals interact with the health care system. In particular, it is necessary to know what clinical management strategies are utilized. All of the resources used in the delivery of the intervention should be considered if individually or collectively they could be large enough to potentially impact on decision-making about the use of the intervention. Small amounts of resources that are consumed by large numbers of individuals could have an important impact on the analysis.

Approaches to the measurement of resource utilization vary along a spectrum of specificity. At one end is the approach that enumerates each and every cost element used in the treatment of a patient. At the other end of the spectrum are gross approaches to the estimation of the cost of components of care, such as assigning a national average figure to the cost of treating a specific disease state. The former approach is referred to as 'micro-costing' and the latter is called 'gross' or 'macro-costing'.[8] The majority of studies utilize micro-costing approaches starting with a detailed inventory and measurement of resources consumed during a treatment. For studies of chemotherapy administration in lung cancer, details of drugs and supplies used, clinic and hospital visits, and personnel time involved in preparation and administration of the drugs are determined, often using time-and-motion studies. Macro-costing uses estimates for units of input or output that are large relative to the intervention being studied. The choice between these two cost approaches depends on the needs of the analysis for precision and freedom from bias, balanced against the complexity and cost of obtaining the cost estimate. Generally, micro-costing is preferred, because it allows others to see the elements of the analysis in sufficient detail that they can assess the relevance of the analysis to their own situation.

OTHER CONSIDERATIONS

Setting

Economic evaluations are generally specific to the health care system in which they are performed. Countries with a single payer system such as Canada, in which the government funds virtually the entire direct cost of medical care, are quite different from countries where health care funding is predominantly through private insurers.[8] With multiple payers, market forces prevail, and the charges for medical care are the result of the market, government regulations, taxation law and other factors. As a result, the charges for care may bear little resemblance to the actual resource costs. In European countries, a co-payment system is common, and requires patients to pay for some of their care, while universal access to care is provided. The differences between health care systems make it difficult to translate the results of an economic evaluation from one setting to another. Transparent and explicit presentation of the components of the evaluation is necessary in order to attempt such interpretations.

Sensitivity analysis

The standard statistical techniques used in clinical trials cannot be used to look for differences between the arms of an economic analysis.[9,10] Economic endpoints often require larger sample sizes than clinical studies owing to variation in the economic parameters, such as length of hospital stay, which is not controlled for in a clinical study. Therefore it is necessary to undertake detailed sensitivity analyses to assess how sensitive the results are to varying the estimates of resource use and effectiveness over a range of plausible values. No matter how accurately costs and benefits have been quantified and valued, it is likely that certain assumptions have been made that may be subject to criticism. For an economic evaluation to be considered sound, it is necessary to test the effects of changes to the assumptions. If altering the value of a key parameter changes the conclusion of the study then it is considered sensitive to that parameter, and the conclusion is not 'robust'. The question being answered by a sensitivity analysis is not whether all estimates of resource use and survival are accurate, but rather whether any errors would have a meaningful impact on the results.

ESTIMATING THE COSTS OF LUNG CANCER CARE IN CANADA

Statistics Canada has undertaken a detailed costing of the diagnostic and therapeutic approaches to lung cancer in Canada, and has developed information at the population level on the economic burden of lung cancer from the perspective of the government as the payer in a universal health care system.[6,7,11] This POpulation HEalth Model (POHEM) will ultimately provide a comprehensive microsimulation of Canadian health, including such important diseases as lung, breast, colon and prostate cancer, cardiovascular disease, dementia, arthritis, and osteoporosis. The model integrates risk factors for disease, diagnostic and therapeutic approaches, health care resource utilization, and direct medical care costs. The lung model assigns a histological cell type (small cell versus non-small cell) and stage to each patient in a simulated lung cancer population.[6,7] It then describes the treatment appropriate for cell type and stage, and the anticipated progress and survival of the cancer in response to treatment. Costs are assigned according to tumor cell type and treatment option.

To develop this model, it was necessary to access multiple databases including the Canadian Cancer Registry, for information on cancer incidence, tumor cell type and patient demographics, and several provincial cancer registries for stage distribution. Questionnaire surveys of Canadian oncologists were undertaken to obtain information not accessible from provincial databases, such as diagnostic tests used or follow-up practices. Information on duration of hospitalization for diagnostic work-up and initiation of therapy was obtained from Statistics Canada's national person-oriented hospital morbidity database. Costs for hospital outpatient chemotherapy treatment were extracted from an economic analysis done by the National Cancer Institute of Canada following a clinical trial (BR5), which compared chemotherapy and best supportive care in advanced non-small cell lung cancer (NSCLC).[12]

Costs were initially determined in 1988 Canadian dollars, but have been updated periodically since the original report.[6,7] The economic analysis was performed from the perspective of the government as payer in a universal health care system. Since the fees paid for physicians' assessments, laboratory and surgical procedures vary from province to province in Canada, the fee schedule operative in the province of Ontario under its health insurance plan was used as the standard. Statistics Canada's 'Hospital Statistics': Preliminary Annual Report was used to determine the average cost of hospitalization by type of hospital.[13] The per diem rate for a Canadian teaching hospital at the time of this analysis was C$818.50.

Hospital costs for non-surgical care of lung cancer cases, including terminal care, were derived from the economic analysis of the National Cancer Institute of Canada clinical trial of best supportive care versus chemotherapy.[14]

Table 17.2 Costs of diagnosis and treatment of NSCLC by stage (in 1988 C$)

Tumor stage and treatment	Diagnostic and preoperative tests	Surgery	Radio-therapy	Hospitalization and clinic	Follow-up first year	Total
Stage I and II						
Surgery alone	1234	1342	—	10 904	630	14 110
Surgery + postoperative radiotherapy	1234	1342	3779	10 904	630	17 889
Radiotherapy alone	1553	—	3748	6 543	630	12 474
Stage IIIa						
Radiotherapy	1518	—	3023	6 543	630	11 714
No radiotherapy	1397	—	103[a]	6 543	330	8 373
Stage IIIb						
Radiotherapy	913	—	1561	6 543	330	9 347
No radiotherapy	683	—	103[a]	5 452	330	6 568
Stage IV						
Supportive care	881	—	—	5 452	—	6 333

[a] Additional radiation consultation to determine that radiotherapy will not be administered. Follow-up costs after the first year are assumed to be similar to those in the first year. Relapse costs (diagnostic tests and hospitalization) are assigned to all stages except non-radiotherapy arms of stages IIIa and IIIb and stage IV, and are estimated to be C$1528. Terminal-care costs of C$10 331 (palliative radiotherapy and hospitalization) are assigned to patients in the year of death.

These costs were inflated by the rate that the national per diem rate for tertiary care facilities had inflated during the same time period. More details of the costing methodology are included in previous publications.[6,7,11]

A summary of the estimated cost of diagnosis and treatment for each stage of therapeutic approach for NSCLC is shown in Table 17.2. The cost of diagnosis and initial treatment for stage I and II lung cancer (excluding relapse costs) was C$14 110. The cost of combined-modality therapy (surgery and radiotherapy) for patients in stage I and II was C$17 889. For those who were not surgical candidates, but were treated with radical radiotherapy, the initial cost of diagnosis and treatment was estimated to be C$12 474. The costs of treating stage IIIA and IIIB disease with radiation alone were less, at C$11 714 and C$9347 respectively. The initial cost of diagnosis and care of stage IV (metastatic disease) patients was C$6333. Further significant costs are incurred by these patients when they relapse and

Table 17.3 Costs of diagnosis and treatment of SCLC (in 1988 C$)

Tumour stage and treatment	Diagnostic and staging tests	Radio-therapy	Chemo-therapy	Hospitalization and clinic[a]	Follow-up	Total
Limited disease						
Chemotherapy + radiotherapy	1088	4065	5428	8110	—	18 691
Extensive disease						
Chemotherapy + radiotherapy	1088	1592	3818	7027	—	13 525
Palliative care	1088	—	—	3272	379	4 739

[a]Follow-up costs in the first year are included in clinic costs. Assume follow-up costs after the first year are C$944. Assume the chemotherapy/radiotherapy arms of limited and extensive disease can relapse. Relapse costs (diagnostic tests and hospitalization) are determined to be C$1590. Assume that terminal-care costs are assigned to patients in the year of death. Terminal-care costs for limited disease (palliative radiotherapy and hospitalization) are C$10 544. For extensive disease (hospitalization), they are C$9387.

enter the terminal-care phase of their illness (the last three months prior to death), with costs equaling C$10 331.

Based on the fact that there were 12 549 NSCLC patients in Canada in 1988, and assuming that all would have access to appropriate care as defined in the treatment algorithms, the total cost of treatment for a cohort of patients with NSCLC followed over five years would be C$240 236 000.[11] The average cost per case would be C$19 781.

A similar analysis for the 3075 small-cell lung cancer (SCLC) cases according to disease stage revealed that patients with limited-stage disease treated with combined-modality therapy would incur costs of approximately C$18 500 (Table 17.3). Patients with extensive disease received less radiotherapy and less chemotherapy, and therefore incurred fewer costs. The total cost per case estimated in the POHEM was C$13 525. The terminal-care costs for extensive disease patients were estimated to be C$9387, and these costs would be added to those of the treatment-related costs during the year of the patient's death. Overall, the total burden incurred in managing all cases of SCLC diagnosed in 1988 over five years would total C$79 913 000.[11] The average cost per case was estimated to be C$25 988.

Rosenthal et al[15] conducted an institution-based evaluation of direct health care costs for SCLC. They estimated that the cost per case was A$18 234 for limited stage and A$13 177 for extensive stage, with an average cost per case of A$14 413, using 1990 Australian dollars.

Figure 17.1 shows the cost components of lung cancer management. It illustrates the value of this type of cost analysis, in that it immediately makes apparent the major sources of expenditure in the health care system for the management of

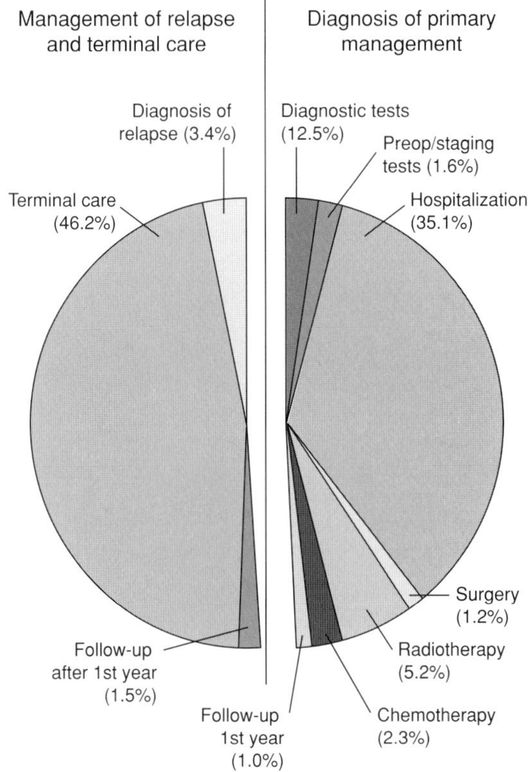

Figure 17.1
Cost components of lung cancer management (1992).

lung cancer patients. For all stages of lung cancer, the use of acute-care hospital beds accounts for more costs than diagnostic tests, medications and physician fees combined. Hospitalization during initial diagnosis and management made up 35.8% of the total five-year costs, and the cost of terminal care utilizing acute-care hospital beds was 38.7% of the total cost. Therefore, assuming the goal is to make the health care system more cost-efficient, strategies need to be developed that will result in the devolution of inpatient care to ambulatory care. This can be accomplished through ambulatory diagnostic assessment units for patients with a presumptive diagnosis of lung cancer and by the provision of a greater amount of palliative care within the home environment or through palliative-care units.

The POHEM also provides a framework within which to assess new interventions for their cost-effectiveness. The costs of the survival benefit associated with new treatments, such as chemotherapy for stage IV NSCLC, are compared against the costs and benefits of standard treatment. Recent practice guidelines in Canada recommend that cisplatin-based chemotherapy be offered as a treatment option for medically suitable patients to improve survival, symptom control and quality of life.[16] Cost-effectiveness analyses are important in a time of fiscal restraint in health care budgets, since there are many physicians and health care administrators who question whether it is appropriate to offer relatively expensive and toxic agents that only modestly impact survival.

The National Cancer Institute of Canada was the first to demonstrate in a cost analysis that chemotherapy administration might actually reduce the overall costs to the health care system, primarily by reducing the average length of hospital stay for terminal care. Jaakkimainen et al[14] undertook an economic analysis of the National Cancer Institute of Canada clinical trial (BR5) that compared the use of vindesine–cisplatin (VP) chemotherapy and the combination of cyclophosphamide, doxorubicin (Adriamycin) and cisplatin (CAP) versus best supportive care (BSC) in patients with stage IV NSCLC.[12] This study, which used primary survival data from all patients entered in the trial and estimated costs from the two largest institutions contributing patients to the trial, demonstrated that CAP was a dominant treatment strategy, prolonging life and lowering costs. On average, survival was increased by eight weeks, while costs decreased by C$949 per CAP-treated patient. This translated to a saving of C$6172 per life-year gained, and was attributable to the reduction in hospitalization rates in those who received CAP chemotherapy. Patients who received VP chemotherapy also had fewer terminal-care hospital bed days compared with BSC, but hospitalization for administration of high-dose cisplatin chemotherapy and the cost of the drugs made this a more expensive treatment approach. With an increased survival of 12.8 weeks and an additional cost of C$3638 per patient, the cost-effectiveness ratio was C$14 778 per life-year saved (LYS). The results of this study underscored the need for ambulatory administration strategies for chemotherapy delivery.

We are now faced with a proliferation of promising new drugs with encouraging activity in NSCLC. Each of these drugs is, however, significantly more expensive than the older drugs. By using the POHEM, information on the costs of the old 'standard' therapies and their outcomes can be compared with the costs of the new agents and their survival benefits. Based on data from a randomized trial of vinorelbine alone compared with the combinations of vinorelbine–cisplatin and vindesine–cisplatin,[17] estimates of the cost-effectiveness of these regimens relative to BSC were made in the POHEM.[18] Vinorelbine was a dominant strategy, saving C$1447 per case. Vinorelbine–cisplatin was also a dominant strategy as an ambulatory regimen, saving C$473 per case, and was more cost-effective than the same chemotherapy given as an inpatient regimen (C$5551 per LYS).

Hillner and co-workers[19,20] also undertook a cost-effectiveness analysis of vinorelbine–cisplatin and vindesine–cisplatin compared with vinorelbine alone in stage IV, based on the same clinical trial reported by Le Chevalier et al.[17] They used American costs (charges) and found that vinorelbine–cisplatin cost US$17 700 per LYS relative to vinorelbine. Vindesine–cisplatin had a cost-effectiveness ratio of US$22 100 per LYS relative to vinorelbine. Nonetheless, even in this comparison against vinorelbine alone as opposed to BSC, the combination of vinorelbine–cisplatin was seen to be cost-effective.

Evans[21] undertook an economic evaluation of the use of gemcitabine in the management of patients with stage IV lung cancer. Based on phase II survival data from the large EO 18 trial[22] and estimates of drug costs per treatment cycle ranging from C$800 to C$1800, gemcitabine was observed to be cost-effective over a range of sensitivity analyses. At the greatest cost per cycle (C$1800) and with survival reduced by 50% compared with the EO 18 result, the cost per life year gained was estimated to be C$16 230.

Earle et al[23] undertook a similar analysis of paclitaxel alone compared with BSC, based on the data from two phase II clinical trials.[24,25] The total costs of administering three cycles of chemotherapy were C$8143 and C$3375 more than the strategy of BSC. However, on the basis of the difference in survival duration between stage IV patients treated in the BSC arm of a previous National Cancer Institute of Canada Trial and those represented in the pooled phase II survival results, the cost per life-year gained was C$4778.

All of the chemotherapy regimens that have been evaluated in the POHEM and updated to current costs are summarized in Table 17.4. For all of these various regimens, physicians' fees, and the personnel costs associated with drug preparation and delivery were measured at the Ottawa Regional Cancer Centre. The laboratory and imaging studies necessary to monitor patients on treatment were extracted from the treatment protocols described in the medical literature. The frequency and cost of treatment-associated complications were estimated on the basis of trial data, where available.

As noted in Table 17.4, vinblastine–cisplatin, vinorelbine–cisplatin and etoposide (VP-16)–

Table 17.4 Comparison of costs of best supportive care versus chemotherapy treatment of stage IV NSCLC (in 1995 C$)

	BSC	VLB–P	NVB	NVB–P	VDS–P	VP-16–P	TAX[a]	GEM[b]	TAX–P[c]
Chemotherapy cost (C$)	—	1 920	3 750	4 830	8 410	3 560	6 020	5 058	7 830
Average cost/case (C$)	28 270	25 410	27 220	28 200	31 900	27 140	29 480	28 491	31 160
Average survival (years)	0.49	0.76	0.77	0.93	0.76	0.97	1.15	0.90	1.0610
Average years saved[d]	NA	0.27	0.28	0.44	0.27	0.48	0.67	0.41	0.57
Cost per life year saved (C$)	NA	D	D	D	13 500	D	1814	530	5034

BSC, best supportive care; VLB–P, vinblastine–cisplatin; NVB, vinorelbine (Navelbine); NVB–P, vinorelbine–cisplatin; VDS–P, vindesine–cisplatin (inpatient); VP-16–P, etoposide–cisplatin; TAX, paclitaxel (Taxol); GEM, gemcitabine; TAX–P, paclitaxel–cisplatin (generic + outpatient); NA, not applicable; D, dominant strategy.

[a]Assume 3 treatment cycles per patient at a drug cost of C$1509 (generic) per treatment cycle (200 mg/m^2).

[b]Assume 3.3 treatment cycles per patient at a drug cost of C$1038 per treatment cycle.

[c]Paclitaxel at 135 mg/m^2 (3 h); cisplatin at 75 mg/m^2 (includes toxicity cost of C$737).

[d]Compared with best supportive care.

cisplatin were all found to decrease the cost of treatment per patient compared with BSC, while increasing survival relative to BSC. Therefore these chemotherapy regimens should be considered dominant treatment strategies. This important observation is true in the Canadian health care environment, but it may not be reflective of reality in other health care environments. If patients with NSCLC are not currently hospitalized for their diagnostic or terminal care, as they were in Canada at the time of this analysis, then there will not be any potential to decrease health care costs, but only to increase expenditures due to the cost of the drugs.

The important influence of the health care environment on the outcome of economic analyses is seen in the report of Lappas et al.[26] They undertook a pharmacoeconomic analysis of the impact of paclitaxel–carboplatin and vinorelbine–cisplatin. To obtain survival outcome data, they performed a meta-analysis of all available clinical trial literature. US Medicare reimbursement figures were used to determine the total expected cost. This was determined to be US$19 322 and US$20 790 for paclitaxel–carboplatin and vinorelbine–cisplatin respectively. Treatment with the vinorelbine-containing regimen was 7% more costly than the paclitaxel-containing regimen. Lower administration costs and less frequent adverse event management costs led to the lower overall cost and to the recommendation that paclitaxel–carboplatin be the preferred choice from an American pharmacoeconomic perspective. As can be seen from

Table 17.4, estimates of the cost per case are greater for paclitaxel–cisplatin in the Canadian environment than for vinorelbine–cisplatin, even though generic pricing is in effect for paclitaxel in Canada. The paclitaxel–carboplatin combination would be even more expensive on a cost per case basis, because the current cost of carboplatin greatly exceeds that of cisplatin. Relative to BSC, paclitaxel–cisplatin is a cost-effective intervention at C$5034 per LYS, but vinorelbine–cisplatin is a dominant strategy.

The cost-effectiveness analyses illustrated above can be converted to cost–utility estimates by assigning utilities to each of the chemotherapy regimens and to BSC. Oncologists working as part of the Ontario Practice Guideline Initiative have estimated utilities for the different chemotherapy regimens. The scale used ranged from 0 to 1, where 0 represents death and 1 is perfect health. The utilities for the chemotherapy regimens ranged from 0.5 to 0.7, with the utility estimate for best supportive care being 0.5. With the incorporation of utilities into the calculation of cost-effectiveness, the chemotherapy regimens actually become more cost-effective compared with best supportive care.

Chemotherapy interventions for stage IV NSCLC can be ranked for their cost-effectiveness based on alternative threshold values.[27] Depending on the value that society is willing to pay for each unit of outcome gained, the ranking of each intervention will vary. In North America, the common threshold is C$50 000 per life-year saved. Using this threshold, paclitaxel followed by paclitaxel–cisplatin, vinorelbine–cisplatin (ambulatory) and gemcitabine would be the preferred regimens. If the threshold was for therapies costing only C$10 000 per life-year gained, vinblastine–cisplatin would be the preferred regimen, followed by vinorelbine–cisplatin given on an ambulatory basis, etoposide–cisplatin and vinorelbine alone

The cost-effectiveness for combined-modality therapy for stage IIIA and IIIB disease has been evaluated using the POHEM.[28] For stage IIIA, combined-modality therapy consisting of pre- and postoperative chemotherapy and radiotherapy, as described by Kris et al,[29] was modeled for patients with clinically evident N2 disease. For patients with stage IIIB disease, the costs associated with delivering two cycles of vinblastine–cisplatin followed by radical radiotherapy (60 Gy in 30 fractions), as reported by CALGB,[30] have been modeled.

Although the incremental cost per case was high, particularly for combined-modality therapy for stage IIIA disease (C$22 963 more than standard radiotherapy), the estimated life-years gained were also substantial and the cost–effectiveness was C$14 958 per life-year gained. The combined-modality approach of vinblastine–cisplatin followed by radical radiotherapy for stage IIIB patients was more expensive than standard Canadian radiotherapy (C$22 303 versus C$13 391). However, the estimated number of life-years gained with combined-modality therapy was large, and resulted in a cost-effectiveness ratio of C$3348 per life-year gained.

Despite evidence of the cost-effectiveness of lung cancer treatment, there remains a reluctance in the medical community, even in North America, to adopt some of these new approaches in the management of lung cancer. Concern has been expressed about the quality of life that accompanies such treatments. However, even when this has been factored into the economic evaluations, the quality-adjusted life-year gained remains in the range that is considered acceptable for health care interventions in Canada.[31] The reluctance of many institutions to provide combined-modality therapy for locally advanced disease or chemotherapy for metastatic disease may relate to the absolute cost of introducing these new treatments. Since there are a large number of patients who potentially could receive these treatments, the total fiscal burden could be quite large. In developing countries, where there is a need to prioritize health care expenditures even more carefully, the absolute cost of care for lung cancer patients may become a significant factor in determining health policy. Choices may need to be made between the introduction of these new strategies and the withdrawal of previously existing treatments for cancer or the treatment of other illnesses. Before such decisions are taken, however, economic data derived from the cost of care in that particular environment need to be determined. Evaluations in North America have dispelled the myth that the treatment of lung cancer is costly and not cost-effective in this health care environment. Although caution must be exercised in extrapolating this to other health care jurisdictions, economic factors should probably not be a barrier to the delivery of current best treatment practices. The comparative cost-effectiveness data presented in this paper may be useful to those who must make the decisions about which regimens or strategies to chose.

REFERENCES

1. Parker SL, Tong T, Bolden S et al, Cancer Statistics 1997. *CA Cancer J Clin* 1997; **47**: 7–26.
2. *Canadian Cancer Statistics 1997*. National Cancer Institute of Canada: Toronto.
3. Fry WA, Menck HR, Winchester DP, The National Cancer Data Base Report on lung cancer. *Cancer* 1996; **77**: 1947–55.
4. Schuette HL, Tucker TC, Brown ML et al, The costs of cancer care in the United States: implications for action. *Oncology* 1995; **9**(11 Suppl): 19–22.
5. Brown ML, Fintor L, The economic burden of cancer. In: *Cancer Prevention and Control* (Greenwald R, Kramer BS, Weed DL, eds). Marcel Dekker: New York, 1995: 69–81.
6. Evans W, Will BP, Bertholot J-M, Wolfson MC, Estimating the cost of lung cancer diagnosis and treatment in Canada: the POHEM model. *Can J Oncol* 1995; **5**: 408–17.
7. Evans WK, Will BP, Berthelot J-M, Wolfson MC, Diagnostic and therapeutic approaches to lung cancer in Canada and their costs. *Br J Cancer* 1995; **72**: 1270–7.
8. Drummond MF, O'Brien B, Stoddart GL, Torrance GW, *Methods for the Economic Evaluation of Health Care Programmes*, 2nd edn. Oxford University Press: Oxford, 1997.
9. Earle CC, Coyle D, Evans WK, Cost-effectiveness analysis in oncology. *Ann Oncol* 1998; **9**: 475–82.
10. Coyle D, Statistical analysis in pharmacoeconomic studies. A review of current issues and standards. *Pharmacoeconomics* 1996; **9**: 506–16.
11. Evans WK, Will BP, Berthelot J-M et al, The cost of managing lung cancer in Canada. *Oncology* 1995; **9**: 147–52.
12. Rapp E, Pater JL, Willan A et al, Chemotherapy can prolong survival in patients with non-small cell lung cancer: report of a Canadian multicentre randomized trial. *J Clin Oncol* 1988; **6**: 633–44.
13. *Annual Return of Hospitals – Hospital Indicators (1988–89)*. Statistics Canada, Catalogue 83-233: Ottawa, 1993.
14. Jaakkimianen L, Goodwin PJ, Pater JA, Counting the cost of cancer chemotherapy in the National Cancer Institute of Canada randomized trial of non-small cell lung cancer. *J Clin Oncol* 1990; **8**: 1301–9.
15. Rosenthal MA, Webster PJ, Gebski VJ et al, The cost of treating small cell lung cancer. *Med J Austr* 1992; **156**: 605–10.
16. Lopez PJ, Stewart DJ, Newman TE et al, Chemotherapy in stage IV (metastatic) non-small cell lung cancer. *Cancer Prev Control* 1997; **1**: 18–27
17. Le Chevalier T, Brisgand D, Douillard JY et al, Randomized study of vinorelbine and cisplatin versus vindesine and cisplatin versus vinorelbine alone in advanced non-small cell lung cancer: results of European multicenter trial including 612 patients. *J Clin Oncol* 1994; **12**: 360–7.

18. Evans WK, Le Chevalier T, The cost-effectiveness of Navelbine alone or in combination with cisplatin in comparison to other chemotherapy regimens and best supportive care in stage IV non-small cell lung cancer. *Eur J Cancer* 1996; **32A**: 2249–55.
19. Hillner BE, Smith TJ, Cost-effective analysis of three regimens using vinorelbine (Navelbine) for non-small cell lung cancer. *Semin Oncol* 1996; **23**: 25–30.
20. Smith TJ, Hillner BE, Neighbours DM et al, Economic evaluation of a randomized clinical trial comparing vinorelbine, vinorelbine plus cisplatin and vindesine plus cisplatin for non-small cell lung cancer. *J Clin Oncol* 1995; **13**: 2166–73.
21. Evans WK, An estimate of the cost effectiveness of gemcitabine in stage IV non-small cell lung cancer. *Semin Oncol* 1996; **23**: 82–9.
22. Gatzemeier U, Shepherd FA, Le Chevalier T et al, Activity of gemcitabine in patients with non-small cell lung cancer. A multicenter, extended phase II study. *Eur J Cancer* 1996; **32**: 243–8.
23. Earle CC, Evans WK, A comparison of the costs of paclitaxel and best supportive care in stage IV non-small-cell lung cancer. *Cancer Prev Control* 1997; **1**: 282–7.
24. Chang AY, Kim K, Glick J et al, Phase II study of Taxol, Merberone and Piroxantrone in stage IV non-small-cell lung cancer: the Eastern Cooperative Oncology Group results. *J Natl Cancer Inst* 1993; **85**: 388–93.
25. Murphy WK, Fossella FV, Winn RJ et al, Phase II study of Taxol in patients with untreated advanced non-small cell lung cancer. *J Natl Cancer Inst* 1993; **85**: 384–8.
26. Lappas PT, Hainsworth JD, Einarson TR et al, A health economic evaluation of Taxol (paclitaxel) and carboplatin versus vinorelbine and cisplatin combination chemotherapy in the treatment of non-small cell lung cancer: a meta-analysis. *Proc Am Soc Clin Oncol* 1998; **17**: 493a.
27. Bordeleau L, Earle C, Will BP et al, Making a decision framework that incorporates economic data in the choice of chemotherapy regimen for advanced non-small cell lung cancer. Submitted for publication.
28. Evans WK, Will BP, Berthelot J-M, Earle CC, Cost of combined modality interventions for stage III non-small-cell lung cancer. *J Clin Oncol* 1997; **15**: 3038–48.
29. Kris MG, Martini N, Gralla RJ et al, Primary chemotherapy in stage IIIA non-small cell lung cancer with clinically apparent mediastinal lymph node metastases: focus on 5-year survivors. *Lung Cancer* 1993; **9**: 369–76.
30. Dillman RO, Seagren SI, Propert KJ et al, A randomized trial of induction chemotherapy plus high-dose radiation versus radiation alone in stage III non-small-cell lung cancer. *N Engl J Med* 1990; **323**: 940–5.
31. Laupacis A, Feeny D, Detsky A, Tugwell P, How attractive does a new technology have to be to warrant adoption and utilization? Tentative guidelines for using clinical and economic evaluations. *Can Med Assoc J* 1992; **146**: 473–81.

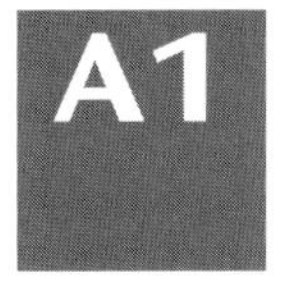

Appendix 1: Surgical techniques in the management of lung cancer

Tsuguo Naruke, Robert J Downey

Contents

INTRODUCTION: PREOPERATIVE, INTRAOPERATIVE, AND POSTOPERATIVE MANAGEMENT

Complete surgical resection, with or without chemotherapy or radiation therapy, offers the best opportunity for a cure to the patient with primary lung cancer. However, while the benefits are real, the risks incurred are also substantial. Patients being considered for pulmonary resection usually present with reduced pulmonary capacity, and often with poor exercise tolerance; then, almost every aspect of a potentially curative lung resection works in concert to worsen a patient's ventilatory capacity further. Large series estimate the overall operative mortality rate for pulmonary resection to range from 2% to 4%.[1,2] Mortality rate estimates increase with the size of the resection: from 1% or less for a wedge resection, to 3% for a lobectomy, and 6–9% for a pneumonectomy. The morbidity associated with these procedures is also considerable: non-fatal complications occur in 41–50% of patients undergoing lobectomy and 36–75% of those undergoing pneumonectomy. The major cause of morbidity and death after pulmonary procedures is respiratory failure with or without pneumonia; myocardial infarction and arrhythmias, bronchopleural fistulae, empyema and pulmonary embolus also occur, but less frequently. In this appendix, we shall review:

- the selection and preparation of the patient appropriate for lung resection;
- the operative techniques of thoracotomy and pulmonary resection;
- routine postoperative management;
- common and uncommon complications encountered following lung resections.

PREOPERATIVE ASSESSMENT AND OPTIMIZATION

Assessment of pulmonary function

A surgeon's evaluation of a patient's tolerance for a planned lung resection begins with first meeting the patient. The most important but least objective factor is a patient's willingness to undergo the work of recovery from a thoracic resection. Evidence provided by the Lung Cancer Study Group[3] suggests that a patient's attitude towards his or her disease is the best predictor of long-term survival. A patient who is unwilling or unable to participate in his or her own recovery should explore reasonable alternative therapies, such as definitive radiation treatment.

Despite the range of preoperative pulmonary function tests that have been investigated in an attempt to estimate the risk that a patient assumes by undergoing a pulmonary resection,[4] current preoperative testings predict only a small percentage of postoperative complications, and most appear to be almost random events visited on the patient. Kohlman et al[5] analyzed, in a study of 476 patients resected over 12 years, the predictive value of 37 preoperative risk factors for morbidity and mortality, and found only three that bore a significant association with mortality: age > 60 years, the planned procedure being a pneumonectomy, and the presence of premature ventricular beats on preoperative EKG. All risk factors analyzed together accounted for only 12% of the risk of mortality. The surgeon's impression of operative risk may very well prove the most useful tool for selecting patients for pulmonary resection.

The patient should be evaluated for the amount and character of sputum production, the effectiveness of cough, and the ability to climb a flight of stairs of fixed height.[6,7] Patients with hypercapnia on preoperative arterial blood gases probably have pulmonary hypertension, and, although likely to do poorly after a pneumonectomy, may be able to tolerate a lobectomy. Pulmonary function tests allow an estimate of the FEV_1, which if taken in combination with lobar perfusion scans, allows prediction of postresectional FEV_1 to within 100 cm^3 (ME Burt, late of Memorial Sloan-Kettering Cancer Center, personal communication). A predicted postresectional FEV_1 of less than 40%, or less than 800 cm^3, should raise concern. Ferguson et al[8] studied the *DL*CO preoperatively in 165 lung resection patients and found it to be the best predictor of postoperative pulmonary complications or death. Maximal exercise oxygen consumption ($M\dot{V}O_2$) measurements have been studied:[9] a patient able to sustain an $M\dot{V}O_2$ of 20 cm^3/kg/min was least likely to have complications, while patients unable to generate an $M\dot{V}O_2$ more than 15 cm^3/kg/min suffered 75% of all postoperative morbidity.

Optimizing preoperative pulmonary function

A full discussion of effective therapies for improving patients' pulmonary function is beyond the scope of this appendix, and is available in several recent detailed reviews of this subject.[5,10] Briefly, improvement of function begins with smoking cessation. Smoke is an airway irritant, leading to excessive mucus production, and airway hyperreactivity;[11,12] even a short abstinence from smoking can improve the effectiveness of mucociliary transport,[13] as well as decreasing the blood levels of carboxyhemoglobin, with an improvement in oxygen transport.[14] The time necessary for these effects to be seen is unclear, but studies of patients undergoing abdominal surgery[15] and coronary artery bypass surgery[16] suggest that eight weeks of smoking cessation is optimal for decreasing pulmonary complications.

The addition of nebulized albuterol[17] and/or mucolytics such as *N*-acetylcysteine (with attention to the possible side-effect of bronchoconstriction[18]) may be of benefit for individual patients. Because of a narrow therapeutic index, methylxanthines are utilized rarely; similarly, despite the fact that patients with demonstrated reversible airflow obstruction will improve with steroids,[19] prednisone or other corticosteroids are added reluctantly because of the possible deleterious effects on wound healing and resistance to infection. Bronchitics with purulent sputum should be treated with oral antibiotics, directed towards the most common bacteria (*Streptococcus pneumoniae*, *Haemophilus influenzae*, and *Moraxella catarrhalis*[20]); appropriate choices of antibiotics for these species include trimethoprim–sulfamethoxazole, ampicillin, or doxycycline.

TECHNIQUES OF SURGICAL RESECTION

Resections: pneumonectomy

Pneumonectomy is most commonly performed in the modern era to resect either primary lung malignancy or metastatic disease to the lung that cannot be removed by a lesser resection. In the era of antibiotics and modern pulmonology, it has become distinctly unusual to perform a pneumonectomy for infectious, inflammatory, or other benign conditions. Any incision that allows adequate exposure to the hilum can be utilized for a pneumonectomy; it cannot be emphasized enough that compromised exposure may lead to an increased risk of vascular injury, and decreased ability to control bleeding once it occurs.

Single-lung anesthesia for either a right or left pneumonectomy is probably best provided by a standard disposable left-sided Robert–Shaw double-lumen endotracheal tube. A bronchial blocker in combination with a single-lumen endotracheal tube is acceptable, although it is prone to being dislodged (usually seemingly during the most difficult parts of the hilar dissection) and does not allow for as rapid inflation and deflation of the lung as a double-lumen tube.

Intraoperatively, prior to a decision being made as to the sequence of division of the vessels and the airway, the hilum should be dissected as completely as possible. The sequence in which the structures are divided depends most importantly on the location of the malignancy, or, for patients with benign disease, the amount of inflammation investing individual structures. Although there may be theoretical concerns that, in a patient with cancer, the venous vessels should be divided first to limit the circulation of malignant cells, it has never been shown that patients who have the pulmonary artery divided first suffer earlier, or more frequent, presentations of metastatic disease. The lung will also not become engorged if the venous vessels are divided first, as occurs with splenectomy. Therefore the vessels may be divided in any order that appears appropriate given the anatomical configuration, the location of the malignancy (if present), and the presence of scarring and adherent lymph nodes.

Should the location of malignant tissue or scarring from prior surgery or inflammatory disease preclude safe isolation of the extrapericardial pulmonary artery, intrapericardial control may be obtained. On the right, the pericardium may be opened anterior to the hilum, with careful attention being paid to the location of the phrenic nerve. Two to three more centimeters of length on the right pulmonary artery should be available, especially if the superior vena cava is mobilized. On the left, the pericardium is also entered anteriorly, but mobilization often requires division of the ligamentum arteriosum, with careful attention to the course of the left recurrent laryngeal nerve. Division of the pulmonary artery may be performed by application of a vascular stapler, ligation, or oversewing with suture. Similar techniques may be used to divide the pulmonary veins.

Dissection of the bronchus should be kept only to the amount necessary to perform a tension-free closure, and to allow complete resection of all malignant tissue; over-dissection risks devascularization. On the right, division of the bronchus prior to division of the vessels may facilitate exposure of the vascular elements of the hilum; however, caution is needed in separating the anterior wall of the bronchus from the posterior wall of the pulmonary artery, since the artery may be injured. The bronchus should be divided close enough to the carina so that a 'long-stump' is avoided, since this will lead to pooling of secretions. However, the bronchus should not be divided flush with the carina, since the cartilaginous rings are very irregular in this area, and will exert significant elastic force that may lead to disruption of the airway closure. It is important to note that a double-lumen tube sitting in either bronchus will exert a significant stenting force; pulling a double-lumen tube back out of the bronchus to sit within the trachea will lead to a more normal elasticity of the bronchus at the time of airway division and closure.

The airway may be either stapled (usually with a TA-30 4.8 stapler) or divided and oversewn (usually with 4-0 Vicryl interrupted staples placed approximately 1 mm apart and encircling one cartilaginous ring). It is the practice at Memorial Sloan-Kettering Cancer Center (MSKCC) to reinforce all pneumonectomy stumps, usually with interrupted 4-0 Vicryl sutures, and the stump with tissue as available – either a pleural flap mobilized off the chest wall, a pericardial fat pad, a pericardial flap, omentum, intercostal muscle or a chest wall muscle (either serratus anterior or even latissimus dorsi). It is important to ensure that the tissue placed over the stump is adequately perfused, since there can be few things less conducive to healing than an acidotic tissue mass. After the airway is closed and no further sutures are to be placed, it should be tested to 30 cm of airway pressure; any leaks should be repaired, usually with interrupted 4-0 Vicryl sutures.

Resections: lobectomy

Lobectomy is the most common resection performed with curative intent for primary lung malignancies, with pneumonectomy reserved for more centrally located disease, and segmentectomies, wedge resections or needle cautery excision reserved for patients with inadequate pulmonary reserve to tolerate more extensive resections. Resection is begun by complete incision of the pleura investing the hilum. Exploration of the intralobar fissure allows exposure, on the right, of the superior segmental artery, the middle lobe artery(ies), and the posterior (recurrent) segmental artery of the upper lobe, and, on the left, of the superior segmental artery of the lower lobe and the lingular arteries of the upper lobe. The 'sump' lymph nodes should be examined by frozen section prior to making a decision about the extent of lung resection needed. With the hilar vessels in view, the fissures may be completed, usually with multiple applications of an Endo-GIA stapler if possible to minimize air leaks off the divided lung.

The pulmonary arterial and venous branches are divided either with application of vascular staples or by double ligature with 2-0, 3-0, or 4-0 silk prior to division. The bronchus is divided after stapling with a TA30-4.8 or TA30-3.5 stapler. Alternatively, the bronchial closure may be performed by interrupted Vicryl sutures. At MSKCC, it is routine to oversew with 4-0 Vicryl all stapled closures of the airway after lower lobectomy because of the increased risk of bronchopleural fistula. After upper or middle lobectomy, chest tube drainage is performed with two 28F chest tubes placed to the apex of the cavity; after lower lobectomy, drainage is by a 28F straight chest tube to the apex, and a 28F right-angle chest tube placed into the costophrenic angle.

Resections: sublobar – segmentectomy, wedge, or precision needle cautery excision

A true segmentectomy is rarely performed today, since many lesions are either subpleural and amenable to a wide wedge resection with multiple applications of staplers, or too deeply set for a segmental resection to allow adequate margins around the hilar structures. Ideally, for a segmentectomy, a lesion should be small (less than 2 cm) and completely surrounded by segmental pulmonary parenchyma. Performing a segmentectomy requires a detailed knowledge of the arterial and bronchial anatomy. After exposure of the hilar anatomy, division (after double ligation with 3-0 or 4-0 silk) of the arterial supply to the segment is usually performed first, since this allows exposure of the adjacent bronchus. Occlusion of the bronchus allows delineation of the segment within the lobe. Either the segmental bronchus can be occluded (best done with a large vascular clip) and the lung inflated, with the residual atelectatic portion of the lung being taken to represent the segment to be removed, or the lung can be inflated, a clip applied to the bronchus, and the lung allowed to deflate with the portion that fails to collapse being taken to represent the segment to be removed. It is often easier to divide the segmental bronchus sharply, and to oversew it with interrupted or continuous 4-0 Vicryl sutures, rather than with a stapler, because of the excessive torsion that this applies to surrounding vascular structures. Stapling devices are then applied along the intersegmental plane as delineated in the partially inflated lung as above.

The usual alternative to a segmentectomy is a wedge resection, which is a non-anatomical resection of lung parenchyma without division of hilar structures. A 2 cm margin of lung parenchyma should be obtained in all directions, to minimize the chances of residual microscopic disease, usually by multiple applications of an Endo-GIA stapler, often in conjunction with a TA30-4.8 stapler. Alternately, precision cautery removal[21,22] may be employed. Manual pressure is applied to the lesion to press it out towards the closest pleural surface. Dissection with cautery through the pleura and the surrounding lung parenchyma is performed, with careful attention to all bleeding sites. If substantial vessels are encountered, they are divided after suture ligation or clipped. Once the lesion has been removed, the parenchyma and the pleura may be approximated with continuous 4-0 Prolene sutures; the tissues are often easily torn, and the sutures are best applied by placing multiple passes with the needle through the surrounding tissues prior to drawing up on the ends of the stitch.

Systematic nodal dissection

Anatomical lung resection with systematic nodal dissection is recognized as the therapy that is most likely to achieve local control for selected patients with lung cancer. The factors affecting the likelihood of achieving this outcome are the sites of the nodes involved, the number of nodes involved, the extent of tumor involvement within the nodes, and the histological type.

The terminology 'radical mediastinal lymph node dissection' was formerly widely used, but is unsatisfactory, since the term 'mediastinal' failed to recognize the importance of the evaluation of N1 nodes, the term 'sampling' suggested that only small parts of any node should be removed, and the term 'radical' implied therapeutic benefit. The terminology 'systematic nodal dissection' is now recommended.[23] The technique of systematic lymph node dissection as discussed in this text is based on studies by Rouviere,[24] Weinberg,[25] Nohl,[26] Borrie,[27] and Naruke,[28,29] among others.

The first lymph node map was introduced in the late 1960s.[28–30] This map was adopted in 1976 by the American Joint Committee for Cancer (AJCC) Staging and End Results Reporting to help in the classification of lung cancer,[31–33] and has been published with the TNM classification of malignancies by the Union Internationale Contre le Cancer (UICC).[34,35] A modified version has been introduced by the American Thoracic Society.[36]

Most recently, in 1997, Mountain and Dresler[37] also published regional lymph node stations modified from Naruke's ATS/LCSG Map, which was introduced for educational use. However, problems persist: for example, there is no category for the previous level 3 pretracheal lymph nodes, and the definition of level 10 along the main bronchus has been altered such that some nodes now belong to a different N stage from the previous versions. Under these circumstances, general approval of a standard map has yet to be reached.

Lymph node nomenclature

Level 1 lymph nodes

These correspond to the upper third of the part of the intrathoracic trachea defined by a horizontal line at the upper border of the subclavian artery and a horizontal line at the center point of the trachea, where the upper border of the brachiocephalic vein ascends to the left, in front of the trachea.

Level 2 lymph nodes

These are located between levels 1 and 4, lateral to the trachea, caudal to level 1 and cranial to the azygos vein.

Level 3 anterior lymph nodes

These are located caudal to level 1 and cranial to the right main pulmonary artery, and their centers appear either on the front side of the tracheal anterior wall or behind the anterior wall line of the superior vena cava. In the American nodal system, level 3 pretracheal nodes are eliminated, and are referred to as either right or left level 4 nodes, in the middle of the trachea.

Level 3 posterior lymph nodes

These are located caudal to level 1 and cranial to the tracheal bifurcation, behind the trachea.

Level 4 lymph nodes

These are located along the right and left lateral tracheal walls and caudal to the superior aspect of the azygos vein, with the centers of the anatomical region lying between the anterior and posterior walls of the trachea.

Level 5 lymph nodes

These are located between the aortic arch and the left pulmonary artery, posterior to the vagus nerve.

Level 6 lymph nodes

These are located between the aortic arch and the left pulmonary artery, anterior to the vagus nerve.

Level 7 lymph nodes

These are located under the tracheal bifurcation.

Level 8 lymph nodes

These are located adjacent to the esophagus but caudal to the tracheal bifurcation, and away from the bronchus.

Level 9 lymph nodes

These are located caudal to the inferior pulmonary vein, within the pulmonary ligament.

Dissection of right mediastinal lymph nodes

Once the hilar pleura has been opened and the phrenic nerve taped, the azygos vein can be dissected. The azygos vein is divided whenever additional exposure is required.

At the apex of the thorax, the subclavian and brachiocephalic arteries are exposed by incision of the pleura, and the right recurrent nerve identified. In dissecting the right superior mediastinum, there is hardly ever a situation where one is forced by lymph node metastases to sacrifice the recurrent nerve, as may be necessary during a left superior mediastinal lymph node dissection. Dissection continues downward, exposing the brachiocephalic artery, the superior vena cava, the pretracheal fascia, and the right wall of the ascending aorta. The small veins flowing into the superior vena cava from mediastinal fatty tissue are ligated and divided.

With this approach, superior mediastinal (level 1), posterior mediastinal (level 3p), paratracheal (level 2), tracheobronchial (level 4) and pretracheal (level 3) nodes may be removed.

The lung is retracted forward and the vagus nerve is exposed and taped. Pulmonary branches of the vagus nerve are cut. Next, the subcarinal space is opened, with care being taken to avoid injury to the descending aorta. After exposure of the pericardium, the subcarinal nodes (level 7) are dissected, as well as the contralateral left main bronchial nodes (level 10).

Finally dissection of lymph nodes in the pulmonary ligament (level 9) is performed, starting from the lowest part of the pulmonary ligament and continuing up to dissect the paraesophageal nodes (level 8).

Dissection of left mediastinal lymph nodes

In operations on the left mediastinum, dissection of subcarinal nodes (level 7) and inferior pulmonary ligament nodes (level 9) is performed prior to dissection of the superior mediastinum. Exposure of the subcarinal region is facilitated by retracting the lung anteriorly. Following the dissection of the pulmonary ligament nodes (level 9), the mediastinal pleura is opened, anteriorly and posteriorly, and the vagus nerve taped. The descending aorta and the esophagus are retracted posteriorly and the tracheal bifurcation exposed. The subcarinal nodes (level 7) and then the left bronchial nodes (level 10) are dissected from along the interior aspect of the left and right main bronchi.

The left superior mediastinum is different from the right superior mediastinum in that the limits of the left are not as well defined. The wall of the left brachiocephalic vein is exposed by incising the overlying pleura. The phrenic and vagus nerves should be taped. The posterior wall of the subclavian artery is exposed. Exposing the side wall of the subclavian artery through the incision may allow dissection of the superior mediastinal nodes (left level 4) between the common carotid and subclavian arteries, but to perform this procedure completely, it is necessary to mobilize the aortic arch by division of the ligamentum arteriosum or to use a trans-sternal approach. If the ligamentum arteriosum is divided, dissection of tracheobronchial (level 4) and subaortic nodes (level 5) becomes easy.

The thoracic duct, located at the deepest point between the left common carotid and the left subclavian arteries, is difficult to see. Damaging the mediastinal branches of the thoracic duet can cause chylothorax; therefore lymphatics and blood vessels as they are encountered should be ligated and divided.

Bronchoplasty or bronchoplastic procedures for lung cancer

Bronchoplasty is indicated for central cancers invading a limited portion of the main airways, is an alternative to pneumonectomy, and is intended to preserve pulmonary function.

Normally, bronchoplastic procedures are performed with single-lung ventilation, using a double-lumen endobronchial tube with a low-pressure cuff (Broncocath, by Mallinckrodt) or a spiral double-lumen endobronchial tube. When reconstruction of the left bronchus is performed, a single-lumen endotracheal tube is used during dissection of the left main bronchus; then a Fogarty balloon is inserted across the operative field into the open bronchus and blown up so as to block the left main bronchus, and, when the reconstruction is almost finished, the balloon is taken out, and two or three stitches are used to complete the whole process.

Bronchoplastic procedures are most commonly indicated for resection of right and left upper lobe tumors. In these cases, the bronchoplastic procedure follows division of the pulmonary vein and artery branches and after mediastinal lymph node dissection. Even with the best possible preoperative judging of the area subject to resection, intraoperative pathological examination of the bronchial stump is essential. Non-absorbable sutures such as Ticron may stretch through the bronchus and cause granulation; the use of absorbable sutures, such as Dexon and Vicryl, led to a drastic decrease in complications. More recently, new materials, including monofilament Maxon and PDS, have proven to be acceptable alternatives. The membranous portion should be utilized to adjust for size differences between the anastomosed bronchi. The appropriate depth of the anastomotic sutures into the bronchus, including cartilage, is approximately 2 mm; this is also the distance between sutures.

In patients who have received neoadjuvant therapy and any other cases in which the bronchial closure is felt to be at risk, a pericardial fat pad, parietal pleural flap, pericardium, azygos vein, or omentum may be used to cover the site, both to promote bronchial healing and to prevent fistulization to the surrounding vascular structures.

After the bronchial anastomosis has been completed, airway pressure is applied as in lobectomy to check for the adequacy of anastomosis; chest tubes are placed, and finally the chest is closed.

Postoperatively, patients often have reduced cough; assistance with clearing of bronchial secretion may be necessary, even using a bronchoscope, particularly during the first four or five postoperative days.

Carinal resection and reconstruction

When lung cancer invades the carina, lobectomy or pneumonectomy with carinal resection is required. Rarely, invasion of the superior vena cava and of the aorta or esophagus lead to en bloc combined resection.

Although the resectable area of trachea varies from case to case, resection of up to 9 rings can be performed.

During preoperative examination, an accurate diagnosis of the sites of tracheal involvement is essential. The most reliable tool for diagnosis of sites of tracheal invasion is the fiberscope; however, assessment by macroscopic findings alone is not always possible, and the final determination rests with pathological examination. If invasion into adjacent organs is possibly present, angiography, esophagography, CT scan, or MRI can be used; however, it is often true that a final determination may only be made at intraoperative examination.

The most important part of intraoperative management lies in airway management. For ventilation, a double-lumen endotracheal tube allowing single-lung ventilation is used, provided that the lumen of the airway is sufficiently large. When a tracheal tube for single-lung ventilation cannot be inserted, the operation has to be performed using a single-lumen endotracheal tube, with the anesthetist taking care to ensure that secretions do not accumulate in the dependent side. Once the airway has been cut, a tube passed across the operative field may be used to maintain ventilation; alternatively, in cases where adequate ventilation cannot be maintained through contralateral lung ventilation alone, high-frequency ventilation may be utilized.

Right sleeve pneumonectomy is most commonly performed in the left lateral decubitus position, through a posterolateral thoracotomy, preferably through the 5th rib bed. Hilar dissection is performed, allowing isolation of the pulmonary vein, pulmonary artery, and the right main bronchus. The bronchus and esophagus should remain undissected as much as possible in order to maintain bronchial perfusion. The left main bronchus should be thoroughly dissected from surrounding tissues so as to relieve the anastomosis from tension; however, care is needed not to divide the bronchial artery to the left main bronchus.

Prior to division of the trachea, a stay suture should be placed on the right side wall of the left main bronchus (usually a 3-0 Ticron or 3-0 Prolene). For the anastomosis, a submucosal suture using absorbable monofilament is used, except for the membranous portion, where a standard total layer suture is employed. Differences in airway caliber can be dealt with by altering the distance between sutures in the membranous portion of the trachea and bronchus.

Adequacy of closure of the anastomosis should be confirmed by application of airway pressure and through flexible bronchofiberscopy. The anastomosis is not usually covered; however, if desired, this may be done with a pericardial fat pad.[41]

Various approaches to left sleeve pneumonectomy have been reported; however, resection with anastomosis of the tracheal bifurcation is most commonly performed through a median sternotomy in supine position. The pericardium is incised anteriorly along the ascending aorta, and again incised in the back, followed by exposing the tracheal bifurcation. After complete lymph node dissection, the right main bronchus is divided, with stay sutures being placed both proximal and distal to the point of division. An endotracheal tube can then be inserted through the right main bronchus or the intermediate trunk. The trachea is then divided.

Suturing of the trachea to the right main bronchus should begin with the membranous portion, since this is located furthest from the surgeon. Differences in caliber can again be accounted for by sliding both sides of the cartilage edge slightly and then suturing, or by wedge resection of the anterior wall of bronchus. A suitable suture material is Maxon, or other absorbable monofilament. Suturing of the cartilaginous portion should begin on the left, since needle placement tends to be difficult owing to the presence of the aortic arch. Prior to suturing of the anterior wall of the anastomosis, the operative field endotracheal tube should be removed, and the per orum tracheal tube advanced to lie within the left main bronchus. After suturing of the anterior wall is completed, the tracheal tube should be pulled back into the trachea. The anastomosis should be checked using an air leak test and bronchoscopy, and then covered with thymus and/or a pericardial fat pad. The median sternotomy is then closed, and, through a left posterolateral incision, left pneumonectomy performed, including dissections of the left upper mediastinal hilar lymph nodes and the subcarinal lymph nodes.

Complications after tracheal resection may be minimized by:

- (i) keeping the resection of the membranous portion to a minimum;
- (ii) limiting resection of the main bronchus;
- (iii) minimizing anastomotic tension;
- (iv) performing proper layer-to-layer anastomosis;
- (v) keeping the suture material out of the lumen;
- (vi) providing tissue cover as needed.

Complications occuring after resection of the tracheal bifurcation include pneumonia, bronchial fistula, anastomotic stenosis, bronchovascular fistula, and empyema. The mortality rate from these complications varies from 11% to 29%.[42,43]

Given the above problems, this is an operative procedure that should be performed either by experienced surgeons or under their instruction.

Thoracoscopic surgery

The standard operative therapy for even relatively early stage lung cancer operation is lobectomy combined with systematic lymph node dissection or sampling.[44,45] Video-assisted thoracic surgical (VATS) techniques cannot simply mimic the techniques of a standard operation, but require modifications. Nevertheless, with only slight technical alterations, lobectomy combined with lymph node sampling can be accomplished with thoracoscopic surgery. However, full standard lymph node dissection is difficult to perform, and currently is practised only by a selected number of well-trained surgeons. Because of this, the indications for VATS lobectomy in lung cancer include procedures in which lymph node sampling is appropriate, such as:

- patients with peripheral tumors less than 2 cm in greatest diameter;
- elderly or high-risk patients with clinical stage IA (T1N0M0) and stage IB (T2N0M0);
- from the oncological point of view, patients with stage IA (T1N0M0) and stage IB (T2N0M0) and, according to complete lymph node sampling, apparently without any sign of mediastinal lymph node metastasis, but with metastases pathologically identifiable at surgery.

At this time, VATS lobectomy should not be attempted on patients with clinical stage II or greater stage, after chemotherapy or radiation therapy because of fibrosis around blood vessels and lymph nodes, or on patients with centrally located tumors. Moderate pleural adhesions are not a contraindication.

Under general anesthesia, the patient is intubated with a double-lumen tube, and flexible bronchoscopy is done through the tube in order to assure proper placement and the lack of involvement of major bronchi by the tumor. The patient is placed in the lateral decubitus position, as in standard posterolateral thoracotomy. A pillow or a towel, folded so as to give an appropriate height, should be placed under the scapular angle of the chest, and the pelvis should be lowered, causing the intercostal space on the operative side to be maximally expanded. After the positions of the trocars and the accessory incision have been marked, the patient should be covered up by a surgical drape. In case of an emergency, instruments for a standard thoracotomy should always be available. In normal practice, two sets of TV monitors should be placed – one each behind the operator and the assistant; however, it is also possible for the two sets to be on the right and left sides of the anesthetist, standing towards the head of the patient.

The lung must be fully collapsed for this procedure. If the lung has not been sufficiently collapsed, intrabronchial suctioning in the mainstem bronchus can be helpful. CO_2 insufflation into the pleural space, although utilized by some, is not necessary. Standard monitoring with an arterial line and pulse oximeter is maintained. If it proves impossible to complete the VATS lobectomy, immediate conversion to standard thoracotomy should be performed.

The first trocar is placed in the 7th intercostal space in the anterior axillary line.

The lung is retracted posteriorly to expose the superior pulmonary vein, and to determine the proper placement of the utility thoracotomy incision. In cases of upper lobectomy and middle or lower bi-lobectomy, incisions are made in the 4th and 5th intercostal spaces respectively. A 6–7 cm utility thoracotomy is made from the mid- to the anterior axillary line. A 1.5 cm incision is made in either the auscultatory triangle or the 5th intercostal space in the posterior axillary line. An additional trocar, to be placed through the 7th intercostal space in the posterior axillary line, is useful when inserting the draining tube after the operation. Through these incisions, the thoracic cavity is examined for the presence of pleural dissemination, lymph node metastasis and pulmonary nodules.

For either a right or left upper lobectomy, the lung should be retracted to the back, and the phrenic nerve encircled with a tape. Double ligature of the superior pulmonary vein is followed by ligature and division of V1 and V2 + V3. With a tape placed under the azygos vein on the right for retraction, dissection and ligature of A3 and A1 + A2 are then done sequentially. A tape is then placed under the upper lobe bronchus, which is divided with an autosuture.

Exposure of the bronchus may be facilitated by sump and lobar lymph node dissection.

To perform a middle lobectomy, the procedure, similar to that for right upper lobectomy, is initiated by division of the middle lobe vein, followed by division of the pulmonary artery and the bronchus.

In lower lobectomy, on either the right or left side, the normal procedure involves division of the pulmonary artery through the interlobar fissure. The pulmonary vein and the bronchus are then divided.

There has been much controversy regarding the necessity of lymph node dissection. Although no final position has so far been reached, it is clear that lymph node dissection improves accuracy of staging, and, for some patients with N2 disease, complete resection may improve survival.[48–59] The great concern is that only a limited number of surgeons are able to perform VATS lobectomy together with VATS systematic nodal dissection. However, there are cases in which the benefit of systematic lymph node dissection is minimal – for example, an early bronchioloalveolar cell carcinoma or a peripheral squamous cell cancer less than 2 cm in diameter. VATS lobectomy is therefore performed for patients who may be able to forego systematic nodal dissection, including those with T1N0M0 lung cancer, elderly patients, and those at increased risk because of cardiopulmonary dysfunction, diabetes and hepatic diseases. Systematic nodal dissection conversely is necessary for those good-risk patients with clinical T1N0M0 lung cancer, if they have proved positive on complete lymph node sampling and have proven sentinel node involvement.

In conclusion, experience at the National Cancer Center Hospital, Tokyo has provided sufficient proof that VATS lobectomy should be among the standard surgical procedures for selected patients with lung cancer. The persuasive facts are that the amount of bleeding is much less than with that in standard thoracotomy, complications are limited to a small number, the procedure is safe, and it has a favorable cost–benefit ratio, given the more rapid recovery.

ROUTINE POSTOPERATIVE CARE

Extubation and postoperative supplemental oxygen

The majority of patients undergoing pulmonary resection are able to leave the operating room extubated, and breathing spontaneously; it is rare that a patient requires reintubation in the immediate postoperative period. If it is anticipated that a patient will require postoperative ventilation, the double-lumen endotracheal tube should be removed and replaced with a single-lumen endotracheal tube of sufficient size to permit the introduction of an adult bronchoscope.

Supplemental oxygen may be necessary during the postoperative period if the arterial oxygen saturation measured by pulse oximetry falls to less than 92%, whether at rest or with exercise. For a patient without desaturation, the routine administration of oxygen is counterproductive, since each additional appliance attached to a patient further limits his or her mobility.

Pain control

A thoracotomy is a painful incision, usually visited on a patient with reduced pulmonary reserve who cannot readily afford the additional burden of a painful chest wall limiting ambulation and effective cough. Following thoracotomy, it is the practice at MSKCC that all patients receive either epidural administration of local anesthetics or opiates or a patient-controlled anesthesia pump (PCA) delivering either morphine or meperidine (pethidine). Epidural opiates are associated with complications that are both numerous and possibly life-threatening;[60,61] these include pruritus, ileus, urinary retention, and respiratory depression. However, in experienced hands, epidural analgesia reliably improves pulmonary function after thoracotomy,[62] and should not be withheld from the patient with severe pain and with markedly impaired pulmonary function. It is clear that the majority of patients tolerate post-thoracotomy pain well with a PCA pump alone, or with the addition of oral ketoralac as an adjunct. Four to five days after thoracotomy, oral medications, such as oxycodone/acetaminophen (Percocet), usually suffice.

Antibiotics

Fortunately, a thoracotomy incision is highly resistant to infection; however, pneumonia and empyema are common, and antibiotics are administered in an attempt to lower the incidence of these complications. There is not a large amount of information on the efficiency of specific antibiotics, but penicillin,[63] cefazolin,[64,65] cephalothin,[66] and tetracycline,[67] among other antibiotics, have been investigated for potential efficacy. Currently, a reasonable practice is to administer a broad-spectrum antibiotic, such as cefazolin, one hour prior to skin incision, and to continue administration for 24–48 hours. At MSKCC, antibiotic coverage is not provided for indwelling chest tubes. Antibiotics may be restarted for clinical signs of infection, such as fever, radiographic infiltrates and leukocytosis, and administration must always be guided by sputum Gram stain and culture results.

It might appear reasonable that sputum cultures obtained at the time of thoracotomy could guide postoperative antibiotic administration, and, indeed, it has been suggested[68] that *Haemophilus influenzae* is the most common organism found in intraoperative sputum cultures obtained. However, the authors point out that the organisms cultured were almost always highly sensitive, and, in particular, susceptible to the antibiotics commonly used in the perioperative period. This suggests that cultures obtained in the postoperative period are more likely to be useful than intraoperatively obtained material.

Fluids, electrolytes, and oral intake

A thoracotomy for pulmonary resection is not usually associated with either intraoperative large fluid loss or 'third space' losses in the postoperative period. Therefore most patients leave the operating room relatively euvolemic, and intravenous fluids consisting of 5% dextrose and 0.45% normal saline at 50–75 cm^3/h, administered until oral intake can be resumed, are usually sufficient to maintain adequate intravascular volume and urine at 0.5–1 cm^3/kg body wt/h. Some surgeons practise a vigorous diuresis with the goal of reducing secretions; however, it is entirely possible that this works only to produce a lower volume of thick tenacious secretions, which may be less desirable than a higher volume of more readily cleared thin secretions. Urine output, heart rate, and blood pressure are almost always reliable guides to intravascular volume; measurement of central venous pressure, although commonly performed, correlates poorly with intravascular volume,[69] and, because of the possibility of disruption of a pulmonary artery closure, many surgeons are reluctant to insert Swan–Ganz catheters after pulmonary resection. The values obtained from a wedged Swan–Ganz catheter balloon should be interpreted cautiously, because it is possible that the inflated balloon may occlude a significant portion of the remaining pulmonary vascular bed, artificially elevating right-sided afterload and decreasing cardiac output.

Chest tube management

Chest tubes allow blood, serum and air to escape from the pleural space, but hinder deep inspiration and movement, and so should be left in place only as long as necessary. It is the practice at MSKCC to place only one apical chest tube for wedge excisions or after pneumonectomy, two apical tubes for an upper lobectomy, and one apical and one basilar right-angled tube for a lower lobectomy.

Following resections less than a pneumonectomy, suction is maintained for the first postoperative night, and then tubes are placed to water seal; longer periods of suction may be appropriate following decortications or reoperations, or for patients who have received neoadjuvant therapy. If, after discontinuing suction, chest radiographs reveal a significant amount of increasing air within the pleural space, suction drainage should be reestablished, usually for 36 hours prior to further attempts at discontinuing suction.

Chest tubes should be removed as soon as there is no air leak and fluid drainage has fallen to below 200 cm^3 per day. After removal, an occlusive dressing is left in place for 36 hours; patients should be advised that, after removal of the dressing, it is not uncommon to have additional drainage that is thin, pink, and self-limited, and occurs on approximately the seventh to tenth postoperative day. Should this occur, patients are advised to apply an absorbent dressing only. A persistently elevated chest tube output in the first 24 hours after surgery (over 200 cm^3/h sustained over 4–6 h) in the absence of a coagulation disorder requires surgical reexploration. Confirmation that the drainage is actually blood can be obtained by drawing a small aliquot off with a needle inserted through the wall of the chest tube; if the hematocrit of the chest tube drainage approximates that of a specimen drawn from a peripheral vein, this is strong evidence for intrathoracic bleeding.

Post-pneumonectomy space drainage allows both monitoring for ongoing bleeding and management of the position of the mediastinum. Shifting of the mediastinal structures into the pneumonectomy cavity may lead to hemodynamic compromise, or, if toward the residual lung, respiratory insufficiency. To 'balance' the mediastinum, a single chest tube should be left in the pneumonectomy cavity. Subsequent management varies among surgeons: some remove the tube in the operating room once the patient has been returned to the supine position and is hemodynamically stable; others remove the tube in the recovery room within the first several days once they can be sure that the patient is not bleeding. If it becomes clear that the mediastinum has moved out of the midline after the chest tube has been removed, air can be either introduced into or aspirated from the pneumonectomy cavity by a needle inserted through the chest wall into the pleural cavity. It is important to note that this is only rarely necessary, but may occasionally relieve the patient with an otherwise-unexplained tachycardia. As potential complications include bleeding into or contamination of the pneumonectomy space, this should not be performed unless necessary.

Atelectasis and pneumonia

Atelectasis, with or without secondary infection, is far and away the most serious complication after thoracic surgery, particularly in patients who are obese, who have continued to smoke, or who are of advanced age. Measures directed toward the minimization of postoperative atelectasis should be initiated prior to surgery, and include preoperative education about the operation and expected postoperative course, smoking cessation, and, for high-risk or very deconditioned patients, an exercise program. The most important steps to be implemented in the postoperative period are deep-breathing techniques, the use of incentive spirometry, early and frequent ambulation, and, possibly, intermittent positive-pressure breathing and bronchoscopy.

Deep inspiratory respiratory maneuvers, with or without an incentive spirometer, have been shown to reduce the occurrence of atelectasis after laparotomy from 30% to 10%.[70] Chest physical therapy (PT) is widely practised, but is of unclear benefit since it is often poorly administered and imposes a considerable physiological load on an already-compromised patient. It has been shown that chest PT increases oxygen consumption and carbon dioxide production to approximately 140% of pretreatment levels;[71] however, the arterial oxygen level was decreased less in patients with baseline hypoxia,[72] suggesting that chest PT should not be withheld from marginal patients, if indicated. At MSKCC, the use of chest physical therapy is limited to patients with atelectasis likely to be due to mucus impaction in a major airway. However, for many patients with major airway obstruction, bronchoscopy is preferred, since it can be performed routinely at the patient's bedside, with results that are often quite gratifying. Tracheal suctioning is also commonly performed, but can be associated with significant hypoxia, is uncomfortable, and, since it is performed blindly without the ability to direct the catheter to specific regions of the airway, has also largely been replaced by bronchoscopy.

REFERENCES

1. Ginsberg RJ, Hill LD, Eagan RT et al, Modern 30 day operative mortality for surgical resections in lung cancer. *J Thorac Cardiovasc Surg* 1983; **86**: 654–8.
2. Deslauriers J, Ginsberg RJ, Dubois P et al, Current operative mortality associated with elective surgical resection for lung cancer. *Can J Surg* 1989; **32**: 335–9.
3. Ruckdeschel J, Piantadosi S, Quality of life in lung cancer surgical adjuvant trials. *Chest* 1994; **106**: 324S–8S.
4. Martinez FJ, Paine III R, Medical evaluation of the patient with potentially resectable lung cancer. In: *Lung Cancer: Principles and Practice*, 1st edn (Pass HI, Mitchell JB, Johnson DH, Turrisi AT, eds). Lippincott-Raven: Philadelphia, 1996.
5. Kohman LJ, Meyer JA, Ikings PM, Oates RP, Random versus predictable risks of mortality after thoracotomy for lung cancer. *J Thorac Cardiovasc Surg* 1986; **91**: 551–4.
6. Bolton JW, Weiman DS, Haynes JL et al, Stair climbing as an indicator of pulmonary function. *Chest* 1987; **92**: 783–8.
7. Olsen GN, Bolton JW, Weiman DS, Hornung CA, Stair climbing as an exercise to predict the postoperative complications of lung resection. Two years' experience. *Chest* 1991; **99**: 587–90.
8. Ferguson MK, Little L, Rizzo L et al, Diffusing capacity predicts morbidity and mortality after pulmonary resection. *J Thorac Cardiovasc Surg* 1988; **96**: 894–900.
9. Bechard D, Wetstein L, Assessment of exercise oxygen consumption as preoperative criterion for lung resection. *Ann Thorac Surg* 1987; **44**: 344.
10. Schulz V, Preoperative treatment of chronic obstructive lung disease. In: *Current Topics in General Thoracic Surgery: An International Series*, Vol 2. *Perioperative Care*, 1st edn (Peters RM, Toledo J, eds). Elsevier: Amsterdam, 1992.
11. Gerrard JW, Cockcroft DW, Mink JT et al, Increased nonspecific bronchial reactivity in cigarette smokers with normal lung function. *Am Rev Respir Dis* 1980; **122**: 577–81.
12. Chalon J, Tayyab M, Ramanathan S, Cytology of respiratory epithelium as a predictor of respiratory complications after operations. *Chest* 1975; **67**: 32–5.
13. Sabanathan S, Eng J, Mearns AJ, Alterations in respiratory mechanics following thoracotomy. *J R Coll Surg Edinb* 1990; **35**: 144–5.

14. Kambam JR, Chen LH, Hyman SA, Effect of short term smoking halt on carboxyhemoglobin levels and P50 values. *Anesth Analg* 1986; **65**: 1186–8.
15. Jackson CV, Preoperative pulmonary evaluation. *Arch Intern Med* 1988; **148**: 2120–7.
16. Warner MA, Offord KP, Warner ME et al, Role of preoperative cessation of smoking and other factors in postoperative pulmonary complications: a blinded prospective study of coronary artery bypass patients. *Mayo Clin Proc* 1989; **64**: 609–16.
17. Conradson TB, Eklundh G, Olofsson B, Arrhythmogenicity from combined bronchodilator therapy in patients with obstructive lung disease and concomitant ischemic heart disease. *Chest* 1987; **91**: 5–9.
18. British Thoracic Society Research Committee, Oral *N*-acetylcysteine and exacerbation rates in patients with chronic bronchitis and severe airways obstruction. *Thorax* 1985; **40**: 832–5.
19. Callahan C, Dittus R, Katz B, Oral corticosteroid therapy for patients with stable chronic obstructive pulmonary disease. *Ann Intern Med* 1982; **96**: 17.
20. Anthonisen N, Manfreeda J, Warren C et al, Antibiotic therapy in exacerbations of chronic obstructive pulmonary disease. *Am J Med* 1991; **91**(Suppl 6A): 87S.
21. Cooper JD, Perelman M, Todd TR et al, Precision cautery excision of pulmonary tumors. *Ann Thorac Surg* 1986; **41**: 51–3.
22. Perelman M, Precision techniques for removal of pathological structures from the lungs. *Surgery* 1983; **11**: 12–16.
23. Goldstraw P, Report on the international workshop on intrathoracic staging. *Lung Cancer* 1997; **18**: 107–12.
24. Rouviere H, *Anatomie des Lymphatiques de l'Homme*. Masson: Paris, 1932.
25. Weinberg JA, Identification of regional lymph nodes in the treatment of bronchogenic carcinoma. *J Thorac Surg* 1951; **22**: 517–26.
26. Nohl HC, *The Spread of Carcinoma of the Bronchus*. Lloyd-Duke: London, 1962.
27. Borrie J, *Lung Cancer: Surgery and Survival*. Meredith: New York, 1965.
28. Naruke T, The spread of lung cancer and its relevance to surgery. *Jpn J Surg* 1967; **68**: 1607–21.
29. Naruke T, Suemasu K, Surgical treatment for lung cancer with metastasis to mediastinal lymph nodes. *J Thorac Cardiovasc Surg* 1976; **71**: 279–85.
30. Naruke T, Suemasu K, Ishikawa S, Lymph node mapping and curability at various levels of metastasis in resected lung cancer. *J Thorac Cardiovasc Surg* 1978; **76**: 832–9.
31. American Joint Committee on Cancer Staging and End Results Reporting, Task Force on Lung Cancer, *Staging of Lung Cancer*. American Joint Committee on Cancer: Chicago, 1979.
32. Martini N, Improved methods of recording data in lung cancer. *Clin Bull Memorial Sloan–Kettering Cancer Center* 1976; **6**: 93–8.
33. Mountain F, *'Cancer of the Lung' Classification and Staging of Cancer by Site*. American Joint Committee on Cancer: Chicago, 1976: 95–108.
34. Sellers AH, *A Brochure of Checklists*. International Union Against Cancer: Geneva, 1980.
35. International Union Against Cancer (UICC), *TNM Atlas. Illustrated Guide to the TNM/pTNM Classification of Malignant Tumors*, 3rd edn. Springer-Verlag: New York, 1990: 134–44.
36. American Thoracic Society, Clinical staging of primary lung cancer. *Am Rev Respir Dis* 1983; **127**: 659.
37. Mountain CF, Dresler CM, Regional lymph node classification for lung cancer staging. *Chest* 1997; **111**: 1718–23.
38. Naruke T, Yoneyama T, Ogata T et al, Bronchoplastic procedures for lung carcinoma. *J Thorac Cardiovasc Surg* 1977; **73**: 927–35.
39. Naruke T, Suemasu K, Bronchoplastic surgery for lung cancer and the results. *Jpn J Surg* 1983; **13**: 165–72.
40. Jensik RJ, Faber LP, Brown CM, Kittle CF, Bronchoplastic and conservative resectional procedures for bronchial adenoma. *J Thorac Cardiovasc Surg* 1974; **16**: 556–65.
41. Tsuchiya R, Goya T, Naruke T, Resection of tracheal carina for lung cancer: procedure, complications and mortality. *J Thorac Cardiovasc Surg* 1980; **99**: 779–87.

42. Jensik RJ, Faber LP, Kittle CF et al, Survival in patients undergoing tracheal sleeve pneumonectomy for bronchogenic carcinoma. *J Thorac Cardiovasc Surg* 1982; **84**: 489–96.
43. Naruke T, Kondo H, Goya T et al, Carinoplasty and surgically related problems. *Lung Cancer* 1993; **9**: 203–12.
44. Naruke T, Goya T, Tsuchiya R, Suemasu K, The importance of surgery to non-small cell carcinoma of the lung with mediastinal lymph node metastasis. *Ann Thorac Surg* 1998; **96**: 440–7.
45. Ginsberg RJ, Rubinstein LV, Randomized trial of lobectomy versus limited resection for T1N0 non-small cell lung cancer. *Ann Thorac Surg* 1995; **60**: 615–23.
46. Noguchi M, Morikawa A, Kawasaki M et al, Small adenocarcinoma of the lung: histologic characteristics and prognosis. *Cancer* 1995; **75**: 2844–52.
47. Asamura H, Nakayama H, Kondo H et al, Lymph node metastasis, recurrence, and prognosis in resected small, peripheral, non-small cell lung carcinomas: Are these carcinomas candidates for video-assisted lobectomy? *J Thorac Cardiovasc Surg* 1996; **110**: 1125–34.
48. Smith RA, The importance of mediastinal lymph node invasion by pulmonary carcinoma in selection of patients for resection. *Ann Thorac Surg* 1978; **25**: 5–11.
49. Rubinstein I, Baum GL, Kalter Y et al, Resectional surgery in the treatment of primary carcinoma of the lung with mediastinal lymph node metastases. *Thorax* 1979; **34**: 33–40.
50. Kirsh MM, Sloan H, Mediastinal metastases in bronchogenic carcinoma. Influence of postoperative irradiation, cell type, and location. *Ann Thorac Surg* 1982; **33**: 459–63.
51. Pearson FG, Delarue NC, Ilves R et al, Significance of positive superior mediastinal nodes identified at mediastinoscopy in patients with resectable cancer of the lung. *J Thorac Cardiovasc Surg* 1982; **83**: 1–11.
52. Mountain CF, The biological operability of stage III non-small cell lung cancer. *Ann Thorac Surg* 1985; **40**: 60–4.
53. Martini N, Fleminger BJ, The role of surgery in N2 lung cancer. *Surg Clin North Am* 1987; **67**: 1037–49.
54. Naruke T, Goya T, Tsuchiya R et al, The importance of surgery to non-small cell carcinoma of lung with mediastinal lymph node metastasis. *Ann Thorac Surg* 1988; **46**: 603–10.
55. Watanabe Y, Shimizu J, Oda M et al, Aggressive surgical intervention in N2 non-small cell cancer of the lung. *Ann Thorac Surg* 1991; **51**: 253–61.
56. Maggi G, Casadio C, Cianci R et al, Results of surgical resection of stage IIIa (N2) non small cell lung cancer, according to the site of the mediastinal metastases. *Int Surg* 1983; **78**: 213–17.
57. Miller DL, McManus KG, Allen MS et al, Results of surgical resection in patients with N2 non-small cell lung cancer. *Ann Thorac Surg* 1994; **57**: 1096–101.
58. Goldstraw P, Manam GC, Kaplan DK et al, Surgical management of non-small-cell lung cancer with ipsilateral mediastinal node metastasis (N2 disease). *J Thorac Cardiovasc Surg* 1994; **104**: 19–28.
59. Riquet M, Manac'h D, Saab M et al, Factors determining survival in resected N2 lung cancer. *Eur J Cardiovasc Thorac Surg* 1995; **9**: 300–4.
60. Bromage PR, Camporesi EM, Durant PAC et al, Nonrespiratory side effects of epidural morphine. *Anesth Analg* 1982; **61**: 490–5.
61. Gustafsson LL, Schildt B, Jacobsen K, Adverse effects of epidural and intrathecal opiates: report of a nationwide survey in Sweden. *Br Anaesth* 1982; **54**: 479–86.
62. Zenz M, Schappler-Scheele B, Neuhaus R et al, Long-term peridural morphine analgesia in cancer patients. *Lancet* 1981; **i**: 91.
63. Frimodt-Moller N, Ostri P, Pedersen IK, Poulsen SE, Antibiotic prophylaxis in pulmonary surgery: a double blinded study of penicillin versus placebo. *Ann Surg* 1982; **195**: 444–50.
64. Kvale PA, Ranga V, Kopacz M, Pulmonary resection. *South Med J* 1977; **70**: 64–8.
65. Truesdale R, D'Allessandri R, Manuel V et al, Antimicrobial vs placebo prophylaxis in noncardiac surgery. *JAMA* 1979; **241**: 1254–6.
66. Ilves R, Cooper JD, Todd TR, Pearson FG.

Prospective, randomized, double blind study using prophylactic cephalothin for major, elective, general thoracic operations. *J Thorac Cardiovasc Surg* 1981; **81**: 813–17.

67. Tarkka M, Polela R, Lepojarvi M et al, Infection prophylaxis in pulmonary surgery: A randomized prospective study. *Ann Thorac Surg* 1987; **44**: 508–13.
68. Wansbrough-Jones MH, Nelson A, New L et al, Bronchoalveolar lavage in the prediction of post-thoracotomy chest infection. *Eur J Cardiovasc Surg* 1991; **5**: 433–4.
69. Shoemaker WC, Monitoring of the critically ill patient. In: *Surgery of the Chest*, 2nd edn (Shoemaker WC, Thompson WL, Holbrook PR, eds). Saunders: Philadelphia, 1990.
70. Baxter WD, Levine RS, An evaluation of intermittent positive pressure breathing in the prevention of postoperative pulmonary complications. *Arch Surg* 1969; **98**: 795–8.
71. Weissman C, Kemper M, Damask MC et al, Effect of routine intensive care interactions on metabolic rate. *Chest* 1984; **86**: 815–18.
72. Pryor JA, Webber BA, Hodson ME, Effect of chest physiotherapy on oxygen saturation in patients with cystic fibrosis. *Thorax* 1990; **45**: 77.

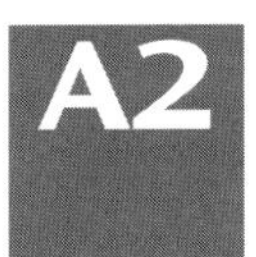

Appendix 2: Chemotherapy*

Cristiana Sessa, Heine H Hansen

Contents

GLOSSARY OF TERMINOLOGY USED IN CLINICAL PHARMACOKINETICS

Absolute bioavailability is the fraction of drug absorbed upon extravascular administration in comparison with the dose administered.

Area under the curve (AUC∞) is a measure of the quantity of unchanged drug absorbed and in the body, calculated as the integral of drug plasma or blood levels over time from zero to infinity.

Bioavailability (F) is the fraction of drug systematically available, defined as both the fraction of the administered dose absorbed and the fraction of absorbed dose reaching systemic circulation in the presence of a first-pass effect.

Central compartment is the sum of all body regions (organs and tissues) in which the drug concentration is in instantaneous equilibrium with that in blood or plasma. Blood or plasma is always part of the central compartment.

Compartment is a mathematical entity that can be described by a definite volume and a concentration of drug contained in it. In pharmacokinetics, experimental data are explained by fitting them to compartmental models.

Cumulative urinary excretion curves are plots of the actual cumulative amounts of drug and/or its metabolites excreted into urine versus time after administration.

Disposition is the loss of drug from the central

*Adapted from Sessa C, Anticancer agents. In: *Textbook of Medical Oncology*, 2nd edn (Cavalli F, Hansen HH, Kaye SB, eds). Martin Dunitz: London, 2000.

compartment due to distribution into other compartments and/or elimination and metabolism.

Dose or concentration dependence refers to a change of one or more of the pharmacokinetic processes of absorption, distribution, metabolism and excretion with increasing dose or concentration.

Elimination (biological) half-life ($t_{1/2}$) of a drug is the time required for the drug levels (in blood, plasma or serum) to decline by 50% after equilibrium (between plasma and tissue) is reached. Loss of drug from the body, as described by the biological half-life, means the elimination of the administered parent drug molecule (not its metabolites) by urinary excretion (renal clearance), metabolism (metabolic clearance) or other pathways of elimination (lung, skin, etc.). It includes $t_{1/2\alpha}$ (distribution) and $t_{1/2\beta}$ (terminal). For drugs with a high tissue distribution (arthracyclines, platinum compounds), $t_{1/2}$ also includes $t_{1/2\gamma}$, which reflects accumulation and slow release from third spare compartment. $t_{1/2}$ may be influenced by dose, variation in urinary excretion (pH), intersubject variation, age, protein binding, concomitant drugs, and liver and renal functions.

Enzyme induction is an increase in enzyme content or rate of enzymatic processes resulting in faster metabolism of a compound. It may increase clearance and decrease biological half-life.

Enzyme inhibition is a decrease in the rate of metabolism of a compound, usually by competition for an enzyme system. It may increase biological half-life and decrease clearance of a drug.

First-pass effect is the phenomenon in which some drugs are already *metabolized* (not chemically degraded) between the site of absorption and reaching systemic circulation. It may occur in the gut wall, mesenteric blood and/or the liver, upon oral and deep rectal administration.

Hepatic clearance (CL_H) is the hypothetical volume of distribution in litres of the unmetabolized drug that is cleared in one minute via the liver. It depends upon intrinsic hepatic clearance and liver blood flow.

Loading dose, **Priming dose** or **Initial dose** is the dose used in initiating therapy so as to rapidly achieve therapeutic concentrations. The need for a loading dose depends upon biological half-life, dosing interval and therapeutic concentration to be achieved.

Mean residence time (MRT) is the average time that the drug stays in the body or plasma.

Nonlinear kinetics or **Saturation kinetics** refers to a change in one or more of the pharmacokinetic parameters during absorption, distribution, metabolism or excretion caused by saturation or overloading because of increasing doses.

Peak concentration (C_{max}) is the maximum concentration of a drug achieved in plasma or in blood after drug administration.

Peripheral compartment is the sum of all body regions (i.e. organs, tissues or parts of them) to which a drug is eventually distributed, but is not in instantaneous equilibrium with the central compartment.

Plasma clearance (CL) can be defined as the volume of plasma that is completely cleared of drug per unit time.

Protein binding is the phenomenon that occurs when a drug combines with plasma protein to form a reversible complex. Some drugs can be displaced from protein binding by other compounds of higher affinity for the protein-binding sites. Protein binding is of clinical significance (e.g. with regard to displacement, volume of distribution and metabolism) when it exceeds 80–90%. It is the unbound drug that is in equilibrium with the biophase (FF).

Renal clearance (CL_R) is the hypothetical plasma volume in litres (volume of distribution) of the unmetabolized drug that is cleared per unit time via the kidney. Renal clearance is affected by renal blood flow, urinary pH, and the net effects of tubular reabsorption and secretion.

Steady-state concentration (C_{ss}) is the concentration of drug in blood and tissue upon multiple dosing when input and output are at equilibrium or during a constant-rate intravenous infusion.

Time to peak concentration (T_{max}) is the time until C_{max} is reached from drug administration.

Total body clearance (CL_b) is an overall measure of the body's drug removal rate. CL_b is the result of all drug removal processes, including renal clearance of the unchanged drug and metabolic clearance. CL_b is the hypothetical volume of distribution in litres of the unmetabolized drug that is cleared per unit of time (l/min or l/h) by any pathway of drug removal (renal, hepatic and other pathways of elimination); it is a proportionality constant relating absorbed dose and steady-state blood, plasma and serum concentration.

Volume of distribution (V_d) is the hypothetical volume of body fluid that would be required to dissolve the total amount of drug at the same concentration as that found in blood or plasma. It is a proportionality constant that relates the amount of drug in the body to the serum or plasma concentration.

ABBREVIATIONS

Drugs

5-CHO-FH_4: 5-formyltetrahydrofolate (leucovorin)
5-FU: 5-fluorouracil

Ara-C: cytarabine
ATRA: all-*trans*-retinoic acid

BLM: bleomycin

CCNU: lomustine
CPT-11: irinotecan
CTX: cyclophosphamide

dFdC: difluorodeoxycytidine (gemcitabine)
DHAD: mitoxantrone

EPI: epirubicin

FT: ftorafur

HMM: hexamethylmelamine
HN_2: mechlorethamine
HU: hydroxyurea

IFO: ifosfamide

LV: leucovorin

MGA: megestrol acetate
MMC: mitomycin C

MPA: medroxyprogesterone acetate
MTX: methotrexate

VCR: vincristine
VLB: vinblastine
VM-26: teniposide
VP-16: etoposide

Other abbreviations

ADA: adenosine deaminase
ADCC: antibody-dependent cell-mediated cytotoxicity
AICAR: aminoimidazole carboxamide ribonucleotide transformylase
ANC: absolute neutrophil count
AP: alkaline phosphatase
AR: androgen receptor
Ara-CTP: cytarabine triphosphate
Ara-U: uracil arabinoside
AST: aspartate transarinase
AUC: area under the curve, concentration × time

BM: bone marrow

CDC: complement-dependent cytotoxicity
CdR kinase: deoxycytidine kinase
CH_2-FH_4: reduced-folate cofactor
CHF: cardiac heart failure
CI: continuous infusion
CL: clearance
CNS: central nervous system
COPD: chronic obstructive pulmonary disease
Cr: creatinine
CR: complete remission
CSF: cerebrospinal fluid
C_{ss}: steady-state concentration
Cyd deaminase: cytidine deaminase
CYP450: cytochrome P450

dATP: deoxyadenosine triphosphate
dCTP: deoxycytidine-5'-triphosphate
dFdCTP: difluorodeoxycytidine triphosphate
dFdU: difluorodeoxyuridine
DHFR: dihydrofolate reductase
DL: dose-limiting
dNTP: deoxynucleotide triphosphate
DPD: dihydropyrimidine dehydrogenase
dTTP: deoxythymidine triphosphate
DVT: deep venous thrombosis

F-DHU: 5-fluorodihydrouracil
FdUMP: 5-fluoro-2'-deoxyuridine 5'-monophosphate
FH_4: reduced folates
FPGS: folylpolyglutamate synthethase
FUMP: 5-fluorouridine 5'-monophosphate
FUTP: 5-fluorouridine 5'-triphosphate

GAR: glycinamide ribonucleotide transformylase
G-CSF: granulocyte colony-stimulating factor
GFR: glomerular filtration rate
GM-CSF: granulocyte–macrophage colony-stimulating factor

H_2O_2: hydrogen peroxide
HAI: intrahepatic arterial infusion
HGPRTase: hypoxanthine–guanine phosphoribosyl transferase
HSR: hypersensitivity reaction
HZ: herpes zoster

IFN: interferon
IL: interleukin
i.t.: intrathecal

LFTs: liver function tests
LVEF: left ventricular ejection fraction

MDR: multidrug resistance
mFBP: membrane folate-binding protein
MMR: mismatch repair
MTD: maximum tolerated dose
MTIC: 5-(3-methyl-1-triazeno)-imidazole-4-carboxamide

NAD: nicotinamide adenine dinucleotide
N&V: nausea and vomiting
NSAID: non-steroidal antiinflammatory drug
NV: normal value

$O_2^{\cdot -}$: superoxide
O^6-**AT**: DNA–O^6-alkylguanine–DNA alkyltransferase
OH: hydroxyl radical

PALA: *N*-phosphonocetyl-L-aspartate
PB: premature beats
PBSC: peripheral blood stem cell support
PDGF: platelet-derived growth factor
PE: pulmonary embolism
PEG: polyethylene glycol
P-gp: P-glycoprotein
PK: pharmacokinetics
PKC: protein kinase C
plt: platelets
PRPP: phosphoribosyl pyrophosphate
PS: performance status
PT: prothrombin time
pts: patients
PTT: partial thromboplastin time

RAR: retinoic acid receptor
RBC: red blood cells
RIA: radioimmunoassay
RNR: ribonucleotide reductase
RT: radiotherapy

TE: thromboembolic
Topo: topoisomerase
TS: thymidylate synthase

VOD: veno-occlusive disease

WBC: white blood cells

ALKYLATING AGENTS

Name, chemistry, relevant features	Mechanism of action	Pharmacology and dose modifications
Mechlorethamine (HN_2) [Mustargen]*	Prototype bifunctional alkylating agent: covalent bond of the alkyl group to N-7 of guanine with formation of DNA-interstrand crosslinks between two guanines located in the opposite strands	Chemical transformation into highly reactive compounds, rapidly bound to tissues. Degradation by spontaneous hydrolysis. PK not studied
Cyclophosphamide (CTX) [Cytoxan] Cyclic phosphamide ester of HN_2	Hepatic CYP450 activation to highly reactive metabolites (acrolein: bladder irritant; phosphoramide mustard: alkylating moiety) causing DNA–interstrand crosslinks	p.o well absorbed. Biphasic plasma disappearance with $t_{1/2\beta}$ = 4–6.5 h after 6–80 mg/kg; high degree of interpatient variation in metabolism; renal excretion of metabolites; only CTX measured in CSF. ↓ dose if Cr CL < 20 ml/min
Ifosfamide (IFO) [Ifex] Analogue of CTX; oxazophosphorine HN_2	In comparison with CTX, slower hepatic activation to acrolein and ifosforamide mustard (which causes DNA–interstrand crosslinks) and higher proportion of inactive dechloroethylated metabolites	High degree of interpatient/intrapatient variability of PK and metabolism. $t_{1/2}$ = 15 h; 55% unchanged drug in urine after single doses (3.8–5 g/m^2). Induction of IFO metabolism after 3 days of i.v. bolus or CI with increased CL due to production of dechloroethylated species; decreased urinary fraction of unchanged IFO after repeated doses. Comparable serum AUCs and urinary fractions of IFO and metabolites after i.v. bolus and CI administration; no effect of dexamethasone on IFO metabolism. CSF: plasma ratio greater for IFO than for CTX; CSF:plasma ratio for ifosforamide mustard greater than that of IFO or any other metabolite; CL_R <25% GFR rate; ↓ dose in renal impairment.

* Drug names given in square brackets denote trade names

Drug interactions	Route, dosage and administration	Toxicity
	LOCAL VESICANT ON EXTRAVASATION i.v.: 0.4 mg/kg (10–12 mg/m^2) every 4–6 weeks	Neutropenia and thrombocytopenia (after about 8 days, for 10–20 days); acute severe prolonged N & V; phlebitis, rare severe allergic reactions; maculopapular rash
Potential, but of unknown clinical relevance with CYP450 enzyme activity inducers (barbiturates) or blockers (glucocorticoids); detoxification with mesna	p.o: 50–100 mg/m^2 daily i.v.: 1000–1500 mg/m^2 every 3 weeks *i.v. high-dose:* 7000 mg/m^2 (MTD) (i.v. hydration + mesna)	DL neutropenia after 8–14 days, recovering within 10 days; N & V (delayed with i.v. therapy); alopecia; haemorrhagic cystitis (prevented by adequate pre- and posthydration) Thrombocytopenia; SIADH (more common at >50 mg/kg); cardiotoxicity (↑ incidence in case of prior anthracyclines, large single infusions, glutathione-depleting agents)
See CTX; ↑ renal damage with nephrotoxic drugs (cisplatin); ↑ CNS toxicities with CNS-active agents (including opioids, some antiemetics); methylene blue to reverse and prevent CNS toxicities	Adequate hydration before, up to 72 h after to avoid haemorrhagic cystitis. i.v.: short (1–3 h infusion) or CI: 1.2–1.5 g/m^2 on days 1–3 or on days 1–5 every 3–4 weeks; 24 h CI: 5 g/m^2 *i.v. high-dose (CI):* 3–4 g/m^2 on days 1–4 (MTD)	DL haemorrhagic cystitis prevented with mesna; myelosuppression with cumulative anaemia; >50% N & V; >80% alopecia; 12% CNS toxicity with confusion, lethargy, seizures; 60% nephrotoxicity (tubular), Similar toxicities, but of ↑ incidence and degree

Name, chemistry, relevant features	Mechanism of action	Pharmacology and dose modifications
Mesna [Uromitexan] Sodium mercaptoethane sulfonate	Selective urinary tract protectant for oxazophosphorine-type alkylating agents through binding of the SH moiety to acrolein	Dimerization in blood to the inactive disulfide dimesna, reduced back to mesna in renal tubules and excreted in urine. 40% and 30% urinary bioavailability of free-thiol mesna after i.v. and p.o. administration; lower more prolonged (between 12 and 24 h) urinary excretion of free-thiol mesna after p.o. than i.v. administration
Thiotepa *N*, *N*', *N*''-triethylene thiophosphoramide Can be administered by any parenteral route	Polyfunctional alkylating agent with three aziridine groups. Intracellular release of aziridine and generation of ethylenimonium ions acting as monofunctional alkylating agents; the different functional groups induce DNA-interstrand crosslinks	40% protein-bound; rapid activation by CYP450 to main metabolite TEPA, less cytotoxic and with longer terminal $t_{1/2}$ (5 h); 24% of dose excreted in 24 h urine Possible metabolic saturation at the highest doses studied (6–7 mg/kg). Advantages of i.t. over i.v. administration still to be verified. After i.v., CSF levels equivalent to those in plasma
Lomustine (CCNU) Chloroethylcyclohexyl-nitrosourea	DNA chloroethylation, with formation of inter- and intrastrand crosslinks between guanine and cytosine on opposite strands; carbamoylation of proteins through isocyanate molecules	Rapid absorption, decomposition and metabolism in liver with parent drug never detectable; C_{max} of metabolites within 3 h. 50% of dose in 12 h urine as degradation products. >30% plasma levels in CSF
Temozolomide [Temodal] Imidazotetrazine derivative; methyl derivative of mitozolamide	Prodrug; converted to cytotoxic MTIC through chemical process. ↑ induction of O^6-alkylguanine adducts with depletion of O^6-AT. Schedule-dependent antitumour activity	100% *F* not affected by food or ranitidine. Rapidly absorbed, with C_{max} at 0.7 h; $t_{1/2\beta}$ = 1.8 h; linear PK. Wide tissue distribution; crosses blood–brain barrier; ratio CSF/plasma AUC = 30%. No accumulation with daily dosing. Clearance not affected by anticonvulsants, H_2 blockers, barbiturates, dexamethasone

Drug interactions	Route, dosage and administration	Toxicity
Incompatible in solution with cisplatin; does not affect the antitumour activity of other cytotoxic agents	*IFO/CTX i.v. short infusion:* 60% daily total dose divided in 3 doses (each 20%) 15 min before (always i.v.), 4 and 8 h later. Double dose if p.o. *IFO CI*: same equal dose (directly mixed), continue up to 12–16 h after the end of IFO	p.o.: N & V if given undiluted; in case of V within 1 h, redose i.v. False ↑ of urinary chetones
Inhibition of pseudocholinesterase activity with ↑ effect of succinylcholine.↑ absorption from body cavities in presence of infiltration/inflammation of mucosa (radiotherapy)	i.v. bolus: 0.3–0.4 mg/kg every 1–4 weeks *i.v. high-dose:* 500–1125 mg/m^2 (MTD 1000 mg/m^2) Intrapleural, intrapericardial: 60 mg at ⩾1 week interval Intravesical: 30–60 mg/week × 4 i.t.: 15 mg at ⩾1 week interval	Dose-related and cumulative myelosuppression with short WBC and longer plt nadir DL mucositis; hyperpigmentation of skin; hepatotoxicity; confusion, somnolence Rare myelosuppression Lower-abdominal discomfort, bladder irritability
↑ myelosuppression with cimetidine	p.o.: 100–130 mg/m^2 (single agent) every 6–8 weeks (empty stomach)	Delayed (after 3–6 weeks) potentially cumulative myelosuppression; acute N & V; mild reversible hepatic toxicity; ↑ risk of second malignancy after long-term therapy
Possible synergism with antitumour agents with similar mechanism of action to deplete O^6-AT. Possible synergism with ionizing radiation	p.o.: 150–200 mg/m^2 on days 1–5 every 4 weeks (fasting, single-dose) Heavily pretreated patients: 150 mg/m^2 on days 1–5 every 4 weeks Non-heavily pretreated patients: 200 mg/m^2 on days 1–5 every 4 weeks	DL myelotoxicity (mainly anaemia and thrombocytopenia), with nadir about day 22 and recovery in 7–14 days; 50% N & V; 30% fatigue and malaise

Name, chemistry, relevant features	Mechanism of action	Pharmacology and dose modifications
Procarbazine An *N*-methylhydrazine: structure similar to MAO inhibitors	Prodrug; generates several reactive free radicals, with direct damage to DNA through auto-oxidation, chemical decomposition and CYP450-mediated metabolism. Also generates methyldiazonium with monofunctional alkylating activity. Also DNA methylation mainly at N^7-O^6 of guanine, with extent of O^6 methylation correlated with O^6-AT activity	Completely absorbed, with peak plasma and CSF concentrations in 1 h. Rapidly concentrated and metabolized ($t_{1/2\beta}$ = 10 min) in liver and kidney, with 75% of dose excreted as metabolites in 24 h urine; ↓ dose if liver or renal impairment; guidelines not available
Hexamethylmelamine (HMM) [Hexalen] Triazene ring with dimethylamino groups at each of the three carbons	Still unknown, possibly DNA alkylation; structurally similar to triethylenemelamine	>90% protein-bound; variable p.o. absorption with peak levels after 0.5–3 h. Rapid demethylation by microsomal CYP450 enzymes; $t_{1/2\beta}$ = 3–10 h; 60–70% of dose in 24 h urine as metabolites

Drug interactions	Route, dosage and administration	Toxicity
Inhibition of MAO with ↑ effect of CNS depressants, ↑ effect of sympathomimetic drugs (isoproterenol, ephedrine), tricyclic antidepressants or tyramine-rich foods (dark beer, cheese, red wine, bananas), with hypertensive crisis, tremor, palpitations. Antabuse-like activity with severe GI toxicity, headache, if concomitant alcohol. Possible interaction with antitumour agents through (1) inhibition of CYP450 enzyme system; (2) depletion of O^6-AT	p.o.: 100 mg/m^2 on days 1–14 every 4 weeks in combination; (lower initial doses with daily increase to ↓ GI toxicity)	DL delayed myelosuppression (mainly thrombocytopenia after up to 4 weeks); acute GI toxicity (N & V, diarrhoea), with tolerance after continued administration; 'flu-like syndrome at the beginning of treatment; allergic reactions with skin rash and pulmonary infiltrates (controlled with low-dose cortisone); CNS disturbances (paraesthesia, headache, insomnia). Late toxicities; azospermia, anovulation
Possible with CYP450 enzyme inducers (phenobarbitone) with ↓ antitumour effect. Severe orthostatic hypotension with concomitant MAO inhibitors	p.o.: single agent, 260 mg/m^2 on days 1–14; combination, 150–200 mg/m^2 on days 1–14 every 4 weeks (four divided daily doses)	DL N & V, ↓ if taken after meals. Cumulative central (somnolence, mood disorders, hallucinations) dizziness and peripheral (mainly sensory) neurotoxicity. Reversible mild leukopenia

PLATINUM COMPOUNDS

Name, chemistry, relevant features	Mechanism of action	Pharmacology and dose modifications
Cisplatin (DDP) *cis*-Diamminedichloro-platinum(II) Inorganic planar coordination complex	DNA binding of aquated species, with formation of DNA inter- and intrastrand crosslinks. Binding to SH groups of critical enzymes. Mechanisms of resistance include ↓ cellular drug accumulation, cytosolic inactivation by thiol-containing compounds, enhancement of DNA repair, overexpression of some proto-oncogenes and loss of DNA MMR activity	Active species produced within the cell by aquation hydrolysis. 90% protein-bound; poor CSF penetration. Triphasic disappearance of total platinum with $t_{1/2\gamma} = 5.4$ days and high tissue distribution. 90% renal excretion, mainly by glomerular filtration; 40% of dose excreted in 24 h urine. Mannitol and higher hydration to ↑ diuresis in case of mild renal impairment (Cr CL 50–70 ml/min)
Carboplatin (CBDCA) 1,1-Cyclobutane-dicarboxylato(2−)-*O*, *O*′]-platinum(II) Second-generation platinum compound; 10-fold more water-soluble than cisplatin	Same as that of cisplatin; slower reactivity with DNA and lower potency than cisplatin. Mechanisms of resistance possibly similar to those of cisplatin	Lower relative rate of activation than cisplatin. 60–80% protein-bound; $t_{1/2}$ of ultrafilterable platinum of 170 min. Triphasic disappearance of total platinum, with $t_{1/2\beta} = 1.5$ h and $t_{1/2\gamma} = 5.8$ days. 30% plasma levels in CSF after i.v. treatment. 70% of dose in 24 h urine; plasma clearance of ultrafilterable species correlated to GFR; if impaired renal function, doses are based on Cr CL as estimate of GFR to avoid severe myelotoxicity

Drug interactions	Route, dosage and administration	Toxicity
Delayed excretion of drugs eliminated through kidneys (MTX, BLM, IFO); ↑ renal toxicity with concomitant nephrotoxic drugs (aminoglycosides, amphotericin B); ↓ renal toxicity with concomitant SH-containing agents (sodium thiosulfate, amifostine, glutathione). ↑ incidence of peripheral neuropathy when administered with taxanes	*Standard dose:* i.v. (30–60 min infusion): 50–100 mg/m^2 every 3 weeks; 20 mg/m^2 on days 1–5 every 3 weeks (with pre-post hydration to ↑ diuresis and prevent renal toxicity) *High-dose:* i.v. (60 min infusion): 120 mg/m^2 single day every 3 weeks; 40 mg/m^2 on days 1–5 every 3 weeks (with hypertonic saline; nephroprotective agents).i.p.: 90–270 mg/m^2 (with pre–post hydration)	Dose-dependent, early (after 1–24 h) severe and delayed (after 24–120 h) N & V; acute tubular damage with hypomagnesaemia; cumulative subclinical tubular damage with ↓ Cr CL; cumulative peripheral sensory neuropathy (paraesthesias, sensory loss), slowly reversible; 30% irreversible Same toxicities but of ↑ incidence and degree; dose-dependent high-frequency hearing loss and myelotoxicity (anaemia). Rare, focal encephalopathy and retinal toxicity
Dose modifications: *Calvert formula:* (GFR as estimated by ^{51}Cr-EDTA or 24 h urine collection). Total dose (mg) = target AUC × (GFR + 25); pretreated pts AUC, 4–6 mg/ml/min; untreated pts AUC, 6–8 mg/ml/min *Egorin formula:* Dose (mg/m^2) = 317 × {[(pretreatment plt count − plt nadir desired)/ pretreatment plt count] × 100 − *} × (BSA/Cr CL) + 447 Pretreated pts * = 92.4 Untreated pts * = 82.1	*Standard dose:* i.v. (30–60 min infusion): Untreated pts/ Calvert formula; single agent, AUC 6–8 mg/ml·min every 3–4 weeks; combination, AUC 4–5 mg/ml·min every 3–4 weeks (without hydration) *High dose:* i.v. (60 min infusion): Single agent, 2000 mg/m^2 (MTD) (with hydration); combination, AUC 11–20 mg/ml·min	DL cumulative thrombocytopenia after 2–3 weeks, recovering within 2 weeks; moderate N & V after 6–12 h; allergic reactions after very high cumulative doses; no cross-reactivity with cisplatin; transient ↑ hepatic enzymes Myelotoxicity; peripheral neuropathy; hepatotoxicity; nephrotoxicity with loss of serum electrolytes

ANTITUMOUR ANTIBIOTICS

Name, chemistry, relevant features	Mechanism of action	Pharmacology and dose modifications
Bleomycin sulfate (BLM) Mixture of sulfur-containing glycopeptides; formed by a DNA-binding fragment and an iron-binding portion. Activation through O_2 binding. 1 mg = 1 U of inhibitory activity in vitro	DNA binding, with production of single- and double-strand breaks; DNA damage affected by specific repair enzymes, glutathione, ionizing radiation. BLM inactivated by BLM hydrolase pulmonary toxicity as a result of low enzyme concentration and high O_2 tension	10% protein-bound; $t_{1/2}$ = 2–3 h. Rapid tissue inactivation, lower in skin and lung, with 50% of dose in 24 h urine, mainly as inactive species. C_{max} with i.m. administration after 30–60 min, 1/3 of those after i.v. ↓ excretion and ↑ toxicity if renal impairment; ↓ dose by 50% if Cr CL ≤ 30 ml/min
Mitomycin C (MMC) Possible preferential activation in hypoxic environment	Activation to bifunctional alkylating agent, with formation of DNA interstrand crosslinks and oxygen free radicals. Activation by chemical reducing agents, enzymatic reduction, exposure to acidic pH	Rapid plasma disappearance as a result of tissue distribution and liver metabolism; $t_{1/2\beta}$ = 25–90 min; <10% of dose in 24 h urine; 23% hepatic extraction with HAI administration. PK unchanged if liver/renal impairment

ANTIMICROTUBULE AGENTS: VINCA ALKALOIDS AND TAXANES

Name, chemistry, relevant features	Mechanism of action	Pharmacology and dose modifications
Vinblastine sulfate (VLB) [Velban] Sulfate salt of a dimeric alkaloid from *Vinca rosea*; formed by two multi-ringed units (catharanthine and vindoline) with methyl side-chain on vindoline	Binding to a specific site on tubulin with prevention of polymerization, inhibition of microtubule assembly and mitotic spindle formation. Involved in MDR phenomenon through P-gp overexpression	80% protein-bound. Rapidly distributed into tissues with triphasic disappearance ($t_{1/2\gamma}$ = 19–25 h). Partially metabolized in liver to desacetyl VLB; 80% of dose excreted unchanged in bile; ↓ dose if obstructive liver disease

Drug interactions	Route, dosage and administration	Toxicity
↑Risk of pulmonary toxicity with hyperoxia, concomitant RT, nephrotoxic drugs with ↓ excretion of BLM	i.v. bolus: 10–20 mg/m^2/week (i.m., s.c. with antipyretics/ steroids to prevent fever) i.v. CI: 5–10 mg/m^2 on days 1–4 every 3 weeks Intrapleural: 60–120 U (50% of dose in the systemic circulation). Avoid NSAIDs against chest pain	i.v.: acute DL stomatitis; 50% fever and chills; 50% cumulative skin hyperpigmentation. Mild to moderate alopecia. Rare, HSR and Raynaud's phenomenon. Low-dose hypersensitivity pneumonitis responsive to steroids. 10% late chronic pneumonitis up to irreversible interstitial fibrosis (dry cough, dyspnoea, rales, basilar infiltrates); ↑ incidence for cumulative dose >250 U, age >70 years, COPD, thoracic RT, hyperoxia during surgical anaesthesia; role of steroids uncertain
↑ Risk of cardiotoxicity with concomitant DOX	LOCAL VESICANT ON EXTRAVASATION i.v. bolus: single agent, 20 mg/m^2 every 6–8 weeks; combination, 10 mg/m^2 every 6–8 weeks. Intravesical: 20 mg × 3/week	Delayed (after 3–8 weeks) cumulative leuko- and thrombocytopenia, cumulative anaemia; partial alopecia. Microangiopathic haemolytic anaemia with renal and cardiac failure; ↑ risk for cumulative dose >50 mg, exacerbated by RBC transfusions, rarely reversible, steroids ineffective. Rare, interstitial pneumonitis
	LOCAL VESICANT ON EXTRAVASATION i.v. (bolus): 4 mg/m^2 for starting, increased to 6 mg/m^2/ week	DL leukopenia after 5–10 days, recovering within 7–14 days; neurotoxicity with constipation and abdominal pain (prophylactic lactulose); less frequent, peripheral neuropathy, jaw pain, urinary retention (↑ incidence if underlying neurological problems); stomatitis and mild alopecia

Name, chemistry, relevant features	Mechanism of action	Pharmacology and dose modifications
Vincristine sulfate (VCR) [Oncovin] Sulfate salt of a dimeric alkaloid from *Catharanthus rosea*; as VLB with formyl side-chain on vindoline	Same as that of VLB	48% protein-bound. Rapidly distributed into tissues with triphasic disappearance. Liver metabolism with 70% of dose in 72 h faeces; ↓ dose if liver impairment (50% for bilirubin up to 3 mg/ml)
Vindesine (DVA, VDS) [Eldisine] Desacetyl vinblastine amide; synthetic derivative of VLB	Same as that of VLB	Rapidly distributed into tissues with triphasic elimination ($t_{1/2\gamma}$ = 20 h). Elimination through hepatic metabolism; ↓ dose if liver impairment
Vinorelbine [Navelbine] Semisynthetic derivative of VLB with structural modifications on the catharanthine ring	Same as VLB; ↓ activity on axonal microtubules with possibly ↓ neurotoxicity	80% protein-bound. Rapid tissue distribution with triphasic disappearance ($t_{1/2\gamma}$ = 18 h). High liver uptake and metabolism; main excretion non-renal. 27% ± 14 mean *F* after p.o.: C_{max} after 1.5 h and large first-pass effect. ↓ Dose by 50% for bilirubin >2 × NV

Drug interactions	Route, dosage and administration	Toxicity
↑ Accumulation of MTX in tumour cells	LOCAL VESICANT ON EXTRAVASATION i.v. (bolus): 0.4–1.4 mg/m^2 (maximum 2 mg total dose) per week i.v. (CI): single agent, 0.5 mg/m^2 on days 1–5	DL cumulative neurotoxicity, with peripheral neuropathy (paraesthesias, loss of deep tendon reflexes); less frequent, autonomic effects with abdominal pain and constipation; ↑ incidence if underlying neurological problems; 20% alopecia. Rare SIADH
	LOCAL VESICANT ON EXTRAVASATION i.v. (bolus): 3 mg/m^2/week for 2–3 weeks every 4 weeks	DL leukopenia with short nadirs; cumulative peripheral neurotoxicity with paraesthesias, proximal muscle weakness, fatigue; 90% alopecia
	LOCAL VESICANT ON EXTRAVASATION i.v. (5–10 min infusion): single agent, 30 mg/m^2/week with ↓ dose according to myelotoxicity; combination, 25 mg/m^2 on days 1 and 8 every 3–4 weeks	DL non-cumulative neutropenia (90%; 36% grade 4) after 7–10 days, recovering within 7–14 days; 25% neurotoxicity with decreased deep tendon reflexes; 35% constipation and paraesthesias; 40% N & V (2% severe); 12% alopecia; 10% chemical phlebitis

Name, chemistry, relevant features	Mechanism of action	Pharmacology and dose modifications
Paclitaxel [Taxol] Diterpene from bark of *Taxus brevifolia* Poor water-solublility; vehicle of 50% polyoxyethylated castor oil (Cremophor EL) and 50% ethanol	Promotes microtubule assembly of tubulin dimers and stabilizes microtubule dynamics, with inhibition of cell proliferation, blockade of mitosis and induction of apoptosis. Resistance related to P-gp overexpression and mutations of tubulin, slower rate of microtubule assembly, and overexpression of Bcl-2. ↑ in vitro cytotoxicity after longer exposure time. P-gp-mediated resistance possibly overcome by prolonging infusion time. In vitro sensitizing effect to ionizing radiation. Effective in vitro concentrations (≥0.1 μmol/l) at the end of infusion in clinical studies.	>90% protein-bound. Rapid substantial tissue uptake, with triphasic plasma disappearance (20 h) and extensive liver metabolism at the level of the taxane ring through specific CYP450 enzymes (CYP2C8 and CYP3A4); main metabolite inactive 6-OH-paclitaxel. High biliary secretion and low intestinal absorption of paclitaxel and metabolites. Nonlinear PK in humans, mainly caused by Cremophor EL; C_{max} and AUC not proportional to dose, because of saturable distribution, metabolism and elimination. Neutropenia related to the time for which plasma concentrations of ≥0.05–0.1 μmol/l are maintained. Does not cross blood–brain barrier. ↓ dose to 75–100 mg/m^2 (3 h infusion) if liver enzymes >2 × NV or bilirubin >1.5 mg/ml; no need of dose ↓ in pts with renal impairment. After i.p. treatment, low V_d, slow peritoneal CL, prolonged significant i.p. and plasma concentrations. 11% oral *F* in mice, enhanced by cyclosporin A and SDZ PSC 833.

Drug interactions	Route, dosage and administration	Toxicity
In vitro effects on metabolism of concomitant CYP450 isoenzyme substrates (cyclosporin, steroids, macrolide antibiotics, benzodiazepines, barbiturates, antiepileptic drugs, fluconazole). In vivo ↓ CL if paclitaxel (24 h infusion) given after cisplatin and if paclitaxel (3 h infusion) coadministered with R-verapamil. ↑ incidence of CHF with paclitaxel (3 h infusion) and DOX (bolus) for >380 mg/m² cumulative dose of DOX, possibly because of ↓ CL of DOX and doxorubicinol. ↑ stomatitis if paclitaxel (24 h infusion) given before DOX (48 h infusion). ↑ peripheral neuropathy if paclitaxel given with cisplatin. ↓ C_{ss} and ↓ systemic toxicity in pts receiving 96 h infusion paclitaxel with concomitant enzyme-inducing antiepileptic drugs. ↑ antitumour activity and tolerability if paclitaxel (3 h infusion) given on day 4 after etoposide on days 1–3.	*Premedication:* steroids, histamine H_1- and H_2-receptor antagonists (day −1, day 1). *Standard dose:* i.v. (3–24 h infusion): good-risk pts 175–200 mg/m²; poor-risk pts 135–175 mg/m² every 3 weeks	DL non-cumulative neutropenia (50% grade 4) after 7–10 days, recovering in 1 week; total alopecia (within 2–4 weeks); 60% dose-dependent myalgia (8% severe) after 2–3 days for 3–4 days; 60% dose-dependent cumulative peripheral neuropathy (3% severe), slowly reversible; 41% HSR (<2% severe); 12% hypotension; 23% ECG abnormalities (sinus bradytachycardia, PB), usually asymptomatic, not requiring interventions; radiation-recall skin reaction. Schedule-dependent neutropenia and mucositis, ↑ with 24 h infusion. DL peripheral neuropathy
	High-dose (+G-CSF) (3 h infusion): good-risk pts 250 mg/m²; poor-risk pts 200 mg/m² every 3 weeks i.v. (3 h infusion) each week: 60–70 mg/m²	DL cumulative peripheral neuropathy; nail disorders
	i.v. (96 h CI): 140 mg/m² (without premedication)	DL mucositis
	i.p. 82.5–125 mg/m² every 3 weeks	Abdominal pain

Name, chemistry, relevant features	Mechanism of action	Pharmacology and dose modifications
Docetaxel [Taxotere] Semisynthetic derivative from needles of *Taxus baccata* More water-soluble than paclitaxel; Tween 80 in the solution	Same as that of paclitaxel. Schedule-independent antitumour activity. In vitro sensitizing effect to ionizing radiation. Same mechanisms of resistance	>90% protein-bound. Linear PK up to 115 mg/m^2 with triphasic plasma disappearance ($t_{1/2\beta}$ = 38 min and $t_{1/2\gamma}$ = 12 h). Extensive liver metabolism with successive oxidations on the C-13 side-chain and production of inactive metabolites. High interpatient variability of metabolism and PK. 74% of dose excreted in faeces as metabolites, 5% in urine. 27% ↓ of docetaxel CL in pts with ↑ transaminases; docetaxel CL shown to be independent predictor of severe and febrile neutropenia in population PK study. ↓ dose by 25% if AP > 2.5 × NV and transaminases > 1.5 × NV; discontinue therapy if ↑ bilirubin, AP > 6 × NV, transaminases >3.5 × NV

Drug interactions	Route, dosage and administration	Toxicity
Specific substrates of CYP450-3A isoenzymes (erythromycin, ketoconazole, nifedipine) could modify docetaxel CL	*Premedication:* dexamethasone 8 mg twice a day for 3 days (from day −1) i.v. (1 h infusion): single agent, 100 mg/m^2 every 3 weeks; combination, 75–100 mg/m^2 every 3 weeks	DL non-cumulative neutropenia (80% grade 3–4, 11% febrile neutropenia) after 8 days, recovering within 1 week; total alopecia (within 2–4 weeks); 62% asthenia (15% severe); 50% cumulative neurosensory; 47% skin reactions; 39% diarrhoea, 21% acute HSR (7% severe); 61% fluid retention (13% severe) due to capillary protein leak syndrome, after a median cumulative dose of 400 mg/m^2. Steroids useful to ↓ severity of skin reactions and of fluid retention (64% overall incidence, 6% severe) after a median dose of 800 mg/m^2, and to avoid severe HSR (2%).
	Weekly: 36 mg/m^2/week × 6 every 8 weeks	DL toxicities fatigue and asthenia; rare peripheral oedema and neuropathy; uncommon mild neutropenia

ANTHRACYCLINES AND ANTHRACENEDIONES

Name, chemistry, relevant features	Mechanism of action	Pharmacology and dose modifications
Doxorubicin (DOX) [Adriamycin] Hydroxydaunorubicin anthracycline antibiotic constituted by water-soluble aminosugar (daunosamine) linked to planar anthraquinone nucleus (adriamycinone), site of electron transfer reactions	Cytotoxicity due to: (1) DNA intercalation of aglycone between base pairs, with inhibition of nucleic acid synthesis; (2) Topo II inhibition; (3) Generation of hydroxyl radicals (relevant mainly for cardiac toxicity) through (a) redox cycling of quinone with production of $\dot{O_2^-}$, H_2O_2 and OH^-, which bind to DNA and cell membrane lipids; (b) formation of drug-metal (Fe^{2+}, Cu^{2+}) complexes that catalyse and bind to DNA and cell membranes. Cardiomyopathy possibly related to (3) because of destruction of detoxifying glutathione peroxidase by DOX and relative deficiency of scavenging enzymes in heart. Involved in MDR phenomenon through P-gp overexpression and Topo II alterations	75% protein-bound, with rapid tissue distribution; triphasic plasma disappearance ($t_{1/2\gamma}$ DOX and metabolites: 25–28 h). Main metabolite doxorubicinol produced by ubiquitous (mainly liver) aldoketo reductase, less active than DOX; 7-deoxyaglycones, inactivation species produced mainly in liver, conjugated and excreted into bile and urine. 40% of dose excreted in bile and 5% in 7-day urine; ↓ dose if severe liver impairment (↓ dose by 50% if bilirubin $>$ 1.25–1.5 $\times$ NV). Guidelines in case of abnormal transaminases missing, ↓ dose by 25% if ↑ AST

Drug interactions	Route, dosage and administration	Toxicity
Compatible with i.v. BLM, VLB, VCR, CTX; incompatible with dexamethasone, 5-FU, heparin. ↑ CL with CYP450 enzyme activity inducers; ↓ CL with MDR modulators through P-gp inhibition. ↑ risk of cardiotoxicity with MMC, CTX, paclitaxel, calcium antagonists; ↓ risk of cardiotoxicity with iron chelator ICRF 187 (dexrazoxane)	LOCAL VESICANT ON EXTRAVASATION i.v. (bolus): single agent, 60–75 mg/m^2 every 3 weeks; combination, 50–60 mg/m^2 every 3 weeks	DL neutropenia after 10–14 days recovering in 1 week; acute dose-dependent N & V; total alopecia within 3 weeks; hyperpigmentation of skin; radiation recall; venous flare reactions; rare stomatitis
	Cumulative dose (<10% cardiomyopathy): ≤450 mg/m^2; 300–400 mg/m^2 if combination CT, prior mediastinal RT, age >70 years, pre-existing heart disease. i.v. (72–96 h) CI (central i.v. line): 60 mg/m^2 every 3 weeks; cumulative dose ≤700 mg/m^2	*Cardiotoxicity* *Dose-independent acute* (after hours or days): arrhythmias (with non-specific ST segment and T-wave changes, AV blocks, A tachyarrhythmias); more rarely acute pericarditis–myocarditis. *Dose-related cumulative delayed irreversible chronic cardiomyopathy with CHF* responsive to diuretics, digitalis, ACE inhibitors. Serial determinations of LVEF by MUGA/ECHO to minimize the risk of cardiotoxicity (baseline, 300, 450 mg/m^2, then after each dose). Discontinue treatment if ≥10% ↓ of baseline to a level below normal. Endomyocardial biopsy findings predictive of subsequent CHF
	i.v. (bolus) weekly: 20 mg/m^2 per week; cumulative dose ≤700 mg/m^2	More frequent stomatitis

Name, chemistry, relevant features	Mechanism of action	Pharmacology and dose modifications
Doxorubicin HCl liposome [Caelyx, Doxil] DOX encapsulated in pegylated (STEALTH) liposomes	Longer circulation times; higher concentrations in tumour tissues in animal models than DOX, possibly owing to enhanced permeability and retention	$t_{1/2}$ = 55 h. Mainly eliminated by liver metabolism; ↓ dose if liver impairment; guidelines not available
Epirubicin (EPI, 4'-epidoxorubicin) [Farmorubicin] Epimer of DOX with 4'-OH on daunosamine in equatorial rather than axial position ↑ lipophilicity, ↑ β-glucuronidation to inactive compounds with ↓ cardiotoxicity, ↑ plasma CL and ↓ potency	(1) and (2) same as those of DOX; (3) less prominent owing to ↓ glucuronide production escaping redox cycling and free-radical formation. Involved in MDR phenomenon	Extensive liver metabolism with EPI and 13-OH derivative (epirubicinol) with formation of glucuronides that are rapidly excreted. Triphasic plasma disappearance with $t_{1/2\gamma}$ = 40 h; 50% of dose excreted in the bile in 4 days and <20% into urine; ↓ dose only if severe liver impairment; guidelines not available

Drug interactions	Route, dosage and administration	Toxicity
No drug interaction studies. DO NOT MIX WITH OTHER DRUGS	IRRITANT ON EXTRAVASATION i.v. (30 min infusion): 35–50 mg/m^2 every 4–5 weeks Cumulative dose not defined	Dose-dependent cumulative skin toxicity with palmar–plantar erythrodysaesthesia, possibly due to preferential accumulation in flexure, pressure areas, palms (20% at 50 mg/m^2 but 6% grade 4), ↓ incidence at ≥4-week intervals and by avoiding pressure, high temperature for 1 week after treatment. Pyridoxine possibly useful
	Standard dose, i.v. (10–15 min infusion): single agent, 90 mg/m^2 every 3 weeks; combination, 75 mg/m^2 every 3 weeks; cumulative dose (<10% cardiomyopathy) ≤900 mg/m^2 *High dose*, i.v. (30–60 min infusion): days 1–2; total dose single agent, 120–150 mg/m^2; combination, 120 mg/m^2 + colony-stimulating factor, 200 mg/m^2 + PBSC	Acute side-effects comparable to those of DOX, with dose ratio of DOX : EPI of 1 : 1.2 for haematological, 1 : 1.5 for non-haematological toxicities, 1 : 1.8 for cardiotoxicity. *Dose-related cumulative delayed cardiotoxicity:* as for DOX; serial LVEFs by MUGA/ECHO (at baseline, 300–400 mg/m^2, 600–700 mg/m^2, then after each dose) to mimimize the risk of cardiotoxicity (4% at ≤950 mg/m^2, 15% at 1000 mg/m^2). Recommended maximum cumulative dose 900 mg/m^2. RT to mediastinum and to thoracic spine risk factors for CHF. Criteria for discontinuation as for DOX. DL mucositis; 90% grade 4 neutropenia; severe N & V; total alopecia

Name, chemistry, relevant features	Mechanism of action	Pharmacology and dose modifications
Mitoxantrone (DHAD) [Novantrone] Synthetic dihydroxyanthracenedione constituted by a tricyclic planar hydroxyquinone analogue and two identical aminoalkyl side-chains	(1) and (2) same as those of DOX; (3) less prominent owing to lack of redox cycling and ↓ potential of cardiotoxicity. Involved in MDR phenomenon	78% protein-bound. Rapid tissue distribution, with triphasic plasma disappearance ($t_{1/2\gamma}$ = 23–42 h). Primary hepatobiliary elimination, with 25% of dose in faeces of 5 days; ↓ dose if severe liver impairment; guidelines not validated

TOPOISOMERASE II INHIBITORS: EPIPODOPHYLLOTOXINS

Name, chemistry, relevant features	Mechanism of action	Pharmacology and dose modifications
Etoposide (VP-16) [Vepesid] Semisynthetic derivative of podophyllotoxin with epipodophyllotoxin linked to a glucopyranoside with a methyl group; made more water-miscible by organic solvents (Tween 80, polyethylene glycol)	Topo II inhibition with stabilization of the DNA–Topo II complex and production of DNA double-strand breaks. Cytotoxicity phase- and schedule-dependent; lower repeated doses more effective than higher single. Involved in MDR phenomenon through P-gp overexpression and Topo II alterations (↓ activity, point mutations)	95% protein-bound; biphasic disappearance with $t_{1/2\beta}$ = 6–8 h; linear PK also at high doses; 40% of dose (mainly parent compound) in 48 h urine; <10% biliary excretion; hepatic metabolism with production of less active compounds. Dose-dependent, variable p.o. *F* (50–70%) up to 200 mg total dose; lower at >200 mg. Measurable CSF levels of parent compound and metabolites after high doses. ↓ Dose if ↓ Cr CL, ↓ albumin, age >65 years to avoid severe neutropenia

Drug interactions	Route, dosage and administration	Toxicity
	i.v. (10–15 min infusion): single dose, 12–14 mg/m² every 3 weeks; combination, 10 mg/m² every 3 weeks; Cumulative dose (<10% cardiomyopathy); ≤160 mg/m², ≤120 mg/m² if risk factors. *High dose:* 60–80 mg/m²	DL neutropenia after 12 days, with recovery in 1 week; 30% grade 1–2 N & V; 15% alopecia; rare mucositis. *Cumulative delayed cardiotoxicity:* as for DOX after higher cumulative equitoxic doses. Similar treatment and monitoring

Synergistic interaction with cisplatin and Topo I inhibitors. ↓ CL if given with cisplatin, high-dose carboplatin, cyclosporin A; ↑ CL with concomitant anticonvulsant therapy	i.v. (30–60 min infusion): 100–120 mg/m² on days 1–3; on days 1–5 every 3–4 weeks *i.v. high dose* (500 mg/h infusion): single agent, 60 mg/kg (preparatory for BMT), 3000 mg/m² (MTD); combination, 400–800 mg/m² on days 1–3; i.v. (72 h CI): 150 mg/m²/day. p.o.: 100 mg (50 mg × 2) per day: untreated, good-risk pts, days 1–14 (21); pretreated, poor risk pts, days 1–10 every 4 weeks	DL non-cumulative neutropenia after 10–12 days, recovering within 7–10 days; N & V; less frequent, exacerbation of pre-existing VCR neuropathy; diarrhoea. Rare hypotension, flushing *High dose*: DL myelotoxicity; mucositis; severe N & V p.o.: DL neutropenia after 3 weeks, recovering in 1 week; mild-to-moderate N & V; total alopecia after repeated cycles ↑ Risk of secondary monoblastic leukaemia with balanced 11q23 translocations, short latency period, no preleukaemic phase for cumulative doses of ≥2 g/m². High-dose cisplatin, alkylating agents and RT as additional risk factors

Name, chemistry, relevant features	Mechanism of action	Pharmacology and dose modifications
Etoposide phosphate [Etopophos] Water-soluble prodrug of etoposide, completely converted to etoposide in vivo	Same as that of etoposide	Same as those of etoposide
Teniposide (VM-26) [Vumon] As etoposide, but with a thenylidene group on the glucopyranoside	Same as that of etoposide	>99% protein-bound; triphasic disappearance with $t_{1/2\gamma} = 20$ h; ≤20% of dose in 24 h urine; ↓ CL_R than etoposide; mostly unknown metabolism. ↓ dose if liver impairment

TOPOISOMERASE I INHIBITORS: CAMPOTHECIN ANALOGUES

Name, chemistry, relevant features	Mechanism of action	Pharmacology and dose modifications
Irinotecan (CPT-11) [Campto] Hydrochloride trihydrate; water-soluble, semisynthetic derivative of camptothecin	Topo I inhibition, with production of single-strand DNA breaks. Converted by a carboxylesterase to SN38, 250–1000-fold more potent, subsequently inactivated by glucuronidation to SN38G; pH-dependent hydrolysis in equilibrium between lactone (closed ring) and carboxylate (inactive open ring) for both CPT-11 and SN38. CYP3A-mediated pathway with production of APC, 500-fold less potent than SN38, and NPC. Antitumour activity not schedule-dependent	CPT-11 >60% protein-bound; SN38 >90% protein-bound. High interpatient variability of PK of CPT-11 and SN38 due to differences in the metabolic pathways; possible pharmacogenetic differences in SN38 glucuronidation rate. CPT-11 $t_{1/2\gamma} = 13.5$ h; SN38 concentrations lower than CPT-11, $t_{1/2\gamma} = 23.5$ h; 28% total urinary excretion, with CPT-11 and SN38 as main products; 24% faecal excretion. For both, linear PK up to 400 mg/m^2, unchanged after repeated cycles; plasma AUC of metabolites 40% of total AUC. Relationship between AUC of CPT-11 and SN38 and % ↓ of ANC. CPT-11 CL affected by liver function; guidelines not available

Drug interactions	Route, dosage and administration	Toxicity
Same as those of etoposide	i.v. (5 min infusion) (solution of higher concentration than for etoposide): 50–100 mg/m^2 on days 1, 3 and 5 *i.v. high-dose:* highest safe dose: 1000 mg/m^2 (2 h infusion) on days 1 and 2	Comparable to those expected from etoposide. 3% anaphylactic type reactions (chills, rigours, bronchospasm, dyspnoea); 2% flushing; 3% skin rashes
	i.v. (30–60 min infusion): single agent, 60 mg/m^2 on days 1–5 every 3–4 weeks	DL neutropenia after 7–10 days, recovering within 1 week; moderate N & V; transient alopecia; mucositis; chemical phlebitis. Secondary leukaemias as after etoposide

In vitro additive or synergistic effect with cisplatin, Topo II inhibitors (given after Topo I inhibitors), radiation, TS inhibitors. In vitro ↓ CYP3A metabolism with CYP3A substrates (loperamide, ketoconazole, ondansetron)	i.v. (⩾30 min infusion): good-risk pts, 350 mg/m^2 every 3 weeks; poor-risk pts, 300 mg/m^2	Early infusion-related symptoms: abdominal cramps, diarrhoea (preventable by atropine), 20% severe N & V; 100% alopecia; fatigue. Late toxicities: DL diarrhoea (severe) after 5 days for 5–7 days (treat with loperamide and rehydration); 20% severe neutropenia after 9 days, of worse prognosis in case of concomitant diarrhoea

Name, chemistry, relevant features	Mechanism of action	Pharmacology and dose modifications
Topotecan [Hycamtin] 9-Dimethylaminomethyl-10-hydroxycamptothecin; water-soluble semisynthetic derivative of camptothecin	Topo I inhibition, with production of single-strand DNA breaks. pH-dependent hydrolysis with predominance of lactone (active species) at pH < 7.0; less-active open ring. Active *N*-desmethyl metabolite in plasma produced by CYP. Higher antitumour activity in experimental models after CI/repeated than single bolus administrations	50% of drug as carboxylate (80% after 18 h) at the end of short infusion; wide tissue distribution; biphasic disappearance of lactone ($t_{1/2\beta}$ = 3 h), with linear PK highly variable. Main renal excretion (40% total drug in 24 h urine). 32–42% p.o. *F*; peak plasma concentrations after 45 min; 30–40% penetration into CSF in children; positive correlation between total AUC and % ↓ of ANC. ↓ dose by 50% if Cr CL between 20–39 ml/min, no data in case of Cr CL <20 ml/min; no need for ↓ dose if liver impairment

ANTIMETABOLITES

Antifolates

Name, chemistry, relevant features	Mechanism of action	Pharmacology and dose modifications
Leucovorin (LV, folinic acid) 5-CHO-FH_4; reduced form of folic acid (racemic mixture); active L-LV	Provides cells with FH_4 depleted because of DHFR inhibition by MTX	90% absorption after p.o. up to <50 mg total dose, then 75%; t_{max} = 30 min. Crosses blood–brain barrier, rescue delayed for ⩾24 h after i.t. treatment

Drug interactions	Route, dosage and administration	Toxicity
Same as those of CPT-11. ↑ neutropenia if topotecan given after cisplatin; ↑ CL with concomitantly administered phenytoin	i.v. (30 min infusion): single agent, 1.5 mg/m^2 on days 1–5 every 3 weeks; combination, 0.75 mg/m^2 on days 1–5 every 3 weeks	Short-term administration (p.o., i.v.): DL neutropenia (60% grade 4) after 8–10 days, recovering in 1 week; 40% anaemia after 5–8 days; 42% diarrhoea; dose-related cumulative alopecia; 57% cumulative fatigue; 60% mild-to-moderate N & V
	i.v. CI: (24, 72, 120 h) every 3 weeks	DL mucositis, neutropenia Prolonged i.v. administration: cumulative neutropenia
	p.o.: 2.3 mg/m^2 on days 1–5 every 3 weeks	Prolonged p.o. administration: diarrhoea

	With MTX: see high-dose MTX *With 5-FU* (short infusion): 20–200 mg/m^2 on days 1–5	

Name, chemistry, relevant features	Mechanism of action	Pharmacology and dose modifications
Methotrexate (MTX) Folic acid analogue; 4-amino, 10-methyl analogue of aminopterin	Tight-binding inhibitor of DHFR, with depletion of intracellular FH_4, necessary for synthesis of purines (through GAR and AICAR transformylases) and thymidylate (through TS), with inhibition of DNA and RNA synthesis. MTX and FH_2 polyglutamated by FPGS, higher in some tumours than in normal cells. DHFR, GAR, AICAR and TS directly inhibited by polyglutamates. MTX enters cells through reduced folate carrier and mFBP, with higher affinity for FH_4 than for MTX. Mechanisms of resistance to MTX include impaired membrane transport, defective polyglutamation and alteration of DHFR due to ↑ expression or ↓ binding affinity. High-dose therapy based on different distribution of transport carrier systems between tumour and normal cells, with passive diffusion of MTX into tumour cells and selective rescue of normal cells by LV. LV intracellularly converted to 10-CHO-FH_4, which competes with polyglutamated species for DHFR; the dose of LV to rescue normal cells depends on MTX concentration. MTX cytotoxicity depends on drug concentration and duration of exposure. Therapeutic concentrations: 1×10^{-6} M	60% protein-bound; triphasic plasma disappearance, with $t_{1/2\beta} = 2–3$ h and $t_{1/2\gamma} = 8–10$ h, longer if ↓ Cr CL and third-space fluid collections with potential ↑ toxicity. 60–100% urinary excretion after high-dose MTX through glomerular and tubular processes with drug CL_R comparable to Cr CL; 40% of drug in 24 h urine as 7-OH-MTX, poorly soluble in acidic pH. Dose ↓ if Cr CL $\leqslant$ 80 ml/min; discontinue if $<$50 ml/min. Biliary excretion $<$10% drug clearance; no need of ↓ dose if liver impairment. Well absorbed after p.o. doses of $\leqslant$25 mg/m^2, but erratic *F* at higher doses. After high dose (8 g/m^2), therapeutic concentrations achieved in CSF and maintained much longer than with i.t. After i.t. administration, $t_{1/2\beta}$ = 12–18 h, with delayed clearance and ↑ myelo-neurotoxicity if active meningeal disease. High-dose or i.t. treatment for meningeal prophylaxis; through Ommaya reservoir for treatment of disease

Drug interactions	Route, dosage and administration	Toxicity
↑ toxicity with salicylates, sulfonamides, phenytoin because of protein-binding displacement; with probenecid, penicillins, cephalosporins, aspirin, NSAIDs because of inhibition of tubular secretion With antitumour agents: ↑ therapeutic activity of 5-FU, VCR or Ara-C if MTX given first;	i.v. (bolus): 30–50 mg/m²/week *High-dose:* (1) i.v.: fluids and urinary alkalinization; (2) MTX plasma levels monitoring; (3) LV rescue (1) Urinary pH > 7, ↑ diuresis at least 12 h before and ≥48 h after MTX; Cr CL > 60 ml/min; (2) To guide duration and amount of (3); (3) Started 2–24 h after MTX until MTX levels are $<5 \times 10^{-8}$ M *Schedule:* 50–250 mg/kg 6 h infusion (Jaffe regimen) *Rescue:* start 2 h from the end of MTX with LV 15 mg/m² i.m. every 6 h × 7, then according to MTX level at 48 h for 8 doses: *MTX level at 48 h* (M) — *LV (mg)* $\geq 5 \times 10^{-7}$ — 15 $\geq 1 \times 10^{-6}$ — 100 $\geq 2 \times 10^{-6}$ — 200 Repeat after 48 h and continue up to $<5 \times 10^{-8}$ M p.o.: 15–20 mg/m² × 2/week i.t., *do not use preservative-containing solutions:* 12 mg total dose every 2–7 days	Leukothrombocytopenia after 4–14 days; stomatitis; diarrhoea; ↑ toxicity in dehydrated, malnourished patients *High-dose:* Acute: reversible nephrotoxicity; N & V; maculopapular rash (up to 5 days after); oral stomatitis (after 3–7 days) preceding myelotoxicity, both reversible within 2 weeks; ↑ liver enzymes reversible within 2 weeks; fever Transient encephalopathy with paresis, aphasia and seizures within 6 days, recovering in 72 h p.o.: *Chronic toxicities*: hepatic fibrosis, interstitial infiltrates i.t.: *acute* chemical arachnoiditis; 10% *subacute* neurotoxicity (motor paralysis, cranial nerve palsies); *chronic* demyelinating encephalopathy (dementia, limb spasticity; ↑ with concomitant cerebral RT)

5-Fluoropyrimidines

Name, chemistry, relevant features	Mechanism of action	Pharmacology and dose modifications
5-Fluorouracil (5-FU) Uracil analogue with fluorine atom substituted for H at C-5 of the pyrimidine ring	Intracellular activation to: (1) FdUMP, with inhibition of TS (ternary complex with CH_2–FH_4) and inhibition of DNA synthesis and repair; (2) FUMP, metabolized to FUTP, with incorporation into RNA, altering RNA functions; (3) FdUMP phosphorylated to FdUTP, with incorporation into DNA. (1) is probably the principal mechanism, with long $t_{1/2}$ (6 h) of ternary complex. Resistance due to deletion of activating enzymes, relative deficiency of CH_2–FH_4, alterations in TS, ↑ activity of catabolic enzymes. Pattern of 5-FU metabolism different in different normal tissues and tumour types. Mechanism of cytotoxicity also related to drug concentration and time of exposure	Erratic *F*, also because of first-pass effect. After i.v. bolus $t_{1/2\beta}$ = 6–20 min, with <1 μM (cytotoxic concentration) within few hours; nonlinear PK at higher doses, with ↓ non-renal CL due to saturation of catabolism. Crosses blood–brain barrier; T_{max} = 30 min. Rapid catabolism (50% of dose) in liver and in tissues to F-DHU by DPD; DPD-deficient persons with ↑ risk of life-threatening toxicity. Main biliary excretion of 5-FU and catabolites; extensive catabolism also extrahepatic with need of ↓ dose only if severe liver impairment. 50% of dose cleared through liver first-pass after HAI or i.v. portal infusion. After i.p. treatment, 300:1 gradient between i.p.:i.v. concentrations due to slow peritoneal absorption and rapid liver metabolism with low systemic toxicity. Improvement of therapeutic index by adapting 5-FU dose to AUC in H & N pts receiving 5-FU (96 h infusion) and cisplatin in a multicentric randomized study

Drug interactions	Route, dosage and administration	Toxicity
Incompatible in solution with any acidic agent; incompatible with diazepam, Ara-C, DOX, MTX. *With LV:* stabilization of the FdUMP–TS–folate ternary complex. *With dipyridamole* (inhibitor of thymidine uptake): ↓ dTTP and ↑ FdUMP. *With PALA* (inhibitor of aspartate transcarbamylase, enzyme in de novo pyrimidine synthesis) given before 5-FU: ↑ FUTP formation and incorporation into RNA. *With MTX* (if given before 5-FU): ↑ FUMP and FUTP. *With IFN* and *with cisplatin:* mechanism of synergism still uncertain. *With allopurinol* (300 mg three times daily) (selective inhibition of 5-FU anabolism in normal tissues): to prevent toxicity. *With delayed high-dose uridine:* to prevent myelosuppression	i.v. (bolus) single agent: 400–500 mg/m^2 (12 mg/kg) on days 1–5 every 3–4 weeks; 500 mg/m^2/week (15 mg/kg). Maximum recommended daily dose 800 mg *Combination with LV:* *Low dose:* i.v. (bolus): 425 mg/m^2 on days 1–5 immediately after LV (bolus) 20 mg/m^2 on days 1–5 every 4–5 weeks *High dose:* i.v. (bolus): 375 mg/m^2 on days 1–5, 1 h after LV (30 min infusion) 500 mg/m^2 on days 1–5 every 3 weeks i.v. (CI): 1000 mg/m^2 on days 1–5 every 3–4 weeks prolonged (CI): 200 mg/m^2/day until toxicity (×4–5 weeks) HAI or i.v. portal infusion i.p.: 500 mg/l p.o.: not recommended	Toxicity and clinical efficacy partly related to schedule of administration. DL neutropenia (31% grade 3–4) after 9–14 days; 70% stomatitis; 6% diarrhoea (i.v. fluids and ↓ dose at subsequent cycles if >3 movements/day). Less frequent, skin hyperpigmentation; radiation recall with erythema; moderate alopecia; ocular toxicity with lacrimation. Rare, neurological disturbances with somnolence and cerebellar ataxia (more frequent after high-dose and LV combination). Cardiac toxicity with chest pain; ECG changes consistent with myocardial ischaemia; ↑ serum enzymes (↑ risk in pts with pre-existing heart disease) *i.v. + LV:* ↑ frequency of myelosuppression, stomatitis and neurological disturbances *CI:* DL stomatitis and diarrhoea; slowly reversible hand–foot syndrome (34% grade 3–4); incidence related to duration of infusion, pyridoxine (50–150 mg/day) possibly useful; 20% epigastric pain and gastric ulcerations; ↑ frequency of cardiac toxicity *HAI or i.v. portal:* mild mucositis and GI symptoms; biliary sclerosis with cholestatic jaundice; catheter-related complications (thrombosis of the gastroduodenal artery with necrosis of intestinal epithelium, haemorrhage, perforation)

Name, chemistry, relevant features	Mechanism of action	Pharmacology and dose modifications
UFT Ftorafur (FT) and uracil in a molar ratio of 1:4. FT is 5-FU linked to a furan ring (dehydroxylated ribose sugar)	FT activated to 5-FU in liver. Inactivated to F-DHU by DPD. Uracil supposed to inhibit subsequent catabolism in liver, with possibly higher concentrations in tumour than in blood or normal tissues	Rapid variable absorption; t_{max} = 0.3–3 h; after 5 days AUC and C_{ss} of 5-FU after UFT equivalent to those achieved with CI of 5-FU; nonlinear PK at doses >900 mg/m^2; no PK modifications after repeated doses. Higher concentrations of 5-FU in tumour than in normal tissues and in plasma in humans

Cytidine analogues

Name, chemistry, relevant features	Mechanism of action	Pharmacology and dose modifications
Cytarabine (cytosine arabinoside; Ara-C) Deoxycytidine antagonist with arabinose instead of deoxyribose	Activated to Ara-CTP in tumour cells by sequential kinase activity; degraded to inactive Ara-U by widely distributed deaminases. Ara-CTP acts by inhibiting DNA polymerase and DNA repair and by incorporation into DNA. Possible differentiating effects on leukaemic cells at lower doses. Cytotoxicity dependent on duration of exposure and rate of DNA synthesis. Entry into cells facilitated by nucleoside transport system at standard doses, by passive diffusion at ↑ doses. Resistance due to deficiency of CdR kinase, ↑ of dCTP pools, ↑ cytidine deaminase activity, ↓ nucleoside transport sites, ↓ intracellular retention of Ara-CTP.	After i.v. bolus, C_{max} = 10 μM after 100 mg/m^2; proportionally higher up to 3 g/m^2 (2 h infusion) (> 100 μM). Rapid plasma elimination, with $t_{1/2\alpha}$ = 7–20 min and $t_{1/2\beta}$ = 30–150 min. 70% of dose in urine as Ara-U; Ara-U predominates in plasma, with $t_{1/2\beta}$ = 3–6 h. After CI of 0.1–2 g/m^2 daily, proportional increase of C_{ss} up to 5 μM; rapid increase of plasma levels with toxicity at higher doses due to saturation of deamination. After s.c. bolus or CI, >2-fold higher AUC than after i.v. bolus. Crosses blood–brain barrier, with C_{ss} CSF 20–40% of those in plasma within 24 h of CI. After 50 mg/m^2 i.t., peak concentrations of 1 mM, with >0.1 μM for 24 h. Drug concentration and duration of exposure primary determinants of toxicity. At high dose, ↓ dose if ↑ Cr because of ↑ risk of neurotoxicity

Drug interactions	Route, dosage and administration	Toxicity
Severe myelosuppression and CNS toxicity with concomitant halogenated antiviral agents.	p.o.: 300 mg/m^2 on days 1–28 every 5 weeks; if LV given in combination: 30 mg three times daily on days 1–28 every 5 weeks (daily dose divided into 3 doses given every 8 h)	DL GI toxicity (2% diarrhoea, 3% N & V, 5% anorexia); 3.5% asthenia; fatigue; leukopenia at the MTD and with shorter more intense schedules. ↑ toxicity of single dosing

Synergism with antitumour agents producing DNA breaks because of inhibition of DNA repair (alkylating agents, cisplatin, etoposide); synergism with RNR inhibitors (thymidine, HU, fludarabine) because of ↓ dCTP pools. ↑ Cytotoxicity with IL-3 or GM-CSF recruiting cells into S phase	i.v. (bolus): 100 mg/m^2 twice daily on days 1–5(7)	DL myelosuppression with leukothrombocytopenia after 7–14 days, recovering within 2–3 weeks. Frequent acute GI toxicity (N & V, abdominal pain, diarrhoea); stomatitis and intrahepatic cholestasis. Flu-like syndrome with rashes
	Low dose s.c. or i.v. (bolus or CI): 5–20 mg/m^2/day × 2–3 weeks	DL myelosuppression
	High dose (3 h infusion >200 mg/m^2): 2–3 g/m^2 twice daily on days 1–6 i.v. CI: 100–200 mg/m^2 on days 1–5(7); s.c. bolus (mainly for maintenance): 100 mg/m^2 twice daily on days 1–5; s.c. CI: 200 mg/m^2 on days 1–5	*High dose*: 20% neurotoxicity with reversible cerebellar and cerebral dysfunction; ↑ risk if >36 g/m^2 total dose, >50 years old, ↑ Cr; repeat neurological examination daily; ↓ incidence with longer infusion. Severe myelotoxicity, mucositis, total alopecia. Conjunctivitis (prophylactic steroid drops up to 7 days after), with slowly reversible visual acuity problems. Rare, pulmonary toxicity with non-cardiogenic oedema
	i.t.: 30 mg/m^2 × 2/week until CR, then one additional dose	Fever, seizures and headache

Name, chemistry, relevant features	Mechanism of action	Pharmacology and dose modifications
Gemcitabine (dFdC) [Gemzar] 2',2'-Difluorodeoxy-cytidine; fluorine-substituted Ara-C analogue	Intracellularly activated to dFdCTP by CdR kinase with accumulation and prolonged retention. Inhibition of DNA synthesis through incorporation into DNA (masked chain termination) and inhibition of RNR with depletion of dNTPs, which compete with dFdCTP for incorporation into DNA (self-potentiating mechanism). Depletion of dNTPs leads also to (1) ↑ rate of dFdC phosphorylation and (2) ↓ activity of Cyd deaminase (self-potentiating mechanisms)	Low protein binding; linear PK; for 30 min infusion, biphasic disappearance, with $t_{1/2}$ = 8 min, due to tissue inactivation by cytidine deaminase (mainly liver and kidney) to dFdU; 77% of dose as dFdU in 24-h urine. Saturable accumulation process of dFdCTP. ↑ intracellular concentrations possibly achieved by longer drug exposure

MISCELLANEOUS

Name, chemistry, relevant features	Mechanism of action	Pharmacology and dose modifications
Hydroxyurea (HU)	Enters cells by passive diffusion. Inhibits RNR, with depletion of ribonucleotides and inhibition of DNA synthesis and repair. Radiation sensitizer	Well absorbed; t_{max} = 1 h; 50% of dose transformed in liver and excreted in urine and as respiratory CO. $t_{1/2}$ = 3.5–4 h. Degraded by urease of intestinal bacteria; metabolism unknown; possibly renal as main route of excretion. Crosses blood–brain barrier and third-space fluids with peaks in 3 h. ↓ Dose if renal impairment; guidelines not available
All-*trans*-retinoic acid (ATRA, tretinoin) Natural retinoid; metabolite of retinol (vitamin A); differentiating agent	Differentiating effect through binding to cytosolic and nuclear receptors (RARs) with induction of transcription of genes involved in growth inhibition and differentiation. ATRA most active among natural retinoids in reversing changes of epithelial-derived malignancies	>95% protein-bound; t_{max} = 1–2 h; high interpatient variability of absorption and plasma levels of ATRA. $t_{1/2}$ < 1 h; ATRA undetectable after 10 h; metabolized by CYP450 to 4-oxo-ATRA, subsequently glucuronidated. 60% renal excretion; ↑ clearance of ATRA with chronic dosing within 2 weeks, due to ↑ catabolism through CYP450 isoenzymes and ↑ tissue sequestration

Drug interactions	Route, dosage and administration	Toxicity
Cytotoxicity reversed by exogenous deoxycytidine; in vitro/in vivo synergistic effect of concomitant cisplatin and ionizing radiation	i.v. (30 min infusion): 1000 mg/m^2 per week × 7 followed by 1 week rest, then weekly × 3 every 4 weeks; 1000 mg/m^2/week × 3 every 4 weeks	DL non-cumulative myelotoxicity (25% grade 3–4 neutropenia, 5% thrombocytopenia); 10% grade 3–4 ↑ liver enzymes; 65% mild-to-moderate N & V; 8% diarrhoea: 29% mild 'flu-like syndrome; 25% maculopapular rash; 30% peripheral oedema. ↑ Non-haematological side-effects after more frequent administrations
Modulation of Ara-C activity, with ↑ production of Ara-CTP and incorporation into DNA. Antagonist effect with 5-FU, with ↓ FdUMP due to inhibition of RNR. Additive effect with 5-FU and LV because of ↓ dUMP pool competing with FdUMP for binding to TS	p.o.: 20–30 mg/kg daily; discontinue if WBC $<2.5 \times 10^9$/l or plt $<100 \times 10^9$/l Radiosensitizer: 80 mg/kg every 3 days from at least 7 days before radiation	DL leukopenia, after a median of 10 days, recovering at discontinuation; maculopapular rash and facial erythema; LFT abnormalities; drowsiness; transient renal function abnormalities. Radiation recall reaction (when used as radiosensitizer)
↑ Catabolism by CYP450 inducers; longer $t_{1/2}$ with co-administration of CYP450 inhibitors (ketoconazole); unproven clinical relevance	p.o.: 40–45 mg/m^2 daily. *Intermittent schedule:* days 1–7 followed by 1 week pause	50% headache due to ↑ intracranial pressure; skin and mucosal toxicity (dryness, itching, peeling, cheilitis); i.v. steroids effective. 30% bone pain; arthralgia; ↑ LFTs slowly reversible. TERATOGENIC: AVOID PREGNANCY

CHEMOPROTECTANTS

Name, chemistry, relevant features	Mechanism of action	Pharmacology and dose modifications
Dexrazoxane (ICRF 187) [Zinecard] Bispiperazinedione; cyclic derivative of EDTA Cardioprotective agent	*Cardioprotection:* intracellular hydrolysis to ring-opened chelating agent with removal of Fe^{2+} and Cu^{2+} from DOX complexes and ↓ of O_2 free-radical generation *Cytotoxicity:* Topo II inhibition	Minimal tissue binding; $t_{1/2\alpha}$ = 15 min; $t_{1/2\beta}$ = 140 min *Indication:* continuation of DOX after ≥ 300 mg/m^2 cumulative dose in pts in whom continued therapy is indicated. Cardioprotection observed in >65 years old and in pts with LVEF low or normal
Amifostine (WR2721) [Ethyol] Ethanethiol, thiophosphate compound *Indications:* to decrease cisplatin cumulative renal toxicity and the risk of neutropenia-related infections due to cisplatin and CTX	Prodrug: dephosphorylated in normal tissues by AP to free thiol (WR1065) which acts: (1) By binding to reactive molecules of alkylating and platinum agents; (2) As a free-radical scavenger. Higher uptake and metabolism in normal versus tumour cells due to higher pH and AP concentration	Cleared from plasma within 10 min; retained in normal tissues; $t_{1/2}$ = 9 min; 4% urinary excretion. High concentration of WR1065 in bone marrow, declining within 2.5 h

ENDOCRINE THERAPIES

Name, chemistry, relevant features	Mechanism of action	Pharmacology and dose modifications
Medroxyprogesterone acetate (MPA) [Provera] **Megestrol acetate (MGA)** [Megace]	Binding to specific cytosol receptors. Anti-oestrogenic effects due to decrease of oestrogen receptor and decrease of gonadotophin secretion. Direct cytotoxic activity	*MPA:* 95% protein-bound; good F; 70% first-pass effect with conjugation. p.o.: 16 days duration of action. i.m.: 4–6 weeks with C_{ss} after 10 days and of high interpatient variability, $t_{1/2}$ = 60 h. Main biliary and urinary excretion *MGA:* t_{max} = 2–5 h, 1–3 days duration of action; $t_{1/2}$ = 15–20 h; 56–78% renal excretion

Drug interactions	Route, dosage and administration	Toxicity
↓ Incidence and severity of DOX cardiomyopathy. Does not influence PK of DOX. Do not mix with other drugs during infusion	i.v. (15 min infusion): 30 min before DOX (from the start of infusion). Dosage ratio to DOX: 10 : 1 (500 mg/m^2 : 50 mg/m^2)	↑ Degree of myelotoxicity caused by chemotherapy
Hypotension with antihypertensive drugs	i.v. (15 min infusion): 910 mg/m^2 followed by cisplatin (>100 mg/m^2) (keep patients in supine position). Antiemetic prophylaxis with steroids and 5-HT_3 antagonists	DL toxicities: emesis (92%) and hypotension at the end of infusion, lasting 5 min. Less frequently: sneezing, warm flush, mild somnolence; hypocalcaemia

High dose not advisable if liver impairment. Guidelines not available	*MPA:* p.o.: 1000 mg on days 1–28, then 500 mg; i.m.: 1000 mg on days 1–5 for 4 weeks, then 500 mg × 2/week. *MGA:* p.o.: 160 mg daily	Hot flushes; vaginal bleeding; weight gain; depression; mild fluid retention; acne *After MPA:* tremor; cramps; cushingoid facies, thrombophlebitis; glucose intolerance; hypertension *After i.m. MPA:* gluteal abscess

Index